AF615813

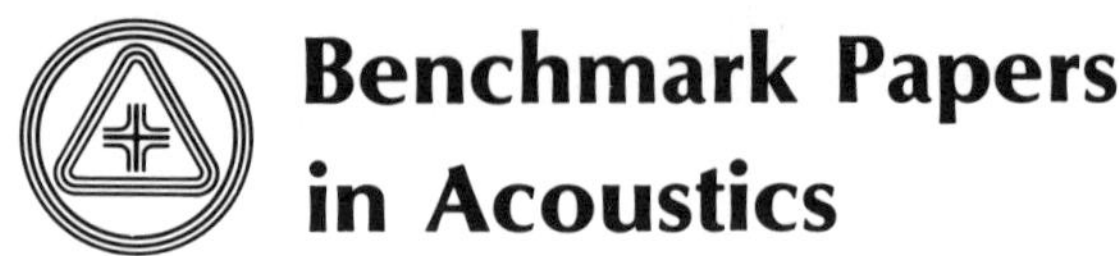

Benchmark Papers in Acoustics

Series Editor: R. Bruce Lindsay
Brown University

Volume

1 UNDERWATER SOUND/*Vernon M. Albers*
2 ACOUSTICS: Historical and Philosophical Development/*R. Bruce Lindsay*
3 SPEECH SYNTHESIS/*James L. Flanagan and Lawrence R. Rabiner*
4 PHYSICAL ACOUSTICS/*R. Bruce Lindsay*
5 MUSICAL ACOUSTICS, PART I: Violin Family Components/*Carleen M. Hutchins*
6 MUSICAL ACOUSTICS, PART II: Violin Family Functions/*Carleen M. Hutchins*
7 ULTRASONIC BIOPHYSICS/*Floyd Dunn and William D. O'Brien, Jr.*
8 VIBRATION: Beams, Plates, and Shells/*Arturs Kalnins and Clive L. Dym*
9 MUSICAL ACOUSTICS:Piano and Wind Instruments/*Earle L. Kent*
10 ARCHITECTURAL ACOUSTICS/*Thomas D. Northwood*
11 SPEECH INTELLIGIBILITY AND SPEAKER RECOGNITION/*Mones E. Hawley*
12 DISC RECORDING AND REPRODUCTION/*H. E. Roys*
13 PSYCHOLOGICAL ACOUSTICS/*Earl D. Schubert*

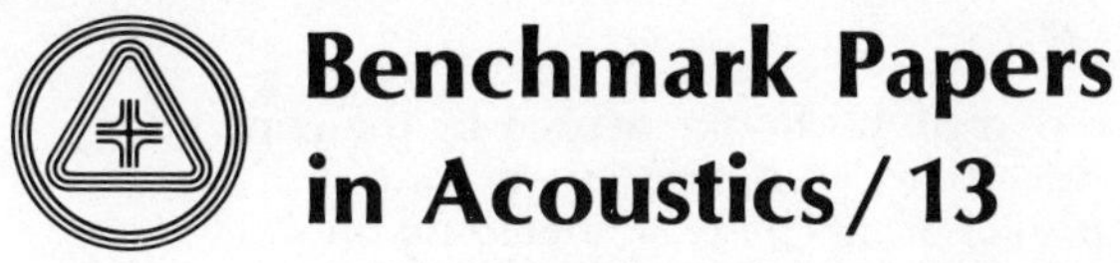

A BENCHMARK ® Book Series

PSYCHOLOGICAL ACOUSTICS

Edited by

EARL D. SCHUBERT

Stanford University

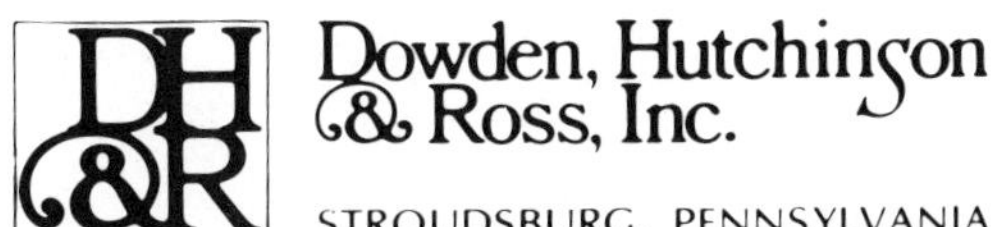

Benchmark Papers in Acoustics, Volume 13
Library of Congress Catalog Card Number: 78-23369
ISBN: 0-87933-338-3

81 80 79 1 2 3 4 5
Manufactured in the United States of America.

LIBRARY OF CONGRESS CATALOGING IN PUBLICATION DATA
Main entry under title:
Psychological acoustics.
(Benchmark papers in acoustics, v. 13)
Includes bibliographies and index.
1. Auditory perception—Addresses, essays, lectures.
I. Schubert, Earl D., 1916-
BF251.P79 152.1'5 78-23369
ISBN 0-87933-338-3

Distributed world wide by Academic Press,
a subsidiary of Harcourt Brace Jovanovich,
Publishers.

SERIES EDITOR'S FOREWORD

The "Benchmark Papers in Acoustics" constitute a series of volumes that make available to the reader in carefully organized form important papers in all branches of acoustics. The literature of acoustics is vast in extent and much of it, particularly the earlier part, is inaccessible to the average acoustical scientist and engineer. These volumes aim to provide a practical introduction to this literature, since each volume offers an expert's selection of the seminal papers in a given branch of the subject, that is, those papers that have significantly influenced the development of that branch in a certain direction and introduced concepts and methods that possess basic utility in modern acoustics as a whole. Each volume provides a convenient and economical summary of results as well as a foundation for further study for both the person familiar with the field and the person who wishes to become acquainted with it.

Each volume has been organized and edited by an authority in the area to which it pertains. In each volume there is provided an editorial introduction summarizing the technical significance of the field being covered. Each article is accompanied by editorial commentary, with necessary explanatory notes, and an adequate index is provided for ready reference. Articles in languages other than English are either translated or abstracted in English. It is the hope of the publisher and editor that these volumes will constitute a working library of the most important technical literature in acoustics of value to students and research workers.

The present volume, *Psychological Acoustics*, has been edited by Earl D. Schubert, Professor of Hearing Science at Stanford University and a member of the faculty of the Medical Center of that institution. In its 36 carefully chosen seminal articles it covers thoroughly the development of the field of psychacoustics during the last half century, a period of remarkable activity in a branch of acoustics of great importance to every human being. Each of the six groups of articles into which the work is divided is prefaced by a commentary explaining the significance of the papers in the group and their relation to other research in the field. Each group is also accompanied by detailed bibliography of other important writings. The historical background is not neglected, and the early work of Ohm, Helmholtz, and Rayleigh comes in for attention. There is much judicious emphasis on the many technical problems which still persist in the field of hearing research, with many suggestions for important future investigation. Both in its coverage and in its method of presentation this volume should command the enthusiastic attention of all workers in acoustics.

R. BRUCE LINDSAY

PREFACE

The study of psychological acoustics is twofold. It is, as implied, a branch of the study of psychology and, as such, emphasizes the responses to acoustic stimuli as they integrate with the total response pattern of the organism. But up to this point, most of our knowledge of how the auditory system processes signals has come from taking the system into the laboratory. Perhaps a similar volume written fifty years hence would be concerned primarily with processing music, environmental sound, and especially interesting speech signals. But at present the papers that have contributed to the advancement of knowledge in psychological acoustics deal necessarily with the engineering aspects of auditory processing, using the perceptual response as the quantifying index.

Even with this restriction, selecting papers for this volume has been difficult. In order to set the papers into some meaningful context, a set of six main topics has been chosen to encompass the major areas of endeavor in psychological research in audition. On occasion, the assignment of a paper to one of these areas rather than another is quite arbitrary. I hope that in each case this has been satisfactorily explained in the text. In the practical world, the choice may of necessity be influenced also by consideration of brevity where any one of a number of papers might meet the criterion of usefulness equally well.

Practical considerations have also dictated the inclusion of only parts of some classical papers rather than the entire work. The criterion in this instance has been subsequent usefulness (such as citation) of the material rather than any judgment about lower merit of the material omitted. It may, indeed, have been most instructive at the time it was published, but not the catalyst for subsequent work to the same degree as the part selected.

I am indebted to those writers whose work appears in whole or in part; and, since the work is essentially historical, I am also indebted to those whose ideas have appeared in works not directly represented here.

That the effort maintained any semblance of order or cohesiveness is attributable to the good offices of my wife, Mid, who searched out the difficult articles, typed the manuscript, and in general kept things on course—and even nearly on schedule—throughout.

EARL D. SCHUBERT

CONTENTS

Series Editor's Foreword v
Preface vii
Contents by Author xiii

Introduction 1

PART I: SENSITIVITY OF THE EAR

Editor's Comments on Papers 1 Through 5 8

1 **SIVIAN, L. J., and S. D. WHITE:** On Minimum Audible Sound Fields 17
Acoust. Soc. Am. J. **4**:288–296, 305–307, 312–314, 320–321 (1933)

2 **WIENER, F. M., and D. A. ROSS:** The Pressure Distribution in the Auditory Canal in a Progressive Sound Field 32
Acoust. Soc. Am. J. **18**:401–408 (1946)

3 **BROGDEN, W. J., and G. A. MILLER:** Physiological Noise Generated under Earphone Cushions 40
Acoust. Soc. Am. J. **19**:620–623 (1947)

4 **DIERCKS, K. J., and L. A. JEFFRESS:** Interaural Phase and the Absolute Threshold for Tone 44
Acoust. Soc. Am. J. **34**:981–984 (1962)

5 **SWETS, J. A.:** Is There a Sensory Threshold? 48
Science **134**:168–177 (1961)

PART II: CLASSICAL PSYCHOACOUSTICS

Editor's Comments on Papers 6 Through 11 60

6 **RIESZ, R. R.:** Differential Intensity Sensitivity of the Ear for Pure Tones 69
Phys. Rev. **31**:867–872 (1928)

7 **SHOWER, E. G., and R. BIDDULPH:** Differential Pitch Sensitivity of the Ear 75
Acoust. Soc. Am. J. **3**:275–280, 287 (1931)

8 **MILLER, G. A.:** Sensitivity to Changes in the Intensity of White Noise and Its Relation to Masking and Loudness 82
Acoust. Soc. Am. J. **19**:609–619 (1947)

9 **GARNER, W. R.:** The Effect of Frequency Spectrum on Temporal Integration of Energy in the Ear **93**
Acoust. Soc. Am. J. **19**:808–815 (1947)

10 **STEVENS, S. S., J. VOLKMANN, and E. B. NEWMAN:** A Scale for the Measurement of the Psychological Magnitude Pitch **101**
Acoust. Soc. J. Am. **8**:185–190 (1937)

11 **STEVENS, S. S.:** A Scale for the Measurement of a Psychological Magnitude: Loudness **107**
Psychol. Rev. **43**:405–416 (1936)

PART III: PITCH MECHANISMS AND PITCH PERCEPTION

Editor's Comments on Papers 12 Through 18 **120**

12 **FLETCHER, H.:** The Physical Criterion for Determining the Pitch of a Musical Tone **135**
Phys. Rev. **23**:427–437 (1924)

13 **SCHOUTEN, J. F.:** The Perception of Subjective Tones **146**
K. ned. Akad. Wet. Proc. **41**:1086–1093 (1938)

14 **LICKLIDER, J. C. R.:** A Duplex Theory of Pitch Perception **155**
Experientia **7**:128–133 (1951)

15 **MILLER, G. A., and W. G. TAYLOR:** The Perception of Repeated Bursts of Noise
Acoust. Soc. Am. J. **20**:171–177, 181–182 (1948)

16 **DAVIS, H., S. R. SILVERMAN, and D. R. McAULIFFE:** Some Observations on Pitch and Frequency **170**
Acoust. Soc. Am. J. **23**:40–42 (1951)

17 **DOUGHTY, J. M., and W. R. GARNER:** Pitch Characteristics of Short Tones. I. Two Kinds of Pitch Threshold **173**
J. Exp. Psychol. **37**:351, 354–356, 365 (1947)

18 **CHIH-AN, L., and L. A. CHISTOVICH:** Frequency-Difference Limens as a Function of Tonal Duration **176**
Sov. Phys. Acoust. **6**:75–80 (1960)

PART IV: SEPARATION OF SIMULTANEOUS SIGNALS

Editor's Comments on Papers 19 Through 24 **184**

19 **MAYER, A. M.:** Researches in Acoustics **193**
Philos. Mag. **2**:500–507 (1876)

20 **WEGEL, R. L., and C. E. LANE:** The Auditory Masking of One Pure Tone by Another and Its Probable Relation to the Dynamics of the Inner Ear **201**
Phys. Rev. **23**:266–276 (1924)

21 **EGAN, J. P., and H. W. HAKE:** On The Masking Pattern of a Simple Auditory Stimulus **212**
Acoust. Soc. Am. J. **22**:622–630 (1950)

22 **FLETCHER, H.:** Auditory Patterns 221
Rev. Mod. Phys. **12**:47–56 (1940)

23 **ZWICKER, E., G. FLOTTORP, and S. S. STEVENS:** Critical Band Width in Loudness Summation 231
Acoust Soc. Am. J. **29**:548–557 (1957)

24 **GREEN, D. M.:** Application of Detection Theory in Psychophysics 241
IEEE Proc. **58**:713–723 (1970)

PART V: TIME RESOLUTION

Editor's Comments on Papers 25 Through 31 254

25 **HAAS, H .:** The Influence of a Single Echo on the Audibility of Speech 264
Audio Eng. Soc. J. **20**:146–159 (1972)

26 **RONKEN, D. A.:** Monaural Detection of a Phase Difference between Clicks 278
Acoust. Soc. Am. J. **47**, Pt.2:1091–1099 (1970)

27 **MILLER, R. L.:** Masking the Effect of Periodically Pulsed Tones as a Function of Time and Frequency 281
Acoust. Soc. Am. J. **19**:798–807 (1947)

28 **ELLIOTT, L. L:** Backward and Forward Masking of Probe Tones of Different Frequencies 297
Acoust. Soc. Am. J. **34**:1116–1117 (1962)

29 **PLOMP, R.:** Rate of Decay of Auditory Sensation 299
Acoust. Soc. Am. J. **36**:277–282 (1964)

30 **CRAIG, J. H., and . L. A. JEFFRESS:** Effect of Phase on the Quality of a Two-Component Tone 305
Acoust. Soc. Am. J. **34**:1752–1760 (1962)

31 **HIRSH, I. J.:** Auditory Perception of Temporal Order 314
Acoust. Soc. Am. J. **31**:759–767 (1959)

PART VI: ADVANTAGES OF THE BINAURAL SYSTEM

Editor's Comments on Papers 32 Through 36 324

32 **STEVENS, S. S., and E. B. NEWMAN:** The Localization of Actual Sources of Sound 333
Am. J. Psychol. **48**:297–306 (1936)

33 **WALLACH, H., E. B. NEWMAN, and M. R. ROSENZWEIG:** The Precedence Effect in Sound Localization 343
Am. J. Psychol. **62**:315–316, 324–336 (1949)

34 **JEFFRESS, L. A., H. C. BLODGETT, T. T. SANDEL, and C. L. WOOD, III:** Masking of Tonal Signals 357
Acoust. Soc. Am. J. **28**:416–426 (1956)

35 **KOCK, W. E.:** Binaural Localization and Masking 368
Acoust. Soc. Am. J. **22**:801–804 (1950)

36 **LEVITT, H., and L. R. RABINER:** Binaural Release from Masking for Speech and Gain in Intelligibility **372**
Acoust. Soc. Am. J. **42**:601–608 (1967)

Author Citation Index **381**
Subject Index **387**

About the Editor **391**

CONTENTS BY AUTHOR

Biddulph, R., 75
Blodgett, H. C., 357
Brogden, W. J., 40
Chih-an, L., 176
Chistovich, L. A., 176
Craig, J. H., 305
Diercks, K. J., 44
Davis, H., 170
Doughty, J. M., 173
Egan, J. P., 212
Elliott, L. L., 297
Fletcher, H., 135, 221
Flottorp, G., 231
Garner, W. R., 93, 173
Green, D. M., 241
Haas, H., 264
Hake, H. W., 212
Hirsh, I. J., 314
Jeffress, L. A., 44, 305, 357
Kock, W. E., 368
Lane, C. E., 201
Levitt, H., 372
Licklider, J. C. R., 155
Mayer, A. M., 193
McAuliffe, D. R., 170
Miller, G. A., 40, 82, 161
Miller, R. L., 281
Newman, E. B., 101, 333, 343
Plomp, R., 299
Rabiner, L. R., 372
Riesz, R. R., 69
Ronken, D. A., 278
Rosenzweig, M. R., 343
Ross, D. A., 32
Sandel, T. T., 357
Schouten, J. F., 146
Shower, E. G., 75
Silverman, S. R., 170
Sivian, L. J., 17
Stevens, S. S., 101, 107, 231, 333
Swets, J. A., 48
Taylor, W. G., 161
Volkman, J., 101
Wallach, H., 343
Wegel, R. L., 201
White, S. D., 17
Wiener, F. M., 32
Wood, C. L., III, 357
Zwicker, E., 231

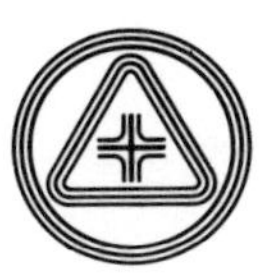

PSYCHOLOGICAL ACOUSTICS

INTRODUCTION

Psychological acoustics deals with the attempt to understand fully the auditory system's perceptual responses to sound. Because the system deals with signals that are fleeting in time for the most part and because the usual "output" of the system is of a highly pragmatic nature and usually difficult to quantify, progress toward a completely satisfactory description of the operation of the system has been disappointingly slow until fairly recently. The process of quantifying the behavior of the system has in the more distant past been slowed even further by the difficulty of controlling acoustic signals with the precision required.

In fact, until the last three or four decades, the study of the psychological reactions of the auditory system was severely curtailed because the system's ability to process sounds exceeded our own capability to manipulate, control, and specify the behavior of sound sources. The fact is that the auditory system is so versatile in its analysis of simultaneously present sounds that, even with modern methods of fabricating and controlling signal sources, we cannot hope to imitate some of its most relevant behavior in sufficiently practical ways to make study of some aspects feasible.

As the prime illustration of this state of affairs, our inability to rival auditory performance in the analysis of everyday speech has thwarted efforts to automate the transcription of speech even under favorable conditions of signal and noise. The auditory system accomplishes the task even in the presence of other signals that seem acoustically too similar to be excluded from the analysis. We cannot, in addition, say why two musical instruments or two voices occupying essentially the same areas of the spectrum, having essentially the same temporal patterns, and coming from the same direction still usually impress the ear unmistakably as two simultaneous but separate sounds, and only rarely as some inseparably fused combination of the two. Even in the presence of interfering signals having energy at least equal to that of the desired signal, the system reports the presence and the changing behavior of a familiar acoustic signal source.

Such difficulties in matching the level of our experiments to the level of performance of the system, fortunately, have not brought the study of psychological acoustics to a complete standstill. On the contrary, it has flourished in its own admittedly limited sphere.

Helmholtz's *Sensations of Tone* in 1863, from the title and indeed from much of the content, was the first major scholarly treatise on psychological acoustics. It necessarily differs in one extremely important regard from most later attempts: It relies heavily on one auditory system—Helmholtz's own apparently keen hearing—for generating its ideas and reaching its conclusions. This reliance on skillful individual perception is, in fact, characteristic of many studies prior to, and for some time after, Helmholtz's contribution. Even more broadly, it was the modus operandi of psychologists of that period: the analysis of the inherent nature of sensations by concentrated introspection. To a lessened degree, fortunately, this is still one likely technique for the discovery of new auditory phenomena, but the research climate now demands systematization and, one hopes, some form of verification before a finding is generally adopted. Very early in the twentieth century, especially among American psychologists, the drastic change in psychological studies away from expert introspection toward the emphasis on recognizing and compensating for individual differences gradually had its effect on psychological acoustics. The contrast is dramatically demonstrated by comparing the nature of evidence presented in the Helmholtz treatise and its admirable successor some sixty years later: *Hearing: Its Psychology and Physiology* (1938) by S. Smith Stevens and Hallowell Davis.

Historically the early concerns of workers in psychological acoustics centered on establishing the lower boundary of hearing and on systematizing the relations between the psychophysical pairs, frequency and pitch, and pressure and loudness. Even recently, these dimensions still occupy the attention of serious scholars.

Closely allied to the sensitivity of the system is its ability to detect the presence of a signal in the midst of interfering noise. As with many other acoustic and electronic devices, it is this parameter that is being measured when auditory "thresholds" are assessed. On close inspection, it becomes apparent that sensitivity studies, detection experiments, and explorations of masking exhibit a great deal of overlap.

One convenient way of dividing the field of psychological acoustics is into that work concerned with the perception of musical signals, that which deals with the processing of speech of speech sounds, and that which centers on the auditory system's interpretation of other sound sources in the environment. They differ in the requirements they impose on the system. For example, people have a great deal of choice in determining the characteristics of the sources to be used in the realm of music. They essentially tailor musical instruments to their auditory capabilities. To a degree, this can be said also of speech in the sense that it would be folly for any adaptive organism to continue to rely on the production of sounds not readily differentiable by its own auditory system, and within limits we have some choice in determining which sounds function in the language. But in the equally important assignment of processing the sounds of the environment, presumably the auditory system faces the task of discriminating sound changes as best it can in a set of signals over which it has much less control.

This turns out to be a useful way of thinking about the utility of the system, but not yet a very practical way of tracing the development of the field and describing its current status. For the most part, we have not yet progressed to the point in psychoacoustic work of being able to interpret responses to such sophisticated signals. What serves as a better descriptive framework at the moment is the set of parameters that we *can* manipulate independently and that appear to be central to the performance of the auditory system as a sensory channel.

One of the risks attendant on this effort to systematize our description of the system is that most of our laboratory study draws us too far away from study of the auditory system as a sensory system. It tends to shape the entire effort into a somewhat abstract study of an acoustic processing device more nearly from an engineering than from a psychological point of attack. Perhaps we gain early quantification at the risk of unduly prolonged simplification. Schroeder characterized one aspect of the result rather delightfully when he pointed out that we study what the ear "might do if it had been designed by fanciful model builders instead of by pragmatic evolution."

It will be apparent to sensory psychologists that this laboratory orientation is a limitation on the breadth of material that appears here to indicate the progress of psychological acoustics. I will, in spite of this restriction, make at least occasional reference to each of these three spheres of human activity that depend on information from the auditory system.

Inevitably, in a necessarily circumscribed description of one direction of study of a complicated acoustic system, several marginally pertinent areas are slighted. The study of psychological acoustics is itself multidimensional, and at each border of the multidimensional space lies an overlapping area of relevance and interest. Physiological acoustics is covered elsewhere in this same series, which means that the pertinent acoustics, mechanics, and neurophysiology enter here only by implication. The study of defective auditory systems is closely allied to the understanding of the normally operating system but is recognized here only as it has made incidental contributions to understanding normal auditory perception.

Another area that has been extremely useful and one that uses the methods of psychological acoustics is the study of temporary threshold shifts, usually from noise exposure. It has not been included because the perceptual response is not the end result in that area of study but only a means to study the state of the auditory system. A few studies have also elicited altered perceptual responses during a period of temporary threshold shift, but to date these are of only incidental interest. Perhaps the most critical assignment of the auditory system—the perception of speech—is not included in this recital because it is the topic of two separate volumes. (See the list on the beginning page of this volume.)

A few words are in order about the specific topics under which the material has been organized. Sensitivity of the ear has been a special topic of study and interest for a long time. I have already spoken of its central position in the history of the study of audition.

What I mean here by classical psychoacoustics has to do with the measurement of the differential sensitivity of the auditory system to rather long, steady-state signals. For some, perhaps the departure from classical psychoacoustics occurred with Steven's championing of the power law against the logarithmic formulation of Fechner. As H. M. Fowler once pointed out about the general view of the split infinitive, the psychoacoustic world might accurately be divided into those who know the difference between the Stevens law and the Fechner law and care very greatly, those who neither know nor care, and those who know but do not find it a matter of grave concern. I have felt it fair to look on the Stevens reform as a refinement and extension of the old psychoacoustics rather than an attempt to approach the whole problem of the organization of auditory behavior with a more dynamic, and therefore possibly a more realistically generalizable, set of signals. The latter I would view as the new psychoacoustics.

Pitch perception, too, is one of the old standbys in audition, so much so, in fact, that it was impossible to keep that section within bounds without ignoring much of the work done on the perception of musical pitch.

One of the early papers discussed there—the Delezenne work—did spring from an argument about musical perception. That 1826 paper might well have been included as a Benchmark paper, but unless one is certain to preserve the original aura in the translation from the French, a paraphrase is safer. I have opted for the latter.

With improved control of duration and envelope of signals, more of our pitch experience has been paralleled inside the laboratory, and it remains one of the central interests in psychological acoustics.

One might expect that this discussion of the nature of pitch perception would be followed by a section on loudness. The absence of that particular section may be traced to my own bias that, although loudness is relatively easy to measure, specific judgments of loudness are rather rare in the everyday listening world, and that the relevant work on the loudness response can be completely covered in the framework of classical psychoacoustics.

As I have already implied, our ability to respond to simultaneous signals is one of the astounding accomplishments of the auditory system. Undoubtedly the system makes use of both spectral and temporal clues in making this separation, but for convenience most of the section on separation of signals is concerned with spectral resolution, or simultaneous masking.

This leaves to temporal resolution both the temporal aspects of separating signals and the temporal considerations involved in the processing of single, rapidly changing sounds. Increasing recognition of the importance of time pattern resolution is well demonstrated in the sequence of papers assigned to this section. One completely arbitrary choice that should be noted is that I have placed the Haas study on perception of single echos in the section on temporal resolution rather than in the discussion of binaural processing. I have done this to emphasize the fact that to date no one has ascertained how much comparable suppression of echo takes place in monaural listening. That it is less effective than for binaural listening seems apparent. In either case, it is an important aspect of temporal processing.

In the papers explaining the binaural advantages, I have not given much emphasis to investigations of localization. Improved signal selection by the binaural system seems to me the more interesting facet perceptually, particularly since most papers on location of signals by the binaural system deal with lateralization rather than localization.

There are, without doubt, other areas of interest than the ones represented here. The topics chosen appear to furnish a suitable framework for the papers that have, directly or indirectly, constituted the supporting evidence on which the current science of psychoacoustics was built. My aim has been to describe briefly the state of that developing science, introducing each paper as it fits into the evolving picture.

Part I

SENSITIVITY OF THE EAR

Editor's Comments on Papers 1 Through 5

1 **SIVIAN and WHITE**
Excerpts from *On Minimum Audible Sound Fields*

2 **WIENER and ROSS**
The Pressure Distribution in the Auditory Canal in a Progressive Sound Field

3 **BROGDEN and MILLER**
Physiological Noise Generated under Earphone Cushions

4 **DIERCKS and JEFFRESS**
Interaural Phase and the Absolute Threshold for Tone

5 **SWETS**
Is There a Sensory Threshold?

As early in the history of audition as signal levels could be controlled, a question of interest has been, What is the faintest sound that can be detected by the human ear? No satisfactory simple answer can be given. If one attempts a realistic everyday sort of answer, the result is definitely determined by the sound levels of our modern civilization rather than by the ultimate sensitivity of the ear. In fact, the adoption of the term *noise pollution* reminds us how infrequently in everyday listening there is any opportunity to approach the actual limits of auditory sensitivity. But to the scholar in psychoacoustics, the question is of theoretical interest, quite apart from the recognition that prevalent ambient noise levels may well obviate any practical involvement with the problem.

A realistic approach asserts that even in quiet listening environments, input noise is the determining factor. Sivian and White (Paper 1) after they had measured the "minimum audible field"—the sound pressure level required at various frequencies at the position of the observer's head for a tone to be detected half the time—looked at their results and, noting the impressive sensitivity of the system, considered the possibility that under very quiet conditions, input noise resulting from Brownian motion in the air of the ear canal is the limiting noise of the system. However, even in the most sensitive range of the ear, other inherent noises in the system appear to set a limit higher than the Brownian source. Furthermore the question of the possible approach to a Brownian-noise limit seems more appropriately raised for Brownian motion in some element farther downstream in the cochlea—possibly after some filtering but prior to any gain in the system—as Harris (1968) pointed out. But whatever may be the limiting factor, the Sivian and White measurements have been the reference for auditory sensitivity. The entire paper makes interesting reading, but with limitations on space, what is reproduced here is the experimental work and the comparison with "minimum audible pressure" measures taken by others.

In the older literature on hearing, "absolute" and "relative" thresholds were frequently spoken of as two distinctly different concepts, the latter being the one determined by some interfering noise. This was not true of the Sivian and White discussion, but it pervaded particularly early audiometric and psychological reports. With increasing familiarity with the nature of threshold, this difference is more difficult to define. Three relevant considerations have emerged. First, it is very difficult to establish how much of the signal measured at some point external to the system is actually effective in stimulating the ear. Second, when external ambient noise is reduced as far as is practical, physiological noise attributable to blood flow, breathing, implicit muscle activity, and so forth is transmitted to the cochlea at a level high enough to constitute the inherent limiting input noise of the system. Third, first-order auditory (eighth nerve) neurons have an inherent noise level of their own, since they fire spontaneously at a characteristic random rate in the absence of an external signal.

With regard to the first point, the Sivian and White paper is still highly instructive some forty years later. Accounting for the differences in minimum audible pressure and minimum audible field turned out to be more troublesome than they predicted. Even when sound pressure was measured at the eardrum, the required sound pressure level for equal detectability or for equal loudness differed when the source was an earphone on the ear from that required when the ear was not covered by a phone. Munson and Wiener (1952) pursued the point further in their fascinating "search for the missing 6dB," this being the puzzling average difference they found at low frequencies between the sound pressure required for tone detection when the source was an earphone and when it was a loudspeaker, even though sound pressure was measured at the eardrum in both instances. They discovered that only by leaving the phones in place and correcting the speaker level to give the same loudness could they achieve equal measured input (sound pressure level at eardrum) for equal auditory output (equal loudness for speaker signal and phone signal). The reason for this was not apparent at the time but now appears to be closely related to point two. Ten years later Rudmose (1962) was still searching for a satisfactory answer. He presented evidence that the difference in minimum detectability was attributable to higher noise level under an enclosing cushion than in open air given the same low ambient level, but he recognized that this still did not explain the difference in apparent loudness "above threshold" under the two conditions. Still later, Anderson and Whittle (1971) decided that the culprit is vascular noise in the pinna and the walls of the ear canal. But we still have only a partial explanation of the difference between minimum audible pressure under phones and from a loudspeaker.

By either input path, we know at least that the ear in its sensitive range must be a reasonably efficient mechanism, since the mechanical amplitudes involved in the limit are infinitesimal (of the order of a fraction of an Ångstrom). Even with modern instrumentation we seldom measure the minimum level directly. Specifying the sound pressure at the input to the system at an agreed-upon distance above "threshold" has become the standard method for controlled studies. This technique was perfected by Wiener and Ross (Paper 2) and reported in a paper that continues to be of both practical and theoretical interest. Shaw and his colleagues (Shaw, 1966a, b; Shaw and Teranishi, 1968) have extended these measurements so that we now have a highly usable picture of the distribution of sound pressures at the input to the ear, and the possible contribution of the external structures to the shape of the sensitivity curve.

To return to the second point, note that Sivian and White were concerned with "physiological noise" as the limiting factor primarily for the minimum audible pressure measurement—that is, when the ear canal was closed by the receiver (transducer) but reported that it was "quite inaudible" when the enclosed volume was as much as 10 cm^3. But Brogden and Miller (Paper 3), by the simple expedient of increasing the physiological noise, attempted some quantifying of its effects and, by implication, indicated how strongly it might affect absolute sensitivity measurements in otherwise quiet environments. The different effect of physiological noise was a factor Munson and Wiener strongly considered when they encountered the missing 6dB.

Further indications of the effect of this type of internal noise stem from the deductions of Diercks and Jeffress (Paper 4) about the nature of noise interference when binaural absolute sensitivity is being measured. Because of their analysis and the work of Egan (1965) on detection of signals when the interfering noise is sensibly identical at the two ears, we know that for both absolute and relative "thresholds," detection with two ears yields an advantage only when there is some difference in the signal and noise relations of the two ears.

The fact that the so-called absolute threshold is also a noise-limited measure generates considerably greater interest in the nature of the inherent noise of the system. Shaw and Piercy (1962) measured the sound pressure levels present under earphone enclosures and demonstrated that at low frequencies (up to 500Hz) the level in a one-third octave band nearly coincides with the minimum audible pressure as measured by Sivian and White. They also showed that with the enclosed volume over the ear held constant, the sound pressure level inside that volume is proportional to the area of skin bounding the cavity. Such findings coupled with the fact that minimum sensitivity can be shown to change with temporary suspension of breathing and is affected by where the signal occurs in relation to heart-beat rhythm support the statement by Brogden and Miller that "a human being is a relatively noisy organism," at least with respect to his own auditory system. A more recent study (Watson et al., 1972) makes use of measurement on normal hearers in a quiet environment to estimate the spectrum of auditory "system noise" between 125Hz and 4kHz. In the low-frequency range, their psychophysically derived estimate agrees well with the spectral level measured in the canal by Shaw and Piercy (1962). In the ear's sensitive range, between 1000Hz and 4000Hz the estimated spectral level of the inherent noise in the system is about -10dB sound pressure level. This situation, combined with point three above, makes the physical situation seem hardly conducive to the use of the "threshold" concept.

It appears that no matter what conditions we arrange for taking absolute sensitivity measures, and no matter at what frequency, the problem is that of ascertaining at what point the designated signal is above some inherent noise, either of the system itself or in the environment. Yet the problem that remains is whether the listener *behaves* as though he has a response threshold, and this is the problem ably expounded in the paper by Swets (Paper 5).

In spite of the foregoing evidence, it is difficult to hold rigidly to the view that some noise floor completely determines the sensitivity curve. Equal loudness contours maintain roughly the same shape for some distance above the minimum audibility curve and must therefore be at least partly determined by transmission properties of the system, not by the spectrum of a masking noise. Thus, quite apart from its minimum level, the shape of the sensitivity curve over the audible range is of special interest. Its gross characteristics can be satisfactorily accounted for, as Zwislocki (1965, 1975) pointed out, by the baffle effect of the head and pinna, the resonance of the canal, and the transmission characteristics of the middle ear mechanism. Whether remaining discrepancies are to be attributed to details of neural coding and neural density or whether more exact knowledge of the transduction process in the cochlea will necessitate some revamping of our current reconstruction of the whole curve from its component parts is still open to conjecture.

Even if we account satisfactorily for the shape and the level of the curve, establishing the frequency limits of sensitivity presents some difficulties at both the high and the low frequency end. Where does the curve end? Wegel (1922), supported later by Fletcher (1929), argues that the rational method of determining the upper and lower frequency limits was to locate the point at each end where the threshold of audibility intersects the threshold of feeling or pain. This is scarcely an appealing criterion for the auditory psychologist for reasons that should become clearer in the ensuing discussion.

At the low end, there is the problem of presenting a pure sinusoidal signal. At the time of earliest reported curiosity about this question, concern for such details was quite impossible. Savart's (1830) sound source was his toothed wheel, and his best frequency-measuring tool was an auditory pitch match to the frequency of the monochord.* But Savart, aware of some earlier estimates of the limit of tonality at the lower end of about fifteen cycles per second and of estimates at the upper end plagued by inability to control the intensity of the source, essentially verified the opinion that the lower limit of tonality was about fifteen impulses per second from his wheel, and that at around 12,000 to 15,000 impacts per second, the decrease in intensity caused the tone to become inaudible.

Many attempts have been made to pursue the low end to its limit. The most successful of these indicate that subjects report experiencing sensation of feeling or pulsation without the experience of sound when presented with sinusoids at frequencies of 10Hz and lower. A thorough exploration of the lower limit with sinusoids was reported by Yeowart et al. (1967). They succeeded in producing low distortion sinusoids down to a frequency of 1.5Hz under conditions that permitted using the standard psychophysical method of limits to examine the minimum sound pressure level for "audibility." Required sound pressure levels at 1.5Hz and 2Hz were slightly over 130dB. It may be interesting to note that the total pressure change equivalent to 130dB sound pressure level is the same as that experienced in a change in altitude of roughly fifty feet. Our experience with rapid elevators or small aircraft may well sug-

*An English translation of this paper is available as Paper 22 in *Acoustics: Historical and Philosophical Development,* ed. R. B. Lindsay (Stroudsburg, Pennsylvania: Dowden, Hutchinson & Ross, 1973).

gest that the sensation experienced when that pressure change takes place in a period of a second or less is more apt to be tactile than tonal. In fact, the observers in the study reported that from 15Hz down to 5Hz, the auditory part of the sensation no longer appeared to be tonal; they described it as "rough" or "popping." From 5Hz down, the auditory aspect was characterized as "chugging" or "whooshing."

Where, then, is the end of a reasonably homogeneous perceptual continuum that maps the parallel between frequency variation and variation in pitch? Nordmark (1968) favors timing as the mechanism of perception of frequency change throughout the entire lower range. Using pulse trains as the signal, he finds a relatively constant function from five hundred pulses per second down to one pulse per second. This seems a rather satisfying continuum perceptually. It moves relatively smoothly through the various low-frequency stages to where tonality begins, and the stimulus remains unquestionably acoustic throughout the entire range. Unfortunately, since pulses have a broad spectrum, it may help but is not definitive in establishing the lower segment of the sensitivity curve.

How far down, then, does low-frequency energy continue to be the true auditory stimulus? Guttman and Pruzansky (1962) bypassed the difficult problem of producing pure sinusoids in this low range. They used pulses of complex spectrum and asked their observers to judge the failure of pitch height to identify the lower limit of pitch. They report nineteen per second as the region where pitch-height perception appears to give way to a faster-slower judgment. But they set the lower limit of "musical pitch" as about sixty per second, since at that point the subjects' ability to make octave judgments became decidedly poorer than at faster rates. Musical practice, as evidenced by the lowest notes of existing instruments, reinforces the impression that their lower figure is in the right range for the lower limit of pitch. The E-string of the contrabass (41Hz), the lowest note of the piano (27.5Hz), and the sixteen-foot organ pipe (33Hz) attest the belief that musical pitch extends below—but not too far below—their 60Hz limit. Suppose we attempt to bypass this problem by having subjects listen specifically for the lowest sinusoid in a complex tone, even though the others are present. A study by Plomp and Mimpen (1968) required subjects to listen for ("hear out") individual partials of complex tones. At a fundamental of 44Hz, their subjects could not demonstrate that they heard the individual tones of the complex. Perhaps this lower limit of the ear's spectral analysis is a good estimate of the lower limit of musical pitch and, by implication, the lower limit for producing the same fused tonal perceptual response as that for sinusoids of higher frequency.

It should be clear, however, that there is no accepted criterion that firmly establishes the low-frequency limit of the sensitivity curve. At the high-frequency end, the problem presented is quite different. There is general agreement that the place principle of pitch perception holds in this range. Ignoring for the moment the fact that precise control of the sound pressure at the eardrum makes it difficult to specify the curve precisely in this range, we face yet another perceptually-based difficulty. Different signal frequencies over this higher range presumably mean different loci for the maximum amplitude of basilar membrane vibration. At some frequency, we might expect that further increases in frequency will require only increases in sound pressure to create virtually the same amplitude envelope at the basal end of the cochlea with no shift in position of maximum.

A report by Deatherage et al. (1954) offers at least indirect evidence that this process may go as high as 100kHz, at least two octaves above the frequency usually given as the upper limit of hearing. Here again it appears that establishing the upper limit of frequency-pitch covariation would give additional meaning to the specification of the upper limit of the sensitivity curve.

Even earlier Pumphrey (1950) had indicated, from his own apparently skillful listening, that the situation is precisely that which the Deatherage et al. study indicates. Pumphrey set the limit for pitch rise at a frequency of about 15kHz, even though this same pitch could be elicited as the frequency of the driving transducer rose to 100kHz. The young, musically trained subjects of Corso and Levine (1965) confirm the fact that pitch judgments fail as the driving frequency rises beyond 16kHz, even though a pitch sensation is elicited for frequencies as high as 94kHz.

At this high end of the frequency continuum, there seems to be general agreement that the limit of musical pitch and the limit of pitch discrimination with frequency change differ considerably. Musical pitch, it is generally agreed, deteriorates rapidly in the neighborhood of 5kHz. Not only is this the top of the range for scale-oriented instruments, but Ward's rather musical subjects (Ward, 1954), attempting octave settings for tones above 2700Hz, either gave up or performed so erratically that Ward concluded, "Musical pitch simply disappears at about 5500Hz." Corso's listeners (Corso and Levine, 1964), though they still performed at 16kHz with an error of only about 1 percent, still doubled their just noticeable frequency change ($\Delta f/f$) between 4000Hz and 8000Hz. Furthermore, Bachem (1948) concluded from experiments with oscillator tones that the limit for absolute pitch is about 5kHz.

Even the more recently investigated residue pitch could not be elicited when the residue-producing components were in the range of 5kHz (Ritsma, 1962). Why these two differently mediated kinds of pitch would fail at the same point on the frequency continuum, or locus in the cochlea, is not readily apparent. There seems plenty of evidence, as we have just seen, and even as far back as Shower and Biddulph (1931), that pitch change—presumably mediated by movement of the basilar membrane maximum—continues for at least another octave, and possibly more.

Thus, whereas establishing the lower portion of the sensitivity curve is beset with uncertainty, and we are left with two equally equivocal ways of accounting for the measured curve, the primary problem of specifying the exact curve at the high end is simply the difficulty of creating and defining a reproducible signal in a segment of the spectrum where the wavelengths are comparable to the size of the ear structures and the coupling cavities.

REFERENCES

Anderson, C. M. B., and L. S. Whittle. 1971. Psychological noise and the missing 6dB. *Acustica* **24**:261-272.

Bachem, A. 1948. Chroma fixation at the ends of the musical frequency scale, *Acoust. Soc. Am. J.* **20**:704-705.

Corso, J. F., and M. Levine., 1965. Pitch-discrimination at high frequencies by air- and bone-conduction. *Am. J. Psychol.* **78**:557-566.

Deatherage, B. H., L. A. Jeffress, and H. C. Blodgett., 1954. A note on the audibility of intense ultrasonic sound. *Acoust. Soc. Am. J.* **26**:582 (L).

Egan, J. P. 1965. Masking-level differences as a function of interaural disparities in intensity of signal and of noise. *Acoust. Soc. Am. J.* **38**:1043-1049.

Fletcher, H. 1929. *Speech and hearing.* New York: Van Nostrand.

Guttman, N., and S. Pruzansky. 1962. Lower limits of pitch and musical pitch. *J. Speech Hear. Res.* **5**:207-214.

Harris, G. G. 1968. Brownian motion in the cochlear partition. *Acoust. Soc. Am. J.* **44**:176-186.

Munson, W. A., and F. M. Wiener. 1952. In search of the missing 6dB. *Acoust. Soc. Am. J.* **24**:498-501.

Nordmark, J. O. 1968. Mechanisms of frequency discrimination. *Acoust. Soc. Am. J.* **44**:1533-1540.

Plomp, R., and H. M. Mimpen. 1968. The ear as a frequency analyzer, II. *Acoust. Soc. Am. J.* **43**:764-767.

Pumphrey, R. J. 1950. Upper limit of frequency for human hearing. *Nature* **166**: 571.

Ritsma, R. J. 1962. Existence region of the tonal residue *Acoust. Soc. Am. J.* **34**: 1224-1229.

Rudmose, W. 1962. Pressure vs free field thresholds at low frequencies. *Fourth Int. Cong. Acoust., Copenhagen, Paper H52.*

Savart, F. 1830. Ueber die Empfindlichkeit des Gehörorgans. *Ann. Phys. Chem.* **20**: 290-304.

Shaw, E. A. G. 1966a. Ear canal pressure generated by a free sound field. *Acoust. Soc. Am. J.* **39**:465-470.

Shaw, E. A. G. 1966b. Ear canal pressure generated by circumaural earphones. *Acoust. Soc. Am. J.* **39**:471-479.

Shaw, E. A. G., and J. E. Piercy. 1962. Audiometry and physiological noise. *Fourth Int. Congr. Acoust., Copenhagen, Paper H46.*

Shaw, E. A. G., and R. Teranishi. 1968. Sound pressure generated in an external-ear replica and real human ears by a nearby point source. *Acoust. Soc. Am. J.* **44**: 240–249.

Shower, E. G., and R. Biddulph. 1931. Differential pitch sensitivity of the ear. *Acoust. Soc. Am. J.* **3**:275–287.

Ward, W. D. 1954. Subjective musical pitch. *Acoust. Soc. Am. J.* **26**:369–380.

Watson, C. S., J. R. Franks, and D. C. Hood. 1972. Detection of tones in the absence of external masking noise. I. Effects of signal intensity and signal frequency. *Acoust. Soc. Am. J.* **52**:633–643.

Wegel, R. L. 1922. The physical examination of hearing and binaural aids for the deaf. *Natl. Acad. Sci. Proc.* **8**:155–160.

Yeowart, N. S., M. E. Bryan, and W. Tempest. 1967. The monaural M.A.P. threshold of hearing at frequencies from 1.5 to 100 c/s. *J. Sound Vib.* **6**:335–342.

Zwislocki, J. J. 1965. Analysis of some auditory characteristics. In *Handbook of mathematical psychology,* ed., R. D. Luce, R. R. Bush, and E. Galanter, vol. 3. New York: Wiley.

Zwislocki, J. J. 1975. The role of the external and middle ear in sound transmission. In *Human communication and its disorders,* ed. E. Eagles, pp. 45–56. New York: Raven Press.

1

Reprinted from pages 288-296, 305-307, 312-314, and 320-321 of
Acoust. Soc. Am. J. 4:288-321(1933)

ON MINIMUM AUDIBLE SOUND FIELDS*

By L. J. Sivian and S. D. White
Bell Telephone Laboratories, New York

[*Editor's Note:* The table of contents and abstract have been omitted.]

Threshold of Hearing—General Discussion

Ideally, an absolute measurement of the least audible sound would state the stimulus in terms independent of the particular apparatus used to produce it. With this in view, most threshold determinations roughly

* Presented before Acoustical Society of America, at Ann Arbor, Michigan, November 29, 1932.

fall into two classes: the "minimum audible field" (M.A.F.) and the "minimum audible pressure" (M.A.P.). The former is in terms of the intensity of the sound field in which the observer's head is placed; the latter, in terms of the pressure amplitude at the observer's ear drum. This paper is concerned only with steady tones; i.e., with tones sustained over one second or longer. Even with this restriction, the generation and measurement of the stimulus over the audio range of frequencies entail considerable difficulty. Because of the technique required, threshold measurements usually have been made by physicists. However, essentially this is an experiment in physiology and psychology, and the data are subject to a number of nonphysical influences.

The M.A.F. values directly relate to the usual mode of hearing, i.e., with the unaided ear. They are the more applicable when extended to include the effects of binaural hearing and of the listener's orientation with respect to the sound field. The M.A.P. data are of interest in the study of the ear mechanism. At sufficiently low frequencies they can be used in conjunction with drum impedance data, to throw some light on the least audible drum displacements. Given anatomically reasonable assumptions as to the low-frequency mechanism of the ear and the cochlea, the minimum audible forces exerted by the basilar membrane may be surmised. One of the requisites for any such deductions is that the frequency be sufficiently low so that the impedance, as measured looking into the ear drum, is predominantly a stiffness reactance. This probably means frequencies below 600 c.p.s. The M.A.P. becomes indefinite at frequencies so high that the pressure on the ear drum can no longer be assumed to be approximately uniform. There is no direct evidence as to where this occurs. For air in a circular cylinder of 1 cm diameter and having rigid walls, the gravest purely transverse mode of vibration corresponds to a frequency of 20,000 c.p.s. This is the case of one nodal diameter and no nodal circles. From this and from similar indirect considerations, it is thought that up to 10,000 c.p.s. at any rate, the pressure is uniform over the area of the drum, well within the limits of threshold work accuracy.

The methods used for threshold determinations, and more detailed definitions of the stimulus, are given in the following three sections. The threshold data discussed are those in which the stimulus either is a pure sinusoidal wave, or a very narrow frequency band within which the ear sensitivity is substantially constant. The graphs representing the M.A.F. or M.A.P. stimulus as a function of frequency are briefly referred to as M.A.F. or M.A.P. curves, respectively. The M.A.F. curves are supplemented by some data showing the effect of the observer's orientation with respect to the sound field, as given in "azimuth" curves.

THE PRESENT MINIMUM AUDIBLE FIELD (M.A.F.) DETERMINATION

The quantity measured

This is the intensity of a progressive wave which produces a minimum audible field for an observer placed in it. The intensity measured is that of the undistorted free field, prior to placing of the observer into it. Ideally, the field would be that of a progressive plane wave. In that case the pressure p, which is the quantity best suited to direct measurement, and the intensity W are simply related: $W = p^2/\rho c$,

where ρc = air density x sound velocity = 41.2 C.G.S. units at 76 cm barometric pressure and 23°C

p = r.m.s. pressure in bars

W = intensity in ergs per second through 1 cm^2 of wave front.

The same equation applies to a progressive spherical wave. It was impractical accurately to realize either of these sound fields over the range of frequencies to be covered: $f = 60$ cycles to $f = 15{,}000$ cycles, corresponding to wave-lengths of $\lambda = 574$ cm and $\lambda = 2.3$ cm, respectively. "Impractical" is used with reference to extensive threshold measurements in which it was desired to use a number of observers and to avoid the interruptions attendant upon work outdoors.

The sound field

Actually, the data were obtained in the field established at one meter in front of a loud speaking receiver[1] in a highly absorbing acoustic structure (referred to later as the "sound stage"). This structure is of the type developed by Wente and Bedell.* It consists of 12 layers of flannel and muslin, separated by air layers, making a total thickness of 12 inches. The receiver radiates from an area of 3.8 cm diameter, in the center of a cylindrical case 16 cm in diameter. The sound stage, the sound source and an observer are shown in Fig. 1. This arrangement establishes in a limited volume a field approximately like that of a progressive spherical wave. If this zone, especially its horizontal dimensions at the level of the observer's ears, is several times larger than the observer's head, the effect on the latter will be nearly the same as that due to a progressive spherical wave.

* U. S. Patent No. 1,907,712, E. H. Bedell.

The center of the observer's ear-line (i.e., of a straight line about 18 cm long joining the two ears), is at one meter from the source, on the receiver axis. The ear-line nowhere departs from a circular arc by more than 0.5 cm, which is small relative to all but the shortest wavelengths used. The difference between the diffraction effects of a plane

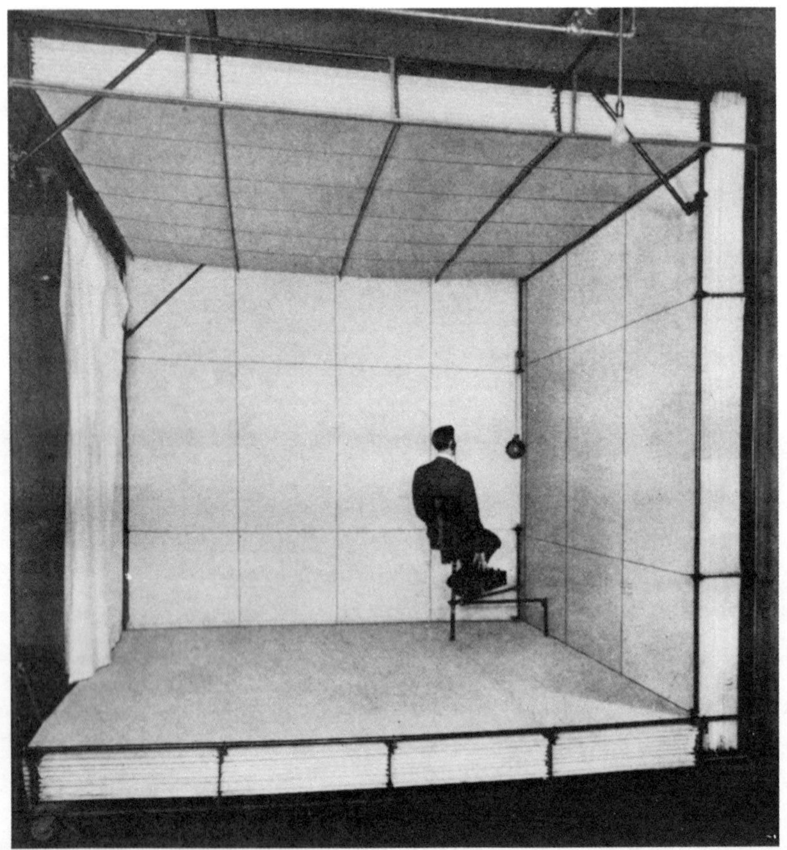

FIG. 1. *The sound stage and sound source, with an observer in position.*

wave and of a spherical wave of one meter radius, is quite small for our purposes. This can further be inferred from the theory of diffraction at a rigid sphere,[2] caused by plane and spherical waves, respectively. Thus Fig. 2 shows the diffraction produced at a 20 cm diameter sphere by two 5500 cycle waves: one plane ($kR=\infty$, $k=2\pi/\lambda$), the other spherical of 1 m radius ($kR=100$, $k=2\pi/\lambda$). The two are seen to be quite similar; the maximum difference of 2.5 db may in part be due to the limits of accuracy with which the zonal harmonics were evaluated. In what follows, no distinction will be made between a plane wave and a spherical wave of 1 m radius, as far as threshold of hearing is concerned.

The sound field was measured by means of a condenser transmitter, whose "field" calibration[3] was obtained with a Rayleigh disk. The sound stage was placed in a corner of a large, carefully sound-proofed room. At no time during the threshold measurements, was either the observer or the operator conscious of sufficient noise to affect the threshold.

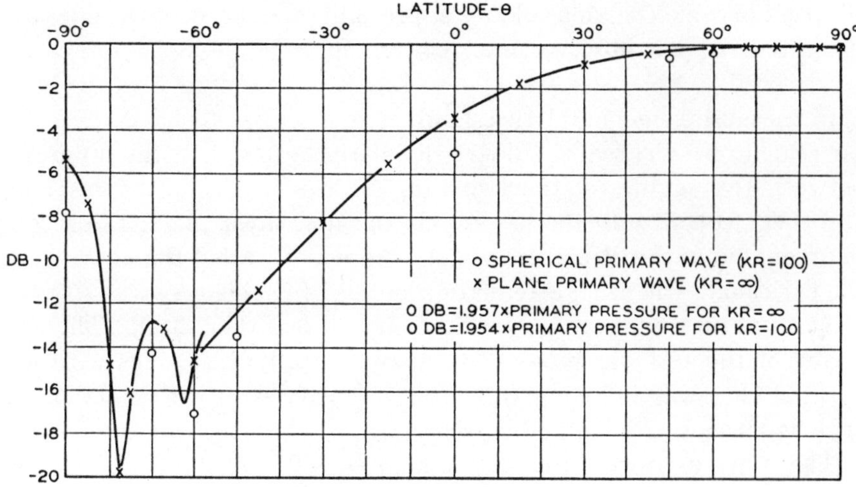

FIG. 2. *Diffraction at a rigid sphere.*

The threshold measurement procedure

The observer was provided with a push button which lighted a small lamp before the operater and which was held down whenever and as long as the tone was audible. The operator allowed the observer to listen to the tone at a level well above threshold, say 30 or 40 db, for a few seconds, and then gradually reduced the intensity by turning up the receiver current attenuator until the observer signalled that he could no longer hear the tone. This level served as a convenient one at which to start interrupting the tone as usually the observer could hear an intermittent tone 10 to 20 db lower.

From this level on down, the operator reduced the sound in steps until threshold was determined, interrupting the tone several times at each attenuator setting. The tone was left on for approximately two seconds, then cut off for about the same length of time, then the tone again, etc. The transition from tone to silence and *vice versa* was made with no audible clicks whatever, by a gradual change in the amplifier filament current. The operator judged from the ability of the observer to follow the interruptions with his key whether or not he heard the tone at each intensity. The sizes of the steps were determined by the operator to give most rapidly an accurate figure for the threshold level and were usually about 5 db at first, becoming smaller down to the 1 db steps of the attenuator as threshold was approached.

The element of fatigue was carefully guarded against. As soon as an observer become conscious of any appreciable fatigue, or if the operator suspected it, that observer was relieved for a while and another observer used.

In measuring monaural threshold, it is essential to have the other ear sealed off. The seal should be definitely better than the difference between the acuities of the two ears. This was effected by inserting absorbent cotton into the ear canal; the first layer plain, the second impregnated with petrolatum which completely sealed the entrance to the ear canal. The usual attenuation obtained in this way was 30 to 34 db, and at no frequency in our range was it less than 20 db. The adequacy of the seal was proved by making threshold settings with and without the seal, and comparing the difference with the acuity difference as measured on an audiometer.

The tones used were 100, 200, 300, 400, 560, 800, 1100, 1600, 2240, 2700, 3200, 3700, 4200, 5000, 6400, 7600, 9000, 10,000, 12,000, 12,800 and 15,000 c.p.s. The electrical circuit and the sound source were so designed and operated that the tone reaching the observer's ear at levels near threshold was completely free from extraneous frequencies. The first six tones were pure sinusoidal waves. The others were "warble" tones centering about the nominal frequencies given. The "warble" range progressively increased from ± 50 cycles at 1100 c.p.s. to ± 146 cycles at 15,000 c.p.s. For all frequencies the warble was at the rate of 10 times per second. The advantage of using the warble is psychological, in that it reduces fatigue and uncertainty on the part of the observer; and physical, because of smoothing out of the residual standing wave patterns produced by reflections. A few check measurements made by the same individual with and without the warble indicated no other systematic differences between the threshold values in the two cases.

Data were obtained on 14 ears: 10 men's, left and right of 5 observers; 4 women's, right of 4 observers. The men's ages ranged from 18 to 26, except one of 40; the women's, from 20 to 23; the average age, about 23.

All observers had good hearing: "normal" or above normal, throughout the greater part of the frequency range,* as judged by their audiometer audiograms. This group will hereafter be referred to as group A.

The observed M.A.F. values

Fig. 3 gives the M.A.F. values found, logarithmically averaged for the 14 ears in group A. At each frequency the mean deviation from the average is indicated in the figure. The corresponding standard deviations are given together with those for binaural thresholds in Table I.

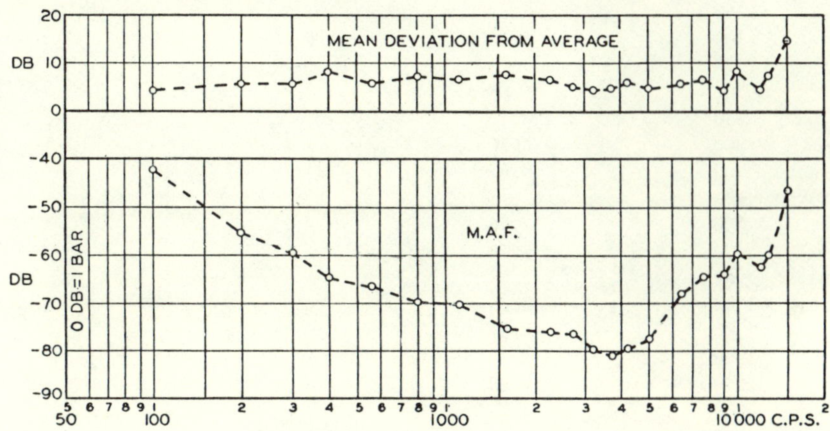

FIG. 3. *Monaural M.A.F., group A.*

It should be borne in mind that this M.A.F. curve is for a group of young people with generally excellent hearing, favored by freedom from fatigue and noise and by the contrast of the intermittent test tone.

Binaural M.A.F.

The binaural M.A.F. data are based on two groups of observers. Group B consisted of the 5 men included in the above group A. Group C consisted of 8 men and 2 women, average age about 24. The two women and three of the men were included in group A above.

The threshold measurements for group C were made under the direction of Mr. W. A. Munson, to whom we gratefully acknowledge our indebtedness for the data.

For group B all measurement conditions were identical with those described in the section on threshold measurement procedure. For two

* The one exception is at 15,000 c.p.s. where one observer's left ear showed abnormally low acuity; at all other frequencies that ear was easily as good as the average of the group.

members of the group data were available binaurally, as well as on each ear separately. These data showed no significant difference between the binaural M.A.F. and the best ear M.A.F. Accordingly for the three others in the group, the best ear M.A.F. was taken to be the binaural M.A.F.

TABLE I. *Standard deviations from average M.A.F.'s.*

Frequency	Group A (db)	Group B (db)	Group C (db)
60			2.5
100	5.1	5.26	
120			3.55
200	6.65	7.8	
240			4.3
300	6.76	7.2	
400	9.83	11.72	
480			4.2
560	7.94	8.2	
800	9.08	9.11	
960			3.35
1100	8.28	8.69	
1600	9.31	10.28	
1920			2.4
2240	7.25	6.74	
2700	6.55	7.85	
3200	6.11	7.05	
3700	5.87	5.85	
3850			3.3
4200	7.62	7.25	
5000	6.34	6.5	
5400			5.8
6400	7.06	6.61	
7600	7.44	6.76	
7800			5.1
9000	5.45	6.76	
10000	11.52	8.97	
10500			5.9
12000	6.49	6.75	
12800	9.31	8.77	
15000	18.2	10.32	12.85

For group C at all frequencies above 240 c.p.s. the measurement conditions were the same as in the section on threshold measurement procedure, except that single frequency tones rather than "warble" tones were employed throughout. At 60, 120 and 240 c.p.s. the sound source arrangement was somewhat different. The source was a moving coil loud speaker, radiating from an 18 inch diaphragm. At these low frequencies the angle of incidence of the sound wave is unimportant, and it was only necessary to insure by direct measurement that the observer's head was placed in a region of substantially uniform pressure.

The results are shown in Fig. 4, for the two groups separately. The mean deviations from the average M.A.F. at each frequency are also shown in this figure, while the standard deviations are given in Table I.

The remark at the end of the section on the observed M.A.F. values, concerning the observers and the test conditions applies to groups B and C as well.

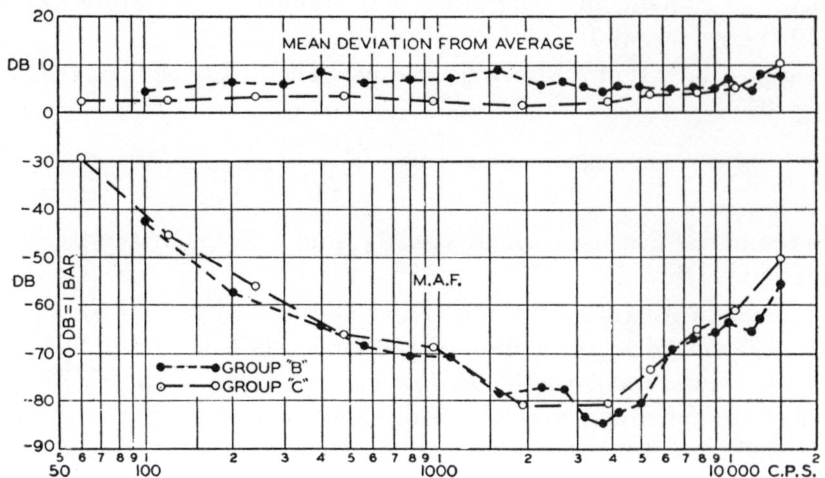

FIG. 4. *Binaural M.A.F., groups B and C.*

[*Editor's Note:* Material has been omitted at this point.]

The theoretical limit of aural acuity

Returning now to the data of Figs. 3 and 4, it may be inquired whether the ear sensitivity is limited by its physiological construction, or whether the limit is imposed by the air as a transmitting medium. Superposed on the average atmospheric pressure there are fluctuations caused by the distribution of thermal velocities of air molecules. What is the spectrum of the resultant thermal-acoustic noise? Is its magnitude compatible with the observed M.A.F.s?

It is interesting to note that in a recent paper by Barnes and Czerny,* a somewhat similar question is raised in regard to differential visual acuity. They conclude that there is some experimental evidence to support the view that the human eye, in that region of the visible spectrum to which it is most sensitive, has a differential sensitivity of

* R. Bowling Barnes and M. Czerny, Zeits. f. Physik **79**, 436–449 (1932).

the same order of magnitude as the fluctuations inherent in a "steady" light due to the shot effect in photon emission.

For purposes of calculation, let us replace the ear with a rigid massless piston, of area S, free to vibrate in an infinite rigid wall and exposed to the atmosphere on one side. Let R_f be its acoustic radiation resistance at the frequency f. Let $P_f^2 \cdot df$ be the square of the thermal-acoustic pressure in the interval df, averaged over S. Then by analogy with the theory* of the J. B. Johnson effect

$$[(S \cdot P_f)^2 \cdot df / R_f] = 4\kappa T \cdot df \tag{1}$$

where κ = Boltzmann's constant, T = absolute temperature, $\kappa T = 4 \times 10^{-14}$ ergs/sec. at $T = 300°$.

Suppose now that S is a circle: $S = \pi a^2$. Then (Rayleigh, *Sound*, Vol. II, §302)

$$R_f = \pi a^2 \cdot \rho c \cdot \left[1 - \frac{J_1(4\pi f a/c)}{2\pi f a/c} \right] \tag{2}$$

where ρc = air density x sound velocity, and J_1 is the first order Bessel function.

On substituting from (2) into (1) we find that in general P_f depends on the value of a, the radius of the circle chosen. In the limit, for $a \gg \lambda$ (λ = sound wave-length), $R_f = \rho c \cdot \pi a^2$ and $P_f = (4\kappa T \cdot \rho c / \pi a^2)^{1/2}$. The case of the ear drum, however, corresponds more nearly to $a \ll \lambda$, up to say 6000 c.p.s. In that case

$$1 - \frac{J_1(4\pi f a)/c}{2\pi f a/c} \doteq \frac{2\pi^2 f^2 a^2}{c^2}$$

whence

$$P_f^2 \cdot df = (8\pi \rho \kappa T/c) \cdot f^2 \cdot df. \tag{3}$$

The r.m.s. pressure $\overline{P}$ in the interval between f_1 and f_2, is

$$\overline{P} = \left[\int_{f_1}^{f_2} P_f^2 \cdot df \right]^{1/2} = \left[\frac{8\pi \rho \kappa T}{3c} (f_2^3 - f_1^3) \right]^{1/2}$$

For example, if $f_1 = 1000$ and $f_2 = 6000$ c.p.s., $\overline{P} = 5 \times 10^{-5}$ bars, or 86 db below 1 bar. In that frequency range, our M.A.F. curve averages about 76 db. In individual cases of particularly excellent hearing, it may average about 85 db. But even then, the above $\overline{P}$ is not likely to be

* H. Nyquist, *Thermal Agitation of Electric Charge in Conductors*, Phys. Rev. **42**, 110 (1928).

audible, if one be permitted to apply the Fletcher-Munson tables* for the loudness of a complex spectrum to levels so near threshold, or even below it. Of course, our computation at best is but a crude approximation. It appears that in the region of maximum ear sensitivity, i.e., 1000 to 6000 c.p.s., the M.A.F. pressures for the average good ear are of the same order, perhaps about three times larger than the r.m.s. thermal-acoustic pressure. For exceptionally good ears, a further increase in physiological sensitivity would be useless in the presence of thermal noise. From this point of view, it is not unlikely that the aural acuity of animals whose outer ear dimensions (drum included) are comparable with those of the human ear, is comparable with human acuity, say in the 1000 to 6000 c.p.s. range.

MINIMUM AUDIBLE PRESSURES (M.A.P.)

Data of the M.A.P. type

The purpose of an M.A.P. determination is to give that pressure *at the drum* which is minimum audible pressure. Several methods have been used, all based on the idea of establishing a known pressure at some measurable level (necessarily, well above threshold). The sound is reduced to threshold by reducing the sound source output by a known amount, usually determined from the required reduction of the electrical input feeding the source. No method has been devised, sufficiently sensitive to admit of direct measurement of the pressure on the ear drum at threshold. In principle, the M.A.P. determination assumes that the pressure is uniform over the area of the drum. This point was touched upon in the first section.

The first step is to produce a known pressure at the drum, which can later be attenuated by measurable amount down to the observer's threshold. Three procedures have been used.

[*Editor's Note:* Material has been omitted at this point.]

DISCUSSION OF M.A.F. AND M.A.P. TYPES OF DATA

From the several M.A.F. and M.A.P. determinations discussed above and the azimuth data on pages 11 and 12, the continuous threshold-frequency curves of Fig. 10 have been derived.

The M.A.F. curves are based primarily upon the data given in the section on the present minimum audible field (M.A.F.) determination. Obviously, the observed points could be fitted about equally well by a number of smooth curves, differing appreciably from one another. In adopting the particular one shown in Fig. 10 (curve 2) some account was taken of the several other M.A.F.-type determinations available.

* To be published in J. Acous. Soc. Am.

This was done quite arbitrarily, according to the authors' judgment of the experimental procedure employed. The number of ears tested in each case also was considered. These two criteria also determined the M.A.P. choice (curve 1, Fig. 10). In this case, of course, data published by others played the larger part; particularly at low frequencies. It has been stressed before that our M.A.F. data apply to young people with good hearing. It is felt that to a lesser extent the same may be said of curve 1, although in drawing it much weight was given to data for observers whose ages were unknown to us.

Now, it so happens that curve 2, Fig. 10, is hardly distinguishable, except at 15,000 c.p.s., from the smooth curve we would select to fit the

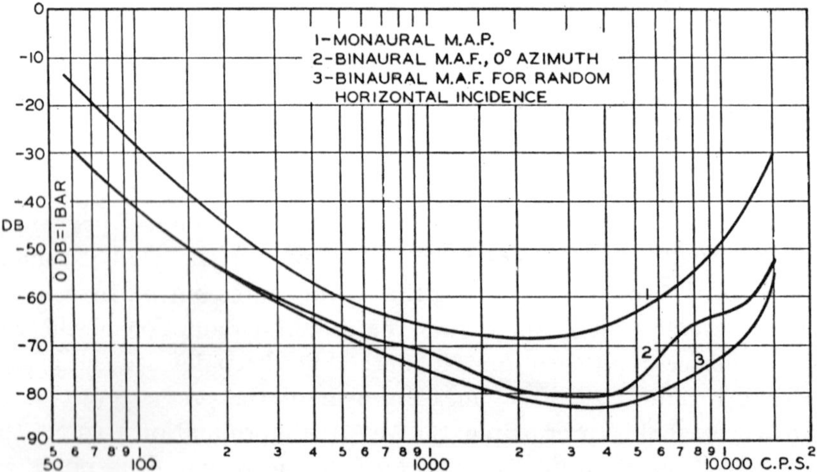

FIG. 10. *M.A.F. and M.A.P. Note: Concerning the ordinate scale for curve I, see note under Fig. 9.*

monaural M.A.F. observations of Fig. 3, also for 0° azimuth; "hardly distinguishable"—bearing in mind the uncertainties of threshold data. Hence for convenience of comparison with the monaural M.A.P. curve, shown in the same figure, we shall in this section use curve 2 as representing either monaural or binaural M.A.F.

The M.A.F. pressures lie below the M.A.P. values throughout the frequency range. At high frequencies the two might well be expected inherently to differ, because of head and pinna diffraction, and wave motion in the auditory canal, even if the physical measurements were perfect in both cases. Thus above say 1000 c.p.s. these effects might produce differences of the order of magnitude seen in Fig. 10. Below 500 c.p.s. they are negligible. The physical pressure measurements involved in M.A.P. determinations become increasily difficult with rising frequency. When method (a) of the section on minimum audible pressure is used, wave motion in the ear canal may vitiate the assumption that the pressure on the ear drum is the same as the sound source would produce in an equal volume but of different shape enclosed by different walls. With the first method under (b), and at higher frequencies with the second method as well, the pressures are measured at points where owing to wave motion they may be quite different from the drum pressures. Purely metric difficulties of the wave motion type probably render most of the M.A.P. data above 4000–5000 c.p.s. open to question. Below say 1000 c.p.s. their effect is negligible.

These factors might account for the large differences between the M.A.F. and M.A.P. values above say 1000 c.p.s., though it is not clear why the differences are all in the same direction. But at lower frequencies the differences are much too large to be explained in this manner. Below 500 c.p.s. we must look for other causes, particularly so because it is just at the lower frequencies that any possible discrepancies due to the possibly older age of the observers used in the M.A.P. work, would disappear. It is well established that in the age range of 20 to 35 years for normal people, there is scarcely any aging effect for auditory acuity below 1000 c.p.s. There are some additional factors, partly metric, partly physiological and psychological, which may affect the M.A.P. results.

[*Editor's Note:* Material has been omitted at this point.]

A definite answer to the question—why do the M.A.F. and M.A.P. curves differ at low frequencies?—cannot now be given. The evidence available indicates that: (1) the correction for drum yielding can account only for part of the discrepancy; (2) part may be due to "physiological noise," particularly from 200 c.p.s. downward; (3) that some such effects as static pressures, higher temperatures, fatigue, etc., play an important part in differentiating open field hearing from hearing with a source tightly fitting on the ear.

REFERENCES

[1] A. H. Inglis, C. H. G. Gray and R. T. Jenkins; *A Voice and Ear for Telephone Measurements,* Bell Sys. Tech. J. April, 1932.

[2] H. T. O'Neil, unpublished, Bell Telephone Laboratories, 1932.

[3] L. J. Sivian, *Absolute Calibration of Condenser Transmitters,* Bell Sys. Tech. J., January, 1931.

[4] Toepler and Boltzmann, Ann. d. Physik u. Chemie **21,** 321 (1870).

[5] Rayleigh, Proc. Roy. Soc. **A26,** 248 (1877); Sci. Papers, **IV,** 117 (1894).

[6] Wead, Am. J. Sci. **26,** 177 (1883).

[7] Webster, *Ludwig Boltzmann's Festschrift;* Barth, Leipzig, p. 866, 1904.

[8] Wien, Pflüger's Arch. f. d. ges. Physiol. **97,** 1 (1903).

[9] Langenbeck, Pflüger's Arch. f. d. ges. Physiol. **226,** 11–46, (1930).

[10] M. Guernsey, Am. J. Psych., October, 1922.

[11] C. E. Lane, Phys. Rev. **19,** 492 (1922).

[12] C. N. Swan, Proc. Am. Acad. Arts and Sci. **58,** 425 (1923).

[13] E. Meyer, Zeits. f. Hals, Nasen u. Ohrenheilkunde, p. 418, 1930.

[14] A. Bühl, Zeits. f. Hals, Nasen u. Ohrenheilkunde, p. 443, 1930.

[15] H. C. Huising, Diss. Univ. Groningen, November, 1932.

[16] Waetzmann and Heisig, Ann. d. Physik [5] **9,** 921 (1931). Waetzmann, Ann. d. Physik [5] **10,** 269 (1931).

[17] C. C. Bunch, Archives of Otolaryngology, 625–636, June, 1929 and 170–180, February, 1931.

[18] H. C. Montgomery, Bell Lab. Rec. 311–313, May, 1932.

[19] H. Abraham, Comptes Rendus **144,** 1099 (1907).

[20] F. W. Kranz, Phys. Rev. **21,** 573 (1923).

[21] Fletcher and Wegel, Phys. Rev. **19,** 553 (1922).

[22] Minton and Wilson, Proc. Nat. Acad. Sci. 9, 273 (1923).

[23] Wegel, Riesz and Blackman, J. Acoust. Soc. Am. **IV,** 6 (1932), abstract.

[24] G. V. Bekesy, Ann. d. Physik [5] **13,** 111 (1932).

[25] J. Troger, Phys. Zeits. **31,** 26 (1930).

[26] L. J. Sivian, unpublished, Bell Telephone Laboratories, September, 1928.

[27] W. A. Munson, unpublished, Bell Telephone Laboratories, July, 1932.

[28] Hahnemann and Hecht, Ann. d. Physik **60,** 454 (1919); **63,** 57 (1920); **64,** 673 (1921); **70,** 283 (1923).

[29] A. L. Thuras, unpublished, Bell Telephone Laboratories, May, 1925.

2

Reprinted from *Acoust. Soc. Am. J.* **18**:401–408 (1946)

The Pressure Distribution in the Auditory Canal in a Progressive Sound Field*

Francis M. Wiener
Psycho-Acoustic Laboratory, Harvard University, Cambridge, Massachusetts

and

Douglas A. Ross
Sanborn Company, Cambridge, Massachusetts

(Received May 29, 1946)

The variation of the sound pressure along the auditory canal was determined experimentally on a number of subjects, male and female, placed in a progressive sound field. This was accomplished by insertion of a small flexible probe microphone at various positions along the auditory canal. The subjects were placed in front of a loudspeaker in a room free from acoustic wall reflections. The free sound field at the subjects' location was essentially that of a plane progressive wave. The measurements were carried out over the significant range of audiofrequencies for various orientations in azimuth of the subjects with respect to the sound source. The sound pressure at the eardrum is found to be greater than the free-field pressure. The average ratio of these two quantities is a function of frequency, and reaches values of about 20 db in the vicinity of 3000 c.p.s. The human ear is thus an effective acoustic "amplifier." The increase in sound pressure at the eardrum over the free-field pressure is caused by a combination effect of diffraction by the head and pinna and resonance in the auditory canal. The measurements of the sound pressures at several other positions along the auditory canal serve to separate these two phenomena to a certain extent and to furnish additional information about the pressure distribution. Most of the data were obtained with a group of male subjects, but measurements on a few women did not show any marked discrepancies.

I. INTRODUCTION

THE acoustic stimulus acting on the ear is best described by specifying the sound pressure at the eardrum. In the past, meaningful measurements of this quantity could not readily be made because the exploring microphones then available were either not small enough or not readily adaptable to insertion into the auditory canal near the eardrum.[1] In the measurements about to be described, a small and flexible probe microphone was used which could be inserted

* This work was begun under Contract OEMsr-658 between the Office of Scientific Research and Development and Harvard University, Cambridge, Massachusetts, where the research is continuing under contract with the U. S. Navy, Office of Research and Inventions (Contract N5ori-76, Report PNR-5).

[1] A curve showing the sound pressure at the eardrum for constant free-field pressure, based mainly on calculations using experimental data on the impedance of the eardrum, is given by G. v. Békésy, Ann. d. Physik **14**, 51 (1932).

deep into the auditory canal without causing discomfort to the subject and without appreciably disturbing the sound field by its presence.

The subjects were placed in front of a loudspeaker in a large anechoic (echo-free) chamber. The free sound field produced at the subjects' location was approximately that of a plane progressive wave. By inserting the probe at various positions along the length of the auditory canal, the distribution of sound pressure was determined as a function of frequency. By Thévenin's theorem, the results obtained under these special conditions, expressed in the form of pressure ratios, can be applied in principle to a variety of other conditions, notably those in which an earphone is worn.

As a second objective of this research, the combined obstacle effect of the human head and auditory canal in a progressive sound field was studied. The ratio of the sound pressure at the eardrum to the free-field sound pressure at a point corresponding to the center of the observer's head was taken to be a measure of this effect.

II. TECHNIQUE

Figure 1 shows the probe tube, which is coupled to a Western Electric Type 640-AA condenser microphone by means of a suitable coupling. The probe consists of a small brass tube, about 2 inches in length, with a piece of plastic tubing of similar length pushed over its free end. The effective area of the microphone is a circle less than 0.1 cm in diameter.

Even with a relatively soft tube of this kind, the experimenter is obliged to approach the subject's eardrum with great caution. To facilitate this procedure, the subject's head was immobilized in a clamp. Figure 2 shows a view of the clamp from behind. It was designed so that the structure would not interfere with the sound field in the neighborhood of the left ear, which was the one used for all the tests. The photograph also shows the method of mounting the microphone and probe tube. Screw and rack-and-pinion adjustments are provided so that the microphone can be moved up or down, or from side to side, or fore and aft. The microphone is also mounted on a vertical swivel joint so that it is possible to change the angle of its approach to the ear canal. Note the marking collar for determining the length of the ear canal. Figure 3 shows a close-up view of the microphone carriage with the probe inserted in the auditory canal.

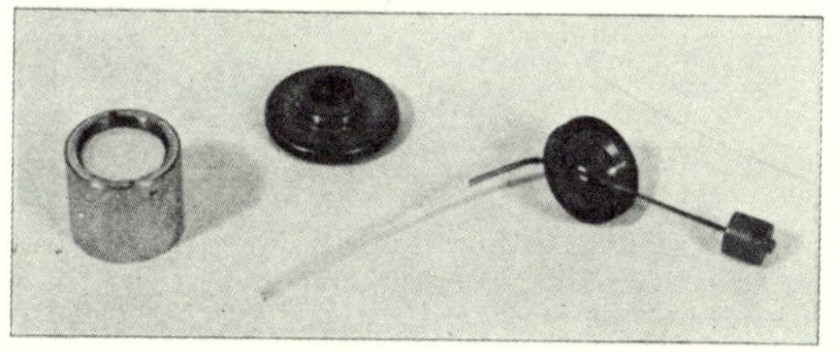

FIG. 1. W. E. Type 640-AA condenser microphone with flexible probe tube and coupling.

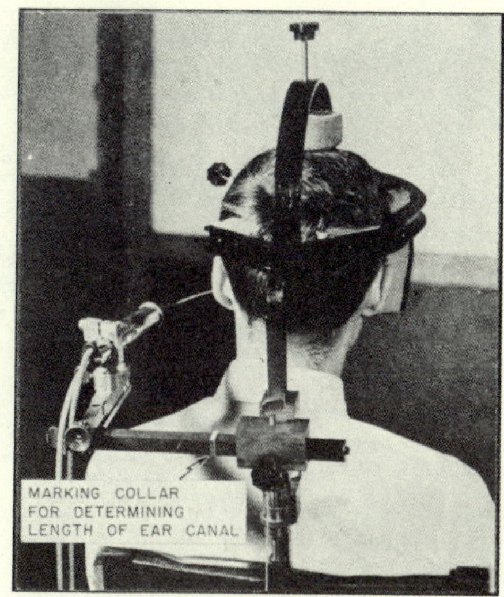

FIG. 2. Rear view of the head clamp and microphone carriage.

Calibration of the probe microphone showed that its sensitivity decreases with frequency at the rate of about 6 db per octave, except for several minor resonant peaks. A simple equalizer with a complementary characteristic was used and a typical calibration curve of the combination is shown in Fig. 4. The signal-to-noise ratio afforded by this instrument is at least 15 db in the range from 200 to 5000 c.p.s. and at least 10 db between 5000 and 8000 c.p.s. The free-field correction is essentially zero for all angles of incidence, and the calibration is independent of even drastic deformations of the flexible tube by bending.

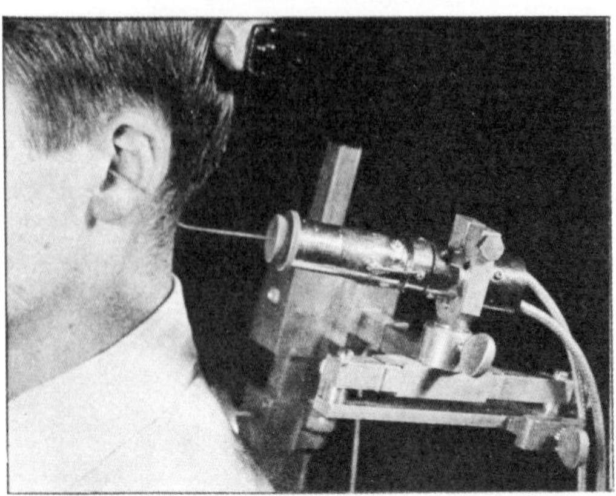

FIG. 3. Close-up view of the probe inserted in the auditory canal.

The sound pressures were measured, as a function of frequency, at the eardrum, at the entrance of the canal, at a point about half-way between these two positions, and also at a point in space corresponding to the center of the line joining the ears of the subject. These measurements were carried out in the frequency range of from 200 to 8000 c.p.s. and for various orientations of the subjects' heads with respect to the sound source. Angles of azimuth of 0, 45, and 90 degrees were explored, where zero azimuth corresponds to the orientation in which the observer faces the source of sound. The results, given later, are expressed in terms of pressure ratios.

It was simple enough, with the help of a beam of light reflected from a perforated concave head mirror, to place the tip of the probe tube in the entrance to the ear canal. The main problem in the placing of the tube was to find out when it was near the eardrum. Preliminary experiments showed that certain characteristic scraping and other readily recognizable noises are produced whenever the tube touches the eardrum, and that, if the drum is touched only gently, no marked discomfort will be experienced. The procedure adopted was to push the tube slowly into the canal, applying intermittent pressure to its springy brass portion so that the tip would move along the canal by minute amounts. Contact with the drum was then recognized by the subject by a series of thumping or scraping sounds of which he informed the experimenter. The tube was then withdrawn just far enough (about 0.1 cm) so that additional gentle thrusts of the tube would not produce any more drum noises. This was the position referred to as being "at the eardrum."

The placement of the tube at the "midpoint" of the ear canal was effected in the following way: A marking collar was provided on the lateral arm of the microphone holder (see Fig. 2). When the drum was reached, the collar was slid up to a stop. The tube was then withdrawn until its tip lay in the plane of the entrance to the canal. The change in position of the marking

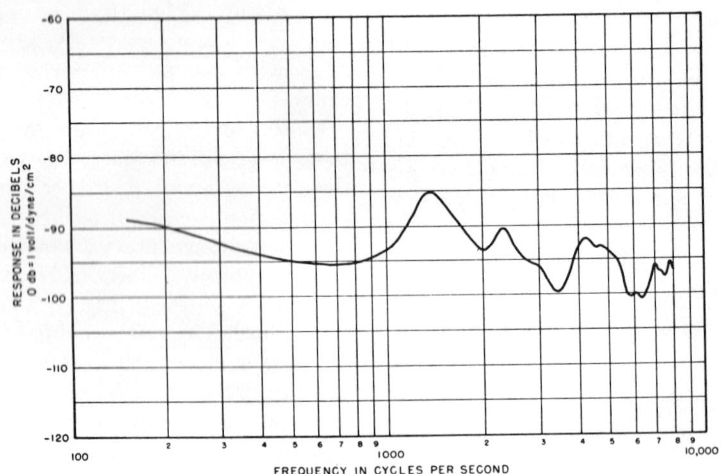

FIG. 4. Response characteristic of the probe microphone with equalizer.

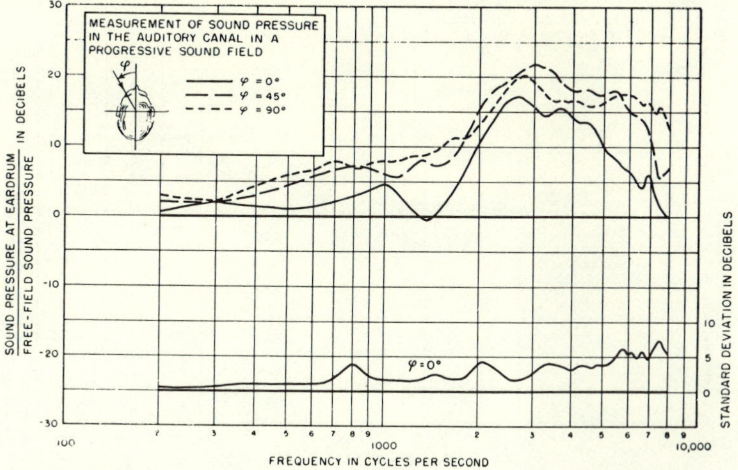

FIG. 5. Ratio of the sound pressure at the eardrum to the sound pressure in the free field at the center of the observer's head. The average of 6–12 male ears is shown for various azimuths as a function of frequency.

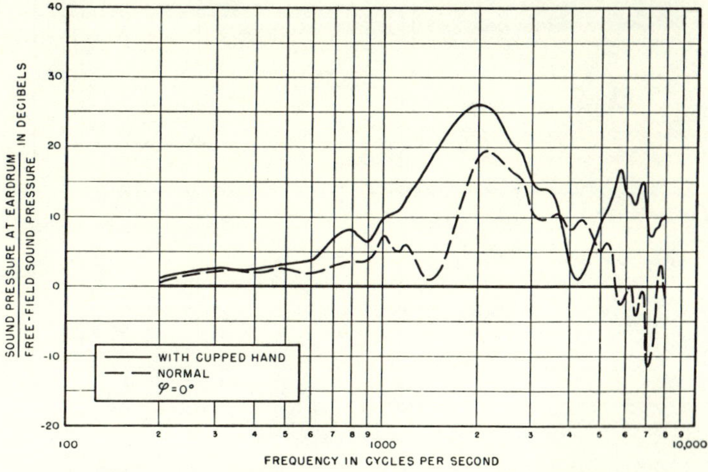

FIG. 6. Showing the increase in sound pressure at the eardrum caused by enlarging the pinna by means of a hand cupped around it.

collar gave the "length" of the auditory canal. The tube was then reinserted a distance equal to half the canal length.

III. RESULTS

Figure 5 shows the ratio of the sound pressure at the eardrum to the free-field pressure averaged for a number of male observers and measured for various azimuths. This ratio may be taken as the combined effect of resonance in the ear canal and diffraction by the head and pinna. The sound pressure at the drum is greater than the free-field pressure, so that over most of the audio-frequency range the ear acts as an acoustic amplifier. A maximum of about 17 to 22 db is reached near 3000 c.p.s. An indication of the variation between individuals is given by the standard deviation plotted as a function of frequency at the bottom of the graph. It can be seen from the graph that the amplification is greater if the ear is turned toward the loud-speaker, i.e., for values of azimuth approaching

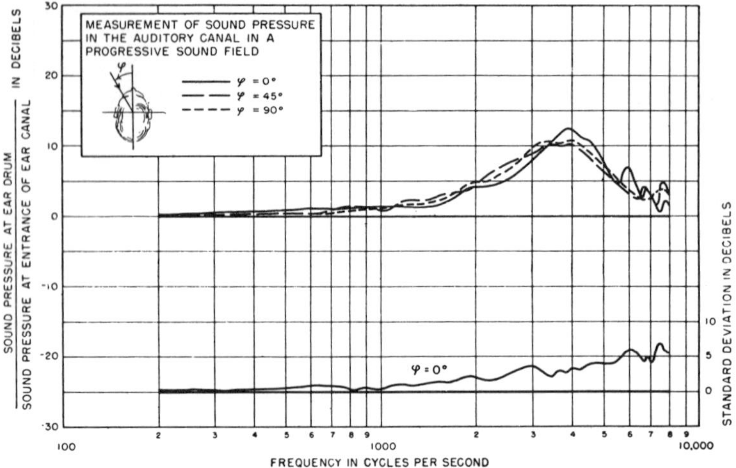

FIG. 7. Ratio of the sound pressure at the eardrum to the sound pressure at the entrance of the auditory canal. (Average of 6–12 male ears.)

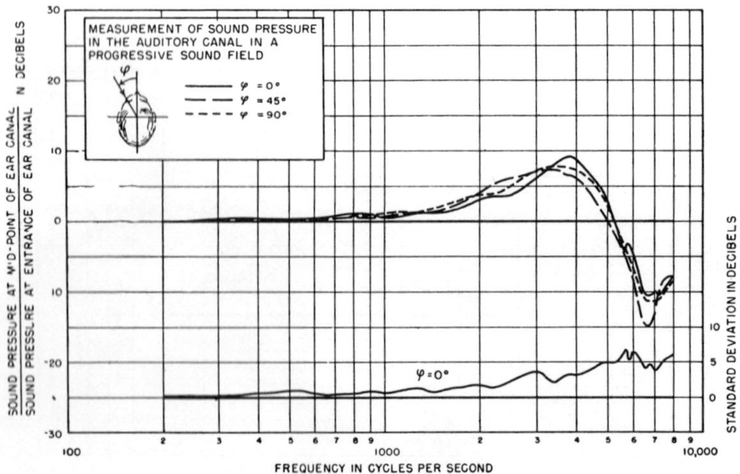

FIG. 8. Ratio of the sound pressure at the midpoint of the auditory canal to the sound pressure at its entrance. (Average of 6–12 male ears.)

90 degrees. It is common experience that faint sounds are heard better if one ear is "cocked" toward the source. The acoustic gain of the ear can be further increased in the important frequency range between 1000 and 3000 c.p.s. if the pinna is effectively enlarged by means of a hand cupped behind the ear, as shown in Fig. 6. Many hard-of-hearing people use this device to reduce their handicap.

Figure 7 shows the average ratio of the sound pressure at the eardrum to the sound pressure at the entrance of the canal. The resonance effect of the ear canal results in a peak of about 10 db near 4000 c.p.s. In the range covered by the tests, this pressure ratio is largely independent of azimuth, as is to be expected. Since the average length of the auditory canal was found to be about 2.3 cm, the peak occurs at a frequency where the length of the canal is approximately equal to one-quarter wave-length.

The results of the measurements made at a point half-way down the auditory canal are shown in Fig. 8 in the form of the ratio of the sound pressure at the midpoint of the canal to

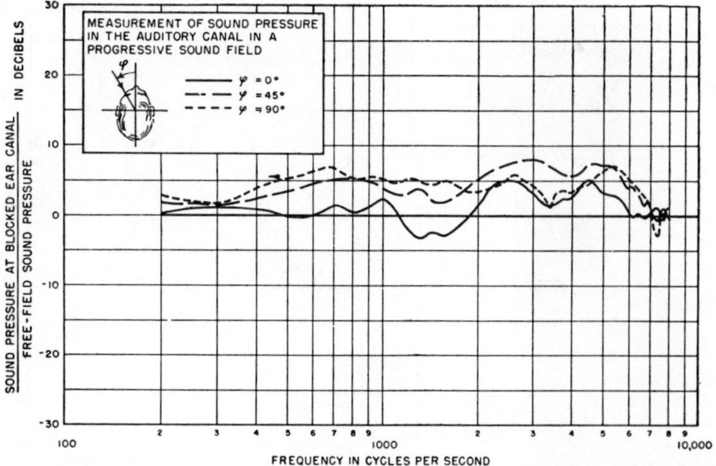

FIG. 9. Ratio of the sound pressure at the blocked auditory canal to the free-field sound pressure.

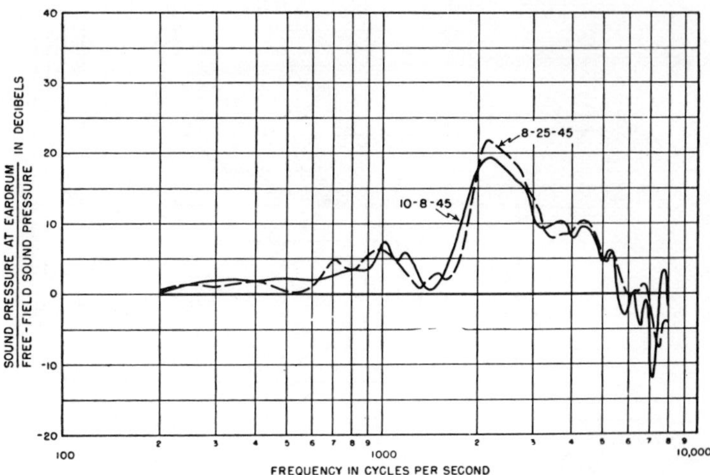

FIG. 10. Showing the results obtained on a given subject over a period of several weeks.

the sound pressure at its entrance. Although this ratio again reaches a peak near 3500 c.p.s., a minimum occurs in the vicinity of about 7000 c.p.s. At this frequency, the sound pressure at the midpoint of the canal is about 15 db below the sound pressure at the eardrum, indicating that a pressure node is set up half-way down the ear canal.

In an effort to separate the obstacle effect caused by the head from the effect of resonance in the ear canal, the canal was plugged by means of a suitable insert tip of the type used for hearing-aid earphones. The opening of the tip was filled with bees-wax. The pressure ratio, as shown in Fig. 9, is a quantitative measure of the obstacle effect due to the head. As is to be expected, this diffraction effect is, on the whole, not unlike that caused by a rigid sphere of comparable dimensions. Diffraction *per se* is seen to account only for a comparatively small part of the acoustic amplification provided by the ear (see Fig. 6).

IV. VALIDITY

Great care was taken to insure the validity of the results outlined above. Measurements were

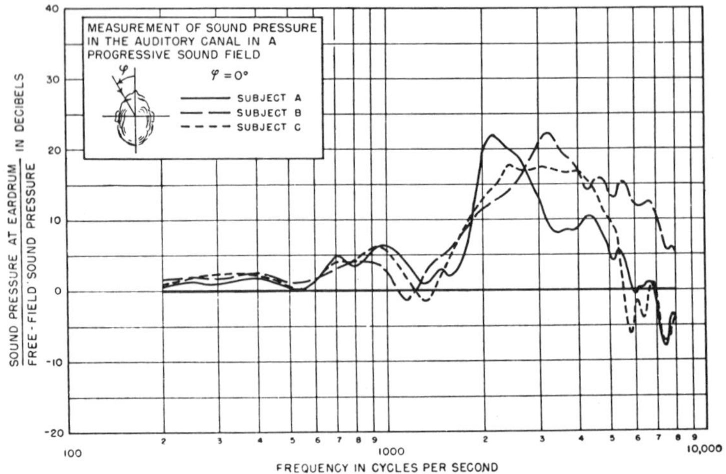

FIG. 11. Showing the variations among three representative observers.

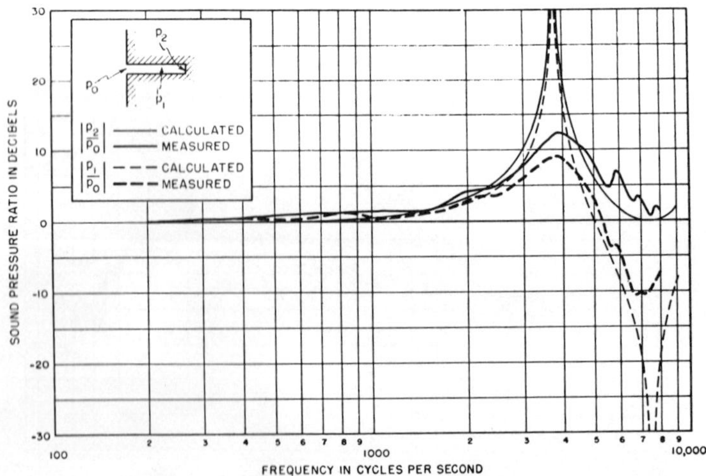

FIG. 12. Showing a comparison between the pressure ratios calculated for an auditory canal with rigid walls and rigid termination, and the pressure ratios obtained from measurements on real ears.

performed on a given subject over a number of weeks, and it was found that the results were repeatable to a satisfactory degree (Fig. 10). Figure 11 gives an estimate of the variations to be expected among individuals.[2] As is typical of many measurements of the psycho-acoustic type, it is clear that the variation among individuals exceeds by far the reliability with which data on a given observer can be obtained.

To test the effect of the prove tube on the sound field in the auditory canal, a second, dummy tube was tied to it and both inserted into the canal. The pressures at the drum were determined and then, without changing the position of the tube, the dummy tube was cautiously removed. The pressure measurements were then repeated. The pressures at the eardrum were found to be the same within ±1 db. The conclusion may be drawn that the presence of a

[2] For further details, see A. S. Filler, D. A. Ross, and F. M. Wiener, "The pressure distribution in the auditory canal in a progressive sound field," December 1, 1945, Psycho-Acoustic Laboratory, Harvard University, Report PNR-5 (available through Publications Board, U. S. Department of Commerce, Washington, D. C.).

single probe tube in the auditory canal does not significantly distort the sound field there.

To determine the possible effect of the presence of the head clamp and microphone carriage on the sound field in the vicinity of the subject's left ear, a wooden sphere whose dimensions approximated the average head was placed in the head clamp. The sound pressure was measured near the surface of the sphere at the location where normally the left ear would have been. Head clamp and chair were then removed and the measurements repeated. For this part of the experiment the sphere was suspended from a fine wire and the microphone was supported by a stand several feet away from the sphere. The differences in sound pressure measured under those conditions were small and comparable to the deviations to be expected from a single repetition of the pressure measurement at the drum on a given individual (see Fig. 10).

The results obtained for the suspended sphere, together with a measurement of the free-field sound pressure, were used to obtain the diffraction effects for the sphere. Comparison with computations from theory showed substantial agreement. It would appear, therefore, that the probe microphone itself does not influence appreciably the sound field near the head (or sphere).

The authors acknowledge with gratitude the help of Mr. A. S. Filler in carrying out the measurements.

APPENDIX

It may be of interest to determine the extent to which the acoustic behavior of the ear canal can be predicted from the simple theory of resonant tubes. For this purpose, let the auditory canal be replaced by a tube with rigid walls of length l, whose transverse dimensions are small compared to a wave-length, and which is terminated rigidly at one end. If the tube is exposed to a sound field and if the sound pressures at the entrance, at the midpoint and at the rigidly terminated end are denoted by p_0, p_1 and p_2, respectively, simple theory asserts that the following relations hold:[3]

$$\left|\frac{p_2}{p_0}\right| = \frac{1}{|\cos kl|}, \tag{1}$$

$$\left|\frac{p_1}{p_0}\right| = \left|\frac{\cos kl/2}{\cos kl}\right|. \tag{2}$$

In these equations, $k=\omega/c$, where ω is the angular frequency and c the velocity of sound in air. In Fig. 12 these relations are plotted against frequency and compared with the experimental values from Figs. 7 and 8. The simple theory predicts correctly the resonant frequency at one-quarter wave-length and the anti-resonant frequency at one-half wave-length. The principal effect of the finite impedance of the eardrum (the walls of the auditory canal can be regarded as rigid) is to broaden and lower the resonant peak and reduce the depth of the anti-resonant minimum. Measurements on an artificial ear canal 2.3 cm in length, with rigid walls and termination agree very closely with the results predicted by theory.

[3] P. M. Morse, *Vibration and Sound* (McGraw-Hill Book Company, Inc., New York, 1936), p. 211.

3

Reprinted from *Acoust. Soc. Am. J.* **19**:620–623 (1947)

Physiological Noise Generated under Earphone Cushions[1]

W. J. BROGDEN[2] AND GEORGE A. MILLER
Psycho-Acoustic Laboratory, Harvard University, Cambridge, Massachusetts

(Received March 25, 1947)

Listeners were required to match the quality and intensity of a low frequency ambient noise to the quality and intensity of the noise which they heard when they held earphones over both ears. A sound-pressure of 55 or 60 db of rumbling, low frequency noise can be generated by the tremor of the tonic contractions of hand and arm muscles.

IN their attempt to account for the differences between the minimum audible pressure and the minimum audible field, Sivian and White[3] suggest that a "physiological noise" is associated with the tight fit of a sound-source to the ear. "Breathing, pulse actions, etc.," cause mechanical vibrations which are transmitted through the head to the walls of the ear-canal. If the canal is tightly closed, an appreciable alternating pressure is established in the cavity, the eardrum is set in vibration, and a low frequency noise is heard. The effect is diminished if the enclosed volume is increased. In a volume of 0.7 cc the physiological noise was "definitely disturbing," with 10 cc, "quite inaudible."

In order to study this effect, we required listeners to match the quality and intensity of a low frequency, ambient noise to the quality and intensity of the noise which they heard when they held earphones over both ears. The listening was done in an anechoic chamber, and the ambient noise was transduced by two loud-speakers (Jensen A-12-PM, mounted in bass reflex cabinets) located to either side of the listener's head. This arrangement avoided the annoying localization effects produced by a single source. Since the listener's hands were occupied in holding the earphone cushions, he controlled the presentation of the ambient noise by a foot-

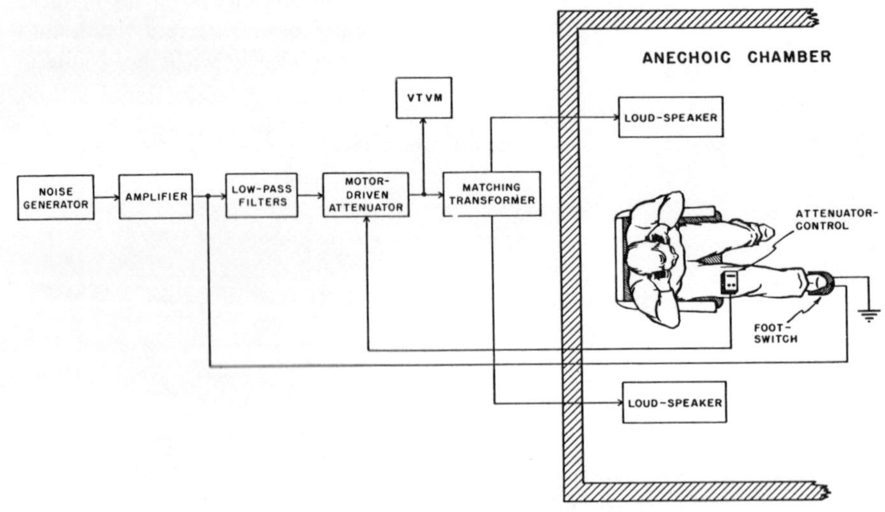

FIG. 1. Schematic diagram of the arrangement of apparatus.

[1] This research was conducted under contract with the U. S. Navy Office of Naval Research (Contract N5ori-76, PNR-31). Members of the Psycho-Acoustic Laboratory who contributed to various phases of this research were S. S. Stevens, F. M. Wiener, and I. J. Hirsh.

[2] Department of Psychology, University of Wisconsin.

[3] L. J. Sivian and S. D. White, "On minimum audible sound fields," J. Acous. Soc. Am. **4**, 288 (1933).

switch. A schematic representation of the test situation is shown in Fig. 1.

QUALITY OF THE NOISE

A rough estimate of the spectrum of the physiological noise was obtained by asking the listeners to compare four different ambient noises with the noise they heard under the earphone cushions. The cushions used were of the circumaural, or doughnut, type and normally enclose a volume of about 22 cc (including the volume of the ear canal). The listener would hold these cushions, which contained dummy phones, over his ears and listen to the noise. Then he would remove the cushions and press his footswitch to produce the ambient noise. After several such comparisons, he would report whether the match was "satisfactory" or "unsatisfactory." He was allowed to set his own criterion for satisfaction. When the report was made, the experimenter changed the spectrum according to a pre-arranged random order, and the listener proceeded with the next comparison (see Fig. 2).

Of the five listeners tested carefully, four selected the lowest pitched noise which the filters would yield, and one preferred slightly the second lowest. Comments like "surprisingly good," or "very close match," were received from the subjects and from several other listeners who heard this lowest noise. This noise, which had the spectrum shown in Fig. 2, was, therefore, adopted for the purpose of matching intensities.

INTENSITY OF THE NOISE

Once we had obtained an ambient noise that sounded quite similar to the physiological noise, the next step was to ask the listeners to adjust the intensity of the ambient noise by means of a motor-driven attenuator until the two noises sounded approximately equivalent in loudness. This equation was made 40 times by each of 5 listeners for 9 different volumes enclosed by the cushion: a supra-aural cushion was used to obtain the smallest volume of 5 cc, and the circumaural cushion was used to obtain volumes of 22, 122, 222, 422, 822, 1222, 1622, and 2022 cc. With the smallest volume data were available for only 4 of the 5 listeners. The manner in which

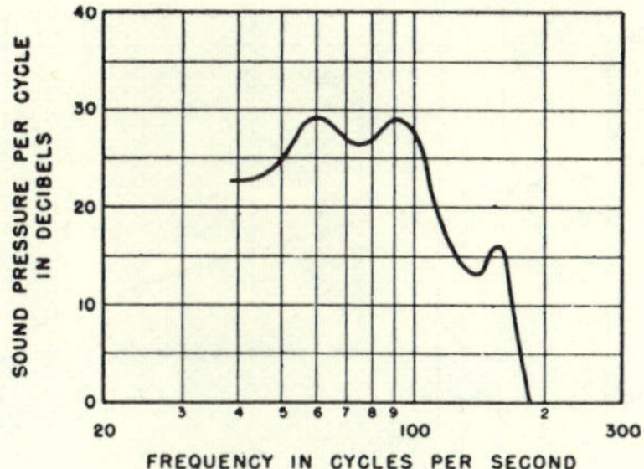

FIG. 2. Spectrum of ambient noise which sounded most similar in quality to physiological noise.

these volumes were produced by extending the length of a tube is shown in Fig. 3.

The results of the loudness matches are shown in Fig. 4 where the intensity of the equivalent ambient noise is plotted in decibels above the threshold for the noise—sensation-level—as a function of the volume of the cavity. The threshold was determined by the method of limits five times for each listener during the course of the loudness matches, and each determination represented the mean of 40 judgments. The minimum audible sound pressure for the spectrum employed was approximately 30 db re 0.0002 dyne/cm². The curve of Fig. 4 represents the empirical equation

$$p/p_0 = 31.7 - 9.5 \log_{10} V,$$

where p is the equivalent ambient sound pressure, p_0 is the pressure at the threshold of hearing, and V is the volume of the closed cavity in cc.

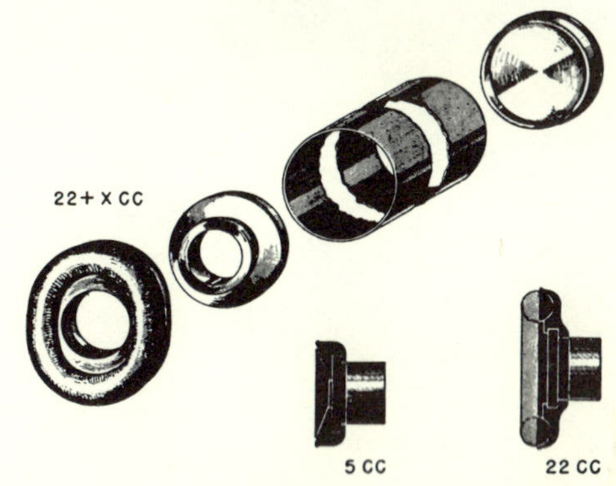

FIG. 3. Arrangement of earphone cushions used to produce cavities of different volumes.

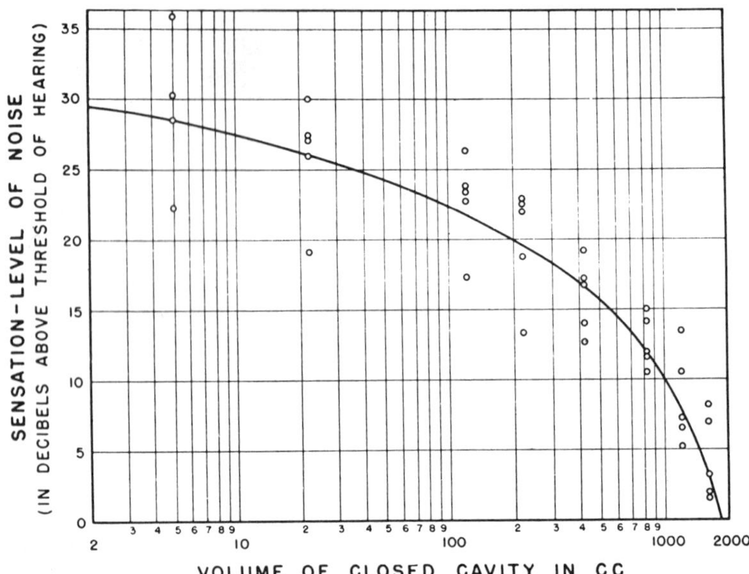

Fig. 4. Sensation-level of ambient noise which sounded equal in loudness to the loudness of the physiological noise.

Three facts are apparent from Fig. 4: the noise decreased as the volume increased, the variability between different listeners was greatest with the smaller cavities, and the intensity of the noise is much greater than that reported by Sivian and White. In the present case the noise could still be heard with a volume of 1622 cc: Sivian's and White's listeners could not hear a noise in a volume of 10 cc. But with this volume our listeners would report hearing a noise 25–30 db above threshold, a sound-pressure level of 55 or 60 db above the standard reference level.

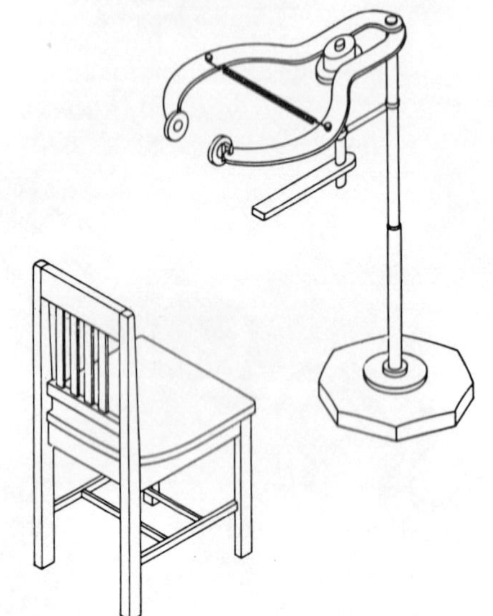

Fig. 5. Device used to position earphones without the use of the hands.

Now a sound pressure of 55 to 60 db of rumbling, low frequency noise is far too much noise to expect from the respiratory and circulatory systems alone. The discovery that so much noise was produced by holding an earphone to the ear was so surprising that we were forced to look for some other source for the sound. The search was quickly rewarded. What our listeners were hearing was the tremor of their own muscles, the muscles of hands and arms which held the earphones to their ears.

In order to demonstrate the importance of the tremor, we devised the caliper-like 'headband' shown in Fig. 5. The arms of the device are forced apart by an elliptical cam, and in this way the listener can quickly remove or replace the earphones without actually touching them with his hands. With the earphones positioned in this way, no physiological noise could be heard in the volume of 22 cc. With the volume of 5 cc the noise is very near threshold, and seems to come and go irregularly. The quality of the noise seemed similar to the quality of the noise produced by the muscles of the hands and arms, but the intensity was so near threshold that loudness-matches were not attempted.

With a good seal enclosing a small cavity at the ears, the pulse is sometimes heard and felt as an intermittent thumping within the head. If this thump is ignored and if the breath is held, it is still possible to detect a faint, low pitched rumble. This rumble seems to be associated with the contractions of the neck muscles which hold the head in place in the apparatus. The rumble can be exaggerated by tensing the muscles of the neck and back. When the jaw muscles are tightened the sound also increases. Or if the fingers are lightly touched to the earphones, the noise becomes prominent. One of the experimenters was even able to produce the noise by wiggling his ears.

In general, then, muscle tremors seem to be the greatest source of physiological noise. The noise of the pulse can be ignored by the listener, and breathing sounds can, to a certain extent, be controlled. It would seem to follow that determinations of the minimum audible pressure at low frequencies should be made with considerable attention to the possible interference of noise from muscles in tonic contraction. The listener should not hold the earphone to his ear with his hand (as is done in most of the standard audiometric tests). A chin rest might serve to reduce the noise from the neck and back muscles. The duration of the tone should be longer than the thump of the pulse, and the time of presentation of the tone should be anticipated by the listener, at least to the extent that would enable him to hold his breath at the proper moment.

These are some of the precautions that suggest themselves as essential when the task is to minimize disturbing factors in meticulous audiometry. A human being is a relatively noisy organism, especially when the vibrations of his contracting muscles are allowed to couple themselves to the walls of the small cavity enclosed under an earphone cushion.

4

Reprinted from *Acoust. Soc. Am. J.* 34:981–984 (1962)

Interaural Phase and the Absolute Threshold for Tone

K. JEROME DIERCKS AND LLOYD A. JEFFRESS
Defense Research Laboratory and Department of Psychology, University of Texas, Austin, Texas
(Received March 29, 1962)

The present study agrees with earlier ones that the binaural absolute threshold is about 3 dB lower than the monaural. It also finds that reversing the interaural phase of the signal lowers the threshold still further. The findings are shown to indicate the likelihood that so-called absolute thresholds are really masked thresholds, with the masking noise present internally and exhibiting a small positive correlation. The close relation of our results to the earlier work of Hirsh on binaural masking phenomena is discussed.

A NUMBER of earlier workers (see Hirsh's[1] and Licklider's[2] reviews, but also Pollack[3]) have found that when subjects have equal monaural thresholds, or where experimental adjustments are made to compensate for differences, the binaural absolute thresholds are in general about 3 dB lower than the monaural. This difference has been taken as suggesting a power summation at the two ears. Since, at least at threshold levels, sound at one ear will not summate acoustically with sound at the other, something else must be responsible. The first thought that comes to mind is that there is some sort of neural summation.

Lorente de Nó[4] found evidence for what is called spatial summation of nerve impulses. If impulses arrive at a certain synapse almost simultaneously via two incoming nerve fibers, the ongoing nerve fiber will fire; if the two impulses arrive at more widely different times, the ongoing fiber will not fire. The time interval between the impulses is critical in determining the action of the synapse.

Since interaural time differences are of great importance in many binaural phenomena, the writers speculated that such differences might also affect the absolute threshold for tone. Specifically they hypothesized that an in-phase signal at the two ears would, by virtue of simultaneity, achieve a lower threshold than would be found when the signals were not simultaneous. Since the earlier workers employed in-phase signals when they found a 3-dB advantage for the binaural threshold, the writers expected that delaying the signal to one ear would reduce the advantage, and so raise the binaural threshold. To make the time difference large, they decided to employ a 250-cps signal and to reverse its phase at one ear. The 2-msec difference resulting should be sufficient to produce an effect if the phenomenon depended upon the spatial summation of neural impulses. Monaural and binaural thresholds were determined and the better ear used as reference.

APPARATUS AND PROCEDURE

The 250-cps tone was turned on and off by an electronic switch having a rise and decay time of 10 msec. Signals were 1 sec in duration and were presented at 2.5-sec intervals. The signals were ordered at the desired intensity levels by means of a bank of preset attenuators. One of the attenuators was adjusted to give no signal as a check on false alarms, and the others to give signals at levels 2 dB apart.

At each experimental sitting, the signals were presented according to four planned haphazard sequences provided by a programming device. Each sequence consisted of 45 signals (5 at each of the 9 intensities) and 5 *Vexierversuchen*. No sequence was repeated during any one experimental sitting. The order in which the sequences were given was arbitrarily selected by the experimenter. Monaural thresholds were determined according to an ABBA pattern for each experimental sitting and the earphones were transposed regularly. Binaural thresholds were determined according to a random order for each experimental sitting and the phones transposed for alternate sittings. A total of

[1] I. J. Hirsh, "Binaural Summation—A Century of Investigation," Psychol. Bull. **45**, 193–206 (1948).
[2] J. C. R. Licklider, in *Handbook of Experimental Psychology*, edited by S. S. Stevens (John Wiley & Sons, Inc., New York, 1951), p. 1030.
[3] I. Pollack, "Monaural and Binaural Threshold Sensitivity for Tones and White Noise," J. Acoust. Soc. Am. **20**, 52–57 (1948).
[4] R. Lorente de Nó, *Symposium on the Synapse* (Charles C. Thomas, Springfield, Illinois, 1939).

TABLE I. Monaural and binaural 250-cps thresholds (in dB *re* 0.002 microbars).

Conditions	JD	RW	GM	MW	Means	Differences
	Subjects					
Monaural[a]	29.7	29.2	31.2	31.2	30.3	
						2.8[b]
Binaural $S0$	25.8	26.3	28.7	30.0	27.5	
						0.9[b]
Binaural $S\pi$	24.8	25.0	27.3	29.5	26.6	

[a] Best ear (mean difference between ears, 1.4 dB).
[b] Significant at 0.01 level.

900 judgements was made by each subject for each monaural threshold, and 1800 judgements for each of the two binaural thresholds.

The subject was seated in a quiet room adjacent to the control room. He was provided with a key which he pressed when he heard the signal. As each signal was produced, the programming device selected the member of a bank of 10 counters corresponding to the selected attenuator, and at the end of each run in a sitting, the scores were read from these. The 50% threshold was computed from these scores, using Müller-Urban weights as modified by Woodworth.[5] Four experienced listeners were employed as subjects for all conditions.

RESULTS

Thresholds (in dB *re* 0.0002 microbar) for each subject for each condition are shown in Table I. The mean difference between the monaural and binaural thresholds for the condition where the sound reaches the two ears simultaneously ($S0$) is 2.77 dB. This value agrees closely with the mean difference obtained by Pollack[3] for a 1000-cps tone. The mean difference between the monaural and binaural thresholds for the condition where the sound is reversed in phase at one earphone ($S\pi$) is 3.67 dB. The mean difference between the binaural in-phase and binaural out-of-phase thresholds is 0.90 dB.

An analysis of variance showed the differences between the monaural and binaural thresholds and between the two binaural thresholds to be significant at the 0.01 level.

DISCUSSION

The results agree with those of earlier workers in that they show the binaural threshold to be about 3 dB below the monaural, but they obviously do not support the hypothesis with which we started. Instead, the out-of-phase binaural condition yields a lower threshold than the in-phase. This finding is reminiscent of results from masking studies where reversing the phase of the signal improves detection, and suggests that the "absolute" thresholds of the present study are in reality masked thresholds, with the masking noise furnished internally.[6]

A study of masking by Hirsh[7] is particularly relevant to the present discussion in that he employed a signal close to the present one in frequency (200 cps) and used noise levels ranging from loud to almost inaudible. He used a variety of interaural phase relations[8–10] and found a hierarchy of thresholds which other experimenters have since verified repeatedly.

Hirsh's hierarchy, with some additions from Jeffress *et al.* and from Blodgett, Jeffress, and Taylor,[11] are as follows, in increasing order of signal detectability: the homophasic and monaural conditions, $N\pi$-$S\pi$, $N0$-$S0$, Nm-Sm (Blodgett *et al.* found them about equal); the mixed conditions, Nu-$S\pi$, Nu-$S0$, $N\pi$-Sm, $N0$-Sm; and best, the antiphasic conditions, $N\pi$-$S0$ and $N0$-$S\pi$. An explanation of the basis for the hierarchy is presented by Jeffress *et al.*[9] Let us borrow from them a few general observations to guide us in our later discussion.

(1) The homophasic conditions provide no interaural interaction to improve signal detection. The same is true of the condition where both signal and noise are monaural. These are therefore the worst conditions.

(2) $N\pi$ and Nu make for more difficult detection

[5] R. S. Woodworth, *Experimental Psychology* (Henry Holt and Company, New York, 1938), pp. 410–418.

[6] The idea that absolute thresholds are really masked thresholds is not a new one. L. J. Syvian and S. D. White, J. Acoust. Soc. Am. **4**, 288–321 (1933), discuss the possibility in connection with thermal agitation of the basilar membrane, and other investigators before and since have considered other sources of "self"-noise.

[7] I. J. Hirsh, "The Influence of Interaural Phase on Interaural Summation and Inhibition," J. Acoust. Soc. Am. **20**, 536–544 (1948).

[8] For convenience in the subsequent discussion let us employ the notation used by Jeffress, Blodgett, Sandel, and Wood,[9] and the terminology used by Licklider[10] in describing the phase relations. They are:

Homophasic conditions:

$N0$-$S0$—Noise in phase at the two ears, signal also in phase;
$N\pi$-$S\pi$—Noise and signal both reversed in phase at one ear relative to the other;

Antiphasic conditions:

$N\pi$-$S0$—Noise reversed in phase, signal in phase;
$N0$-$S\pi$—Signal reversed in phase, noise in phase;

Heterophasic conditions:

Nu-$S0$—Noise uncorrelated, signal in phase;
Nu-$S\pi$—Noise uncorrelated, signal reversed in phase.

For completeness and for later use, let us add the following additional symbols to describe the noise:

$N0$—Noise in phase with a correlation of $+1.0$;
$N\pi$—Noise reversed in phase with a correlation of -1.0;
Nu—Noise uncorrelated (correlation 0.0) (two independent sources);
$N+$—Noise in phase with a low positive correlation;
$N-$—Noise reversed in phase—low negative correlation;
Nx—Internal noise, correlation unknown.

[9] L. A. Jeffress, H. C. Blodgett, T. T. Sandel and C. L. Wood, III, "Masking of Tonal Signals," J. Acoust. Soc. Am. **28**, 416–426 (1956).

[10] J. C. R. Licklider, "The Influence of Interaural Phase Relations upon the Masking of Speech by White Noise," J. Acoust. Soc. Am. **20**, 150–159 (1948).

[11] H. C. Blodgett, L. A. Jeffress, and R. W. Taylor, "Relation of Masked Threshold to Signal-Duration for Various Interaural Phase-Combination," Am. J. Psychol. **71**, 283–290 (1958).

than $N0$ because the noise is more diffuse and locating the signal in it is harder.

(3) The conditions where the signal is monaural and the noise either in phase, $N0$, reversed in phase, $N\pi$, or uncorrelated, Nu, provide some, but not much, interaural assistance in signal detection. They are the poorest of the nonhomophasic conditions.

(4) The antiphasic condition $N0$-$S\pi$ provides the greatest interaural assistance in signal detection of all stimulus conditions involving a tonal signal and a noise masker, with $N\pi$-$S0$, the other antiphasic condition not far behind.

With these facts in mind, let us see whether we can explain the findings of the present experiment in terms of masked thresholds, on the assumption that the masking is provided by internal noise which we will call Nx for the present. If Nx were highly correlated and therefore really $N0$, the order of our three experimental conditions would have been $N0$-$S0$, $N0$-Sm, and $N0$-$S\pi$ with $N0$-$S0$ the worst and $N0$-$S\pi$ best. This was not the case, $S0$ was better than $S\pi$. If Nx were really Nu, we would expect Nu-Sm to be worst, as it was, but, on the basis of Blodgett *et al.*, we should also have expected Nu-$S0$ to be slightly better than Nu-$S\pi$, and the reverse was true. Again if Nx were really $N\pi$, $S\pi$ would have been worse than $S0$; it was not.

These considerations lead us to the conclusion that our Nx must be of the nature of Nu but with a small positive correlation. Let us call it $N+$, and see where this assumption takes us. The small positive correlation will make the $S0$ condition slightly homophasic, $N+$-$S0$, and the $S\pi$ condition, slightly antiphasic, $N+$-$S\pi$. This should favor the $S\pi$ condition, and this is borne out. As far as the monaural signal is concerned, the noise will behave almost as Nu, and this condition should therefore be the worst, as it is. The conclusions make sense, but they are not overwhelmingly convincing; they partake too much of an *ad hoc* argument. Let us see, however, where they lead us when we apply them to other data such as Hirsh's.

Table II presents Hirsh's results for four different noise levels, one (44.1-dB spectral level) loud enough so that the external noise completely dominates the situation, one so weak (−10.9 dB) that the noise can have *almost* no effect, and two levels between. Thresholds are arranged in increasing size from top to bottom and left to right. To make tracing changes in the order of the stimulus conditions easier, their movements, as the noise level changes, are indicated by arrows.

There is a striking change in the hierarchical order of Hirsh's conditions as we go from the −10.9-dB noise to the 44.1 dB. Since the −10.9-dB noise is almost inaudible (effective level only about 6 dB) we should expect the thresholds for this noise to resemble the "absolute" thresholds of the present experiment, and these are placed above for comparison.[12]

TABLE II. Thresholds in SPL for various interaural stimulus conditions.[a]

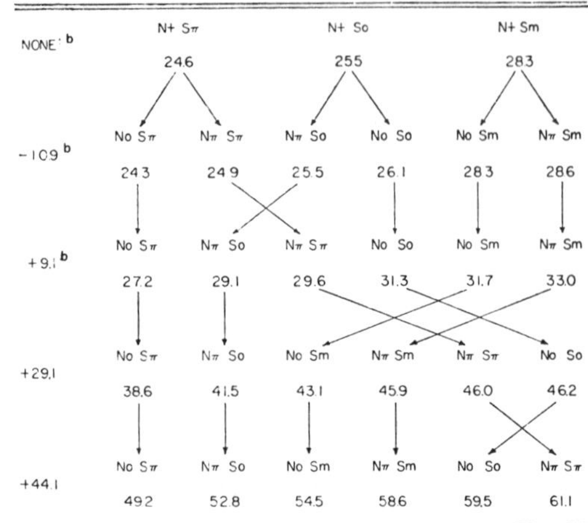

Noise level						
NONE[b]	N+ Sπ		N+ So		N+ Sm	
	24.6		25.5		28.3	
−10.9[b]	No Sπ	Nπ Sπ	Nπ So	No So	No Sm	Nπ Sm
	24.3	24.9	25.5	26.1	28.3	28.6
+9.1[b]	No Sπ	Nπ So	Nπ Sπ	No So	No Sm	Nπ Sm
	27.2	29.1	29.6	31.3	31.7	33.0
+29.1	No Sπ	Nπ So	No Sm	Nπ Sm	Nπ Sπ	No So
	38.6	41.5	43.1	45.9	46.0	46.2
+44.1	No Sπ	Nπ So	No Sm	Nπ Sm	No So	Nπ Sπ
	49.2	52.8	54.5	58.6	59.5	61.1

[a] The upper row of figures and stimulus conditions are for the present experiment. The remainder of the Table is taken from Hirsh.[7] To bring out the striking correspondence between our results and Hirsh's, we have subtracted 2 dB from each of the means of Table I before presenting them here.

[b] Level of external noise expressed as spectral level.

Now let us try to explain why the hierarchy which Hirsh obtained with the −10.9-dB noise was so strikingly different from the one for +44.1 dB. The −10.9-dB noise is obviously having some effect, since reversing its phase changes the thresholds slightly. However, the dominant factor is the phase of the signal. This fact tells us that the −10.9 dB noise is not enough to overcome the effect of the self-noise. We conclude then that when Hirsh adds $N0$ he is increasing the correlation already present in the self-noise, and when he adds $N\pi$, he is decreasing it, but not reversing its sign. This means that for the −10.9-dB noise $N0$-$S0$ is homophasic, and that $N\pi$-$S0$, too, is homophasic, although only slightly so. It also means that $N0$-$S\pi$ is antiphasic, and that $N\pi$-$S\pi$ is also antiphasic, although only slightly so. The thresholds associated with these stimuli tell us that a slightly antiphasic condition lowers the threshold more, relative to the uncorrelated conditions, than the corresponding homophasic condition raises it. Data from Robinson and Jeffress[13] bear

[12] The figures listed in the table for the present experiment are the means taken from Table I, but with 2 dB subtracted from each. This was done to bring out the close numerical agreement between our findings and Hirsh's. Without the correction the relative agreement would have been the same, but the numerical similarity would not have been so striking. Probably, since our results were obtained with no external noise, and at 250 cps, the correction factor should have been slightly greater than 2 dB. Certainly a 2 or even 3 dB disparity between our results and Hirsh's would not be surprising in view of the use of different psychophysical methods and different subjects.

[13] The reader is asked to believe that it was not until this point in the argument had been reached that the authors realized that data were at hand to test this inference. Reference was immediately made to the results of a study of the effect of correlation on masking [see D. E. Robinson and L. A. Jeffress, J. Acoust. Soc. Am. **33**, 1655 (A) (1961)] to check the prediction. The relevant data are presented in the text.

TABLE III. Effect of interaural correlation on masking. (Data from Robinson and Jeffress.[13])

	Coefficient of correlation for the noise		
	*N*π −0.25	*Nu* 0.00	*N*0 +0.25
Signal in phase (*S*0)	4.9	3.3	2.7[a]
Differences	+1.6	0.0	−0.6
Signal reversed in phase (*S*π)	3.0	3.3	4.5
Differences	−0.3	0.0	+1.2

[a] The upper figure in each cell is the masked threshold expressed as a masking level difference in dB referred to a common homophasic condition. The lower figure is the change in detectibility referred to the uncorrelated noise. Thus the difference +1.6 means that detection has been improved by 1.6 dB over the *Nu-S*0 condition when we go to the *N*π-*S*0 condition using a noise correlation of +0.25.

directly on this point and are presented in Table III. The table reveals that even for a correlation as low as 0.25, the antiphasic condition does in fact improve detection more than the corresponding homophasic condition degrades it.

Now let us attempt to trace the changes which occur as we add more and more external noise to the assumed *N*+ already present. Taking the best condition first, we start with *N*+-*S*π. As we add positively correlated noise *N*0, we simply increase the interaural correlation more and more as we add more noise. The condition is the best of the antiphasic conditions and remains so. If instead of adding *N*0, we add *N*π the outcome is very different. For the −10.9-dB noise, the condition, as we have already found, remains antiphasic, almost *Nu-S*π, but still a slight positive correlation. For the +9.1-dB noise the noise correlation becomes negative and detection deteriorates, and continues to do so as more noise is added. The condition is homophasic and with a high level of external noise the correlation is essentially −1.0. This condition then will provide no binaural assistance to signal detection and so yields the highest threshold.

The next "absolute" threshold provides a slightly homophasic condition, *N*+-*S*0, but very nearly *Nu-S*0. When we add *N*π at −10.9 dB we do not quite reverse the sign of the correlation, but we make the condition closer to *Nu-S*0 and improve things slightly. Adding more noise does reverse the sign of the correlation and our condition becomes slightly antiphasic. Adding still more noise produces the truly antiphasic condition, *N*π-*S*0, which is always, for reasons given by Jeffress *et al.*, inferior to the other antiphasic condition, *N*0-*S*π, but still better than any of the mixed conditions. If instead of adding *N*π to our original *N*+-*S*0 condition, we add *N*0, we make the condition more and more truly homophasic and it ends up just beside *N*π-*S*π, the other homophasic condition. The transposition at +29.1 dB is adventitious; the *N*π-*S*π condition has worsened more in the change from +9.1 to +29.1 dB of noise than the *N*0-*S*0 has, but it started from a more favorable spot and so did not quite reach the right-hand column for a noise level of +9.1 dB.

The next "absolute" threshold, the monaural one, provides the condition *N*+-*Sm*. This is essentially *Nu-Sm*, a condition almost as adverse as *Nm-Sm* and the homophasic conditions. It provides little or no binaural assistance in signal detection. Adding *N*0 will improve it, and even adding *N*π will improve it to some extent. The two conditions *N*0-*Sm* and *N*π-*Sm* move downward together in the table until they are displaced by the two homophasic conditions *N*0-*S*0 and *N*π-*S*π.

SUMMARY

Well-known facts about binaural masking phenomena taken with certain of the principles involved have furnished the basis for relating absolute thresholds to masked thresholds. The results provide a consistent body of data—data which progress in an orderly way as the noise level furnished to the subject varies from no noise to moderately intense noise.

CONCLUSIONS

On the basis of the foregoing discussion we may conclude as follows:

(1) That the so-called "absolute" threshold is in reality a masked threshold with "self"-noise providing the masking.[14]

(2) That the "self"-noise is made up of three components, one unique to one ear, one to the other, and one common to both. The last creates a small positive correlation.

(3) That the fact that the binaural "absolute" thresholds are lower than the monaural threshold is to be accounted for in terms of binaural masking phenomena rather than in terms of energy summation.

(4) That low-level external noise will mix with the "self"-noise and either increase, decrease, or reverse in sign the interaural noise correlation.

(5) That the strikingly different hierarchies of interaural stimulus conditions which Hirsh obtained with different noise levels can be explained in terms of the relative contributions of "self"-noise and external noise to the masking mixture.

ACKNOWLEDGMENT

This work was done under Contract NObsr-72627 with the Bureau of Ships.

[14] *Footnote added in proof.* At the May Meeting of the Society, E. A. Shaw and J. E. Piercy presented a paper describing measurements of noise generated in the external ear by heart action. They estimate that under a standard cushion, the noise in a 1/3 octave band centered at 250 cps amounts to about 26 dB. This is equivalent to about +8 dB spectral level. If this were about the noise level present in our experiment, and in Hirsh's at −10.9 dB spectral level, adding 9.1 dB of noise should produce about 3.5 dB more masking than with the self-noise alone. This value lies within the range of those of Table II.

5

Reprinted from *Science* **134**:168–177 (1961)

Is There a Sensory Threshold?

When the effects of the observer's response criterion are isolated, a sensory limitation is not evident.

John A. Swets

One hundred years ago, at the inception of an experimental psychology of the senses, G. T. Fechner focused attention on the concept of a sensory threshold, a limit on sensitivity. His *Elemente der Psychophysik* described three methods—the methods of adjustment, of limits, and of constants—for estimating the threshold value of a stimulus (*1*). The concept and the methods have been in active service since. Students of sensory processes have continued to measure the energy required for a stimulus to be just detectable, or the difference between two stimuli necessary for the two to be just noticeably different. Very recently there has arisen reasonable doubt that sensory thresholds exist.

The threshold thought to be characteristic of sensory systems has been regarded in the root sense of that word as a barrier that must be overcome. It is analogous to the threshold discovered by physiologists in single neurons. Just as a nervous impulse either occurs or does not occur, so it has been thought that when a weak stimulus is presented we either detect it or we do not, with no shades in between. The analogy with the neuron's all-or-none action, of course, was never meant to be complete; it was plain that at some point above the threshold sensations come in various sizes.

From the start the triggering mechanism of the sensory systems was regarded as inherently unstable. The first experiments disclosed that a given stimulus did not produce a consistent "yes" ("I detect it") response or a consistent "no" ("I do not detect it") response. Plots of the "psychometric function" —the proportion of "yes" responses as a function of the stimulus energy—were in the form of ogives, which suggested an underlying bell-shaped distribution of threshold levels. Abundant evidence for continuous physiological change in large numbers of receptive and nervous elements in the various sensory systems made this picture eminently reasonable. Thus, the threshold value of a stimulus had to be specified in statistical terms. Fechner's experimental methods were designed to obtain good estimates of the mean and the variance of the threshold distribution.

It was also assumed from the beginning that the observer's attitude affects the threshold estimate. The use of ascending and descending series of stimulus energies in the method of limits, to take one example, is intended to counterbalance the errors of "habituation" and "anticipation"—errors to which the observer is subject for extrasensory reasons. Typically, investigators have not been satisfied with experimental observers who were merely well motivated; they have felt the need for elite observers. They have attempted, by selection or training, to obtain observers who could maintain a reasonably constant criterion for a "yes" response.

The classical methods for measuring the threshold, however, do not provide a measure of the observer's response criterion that is independent of the threshold measure. As an example, we may note that a difference between two threshold estimates obtained with the method of limits can be attributed to a criterion change only if it is assumed that sensitivity has remained constant, or to a sensitivity change only if it is assumed that the criterion has remained constant. So, although the observer's response criterion affects the estimate of the threshold, the classical procedures do not permit calibration of the observer with respect to his response criterion.

Within the past ten years methods

The author is associate professor of psychology and a staff member of the Research Laboratory of Electronics, Massachusetts Institute of Technology, Cambridge. This article is adapted from an address delivered at a centennial symposium honoring Fechner, sponsored by the American Psychological Association and the Psychometric Society, held in Chicago in September 1960.

have become available that provide a reliable, quantitative specification of the response criterion. These methods permit isolation of the effects of the criterion, so that a relatively pure measure of sensitivity remains. Interestingly, the data collected with these methods give us good reason to question the existence of sensory thresholds, to wonder whether anything more than a response criterion is involved in the dichotomy of "yes" and "no" responses. There is now reason to believe that sensory excitation varies continuously and that an apparent threshold cut in the continuum results simply from restricting the observer to two categories of response.

The methods that permit separating the criterion and sensitivity measures, and a psychophysical theory that incorporates the results obtained with these methods, stem directly from the modern approach taken by engineers to the general problem of signal detection. The psychophysical "detection theory," like the more general theory, has two parts. One part is a literal translation of the theory of testing statistical hypotheses, or statistical decision theory. It is this part of the theory that provides a solution to the criterion estimation problem and deals with sensitivity as a continuous variable. The second part is a theory of ideal observers. It specifies the mathematically ideal detection performance—the upper limit on detection performance that is imposed by the environment—in terms of measurable parameters of the signal and of the masking noise (*2*).

We shall turn in a moment to a description of the theory and to samples of the supporting data. Before proceeding any further, however, we must note that, although Fechner started the study of sensory functions along lines we are now questioning, he also anticipated the present line of attack in both of its major aspects. For one thing, he regarded Bernoulli's ideas on statistical decision as highly relevant to psychophysical theory (*3*). More important, while advancing the concept of a threshold, he spoke also of what he called "negative sensations"—that is, of a grading of sensory excitation below the threshold. That subsequent workers in the field of psychophysics have shown little interest in negative sensations is apparent from the fact that, 75 years after Fechner's work, Boring could write: "So also a sensation either occurs from stimulation or it does not. If it does not, it has no demonstrable intensity. Fechner talked about negative (subliminal) degrees of intensity, but that is not good psychology today. Above the limen we can sense degrees of intensity, but introspection cannot directly measure these degrees. We are forced to comparison, and there again we meet an all-or-none principle. Either we can observe a difference or we cannot. Introspection as to the amount of difference is not quantitatively reliable" (*4*).

Decision Aspects of Signal Detection

How detection theory succeeds in estimating the response criterion may be described in terms of "the fundamental detection problem." The experimenter defines an interval of time for the observer, and the observer must decide whether or not a signal is present during the interval. It is assumed that every interval contains some random interference, or noise—noise that is inherent in the environment, or is produced inadvertently by the experimenter's equipment for generating signals, or is deliberately introduced by the experimenter, or is simply a property of the sensory system. Some intervals contain a specified signal in addition to the background of noise. The observer's report is limited to these two classes of stimulus events—he says either "yes" (a signal was present) or "no" (only noise was present). Note that he does not say whether or not he *saw* (or *heard*) the signal; he says whether, under the particular circumstances, he prefers the decision that it was present or the decision that it was absent.

There is presumably, coinciding with the observation interval, some neural activity in the relevant sensory system. This activity forms the sensory basis—a part of the total basis—for the observer's report. This "sensory excitation," as we shall call it, may be in fact either simple or complex; it may have many dimensions or few; it may be qualitative or quantitative; it may be anything. The exact, or even the general, nature of the actual sensory excitation is of no concern to the application of the theory.

Only two assumptions are made about the sensory excitation. One is that it is continually varying; because of the ever-present noise, it varies over time in the absence of any signal, as well as from one presentation to the next of what is nominally the same signal. The other is that the sensory excitation, insofar as it affects the observer's report, may be represented as a unidimensional variable. In theory, the observer is aware of the probability that each possible excitatory state will occur during an observation interval containing noise alone and also during an observation interval containing a signal in addition to the noise, and he bases his report on the ratio of these two quantities, the likelihood ratio. The likelihood ratio derived from any observation interval is a real, nonzero number and hence may be represented along a single dimension.

The likelihood-ratio criterion. The observer's report after an observation interval is supposed to depend upon whether or not the likelihood ratio measured in that interval exceeds some critical value of the likelihood ratio, a response criterion. The criterion is presumed to be established by the observer in accordance with his detection goal and the relevant situational parameters. If he wishes to maximize the number of correct responses, his criterion will depend upon the a priori probability that a signal will occur in a given interval. If he chooses to maximize the total payoff, his criterion will depend on this probability and also on the values and costs associated with the four possible outcomes of a decision. Several other detection goals can be defined; the way in which each of them determines the criterion has been described elsewhere (*5*). In any case, the criterion employed by the observer can be expressed as a value of the likelihood ratio. Thus, the observer's decision about an interval is based not only on the sensory information he obtains in that interval but also upon advance information of various kinds and upon his motivation.

Next, consider a probability defined on the variable likelihood ratio—in particular, the probability that each value of likelihood ratio will occur with each of the classes of possible stimulus events: noise alone and signal plus noise. There are, then, two probability distributions. The one associated with signal plus noise will have a greater mean (indeed, its mean is assumed to increase monotonically with increases in the signal strength, but for the moment we are considering a particular signal). Now, if the observer follows the procedure we have described—that is, if he reports that the signal is present whenever the likelihood ratio exceeds a certain criterion and that noise alone is present whenever the likelihood

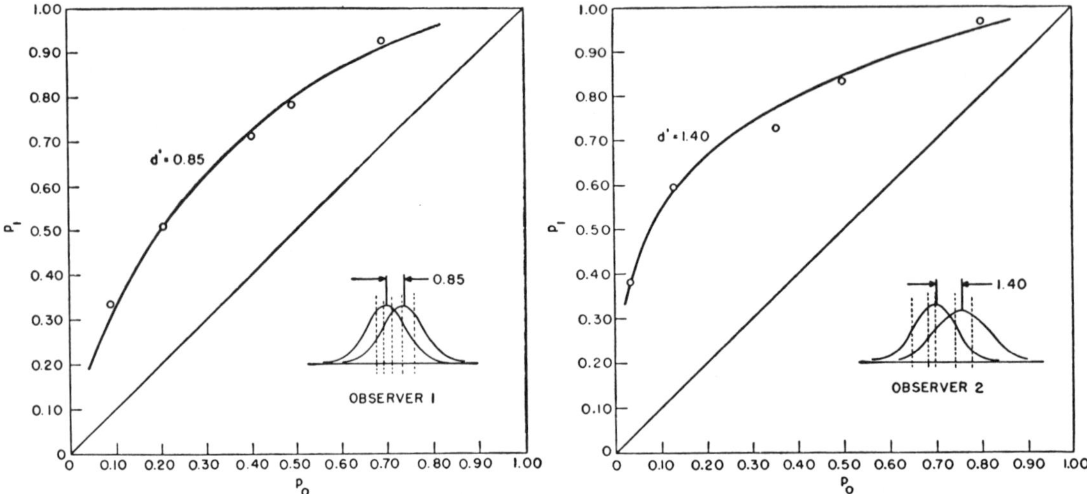

Fig. 1. Two theoretical operating-characteristic curves, with data from a yes-no experiment.

ratio is less than this criterion—then, from the fourfold stimulus-response matrix that results, one can extract two independent measures: a measure of the observer's response criterion and a measure of his sensitivity.

The operating characteristic. The extraction of these two measures depends upon an analysis in terms of the operating characteristic. If we induce the observer to change his criterion from one set of trials to another, and if, for each criterion, we plot the proportion of "yes" reports made when the signal is present (the proportion of hits, or p_1) against the proportion of "yes" reports made when noise alone is present (the proportion of false alarms, or p_0), then, as the criterion varies, a single curve is traced (running from 0 to 1.0 on both coordinates) that shows the proportion of hits to be a nondecreasing function of the proportion of false alarms. This operating-characteristic curve describes completely the successive stimulus-response matrices that are obtained, since the complements of these two proportions are the proportions that belong in the other two cells of the matrix. The particular curve generated in this way depends upon the signal and noise parameters and upon the observer's sensitivity; the point on this curve that corresponds to any given stimulus-response matrix represents the criterion employed by the observer in producing that matrix.

It has been found that, to a good approximation, the operating-characteristic curves produced by human observers correspond to theoretical curves based on normal probability distributions. These curves can be characterized by a single parameter: the difference between the means of the signal-plus-noise and noise-alone distributions divided by the standard deviation of the noise distribution. This parameter has been called *d'*. Moreover, the slope of the curve at any point is equal to the value of the likelihood-ratio criterion that produces that point.

The yes-no experiment. The procedure employed in the fundamental detection problem is often referred to as the "yes-no procedure," and we shall adopt this terminology. Two operating-characteristic curves resulting from this procedure are shown in Fig. 1. The

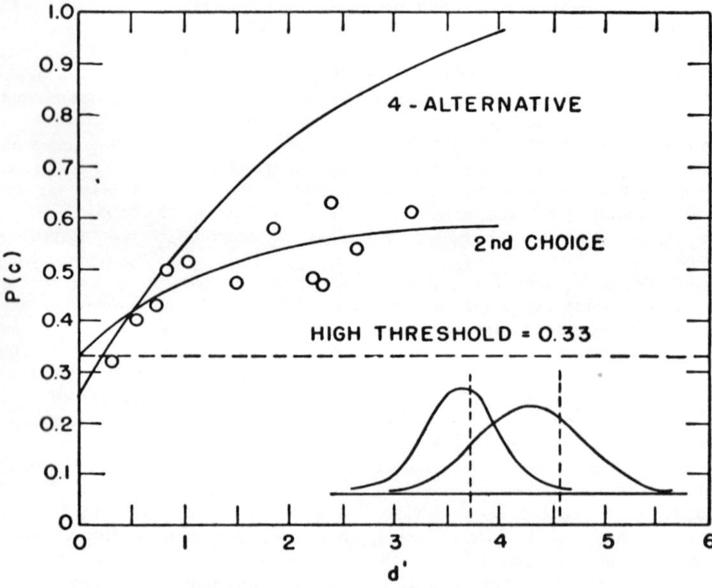

Fig. 2. The results obtained in a second-choice experiment, shown with the prediction from detection theory. [Data from J. A. Swets, W. P. Tanner, Jr., T. G. Birdsall (5)]

data points were obtained in an auditory experiment in which the observers attempted to detect a tone burst in a background of white noise. The curves are the theoretical curves that fit the data best. The inserts at lower right in the two graphs show the normal probability distributions underlying the curves, and the five criteria corresponding to the data points. In this particular experiment the observers changed their criteria from one set of trials to another as the experimenter changed the a priori probability of the occurrence of the signal. The distance between the means of the two distributions is shown as 0.85 for observer No. 1 and as 1.40 for observer No. 2; this distance is equal to d' under the convention that the standard deviation of the noise distribution is unity.

We may note that the curve fitted to the data of the first observer is symmetrical about the negative diagonal, and that the curve fitted to the data of the second observer is not. Both types of curves are seen frequently; the second curve is especially characteristic of data collected in visual experiments. Theoretically, the curve shown in the graph at left will result if the observer knows the signal exactly—that is, if he knows its frequency, amplitude, starting time, duration, and phase. A theoretical curve like the one shown in the graph at right results if the observer has inadequate information about frequency and phase, or, as is the case when the signal is a white light, if there is no frequency and phase information. The probability distributions that are shown in the inserts reflect this difference between the operating-characteristic curves.

Both of the curves shown are based on the assumption that sensory excitation is continuous, that the observer can order values of sensory excitation throughout its range. Two other experiments have been employed to test the validity of this assumption: one involves a variant of the forced-choice procedure; the other involves a rating procedure. We shall consider these experiments in turn.

The second-choice experiment. In the forced-choice procedure, four temporal intervals were defined on each trial, exactly one of which contained the signal. The signal was a small spot of light projected briefly on a large, uniformly illuminated background. Ordinarily, the observer simply chooses the interval he believes most likely to have contained the signal. In this experiment the observer made a second choice as well as a first.

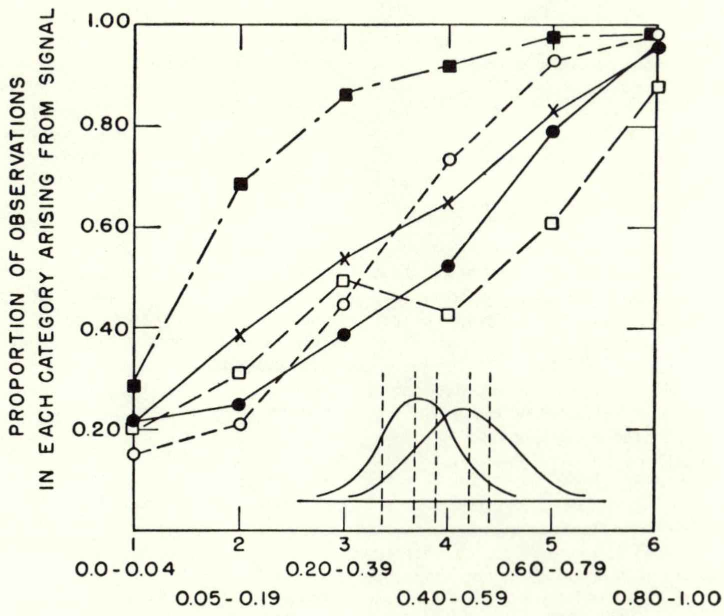

Fig. 3. The results of a rating experiment. [Data from J. A. Swets, W. P. Tanner, Jr., T. G. Birdsall (5)]

The results are shown in Fig. 2. The top curve is the theoretical function relating the proportion of correct first choices to d'; the lower curve is the theoretical relation of the proportion of correct second choices to d'. The points on the graph represent the proportions of correct second choices obtained by experiment. They are plotted at the value of d' corresponding to the observed proportion of correct first choices.

It may be seen that the data points are fitted well by the theoretical curve. The rather considerable variability can be attributed to the fact that each point is based on less than 100 observations. In spite of the variability, it is clear that the points deviate significantly from the horizontal dashed line. The dashed line may be taken as a baseline; it assumes a sensory threshold such that it is exceeded on only a negligible proportion of the trials when noise alone is presented. Should such a threshold exist, the second choice would be correct only by chance. The data indicate that the observer is capable of ordering values of sensory excitation well below this point. Two sensory thresholds are shown in the insert at lower right in Fig. 2. The threshold on the right, at three standard deviations from the mean of the noise distribution, corresponds to the horizontal dashed line in the upper part of the figure. The data indicate that, were a threshold to exist, it would have to be at least as low as the left-hand threshold, at approximately the mean of the noise distribution.

The rating experiment. In the rating procedure, as in the yes-no procedure, a signal is either presented or not presented in a single observation interval. The observer's task is to reflect gradations in the sensory excitation by assigning each observation to one of several categories of likelihood of occurrence of a signal in the interval.

The results of a visual experiment are displayed in Fig. 3. The abscissa represents a six-point scale of certainty concerning the occurrence of a signal. The six categories were also defined in terms of the a posteriori probability of occurrence, but, for our purpose, only the property of order need be assumed. The ordinate shows the proportion, of the observations placed in each category, that resulted from the presentation of the signal.

Five curves are shown in Fig. 3. Four of them correspond to the four observers; the fifth, marked by ×'s, represents the average. It may be seen that the curves for three of the four observers increase monotonically, while that for the fourth has a single reversal. The implication is that the human observer can distinguish at least six categories of sensory excitation.

It is possible to compute operating-characteristic curves from these data, by regarding the category boundaries successively as criteria. The curves (not shown here) are very similar in appearance to those obtained with the yes-no procedure (*5*). By way of illustration, the five criteria used by one of the observers (the one represented by solid circles) are shown in the insert at lower right in Fig. 3.

The experimental invariance of d′. It has been found experimentally, in vision (*5*) and in audition (*6*), that the sensitivity measure d' remains relatively constant with changes in the response criterion. Thus, detection theory provides a measure of sensitivity that is practically uncontaminated by the factors that might be expected to affect the observer's attitude.

It has also been found that the measure d' remains relatively invariant with different experimental procedures. For vision (*7*) and audition (*8*) the estimates of d' from the yes-no procedure and from the four-interval, forced-choice procedure are very nearly the same. Again, consistent estimates are obtained from forced-choice procedures with 2, 3, 4, 6, and 8 intervals (*8*). Finally, the rating procedure yields estimates of d' indistinguishable from those obtained with the yes-no procedure (*9*).

Thus, the psychophysical detection theory has passed some rather severe tests—the quantity that is supposed to remain invariant does remain invariant. This finding may be contrasted with the well-known fact that estimates of the threshold depend heavily on the particular procedure used.

Theory of Ideal Observers

Detection theory states, for several types of signal and noise, the maximum possible detectability as a function of the parameters of the signal and the noise. Given certain assumptions, this relationship can be stated very precisely. The case of the "signal specified exactly" (in which everything about the signal is known, including its frequency, phase, starting time, duration, and amplitude) appears to be a useful standard in audition experiments. In this case, the maximum d' is equal to the quantity $(2E/N_0)^{\frac{1}{2}}$, in which E is the signal energy and N_0 is the noise power in a one-cycle band. An ideal observer for visual signals has also been defined (*10*).

It can be argued that a theory of ideal performance is a good starting point in working toward a descriptive theory. Ideal theories involve few variables, and these are simply described. Experiments can be used to uncover whatever additional variables may be needed to describe the performance of real observers. Alternatively, experiments can be used to indicate how the ideal theory may be degraded—that is, to identify those functions of which the ideal detection device must be deprived —in order to accurately describe real behavior.

Given a normative theory, it is possible to describe the real observer's efficiency. In the present instance, the efficiency measure η has been defined as the ratio of the observed to the ideal $(d')^2$. It seems likely that substantive problems will be illuminated by the computation of η for different types of signals and for different parameters of a given type of signal. The observed variation of this measure should be helpful in determining the range over which the human observer can adjust the parameters of his sensory system to match different signal parameters (he is, after all, quite proficient in detecting a surprisingly large number of different signals), and in determining which parameters of a signal the observer is not using, or not using precisely, in his detection process (*11*).

The human observer, of course, performs less well than does the ideal observer in the great majority of detection tasks, if not in all. The interesting question concerns not the amount but the nature of the discrepancy that is observed.

The human observer performs less well than the ideal observer defined for the case of the "signal specified exactly." That is to say, the human observer's psychometric function is shifted to the right. More important, the slope of the human observer's function is greater than that of the ideal function for this particular case—a result sometimes referred to as "low-signal suppression." Let us consider three possible reasons for these discrepancies.

First, the human observer may well have a noisy decision process, whereas the ideal decision process is noiseless. For example, the human observer's response criterion may be unstable. If he vacillates between two criteria, the resulting point on his operating-characteristic curve will be on a straight line connecting the points corresponding to the two criteria; this average point falls below the curve (a curve with smoothly decreasing slope) on which the two criteria are located. Again, the observer's decision axis may not be continuous. It may be, as far as we know, divided into a relatively small number of categories—say, into seven.

A second likely cause of deviation from the ideal is the noise inherent in the human sensory systems. Consistent results are obtained from estimating the amount of "internal noise" (that is, noise in the decision process and noise in the sensory system) in two ways: by examining the decisions of an observer over several presentations of the same signal and noise (on tape) and by examining the correlation among the responses of several observers to a single presentation (*12*).

A third, and favored, possibility is faulty memory. This explanation is favored because it accounts not only for the shift of the human observer's psychometric function but also for the greater slope of his function. The reasoning proceeds as follows: If the detection process involves some sort of tuning of the receptive apparatus, and if the observer's memory of the characteristics of the incoming signal is faulty, then the observer is essentially confronted with a signal not specified exactly but specified only statistically. He has some uncertainty about the incoming signal.

If uncertainty is introduced into the calculations of the psychometric function of the ideal detector, it is found that performance falls off as uncertainty increases, and that this decline in performance is greater for weak signals than for strong ones (*13*). That is, a family of theoretical uncertainty curves shows progressively steeper slopes coinciding with progressive shifts to the right. This is what one would expect; the accuracy of knowledge about signal characteristics is less critical for strong signals, since strong signals carry with them more information about these characteristics.

It has been observed that visual data (*10*) and auditory data (*14*) are fitted well, with respect to slope, by the theoretical curve that corresponds to uncertainty among approximately 100 orthogonal signal alternatives. It is not difficult to imagine that the product of the uncertainties about the time, location, and frequency of the signals used in these experiments could be as high as 100.

It is possible to obtain empirical corroboration of this theoretical analysis of uncertainty in terms of faulty memory. This is achieved by providing various aids to memory within the experimental procedure. In such experiments, memory for frequency is made unnecessary by introducing a continuous tone or light (a "carrier") of the same frequency as the signal, so that the signal to be detected is an increment in the carrier. This procedure also eliminates the need for phase memory in audition and location memory in vision. In further experiments a pulsed carrier is used in order to make unnecessary memory for starting time and for duration. In all of these experiments a forced-choice procedure is used, so that memory for amplitude beyond a single trial can also be considered irrelevant. In this way, all of the information thought to be relevant may be contained in the immediate situation. Experimentally, we find that the human observer's psychometric functions show progressively flatter slopes as more and more memory aids are introduced. In fact, when all of the aids mentioned above are used, the observer's slope parallels that for the ideal observer without uncertainty, and it deviates as little as 3 decibels from the ideal curve in absolute value (*14*).

Relationship of the Data to Various Threshold Theories

Although there is a limit on detection performance, even ideally, and although the human observer falls short of the limit, these facts do not imply a sensory threshold. We have just seen that the human observer's performance can be analyzed in terms of memory, and, conceivably, additional memory aids could bring his performance closer to the ideal. Moreover, consideration of ideal observers concerns an upper rather than a lower limit. The human observer, while falling short of the ideal, can still detect signals at a high rate. Ideally, any displacement of the signal-plus-noise distribution from the noise-alone distribution will lead to a detection rate greater than chance. Although it is difficult to obtain data near the chance point, the theoretical curves that fit the plots of d' against signal energy for human observers go through zero on the energy scale.

This last-mentioned result, of course, based as it is on extrapolation, cannot stand by itself as conclusive argument against the existence of a threshold. The result also depends on a measure of performance that is specific to detection theory. So we shall not be concerned with it further. It is possible, however, to relate the various threshold theories that have been proposed to the experimental results discussed earlier—results obtained with the yes-no, second-choice, and rating procedures, as shown in Figs. 1, 2, and 3. We shall examine these results in relation to threshold theories proposed by Blackwell (*15*), Luce (*16*), Green (*17*), Swets, Tanner, and Birdsall (*5*), and Stevens (*18*).

Blackwell's high-threshold theory. Blackwell's theory assumes that, whereas the observer may be led to say "yes" when noise alone is presented, only very infrequently is his threshold exceeded by the sensory excitation arising from noise—so infrequently, in fact, that these instances can be ignored. There is a "true" value of p_0—call it p_0'—that for all practical purposes is equal to zero. Corresponding to p_0', there is some true p_1', the value of which depends on the signal strength. Since the observer is unable to order values of sensory excitation below $p_0' \approx 0$, if he says "yes" in response to such a value he is merely guessing and will be correct on a chance basis. The operating-characteristic curve (for a given signal strength) that results from this theory is that of Fig. 4. It is a straight line from (p_0', p_1') through ($p_0 = 1.00$, $p_1 = 1.00$). The insert at lower right shows the location of the threshold. The data of observer 1 shown in Fig. 1 are reproduced for comparison.

This theoretical curve is described by the equation

$$p_1 = p_1' + p_0(1 - p_1') \tag{1}$$

The observed proportion of "yes" responses to a signal (p_1) equals the proportion of true "yes" responses (p_1') plus a guessing factor (p_0) modified by the opportunity for guessing ($1 - p_1'$). The beauty of this high-threshold theory is that, if it is correct, the influence of spurious "yes" responses can be eliminated, the proportion of true "yes" responses being left. The familiar correction for chance success

$$p_1' = \frac{p_1 - p_0}{1 - p_0} \tag{2}$$

is a rearrangement of Eq. 1. The correction serves to normalize the psychometric function so that, whatever the observer's tendency to guess, the stimulus threshold can be taken as the signal energy corresponding to $p_1' = 0.50$.

However, the theory does not agree with the data. The empirical curve shown in Fig. 4, like the great majority of operating-characteristic curves that have been obtained, is not adequately fitted by a straight line. The horizontal line in Fig. 2, which follows from this theory, does not fit the second-choice data shown there. The rating data of Fig. 3 also indicate ordering of values of sensory excitation below a p_0 of approximately zero. Further, yes-no and forced-choice thresholds calculated from this theory are not consistent with each other (*15*).

Luce's low-threshold theory. Luce has suggested that a sensory threshold may exist at a somewhat lower level relative to the distribution of noise—that is, that p_0' may be substantial. Apart from this, the low-threshold theory is like the high-threshold theory, only twice so. Whereas Blackwell's theory permits the observer to say "yes" without discrimination when the sensory excitation fails to exceed the threshold, Luce's theory also permits the observer to say "no" without discrimination when the sensory excitation does exceed the threshold. Thus the operating-characteristic curve of this theory contains two linear segments, as shown in Fig. 5. Again, the data for observer 1 in Fig. 1 are shown for comparison. The location of the threshold indicated by these data is shown in the insert at lower right.

It may be seen that the two-line curve fits the yes-no data reasonably well, perhaps as well as the nonlinear curve of detection theory. Although the calculations have not been performed, it seems probable that this theory will also be in fairly good agreement with the second-choice data of Fig. 2. It provides for two categories of sensory excitation, and two categories would seem sufficient to produce a proportion of correct second choices significantly

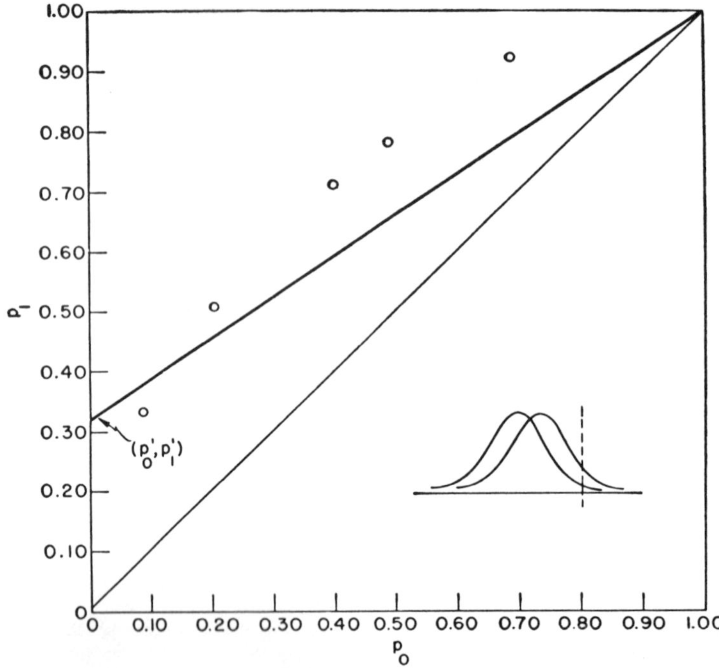

Fig. 4. The results of a yes-no experiment, and a theoretical function from Blackwell's high-threshold theory.

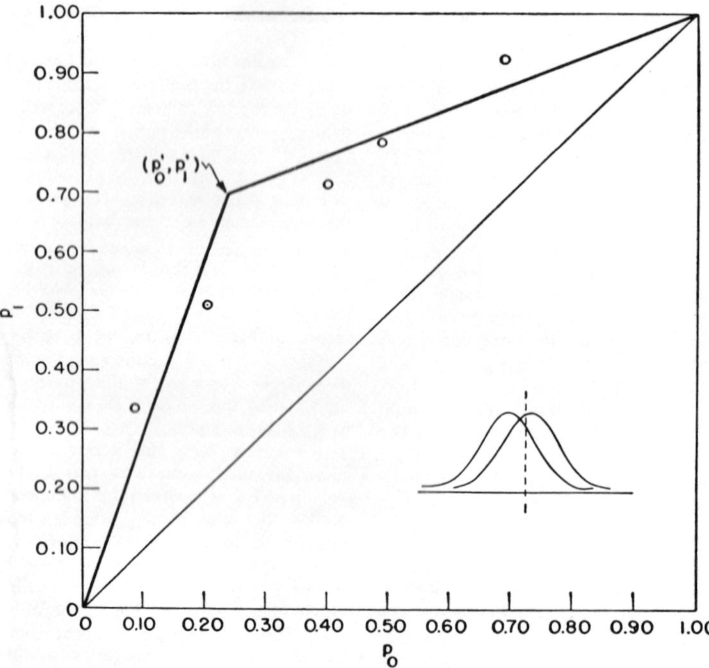

Fig. 5. The results of a yes-no experiment, and a theoretical function from Luce's low-threshold theory.

above the chance proportion. However, on the face of it, a two-category theory is inconsistent with the six categories of sensory excitation indicated by the rating data of Fig. 3. (We may note in passing that the theory raises the interesting question of how another threshold, the one above which a more complete ordering exists, might be measured.)

Green's two-threshold theory. Green has observed that operating-characteristic data, perhaps adequately fitted by Luce's curve of two segments, are certainly better fitted by a curve with three linear segments. This curve, shown in Fig. 6, corresponds to a theory that includes a range of uncertainty between a lower threshold, below which lies true rejection, and an upper threshold, above which lies true detection. The insert at lower right shows the location of the two thresholds.

As is evident from Fig. 6, the curve of three line segments fits the yes-no data at least as well as the nonlinear curve of detection theory. Again, the calculations have not been performed, but it seems very likely that a three-category theory can account for the second-choice data. Even a three-category theory, however, is inconsistent with the six categories of sensory excitation indicated by the rating data.

There is, of course, no need to stop at two thresholds and three categories. A five-threshold theory, with a curve of six line segments, would fit any operating-characteristic data very well indeed and would also be entirely consistent with the second-choice and rating results. However, such a theory is irrelevant to the question under consideration. It is hardly a threshold theory in any important sense. It may be recalled that we considered it earlier as a variant of detection theory.

Swets, Tanner, and Birdsall's low-threshold theory. Tanner, Birdsall, and I proposed a threshold theory that may be described as combining some of the features of Blackwell's and Luce's theories. This theory permits ordering of values of sensory excitation above the threshold but locates the threshold well within the noise distribution. The corresponding operating-characteristic curve is composed of a linear segment above some substantial value of p_0 (say, 0.30 to 0.50) and a curvilinear segment below this value. Inspection of Fig. 1 shows that such a curve fits yes-no data rather well. It is evident that the second-choice data, and rating data exhibiting six categories, could also be obtained without ordering below this threshold.

Stevens' quantal-threshold theory. The quantal-threshold theory advocated by Stevens cannot be treated on the same terms as the other threshold theories. The data of Figs. 1, 2, and 3 are not directly relevant to it. The reason is that, whereas the other threshold theories give a prominent place to noise, collection of data in accordance with the quantal theory requires a serious attempt to eliminate all noise, or at least enough of it to allow the discontinuities of neural action to manifest themselves.

We may doubt, a priori, that noise can in fact be reduced sufficiently to reveal the "grain" of the action of a sensory system. Although the other theories we have examined apply to experiments in which the noise is considerable and, as a matter of fact, are typically applied to experiments in which noise (a background of some kind) is added deliberately, they are not generally viewed as restricted to such experiments. In adding noise we acknowledge its universality. The assumption is that the irreducible minimum of ambient noise, equipment noise, and noise inside the observer is enough to obscure the all-or-none quality of individual nervous elements in a psychological experiment. Noise is added in order to bring the total, or at least that part of it external to the observer, to a relatively constant level, and to a level at which it can be measured.

A recent article reviewing the experiments that have sought to demonstrate a quantal threshold has questioned whether any of the experiments suffices as a demonstration (*19*). Even if we ignore some technical questions concerning curve-fitting procedures and grant that some experiments have produced data in agreement with the quantal-threshold theory, we must observe that obtaining such data evidently depends upon the circumstance of having elite experimenters as well as elite observers (*18*). A relatively large amount of negative evidence exists; several other experimenters have attempted to reproduce the conditions of the successful experiments without success (*19*).

A striking feature of the quantal-theory experiments, in the present context, is the stimulus-presentation procedure employed. Although not contingent upon anything in the theory,

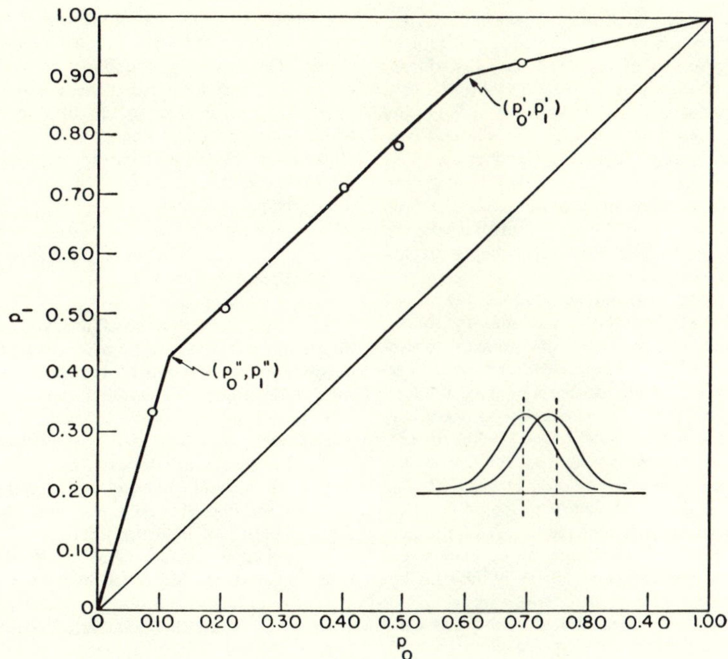

Fig. 6. The results of a yes-no experiment, and a theoretical function from Green's two-threshold theory.

the recommended procedure is to present signals of the same magnitude on all the trials of a series and to make known to the observer that this is the case. This procedure provides an unfortunate protection for the theory; if the observer is likely to make noise-determined "yes" responses, the fact will not be disclosed by the experiment. Licklider has expressed aptly the growing discomfiture over this procedure: "More and more, workers in the field are growing dissatisfied with the classical psychophysical techniques, particularly with the [methods that ask the observer] to report 'present' or 'absent' when he already knows 'present.' It is widely felt that the 'thresholds' yielded by these procedures are on such an insecure semantic basis that they cannot serve as good building blocks for a quantitative science" (*20*). Although the original intent behind the use of this procedure in the quantal-theory experiments was to make the task as easy as possible for the observer, from the point of view of detection theory the procedure presents a very difficult task—it requires that the observer try to establish the response criterion that he would establish if he did not know that the signal was present on every trial.

Thus the advocates of the quantal theory specify a procedure that makes detection theory inapplicable. The result is that, as things stand, the conflict between the two theories cannot be resolved to the satisfaction of all concerned, as it conceivably could be if both theories could be confronted with the same set of data. However, there is reason to hope—since the quantal-theory procedure is not intrinsic to the theory but rests rather on a sense of experimental propriety, which is a relatively labile matter—that such a confrontation will some day be possible.

Is There a Sensory Threshold?

We have considered the data of three experiments—the yes-no, second-choice, and rating experiments—in relation to five competing theories concerning the processes underlying these data. The three sets of data are in agreement with detection theory, a theory that denies the existence of a sensory threshold, and also with the version of a low-threshold theory proposed by Tanner,

Birdsall, and me. Blackwell's high-threshold theory is inconsistent with all three sets of results. Luce's low-threshold theory is consistent with the first, perhaps consistent with the second, and inconsistent with the third. Green's two-threshold theory fits the first two sets of results but not the last. We also considered the only other explicit threshold theory available—the quantal theory, to which the three experiments are not directly relevant.

The outcome is that, as far as we know, there may be a sensory threshold. The possibility of a quantal threshold cannot be discounted, and certainly not on the basis of data at hand. On another level of analysis, there may be what we have termed a low threshold, somewhere in the vicinity of the mean of the noise distribution. The low-threshold theory proposed by Tanner, Birdsall, and me fits all of the data we examined. If the rating experiment can be dismissed (there is now no apparent reason for giving it less than full status), then Luce's and Green's theories, which involve a low threshold, fit the remaining data.

On the other hand, the existence of a sensory threshold has not been demonstrated. Data consistent with the quantal theory are, at best, here today and gone tomorrow, and the theory has yet to be tested through an objective procedure. With respect to a low threshold, we may ask whether demonstration of such a threshold is even conceivable.

It is apparent that it will be difficult to measure a low threshold. Consider the low-threshold theory that permits complete ordering above the threshold in connection with the forced-choice experiment. The observer conveys less information about his ordering than he is capable of conveying if only a first choice is required. We saw in the preceding discussion that the second choice conveys a significant amount of information. Another experiment, in which the observer tried to be incorrect, indicated that he can order four choices (*6*). Thus it is difficult to determine when enough information has been extracted to yield a valid estimate of a low threshold.

Again, it is difficult to imagine how one might determine the signal energy corresponding to the thresholds of Luce's and Green's theories. The determination is made especially difficult by the fact that, in general, empirical operating-characteristic curves for various signal energies are fitted well by the theoretical curves of detection theory. Consequently, the line-segment curves that best fit the data have lines intersecting at a value of p_n that depends upon the signal energy. The implication is that the location of the threshold depends on the signal energy that is being presented.

Implications for Practice

We have, then, the possibility of a threshold, but it is no more than a possibility, and we must observe that since it is practically unmeasurable it will not be a very useful concept in experimental practice. Moreover, even if the low threshold proposed by Tanner, Birdsall, and me did exist, and were measurable, it would not restrict the application of detection theory. We may note that yes-no data resulting from a suprathreshold criterion depend upon the criterion but are completely independent of the threshold value. The same limitation applies to the quantal threshold. It appears that a compelling demonstration of this concept will be difficult to achieve, so that in practice a theory and a method that deal with noise will be required.

Accordingly, with any attempt to measure sensitivity by means of "yes" and "no" responses, a measure of the observer's response criterion should be obtained. The only way known to obtain this measure is to use catch trials—randomly chosen trials that do not contain a signal. The methods of adjustment, limits, and constants in their usual forms, in which the observer knows that the signal is present on every trial, are inappropriate.

A large number of catch trials should be presented. It is not sufficient to employ a few catch trials, enough to monitor the observer, and then to remind him to avoid "false-positive" responses each time he makes one. This procedure merely forces the criterion up to a point where it cannot be measured, and it can be shown that the calculated threshold varies by as much as 6 decibels as the criterion varies in this unmeasurable range (*5*). Precision is also sacrificed when, because highly trained observers are employed, the untestable assumption is made that they do maintain a constant high criterion. Even if all laboratories should be fortunate enough to have such observers, we would have to expect a range of variation of 6 decibels among "constant criterion" observers in different laboratories. To be sure, for some problems, this amount of variability is not bothersome; for others it is.

The presentation of a large number of catch trials—enough to provide a good estimate of the probability of a "yes" response on such a trial—is still inadequate if this estimate is then used to correct the proportion of "yes" responses to the signal for chance success. The validity of the correction for chance depends upon the existence of a high threshold that is inconsistent with all of the data that we examined. It should be noted that the common procedure of taking the proportion of correct responses that is halfway between chance and perfect performance as corresponding to the threshold value of the signal is entirely equivalent to using the chance correction.

In summary, in measuring sensitivity it is desirable to manipulate the response criterion so that it lies in a range where it can be measured, to include enough catch trials to obtain a good estimate of this response criterion, and to use a method of analysis that yields independent measures of sensitivity and the response criterion. One qualification should be added: We can forego estimating the response criterion in a forced-choice experiment. Under the forced-choice procedure, few observers show a bias in their responses large enough to affect the sensitivity index d' appreciably. Those who do show such a bias initially can overcome it with little difficulty. As a result, the observer can be viewed as choosing the interval most likely to contain a signal, without regard to any criterion. For this reason, the forced-choice procedure may be used to advantage in studies having an emphasis on sensory, rather than on motivational or response, processes (*21*).

References and Notes

1. G. T. Fechner, *Elemente der Psychophysik* (1860).
2. The general theory of signal detectability is presented in W. W. Peterson, T. G. Birdsall, W. C. Fox, *IRE Trans. Profess. Group on Information Theory* **PGIT-4**, 171 (1954). Psychophysical theories similar to it have been suggested by M. Smith and Edna A. Wilson, *Psychol. Monographs* **67**, No. 9, Whole No. 359 (1953), and W. N. Munson and J. E. Karlin, *J. Acoust. Soc. Am.* **26**, 542 (1956). The first application of detection theory in psychophysics is described in W. P. Tanner, Jr., and J. A. Swets, *Psychol. Rev.* **61**, 401 (1954).
3. E. G. Boring, *A History of Experimental Psychology* (Appleton-Century-Crofts, New York, ed. 2, 1950), p. 284.
4. E. G. Boring, *The Physical Dimensions of Consciousness* (Century, New York, 1933).

5. J. A. Swets, W. P. Tanner, Jr., T. G. Birdsall, "The evidence for a decision-making theory of visual detection," *Electronic Defense Group, Univ. Michigan, Tech. Rept. No. 40* (1955). This material will appear as "Decision processes in perception," *Psychol. Rev.*
6. W. P. Tanner, Jr., J. A. Swets, D. M. Green, "Some general properties of the hearing mechanism," *Electronic Defense Group, Univ. Michigan, Tech. Rept. No. 30* (1956).
7. W. P. Tanner, Jr., and J. A. Swets, *Psychol. Rev.* **61**, 401 (1954).
8. J. A. Swets, *J. Acoust. Soc. Am.* **31**, 511 (1959).
9. J. P. Egan, A. I. Schulman, G. Z. Greenberg, *ibid.* **31**, 768 (1959).
10. W. P. Tanner, Jr., and R. C. Jones, "The ideal sensor system as approached through statistical decision theory and the theory of signal detectability," proceedings of the Armed Forces–NRC Vision Committee meeting, Washington, D.C., Nov. 1959.
11. W. P. Tanner, Jr., and T. G. Birdsall, *J. Acoust. Soc. Am.* **30**, 922 (1958).
12. J. A. Swets, E. F. Shipley, M. J. McKey, D. M. Green, *ibid.* **31**, 514 (1959).
13. W W. Peterson, T. G. Birdsall, W. C. Fox, *IRE Trans. Profess. Group on Information Theory* **PGIT-4**, 171 (1954).
14. D. M. Green, *J. Acoust. Soc. Am.* **32**, 1189 (1960).
15. H. R. Blackwell, "Threshold psychophysical measurements," unpublished. Also, *Univ. Mich. Eng. Research Inst. Bull. No. 36* (1953).
16. R. D. Luce, *Science* **132**, 1495 (1960).
17. D. M. Green, personal communication.
18. S. S. Stevens, in *Sensory Communication*, W. A. Rosenblith, Ed. (Technology Press and Wiley, New York, in press); ——, *Science* **133**, 80 (1961).
19. J. F. Corso, *Psychol. Bull.* **53**, 371 (1956).
20. J. C. R. Licklider, in *Psychology: A Study of Science*, S. Koch, Ed. (McGraw-Hill, New York, 1959), vol. 1.
21. The preparation of this paper (technical report No. AFCCDD TR 61-10) was supported by the U.S. Army Signal Corps, the Air Force (Office of Scientific Research and Operational Applications Laboratory), and the Office of Naval Research.

Part II

CLASSICAL PSYCHOACOUSTICS

Editor's Comments on Papers 6 Through 11

6 REISZ
Excerpt from *Differential Intensity Sensitivity of the Ear for Pure Tones*

7 SHOWER and BIDDULPH
Excerpt from *Differential Pitch Sensitivity of the Ear*

8 MILLER
Sensitivity to Changes in the Intensity of White Noise and Its Relation to Masking and Loudness

9 GARNER
The Effect of Frequency Spectrum on Temporal Integration of Energy in the Ear

10 STEVENS, VOLKMANN, and NEWMAN
A Scale for the Measurement of the Psychological Magnitude Pitch

11 STEVENS
A Scale for the Measurement of a Psychological Magnitude: Loudness

Boring (1942) remarked about Fechner's struggles with quantification of sensations that it is difficult for moderns to understand the depth of the philosophical schism that separates those convinced of the folly of the assignment of numbers to sensations and those who saw it as a fruitful endeavor. But at least for the last two decades, moderns in audition have been largely spared that struggle by the clear exposition of S. S. Stevens, particularly in the area of the applicability of mathematical rules to the structuring of subjective responses (as early, for example, as 1935 with a short treatise on the "Operational Definition of Psychological Concepts.")

The path has not been without its obstacles and the ideas were not accepted uncritically, however; arguments over the correct procedures to be followed have been frequent and lively. But the general pattern—assignment of magnitudes by repeatable procedures and trial by empirical validation—has been seldom seriously questioned since the conversion of experimental psychologists to the tenets of operational definition (see, for example, Bergmann and Spence, 1944).

What I have chosen to call classical psychoacoustics dealt first of all with the identification of dimensions central to auditory perception. This was followed by an exploration of minimum discriminable differences on the underlying parallel physical continuum and then the scaling of the psychological response. Ordinarily what would be included also is the process of establishing the zero point for such scales in the form of a sensitivity curve. But this latter has been such an interesting and revealing effort in the case of audition that the establishment of the minimum sensitivity curve has been chronicled separately in Part I.

It was obvious to interested observers before psychoacoustics took on any semblance of formal study that pitch and loudness are the two primary attributes for simple tones, but the history of two others, volume and density, as additional tonal attributes is worth at least passing notice for a very important reason. It was during the effort to establish these two as auditory attributes and to structure their relations to pitch and loudness that Stevens made specific to auditory study the principle of operational definition. Thus though volume and density never became household words in audition, they played a very useful role in the early days of experimental psychophysics. By the time timbre and consonance were seriously attacked experimentally, sophistication about measurement of subjective attributes had grown impressively. Pitch and loudness, of course, have been most extensively investigated and stand unquestionably, despite occasional argument about the specific form of the scale, as the primary auditory attributes. (Signal duration, which should have played a larger role from the start, is discussed later.)

The relation of loudness to signal amplitude and pitch to signal frequency was apparent even before the beginnings of laboratory investigation; and specification of the nature of the parallel between amplitude and loudness, frequency, and pitch constituted a large portion of the early research effort in psychological acoustics. It began with the natural step of finding the physical size of the minimally detectable change (Δ) and noting that just noticeable difference (jnd) changed over the usable range of the dimension. This is precisely what Riesz set out to do for the intensity dimension (Paper 6), and Shower and Biddulph made comparable measurements for frequency (Paper 7). It is no accident that both these sets of measurements were made by telephone engineers rather than by psychologists. The decade of the 1930s is definitely within the period when control of the acoustic signal to close enough tolerance for measuring the performance of the auditory system was a problem for most auditory psychologists.

In their 1938 book on hearing, Stevens and Davis combined such measurements on the differential sensitivity of the ear in the frequency and amplitude domain with the information on the upper and lower limits of frequency and intensity into a matrix displaying the total number of tones discriminable by the auditory sense. They divided the auditory area into amplitude-by-frequency rectangles, each half-octave by 10dB, and counted how many discriminably different tones were in each rectangle. This is of some interest, since it demonstrates how intensity and frequency resolution reach their maximum in the middle range on both dimensions. The authors also summed these individual counts within the auditory area and emerged with 330,000 ΔI-by-Δf cells and, by implication, 330,000 tones of differing loudness and pitch. Fletcher (1929) had already found this a useful way to characterize the basic capability of the auditory analyzer. He used Knudsen's (1923) data on just noticeable differences for frequency and intensity to arrive at an estimate of 540,000 auditorally distinguishable tones.

The conviction that the nature of the resolving power of the ear for static signals along these two demonstrably primary dimensions is central to our eventual understanding of the operation of the analyzer still has its strong adherents among those who work in psychological acoustics. That such a view has not been held universally is eloquently attested by a statement Licklider made: "I find myself tending to recast hypothetical auditory mechanisms in such a way as to emphasize the kind of analysis that leads to synthesis (pattern recognition, object construction, concept formation, problem solving) as opposed to the kinds of analysis that lead to scales that correspond to sensory attributes" (1962, p. 30).

Corliss (1967), on the other hand, makes excellent use of the data of Riesz and Shower and Biddulph in unifying a variety of auditory experiments. The heart of the Corliss auditory model is a selector mechanism that behaves like an integrating resonator and has as output an amplitude-sensitive count. If energy content decreases to an amount $e^{-\alpha}$ times its original value within one integrating time interval, a change of a "least count" takes place in the selector output. Psychophysically this resembles the jnd in physical input for a least change in perceptual response. Time enters as the time constant of the system's characteristic bandwidths. Corliss has shown how much of auditory behavior can be accounted for by this model.

There is no intent to imply—in dubbing this discussion classical psychoacoustics—that activity in the area has come to a halt. The two classic studies discussed thus far have only recently been repeated with considerable refinement (Wier et al., 1977; Jestead et al., 1977). Contrary to Riesz's dda in Paper 6, Jestead et al. found the log of $\Delta I/I$ to be the same linear function of sensation level at all frequencies measured; they also found that this held over a sensation-level range from 5dB to 80dB (from just above the listener's threshold to about 80dB above). No such simplification emerged from the Wier et al. study on frequency discrimination, where agreement with Shower and Biddulph (Paper 7) is quite poor; but this might be expected with intervening changes in signals and methods. For reader's interested in bringing their knowledge of auditory tonal discrimination up to date, both these studies are highly recommended.

Any account of auditory experimentation on intensity discrimination is not complete without recognition of Miller's study of perception of intensity changes in white noise (Paper 8). Though it is most often cited for establishing the jnd in intensity for white noise, it is actually a more complete exposition of the psychophysics of white noise as seen at that period.

The salient characteristic of all of these studies I have labeled with the convenient term *classical* is that (with one exception) they have used signals of sufficiently long duration that time is not a dimension of interest in the measurements. It is true that the Shower and Biddulph signals for frequency discrimination changed with time, but they did so so slowly that one might fully expect the same results from static signals.

Gabor (1946) recognized the primary nature of the dimensions of frequency and intensity, particularly the relevance of the measurements of Shower and Biddulph (1931) on the DL for frequency for slowly changing tones and of Bürck, Kotowski, and Lichte (1935) for brief signals. But he emphasized the great importance of the time dimension in "subjective" acoustics and introduced the concept of the time-by-frequency logon as the quantum unit for hearing. In one sense Gabor, who suggested the relevance of a time-frequency uncertainty principle in hearing, was simply expanding an earlier discussion by G. W. Stewart, who, in 1931, discussing an uncertainty principle in acoustics, had called for "redetermination of minimum perceptible differences in frequency as dependent on Δt, and an examination of Δt required for tone perception with varied values of Δf." The measurements of Shower and Biddulph met this request only marginally. Knudsen's earlier work on pitch discrimination had assigned even less importance to the time dimension. Even at the time of Gabor's writing, when Doughty and Garner (1947) attacked one facet of the problem experimentally in attempting to differentiate between "tone pitch" and "click pitch," they emphasized this dichotomous aspect rather than heeding Stewart's injunction to explore the dependence between Δt and Δf in auditory perception. The Doughty and Garner study has been so frequently cited that part of the paper has been included here in the section on pitch (Paper 17). Even their second paper of the series (Doughty and Garner, 1948), though it was titled "Pitch as a Function of Tonal Duration," scarcely touched on the problem of the increase of uncertainty in pitch judgments as duration decreased.

With regard to the time factor in intensity discrimination, the situation is not much different. Garner and Miller (1944) pointed out that in measuring difference limens, "the duration of the comparison tone must be included as one of the parameters." They succeeded in showing that below about 250msec, fineness of intensity discrimination deteriorates, especially for tones of lower intensity—that is, much more rapidly at low intensity (40dB SL) than at higher (70dB SL). Henning (1970) partially verified this principle in two subjects at a single sound pressure level, but we still lack any comprehensive set of data on the relation between intensity discrimination and signal duration. (Comparable data for frequency discrimination are discussed more fully in the section on pitch.)

Gabor's very timely admonition about including time as a primary parameter in audition went largely unheeded for over a decade. Davis (1952) endorsed and adopted the idea of Gabor's logon, but psychoacousticians failed to furnish the kind of data called for much earlier by Stewart. Fletcher's time-pattern theory of hearing (1930), even in its 1953 version and despite its name, took but little recognition of the time-varying nature of most auditory signals.

A welcome exception to this early comparative neglect of the time dimension, however, is the work of Miller and Garner on the integration of signal energy over time by the ear. Although they began the relevant work around 1944, the most concise portrayal of the important measures and the emergent principle is found in Garner's 1947 paper (Paper 9). Miller and Garner's work triggered an enthusiastic series of investigations of one of the very useful time constants of the auditory system. Subsequent work has shown that this integration effect occurs also at above-threshold levels—that is, that signals of about 200msec duration are louder than shorter signals of the same amplitude (Zwislocki, 1960)—and under a large variety of laboratory listening conditions (Blodgett et al., 1958). On a few occasions, enthusiasm has run a bit high, and the approximately 200msec over which integration occurs has been designated as *the* time constant of the auditory system—an extrapolation obviously not compatible with a system that resolves amplitude variations over intervals of milliseconds or less.

Lagging only a little behind the early measurements of auditory discrimination, and certainly complementing them in concept, was the determination of the form of the psychophysical function for pitch and for loudness. One might assume, as Fechner did, that all just noticeable differences are the same subjective size, and settle for supposing that all equal subjective distances are equal numbers of just discriminable steps for any distance along the scale and over any part of its range. Since Weber had established earlier that

$$\frac{\text{necessary change in stimulus}}{\text{size of stimulus}} = \text{a constant,}$$

Fechner's assumption that all just noticeable subjective changes are subjectively equal implies a constant arithmetic change on the subjective dimension for a comparable geometric change on the physical dimension. With the additional assumption that these steps are continuously divisible, integration of the differential form is permissible and led to the formulation

$$\text{psychological value} \propto \log \text{physical value,}$$

an easily understandable form of the Fechner law. As Lewis (1960) points out, the law was "venerated by many investigators, but assailed if not ridiculed by many others" (p. 430).

Empirical justification for the form of the scale is sought for pitch and for loudness in the Stevens, Volkmann, and Newman (Paper 10) and the Stevens (Paper 11) articles reproduced here. The pitch scale of Stevens, Volkmann, and Newman was revised by Stevens and Newman in 1940, with several refinements: the running of additional subjects, an attempt to allow for subjects who needed a zero-pitch reference, and a comparison of fractionation, bisection, and equal sense distances. But the earlier scale is very similar to the revised one, and the psychophysical flavor of the time is more efficiently conveyed in the briefer earlier paper. Along with the equal-loudness contours and the loudness formulation of Fletcher and Munson (1933) for complex signals, these papers represent the cornerstones of classical psychoacoustics.

In 1955, Stevens assembled the evidence from a large number of independent investigators who had asked subjects to change tones and noises of various levels until they seemed half as loud or twice as loud as the original. On the average, subjects changed the sounds by about 10dB to satisfy that criterion. Thus a change of 10 to 1 in intensity (I) corresponds to a change of 2 to 1 in loudness (L), or (since $\log_{10} 2 = 0.3$)

$$L = kI^{0.3}$$

As explained in Paper 11, the unit for this scale is the sone, and the conveniently chosen anchor point (1 sone) is 40dB sound pressure level.

Looking at the equation, one might guess that in conditions under which the subjects made the judgments, loudness grows as the cube root of the sound, but I know of no persuasive psychological or physiological reason why this should be so. Exponents for comparably derived scales for other sensory responses, ranging from judgments of brightness of light to subjective strength of electric shock, vary from 0.3 to 3.5 (Stevens, 1975).

Regarding the loudness scale, Warren and his colleagues (Warren, Sersen, and Pores, 1958) insisted that rather than Steven's $L = kI^{0.3}$, there was good reason to expect the exponent to be 0.5 because of the operation of the inverse square law. He called his rationale the *physical correlate theory of sensory intensity* and asserted that we learn our loudness relations as sources change their distance from us in relatively sound-absorptive environments. In an attempt to minimize subject bias, Warren (1970) presented data that support this notion from 720 subjects who made only one loudness judgment each.

What Stevens might have called classical (rather than modern) psychophysics is the formulation that says psychophysical relations are best expressed as log functions (Stevens, 1961). He insisted instead that the power function (log-log) is the appropriate model for prothetic (subjectively additive) continua and proceeded to show that once power-function exponents had been established within each of two sense modalities, even cross-modal matches could be predicted.

There is no gainsaying the fundamental nature of loudness and pitch in audition. Yet much of the activity in the development of loudness and pitch scales seems activity within a closed system—psychoacoustics for its own sake. Marks (1974, p. 31) has recently cautioned that "scaling cannot stand in isolation from the rest of sensory psychology." But the solution is not so easy as simply adopting the sone and mel scales for plotting subjective responses to all intensity and frequency changes. One frequently makes a judgment of the existence and direction of loudness change but seldom a judgment of the comparative amount of loudness change. What should not be confused here is the auditory clues carried by various aspects of intensity-change patterns that do not entail judgments of loudness. These latter occur much more frequently. The same is true for pitch. Outside the realm of music, judgments of the frequency ratio or the precise pitch distance of a change are rare. On the other hand, awareness of a frequency change is frequently called for in auditory analysis and may or may not be perceived as a change in pitch (movement of vowel formants is an excellent example).

Nevertheless development and refinement of psychophysical scales of loudness and pitch do constitute a large and important segment in the history of psychological acoustics. The only reservation voiced here is some caution in extending these same scales to signals that differ too widely—either on the time dimension or in spectral context—from those on which they were derived.

REFERENCES

Bergmann, G., and K. W. Spence. 1944. The logic of psychophysical measurement. *Psych. Rev.* **51**:1-24.

Blodgett, H. C., L. A. Jeffress, and R. W. Taylor. 1958. Relation of masked threshold to signal-duration for various interaural phase-combinations. *Am. J. Psychol.* **71**:283-290.

Boring, E. G. 1942. *Sensation and perception in the history of experimental psychology.* New York: D. Appleton-Century.

Bürck, W., P. Kotowski, and H. Lichte. 1935. Die hörbarkeit von laufzeitdifferenzen. *Elektr. Nachr. Tec.* **12**:355-367.

Corliss, E. L. R. 1967. Mechanistic aspects of hearing. *Acoust. Soc. Am. J.* **41**: 1500-1516.

Davis, H. 1952. Information theory: 3. Applications of information theory to research in hearing. *J. Speech Hear. Disord.* **17**:189-197.

Doughty, J. M., and W. R. Garner. 1948. Pitch characteristics of short tones. II. Pitch as a function of tonal duration. *J. Exp. Psychol.* **38**:478-494.

Fletcher, H. 1929. *Speech and hearing.* New York: Van Nostrand.

Fletcher, H. 1930. A space time pattern theory of hearing. *Acoust. Soc. Am. J.* **1**: 311-343.

Fletcher, H., and W. A. Munson. 1933. Loudness, its definition, measurement and calculation. *Acoust. Soc. Am. J.* **5**:82-108.

Gabor, D. 1946. Theory of communication. Part 2, The analysis of hearing. *Inst. Electr. Eng. J.* **93**:442-445.

Garner, W. R., and G. A. Miller. 1944. Differential sensitivity to intensity as a function of the duration of the comparison tone. *J. Exp. Psychol.* **34**:450-463.

Henning, G. B. 1970. A comparison of the effects of signal duration on frequency and amplitude discrimination. In *Frequency analysis and periodicity detection in hearing,* ed. R. Plomp and G. F. Smoorenburg, pp. 350-359.

Jestead, W., C. C. Wier, and D. M. Green. 1977. Intensity discrimination as a function of frequency and sensation level. *Acoust. Soc. Am. J.* **61**:169-177.

Knudsen, V. O. 1923. The sensibility of the ear to small differences in intensity and frequency. *Phys. Rev.* **21**:84-103.

Lewis, D. 1960. *Quantitative methods in psychology.* New York: McGraw-Hill.

Licklider, J. C. R. 1962. Periodicity pitch and related auditory process models. *Int. Audiol.* **1**:11-36.

Marks, L. E. 1974. *Sensory processes: The new psychophysics.* New York: Academic Press.

Shower, E. G., and R. Biddulph. 1931. Differential pitch sensitivity of the ear. *Acoust. Soc. Am. J.* **3**:275-287.

Stevens, S. S. 1935. The operational definition of psychological concepts. *Psychol. Rev.* **42**:517-527.

Stevens, S. S. 1961. To honor Fechner and repeal his law. *Science* **133**:80-86.

Stevens, S. S. 1975. *Psychophysics.* New York: Wiley.

Stevens, S. S., and H. Davis, 1938. *Hearing: Its Psychology and Physiology.* New York: Wiley.

Stewart, G. W. 1931. Problems suggested by an uncertainty principle in acoustics. *Acoust. Soc. Am. J.* **2**:325–329.

Warren, R. M. 1970. Elimination of biases in loudness judgments for tones. *Acoust. Soc. Am. J.* **48**:1397–1403.

Warren, R. M., E. A. Sersen, and E. B. Pores. 1958. A basis for loudness judgments. *Am. J. Psychol.* **71**:700–709.

Wier, C. C., W. Jestead, and D. M. Green. 1977. Frequency discrimination as a function of frequency and sensation level. *Acoust. Soc. Am. J.* **61**:178–184.

Zwislocki, J. J. 1960. Theory of temporal auditory summation. *Acoust. Soc. Am. J.* **32**:1046–1060.

6

Reprinted from pages 867-872 of *Phys. Rev.* **31**:867-875 (1928)

DIFFERENTIAL INTENSITY SENSITIVITY OF THE EAR FOR PURE TONES

By R. R. Riesz

Abstract

The ratio of the minimum perceptible increment in sound intensity to the total intensity, $\Delta E/E$, which is called the differential sensitivity of the ear, was measured as a function of frequency and intensity. Measurements were made over practically the entire range of frequencies and intensities for which the ear is capable of sensation. The method used was that of beating tones, this method giving the simplest transition from one intensity to another. The source of sound was a special moving coil telephone receiver having very little distortion, actuated by alternating currents from vacuum tube oscillators. Observations were made on twelve male observers. Average curves show that at any frequency, $\Delta E/E$ is practically constant for intensities greater than 10^6 times the threshold intensity; near the auditory threshold $\Delta E/E$ increases. Weber's law holds above this intensity, the value of $\Delta E/E$ =constant lying between 0.05 and 0.15 depending on the frequency. As a function of frequency $\Delta E/E$ is a minimum at about 2500 c.p.s., the minimum being more sharply defined at low sound intensities than it is at high. This frequency corresponds to the region of greatest absolute sensitivity of the ear. Analytical expressions are given [Eqs. (2), (3), (4) and (5)] which represent $\Delta E/E$, within the error of observation, as a function of frequency and intensity. Using these equations it is calculated that at about 1300 c.p.s. the ear can distinguish 370 separate tones between the threshold of audition and the threshold of feeling.

1. Introduction

In the study of the design and operation of transmission circuits and other apparatus used in the telephone plant, the communications engineer is interested in many phases of the study of speech and hearing. One subject of importance is the investigation of the minimum change in intensity which the ear is able to detect. This information is also of interest to physicists when considering the ear as a physical instrument, to psychologists in formulating relationships between exciting physical stimulus and the resulting sensation and to otologists in the study of normal and abnormal hearing. Since the published data fail to give information over the entire range of frequencies and intensities for which the ear is capable of sensation, the investigation here reported was undertaken with the purpose of covering the range as completely as possible.

The best published information on the sensitivity of the ear to small differences in intensity as well as a good historical survey of the subject is recorded by Knudsen.[1] These data are most conveniently expressed by the ratio, $\Delta E/E$, where ΔE is the minimum preceptible increment in sound intensity and E is the total intensity. This ratio has been variously termed: Weber's constant, Weber-Fechner ratio, intensity sensibility; but in this

[1] The Sensibility of the Ear to Small Differences in Intensity and Frequency, V. O. Knudsen, Phys. Rev. **21**, 84 (1923).

paper it will be called differential sensitivity, a name suggested by N. E Dorsey.

In this investigation the differential sensitivity of twelve observers was measured as a function of intensity and frequency using the method of beating tones. Measurements were made at frequencies of from 35 to 10,000 cycles per second and over an intensity range from the threshold of audition to the threshold of feeling. This practically covers the intensity and frequency range of auditory sensation.[2] As the observers were all of normal hearing, the averaged data may be taken as being representative of the hypothetical average normal ear.

2. Theory of Method Used

The changes in intensity were produced by sending through a special telephone receiver alternating currents whose frequencies were so close together that beats were produced. If two sinusoidal pressure waves, $a_1\cos\omega_1 t$ and $a_2\cos\omega_2 t$, are simultaneously impressed on the ear drum the resultant pressure wave may be expressed as:

$$a = m\cos(\omega_2 t + \Phi)$$

where

$$m^2 = a_1^2 + a_2^2 + 2a_1a_2\cos(\omega_2 - \omega_1)t$$

If $(\omega_2 - \omega_1)$ is small compared with ω_1 and ω_2, there will be a large number of vibrations in each beat cycle and an observer listening to such a sound will not be cognizant of two tones as such but will perceive a single tone whose intensity fluctuates with a frequency $\omega_2 - \omega_1/2\pi$. For beating frequencies such as are used in these experiments, to a close approximation, the amplitude of the resultant wave in the region of maximum intensity is $(a_1 + a_2)$ and the amplitude in the region of minimum intensity is $(a_1 - a_2)$. The difference between maximum and minimum amplitude is then $2a_2$. In the experiments here described the relative values of a_1 and a_2 for just perceptible beats were determined throughout the intensity and frequency range of the ear.

When listening to slow beats such as are used in these experiments, the ear probably does not make simple direct comparisons between the maximum intensity, proportional to $(a_1 + a_2)^2$, and the minimum intensity, proportional to $(a_1 - a_2)^2$. The comparison which the ear does make in such a case is dependent on a number of factors, among which are: the magnitude of the difference between maximum and minimum intensity; the rate of change of intensity, which includes rapidity of fluctuations and mode of transition between maximum and minimum intensity. Throughout these experiments the rapidity of fluctuation was kept constant and the changes between maximum and minimum intensity were made so that to a first approximation the amplitude of the resultant wave varied sinusoidally. Thus

[2] The Frequency-Sensitivity Characteristic of Normal Ears. H. Fletcher and R. L. Wegel, Phys. Rev. 19, 553 (1922).

the second of the above mentioned factors was held constant throughout the experiments and for this type of intensity fluctuation, correlating differential sensitivity with the difference between maximum and mimimum intensity, we have:

$$\frac{\Delta E}{E}=\frac{(a_1+a_2)^2-(a_1-a_2)^2}{(a_1-a_2)^2}=\frac{4a_1a_2}{(a_1-a_2)^2} \tag{1}$$

3. Discussion of Method

Although the type of transition from minimum to maximum intensity using the method of beats is not that usually encountered in actual experience, it possesses the advantage that it produces a simple intensity fluctuation which is not complicated by the possible presence of an undetermined amount of transients. If the transitions from minimum to maximum intensity are made abruptly some of the energy will be scattered to frequencies higher and lower than the impressed frequency. Due to the variation of the absolute sensitivity of the ear mechanism with frequency, these introduced transients may be audible, and influence the observer in deciding when he was just able to detect a fluctuation in intensity. The disturbing effect of transients should therefore be greatest at high and low frequencies and least at intermediate frequencies. Knudsen says that at high frequencies his measurements were disturbed by "contact noises," undoubtedly transients. In using the method of beats, the only frequencies present are the two beating frequencies and if these are kept so close together that the ear is unable to distinguish them separately, it is impossible to conceive of the production of any transients. In this investigation no measurements were made of the magnitude of the effect which transients would introduce.

4. Description of Apparatus

A schematic diagram of the circuit used is shown in Fig. 1. Alternating currents of any desired frequency were generated by two special vacuum tube oscillators. The currents, which were read on ammeters A_1 and A_2, were

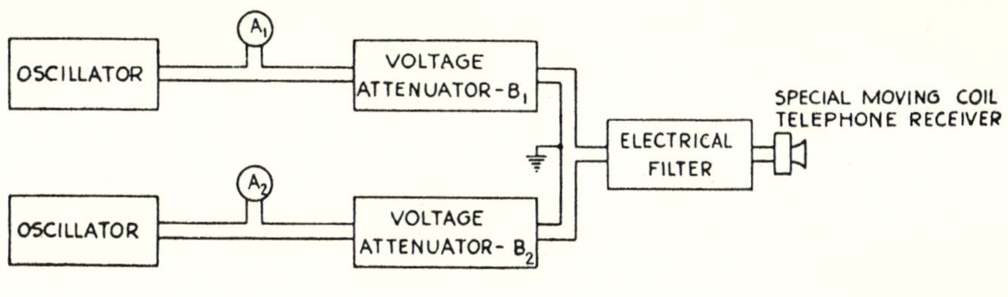

Fig. 1

sent through voltage attenuators B_1 and B_2, whose outputs were in series with the telephone receiver circuit. The attenuators were of the dial type, reading voltage directly on a logarithmic scale and having a range from

1 to 10^{-15}. The filter was necessary to eliminate the effects due to harmonics. Ordinary telephone receivers were found entirely unsuited for this investigation, especially at low frequencies, because of harmonics produced by distortion. A special moving coil receiver was used which was particularly free from distortion. If a pure electrical wave is impressed on the terminals of this receiver the intensity of the harmonics in the acoustic output is less than that of the fundamental in the ratio of $1:10^{-5}$. It was found necessary to make all observations in a sound-proof room.

5. Rapidity of Fluctuations

The differential sensitivity was found to be a function of the rapidity of the intensity fluctuations and a preliminary investigation was conducted to determine the proper rapidity of intensity fluctuation to use. The differential sensitivity for three observers was explored as a function of rapidity of intensity fluctuation at various frequencies and intensities scattered throughout the range of interest. All observers showed practically the same results at all frequencies and intensities. A representative curve of $\Delta E/E$ vs. rapidity of intensity fluctuation is shown in Fig. 2 (the particular fre-

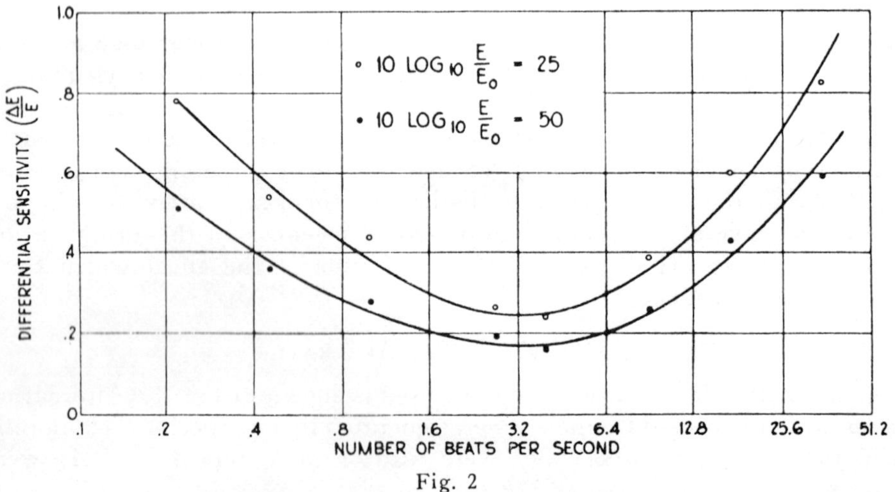

Fig. 2

quency used here was 1000 cycles per second). It is characterized by a broad minimum in the neighborhood of 3 cycles of intensity fluctuation per second. The increase in differential sensitivity is probably due, for faster fluctuations, to the fact that the component tones become so far separated in frequency that they are partially resolved by the ear, for slower fluctuations, to a memory effect. Three cycles of intensity fluctuation per second was adopted as the most logical rapidity to use for all measurements.

6. Experimental Procedure

The weight of the special receiver used being 15 lbs., it was necessary to adjust it to the level of the observer's ear by means of a spring suspension. To further insure uniformity of position the receiver was held against the observer's ear by an elastic strap passing around the head. One oscillator was set at any desired frequency and the other adjusted to give three beats per second. The minimum audible voltage of one attenuator, say B_1, was determined, B_2 being set far below the minimum audible voltage. B_1 was then set at any desired value and B_2 adjusted until the observer signalled that he heard beats. The setting of B_2 was changed each time the observer signalled whether or not the tone seemed to fluctuate. After about 20 such judgments the operator was able to locate with considerable certainty the setting of B_2 for which the observer was just able to detect a fluctuation in intensity. If B_2 was set below this value the fluctuation in intensity was imperceptible. The r.m.s. voltage introduced into the receiver circuit by each oscillator could be calculated from the readings of the ammeters and the settings of the attenuators. At any frequency the r.m.s. alternating pressure on the ear drum is proportional to the voltage introduced into the receiver circuit so that the differential sensitivity can be calculated by Eq. (1). Complete series of measurments were made on twelve male observers at frequencies of 35, 70, 200, 1000, 4000, 7000 and 10,000 cycles per second and at intensities from weak tones near the threshold of audition to very loud tones near the threshold of feeling.

7. Experimental Results

Average curves of differential sensitivity as a function of intensity are shown on Figs. 3 and 4. The crosses are the averages of the twelve observers.

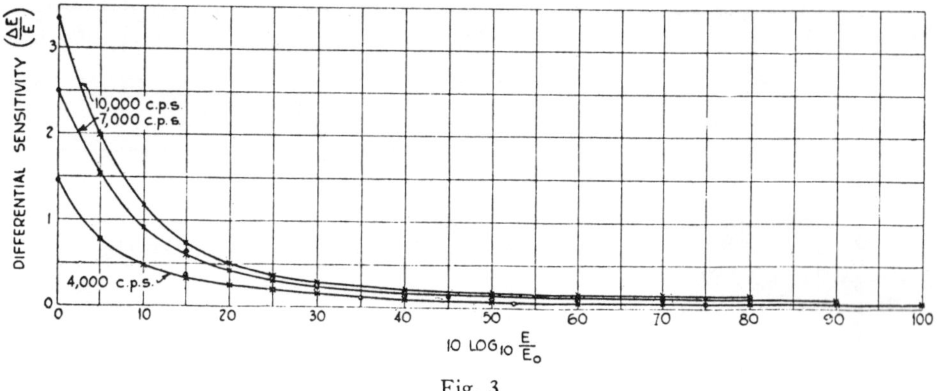

Fig. 3

The intensity is plotted in units of $10 \log_{10}(E/E_0)$ where E_0 is the threshold intensity. If the data are plotted as a function of absolute intensity, the curves will all be shifted along the abscissa by different amounts. The amount of the shift can be calculated from Fletcher and Wegel's curve of the absolute sensitivity of the average normal ear.[2]

Fig. 5 shows curves of differential sensitivity as a function of frequency for various values of the intensity parameter, $10 \log_{10}(E/E_0)$. The spread of the observations for the 12 observers was less than $\pm$ 10% of the average value in every case.

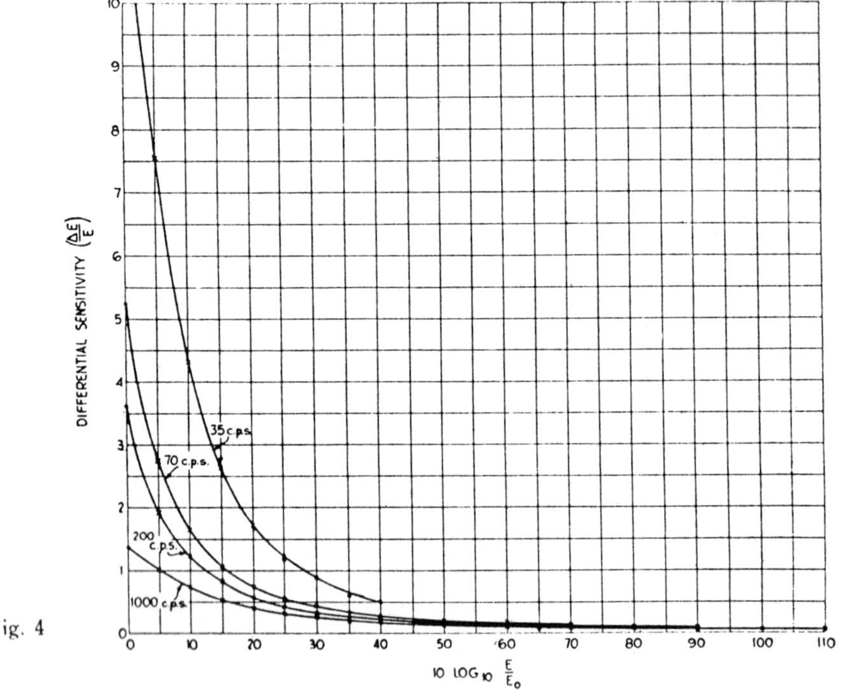

Fig. 4

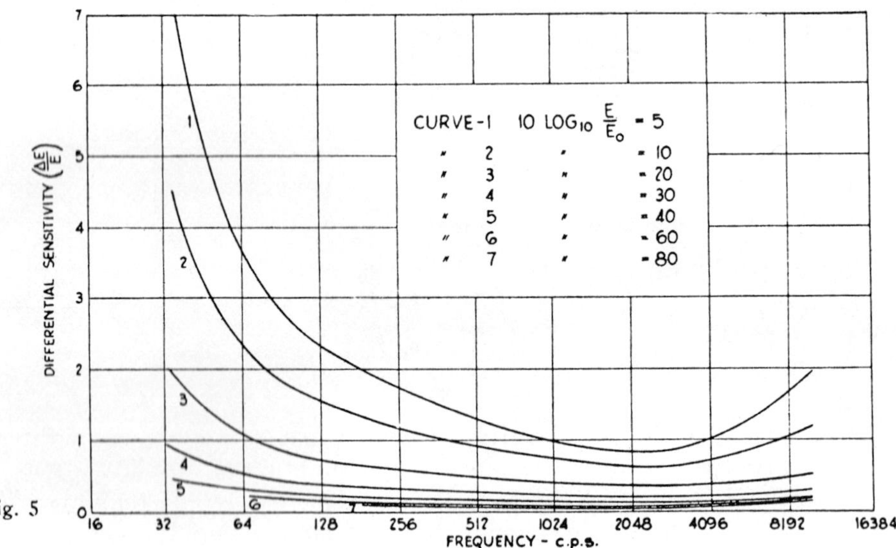

Fig. 5

[*Editor's Note:* Material has been omitted at this point.]

7

Reprinted from pages 275–280 and 287 of *Acoust. Soc. Am. J.* 3:275–287 (1931)

DIFFERENTIAL PITCH SENSITIVITY OF THE EAR

By E. G. Shower and R. Biddulph
Bell Telephone Laboratories

1. Definition

As applied to the ear, differential pitch sensitivity is the minimum change in frequency which is detectable at any one frequency and sensation level. It varies with the frequency and sensation level of the tone and among observers.

2. History

Various investigators have studied this problem. Among the earliest is Delazenne, who reported observations at 60 cycles made in 1827. Later investigations were made by Seebeck at 1029 cycles, Weber at 200, and others who give results but fail to report the frequencies at which the measurements were made. In more recent times Preyer, Luft, Meyer, Stucher, Vance and Knudsen extended the range of the earlier measurements to cover the major portion of the speech frequencies. More complete bibliographies are contained in Vance's report, (1) and in the work of Fletcher (2).

3. Reasons for Further Work

The present investigation was undertaken with the purpose of extending the field covered by the previous measurements. In all cases, with the exception of that of Knudsen (3), no account was taken of the intensity or sensation levels of the tones used, and since tuning forks and vibrating strings were the sources of sound, any technique in which intensity was accounted for would have been hopelessly cumbersome. Knudsen retained a constant sensation level of 40 db above threshold and made measurements at frequencies extending from 62 to 3200 cycles. Upon considering the auditory area it was planned that the present investigation should cover the frequency range 31 to 11700 cycles at sensation levels ranging from 5 db above the threshold to the maximum level which the observer could tolerate at any given frequency.

Since many of the investigators mentioned above report widely varying results, a check by means of a new technique and new type of apparatus would be valuable from the standpoint of the influence of transients, provided the new apparatus were designed with this point in mind. It is obvious that tuning forks and plucked strings will contain harmonics, especially when first excited, and Knudsen reports difficulty from "contact noises" due to the opening and closing of an auxiliary circuit in his vacuum tube oscillator. He indicates that these noises made observations at high frequencies impossible and results at low frequencies questionable.

4. Preliminary Considerations

Upon studying the previous investigations it was decided that the principal difficulties to be overcome in making complete measurements were as follows: Transients inherent in any system in which the frequency is varied, harmonics due to non-linearity of oscillator or receiver, inflexibility of apparatus and the attainment of intensity and frequency ranges sufficient to cover the auditory area.

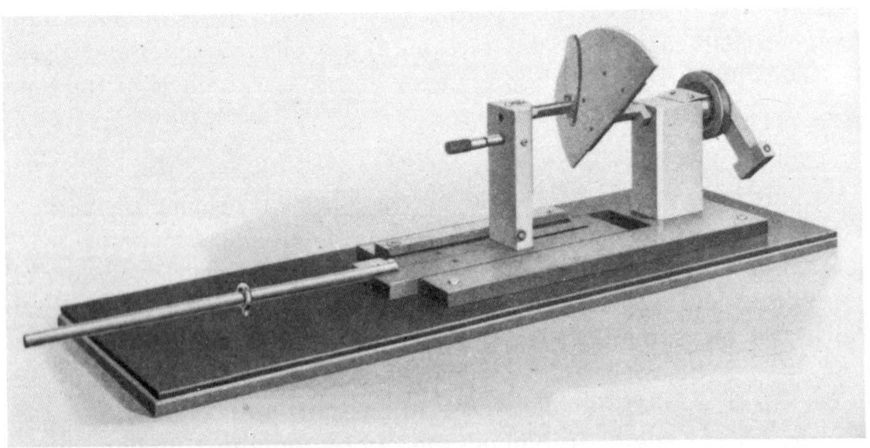

FIG. 1. *Rotary air condenser.*

5. Description of Apparatus

Since it is impossible to vary the frequency of a system without scattering energy into frequency regions other than that being used, a method of variation in which this scattering would be a minimum was sought.

An additional condition imposed upon the frequency changing mechanism was that it should allow the observer to listen to a tone of unvarying pitch for a short interval of time, change the frequency sinusoidally and remain at the new pitch level for another short interval before returning sinusoidally to its original position to complete the cycle. It was considered advantageous to have the length of this cycle variable. The result of this investigation was the design of the special rotary condenser shown in Fig. 1. This condenser is connected across the oscillating circuit of one channel of a heterodyne oscillator. Across the condenser is another condenser of fixed capacity. The frequency of the second oscillator channel is controlled by a precision condenser. For a fixed setting of this condenser and a given setting of the small head on the rotary condenser the output frequency after having been modulated shows a time variation as plotted in Fig. 2.

The crosses mark static measurements of frequency made at the various positions of the rotating head throughout the 360° of its rota-

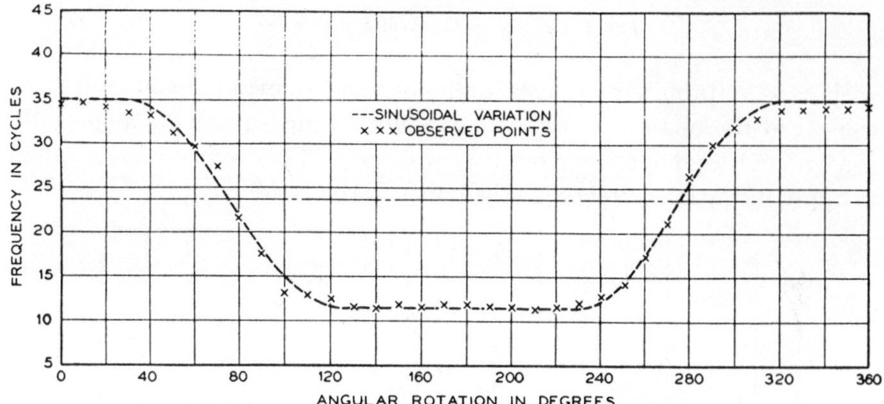

FIG. 2. *Frequency change produced by rotary condenser.*

tion. The dashed curve shows the modified sinusoidal type of variation of the ideal case. It can be seen that the actual case approximates the ideal closely enough for the purpose in mind. For another setting of the small head of the rotary condenser the amplitude of this curve would be changed, whereas a change in the setting of the precision condenser in the variable channel would change the position of the mean ordinate without changing the amplitude.

The frequency variation then, is controlled by the setting of the small head of the rotary condenser and is entirely independent of the other channel. The "base" frequency is controlled by the precision condenser and the frequency thus obtained is amplified and filtered. The filters used are of the band pass type with discriminations of from 70 to 90 db. These filters serve to eliminate harmonics due to non-linearity of the oscillator and amplifier circuits and any extraneous sounds introduced by the power supply. From the filters the output goes to an attenuator and thence through a shielded cable to a sound-proof booth containing the receivers and a signalling push-button for the observer. The general arrangement is shown in Fig. 3.

The receivers used are of the electrodynamic type, designed to handle large amounts of power without excessive distortion. They were fitted

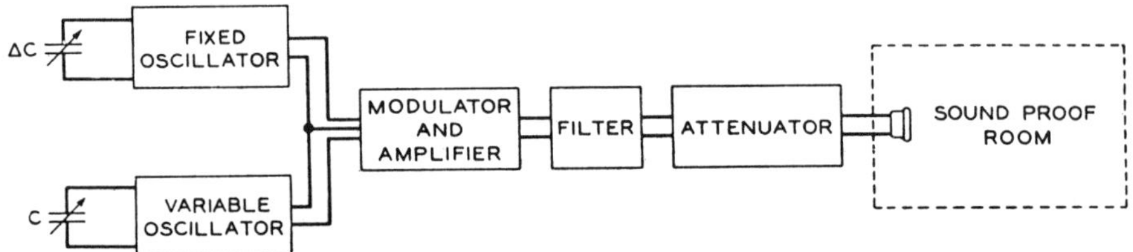

Fig. 3. *General arrangement of apparatus.*

with caps suitable for ear measurements and suspended convenient to the ear of the observer. For bone-conduction measurements a specially constructed loud speaking receiver was used. This receiver is designed to apply vibrations directly to the bones of the head.

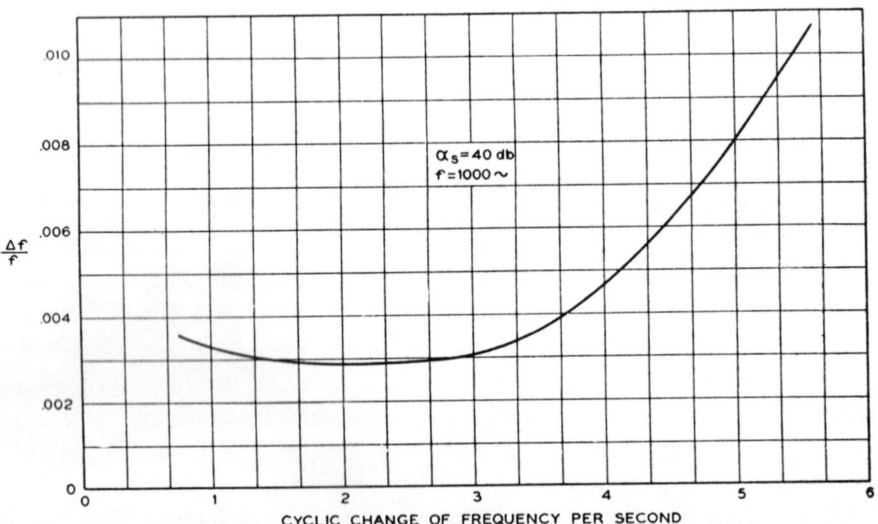

Fig. 4. *Variation of $\Delta f/f$ as a function of the rate of change of Δf.*

6. Technique

In making the measurements the tone was first introduced into the receiver at an unvarying frequency and at a level be easily heard by the observer. The threshold of audibility was determined for the observer and the sensation level set at the desired point. Then the minimum perceptible frequency change was obtained at the various sensation levels by finding the setting of the sliding head of the rotary condenser at which the observer could just detect a variation. These measurements were made as quickly as possible in order to minimize the effect of fatigue, and, as an indication of its presence, a check threshold setting was taken at the end of each run. The observed shift in the threshold was negligible with the exception of some measurements at high frequencies at the highest levels. During all listening tests the observer kept his ear tightly pressed against the receiver cap.

To determine the optimum rate of frequency variation, observations were taken at various frequencies at a sensation level of 40 db using various speeds of the condenser driving motor. The results of these observations are shown in Fig. 4. The curve shows a broad minimum from 2 to 3 variations per second. A value of two per second was chosen and used for subsequent observations.

7. Results

The results are shown in the table below. These are the average $\Delta f/f$ values for ten ears of five men between the ages of 20 and 30 years.

α_s	5	10	15	20	30	40	50	60	70	80	90
Frequency											
31	.1290	.0873	.0702	.0563	.0438	.0406					
62	.0975	.0678	.0546	.0491	.0461	.0426	.0351	.0346			
125	.0608	.0421	.0331	.0300	.0266	.0247	.0270	.0269			
250	.0355	.0212	.0158	.0130	.0109	.0103	.0099	.0098	.0100	.0107	
500	.0163	.0110	.0081	.0067	.0055	.0052	0042	.0035	.0042		
1000	.0094	.0061	.0044	.0039	.0036	.0036	.0036	.0034	.0031	.0030	.0026
2000	.0079	.0036	.0029	.0021	.0019	.0019	.0019	.0018	.0017	.0018	
4000	.0060	.0044	.0038	.0031	.0027	.0023	.0023	.0020			
8000	.0063	.0051	.0045	.0038	.0036	.0029	.0025				
11700	.0069	.0058	.0042	.0038	.0036	.0035	.0030				

These averaged results are plotted in Figs. 5 and 6. In Fig. 5 $\Delta f/f$ is plotted against f with sensation level as parameter. In Fig. 6, f is the parameter with $\Delta f/f$ plotted vs. α_s.

[*Editor's Note:* Material has been omitted at this point.]

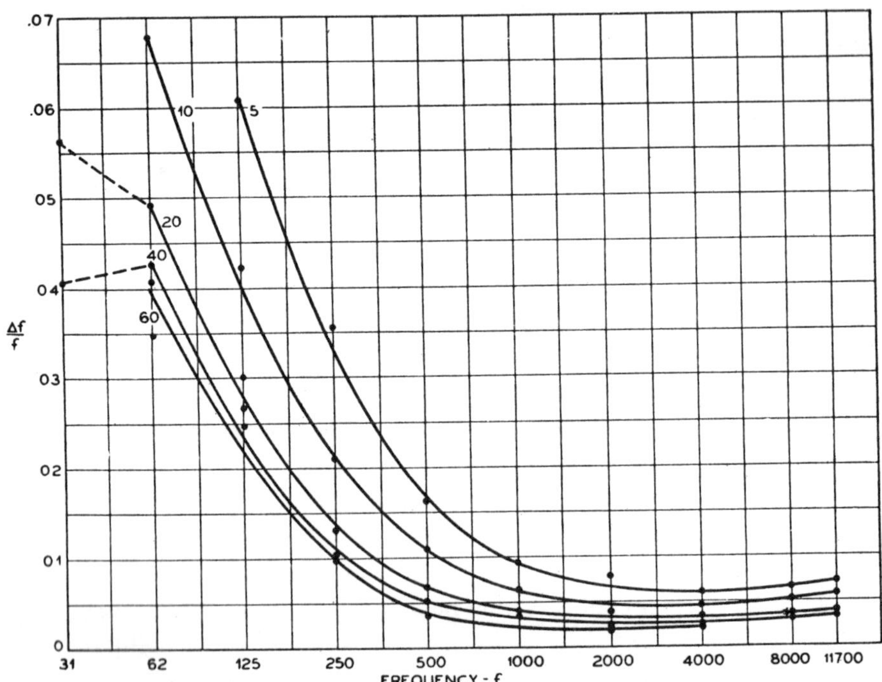

Fig. 5. *Variation of $\Delta f/f$ with frequency—sensation level as parameter.*

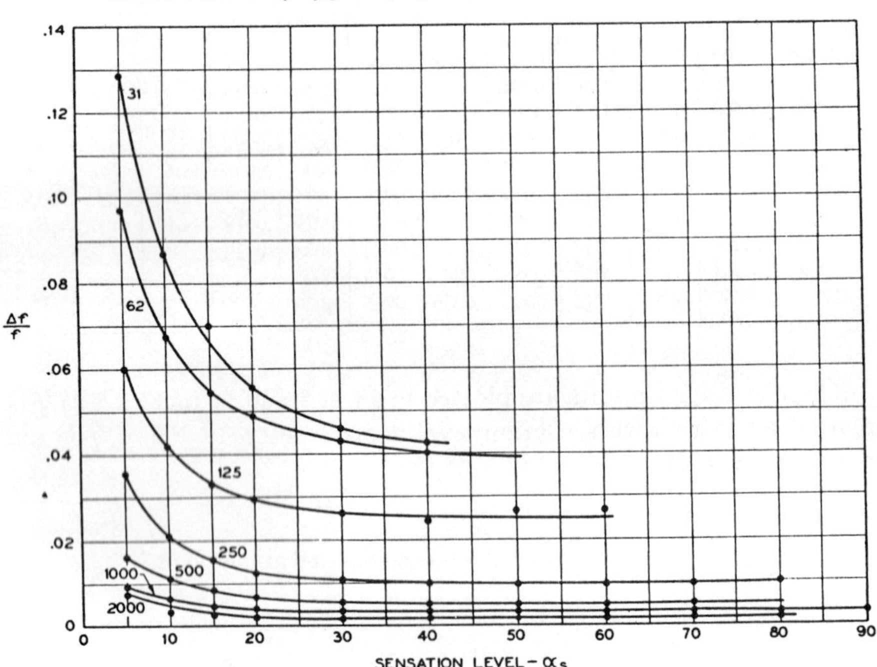

Fig. 6. *Variation of $\Delta f/f$ with sensation level—frequency as parameter.*

BIBLIOGRAPHY

(1) Vance—Variation in Pitch Discrimination within the Vocal Range—Psychological Monograph No. 69–115.

(2) H. Fletcher—B.S.T.J., Vol. II, p. 145, October, 1923.

(3) Knudsen—Phys. Rev. 21, February, 1923, 84.

(4) Loc. cit.

(5) The development given here is due to F. B. Llewellyn. An investigation leading to the same results but conducted along somewhat different lines has been published by J. R. Carson.

(6) H. Fletcher—A Space Time Pattern Theory of Hearing—J.A.S.A., Vol. I, No. 3; April, 1930.

(7) C. E. Dean—Audition by Bone Conduction—J.A.S.A., Vol. II, No. 2, October, 1930, p. 281.

8

Reprinted from *Acoust. Soc. Am. J.* **19**:609–619 (1947)

Sensitivity to Changes in the Intensity of White Noise and Its Relation to Masking and Loudness[1]

George A. Miller

Psycho-Acoustic Laboratory, Harvard University, Cambridge, Massachusetts

(Received March 17, 1947)

Sensitivity to changes in the intensity of a random noise was determined over a wide range of intensities. The just detectable increment in the intensity of the noise is of the same order of magnitude as the just detectable increment in the intensity of pure tones. For intensities more than 30 db above the threshold of hearing for noise the size in decibels of the increment which can be heard 50 percent of the time is approximately constant (0.41 db). When the results of the experiment are regarded as measures of the masking of a noise by the noise itself, it can be shown that functions which describe intensity discrimination also describe the masking by white noise of pure tones and of speech. It is argued, therefore, that the determination of differential sensitivity to intensity is a special case of the more general masking experiment. The loudness of the noise was also determined, and just noticeable differences are shown to be unequal in subjective magnitude. A just noticeable difference at a low intensity produces a much smaller change in the apparent loudness than does a just noticeable difference at a high intensity.

Differential sensitivity to intensity is one of the oldest and most important problems in the psychophysics of audition. But previous experiments have concerned themselves mainly with sensitivity to changes in the intensity of sinusoidal tones, and if we want to know the differential sensitivity for a complex sound, it is necessary either to extrapolate from existing information, or actually to conduct the experiment for the sound in question. This gap in our knowledge is due to expediency, not oversight. The realm of complex sounds includes an infinitude of acoustic compounds, and experimental parameters extend in many directions. Just which of these sounds we select for investigation is an arbitrary matter. Of the various possibilities, however, one of the most appropriate is random noise, a sound of persistent importance and one which marks a sort of ultimate on a scale of complexity.

Although the instantaneous amplitude varies randomly, white noise is perceived as a steady "hishing" sound, and it is quite possible to determine a listener's sensitivity to changes in its intensity.[2] The present paper reports the results of such determinations for a range of noise intensities.

APPARATUS AND PROCEDURE

A white-noise voltage, produced by random ionization in a gas tube, was varied in intensity by shunting the line with known resistances provided by a General Radio Decade Resistance Box. A schematic diagram of the equipment is shown in Fig. 1. The attenuators were used to keep constant the values of source and load impedance, R_0 and R_L, surrounding the shunt resistances, R_1 and R_2, since these values must enter into the computation of the increment which is produced by the insertion of the variable resistance, R_2. The whole system can be represented by the equivalent circuit, also shown in Fig. 1. For this circuit, the size of an increment in voltage ΔE_L is given by

$$\frac{\Delta E_L}{E_L}=\frac{R_0R_2R_L}{R_1[R_0(R_1+R_2+R_3)+R_L(R_1+R_2)]}.$$

If the system does not introduce amplitude distortion after the increments are produced, the increment in sound pressure, expressed in decibels, can be taken as $20\log_{10}(1+\Delta E_L/E_L)$.

Throughout the following discussion the intensity of the noise will be stated in terms of its sensation level—the number of decibels above the listener's absolute threshold for the noise. If the sound-pressure level of the noise is taken to be the level generated by a moving-coil

[1] This research was conducted under contract with the U. S. Navy, Office of Naval Research (Contract N5ori-76, Report PNR-28).

[2] J. E. Karlin, *Auditory tests for the ability to discriminate the pitch and the loudness of noises*, OSRD Report No. 5294 (Psycho-Acoustic Laboratory, Harvard University, August 1, 1945) (available through the Office of Technical Services, U. S. Department of Commerce, Washington, D. C.).

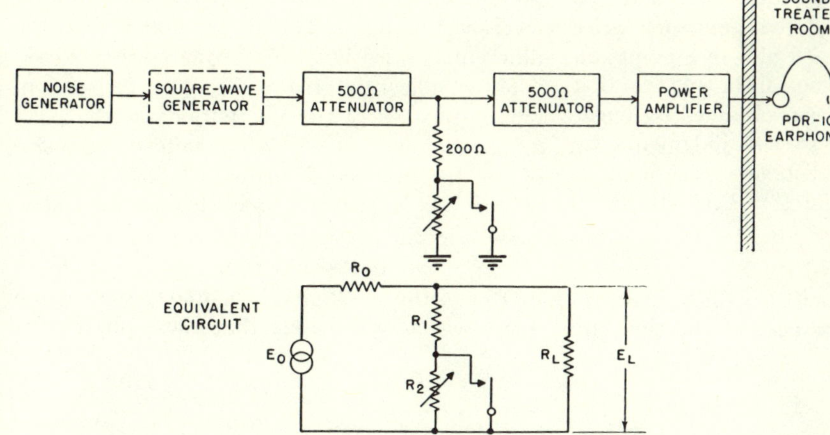

FIG. 1. Schematic diagram of equipment with the equivalent circuit used in the computation of the size of the increment in intensity.

earphone (Permoflux PDR-10) when the voltage across the earphone (measured by a thermocouple) is the same as the voltage required for a sinusoidal wave (1000 cycles) to generate the given sound pressure in a volume of 6 cc, then the absolute threshold for the noise corresponds to a sound pressure of approximately 10 db re 0.0002 dyne/cm². Thus the sensation level can be converted into sound-pressure level by the simple procedure of adding 10 db to the value given for the sensation level. The spectrum of the noise was relatively uniform (±5 db) between 150 and 7000 c.p.s. The measurement and spectrum of the noise transduced by the earphone PDR-10 has been discussed in detail by Hawkins.[3]

Once the sound-pressure level and the relative size of the increment in decibels are known, the absolute value of the increment can be computed. Those interested in converting the decibels into dynes/cm² will find the nomogram of Fig. 2 a considerable convenience. A straight line which passes through a value of ΔI in decibels on the left-hand scale, and through a value of the sound pressure on the middle scale, will intersect the right-hand scale at the appropriate value of ΔP in dyne/cm². When the stimulus is a plane progressive sound wave, its acoustic intensity in watts/cm² is proportional to the square of the pressure: $I = kp^2$.

The peak amplitudes in the wave of a white noise are not constant. It is reasonable to expect, therefore, that the size of the just noticeable difference might vary as a function of the distribution of peak amplitudes in the wave. In order to evaluate this aspect of the stimulus, a second experiment was conducted. The noise voltage was passed through a square-wave generator (Hewlett Packard, Model 210-A) before the increments were introduced. The spectrum and subjective quality of the noise are not altered by the square-wave generator, but the peak amplitudes are "squared off" at a uniform level. The resulting wave form might be described as a square-wave modulated randomly in frequency.

The experimental procedure for determining differential sensitivity was the same as that employed by Stevens, Morgan, and Volkmann.[4] The only difference was the omission of a signal light which they sometimes used to indicate the impending presentation of an increment. The observer, seated alone in a sound-treated room, listened to the noise monaurally through a high quality, dynamic earphone (PDR-10). The listener heard a continuous noise, to which an increment was added periodically. A series of 25 identical increments (1.5 sec. duration at

[3] J. E. Hawkins, "The masking of pure tones and of speech by white noise," in a report entitled *The masking of signals by noise*, OSRD Report No. 5387 (Psycho-Acoustic Laboratory, Harvard University, October 1, 1945) (available through the Office of Technical Services, U. S. Department of Commerce, Washington, D. C.).

[4] S. S. Stevens, C. T. Morgan, and J. Volkmann, "Theory of the neural quantum in the discrimination of loudness and pitch," Am. J. Psychol. **54**, 315–335 (1941).

intervals of 4.5 sec.) was presented, and the percentage heard was tabulated. Four such series were used to determine each of 5 to 8 points on a psychometric function, and from this function the differential threshold was obtained by linear interpolation. Thus 500 to 800 judgments by each of two experienced listeners were used to determine each differential threshold at the 16 different intensities.

RESULTS

The increments in decibels which the two listeners could hear 50 percent of the time are presented in Table I as a function of the sensation level of the noise. It will be noted that the differential sensitivity for "square-wave noise" is not significantly greater than that for random noise. Apparently the fluctuations in the peak amplitude of the wave do not influence the size of the just noticeable increment. The response of the ear is probably too sluggish to follow these brief fluctuations. And since the difference between the two wave forms is essentially a matter of the phase relations among the components, we may conclude that these phase rela-

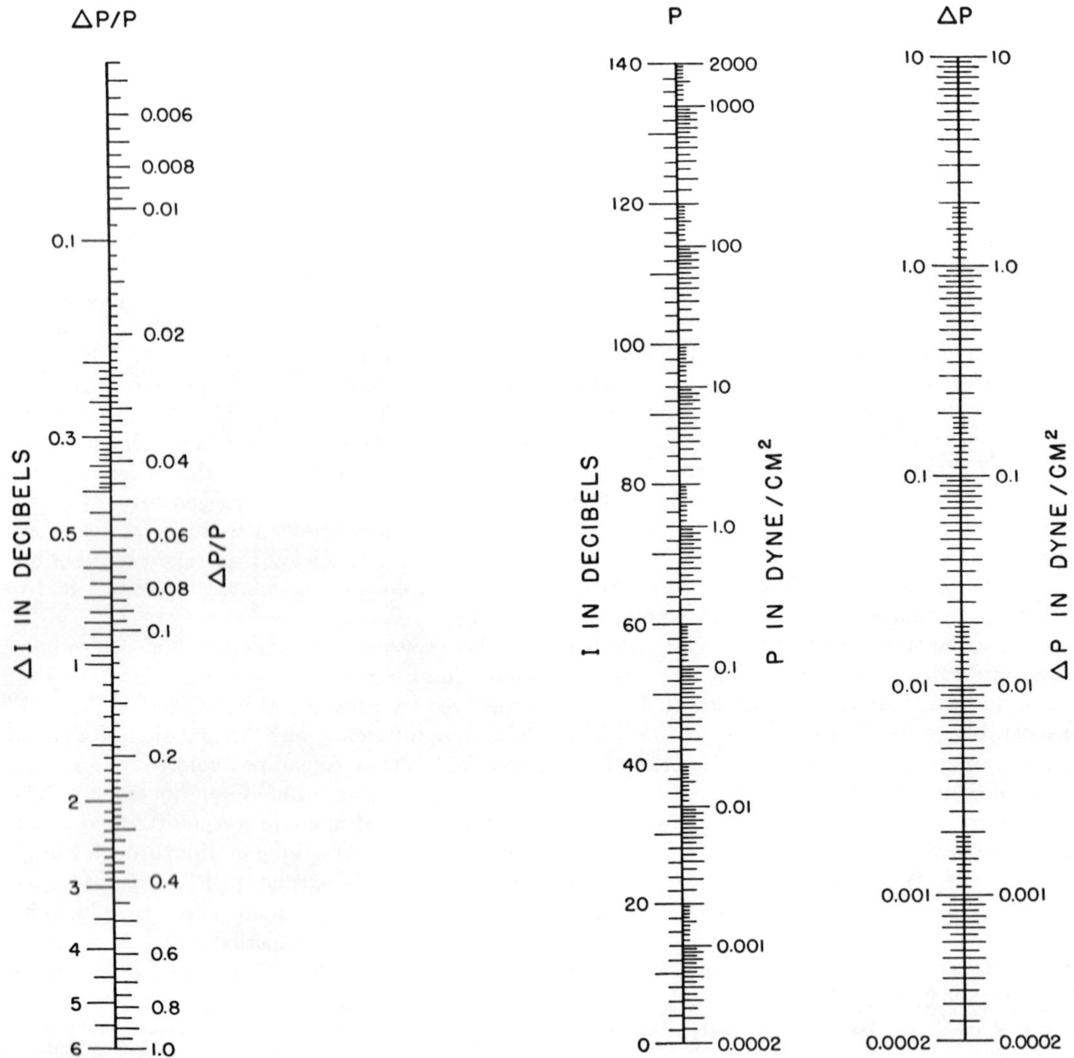

FIG. 2. Nomogram to convert values of $\Delta P/P$ to ΔP when P is known.

TABLE I. Differential sensitivity for intensity of noise. Increments in decibels which two listeners could hear 50 percent of the time, as a function of sensation level.

Sensation level	Random noise GM	Random noise SM	Square-wave noise GM	Square-wave noise SM
3 db	3.20 db	3.20 db		
5	3.00	2.10		
10	1.17	1.17		
12			0.97 db	0.89 db
15	0.85	0.66		
20	0.49	0.55		
25	0.46	0.54		
32			0.40	0.39
35	0.40	0.50		
45	0.42	0.44		
52			0.40	0.46
55	0.39	0.50		
70	0.39	0.47		
82			0.32	0.47
85	0.33	0.48		
100	0.28	0.40		

tions have no important effect on differential sensitivity.

The data indicate that, for intensities 30 db or more above the absolute threshold, the relative differential threshold is approximately constant. At the highest intensities the value is about 0.41 db, which corresponds to a Weber-fraction of 0.099 for sound energy, or 0.048 for sound pressure. The range over which the increment is proportional to the level of stimulation is indicated by the horizontal portion of the solid curve in Fig. 3. The values over this range of intensities agree quite well with the values obtained by Karlin[2] with a group of 50 listeners.

For purposes of comparison, Fig. 3 includes

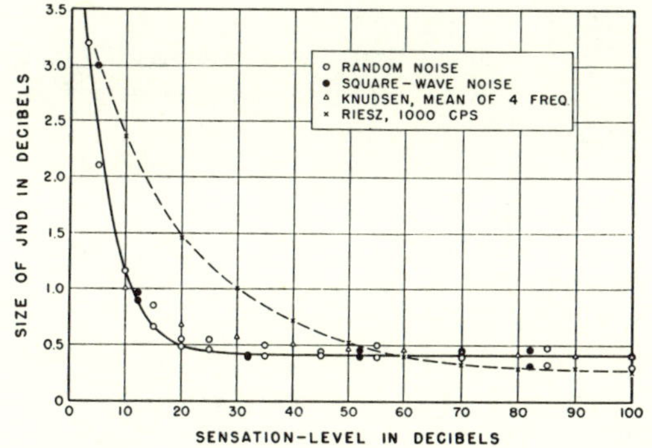

FIG. 3. Increments in intensity heard 50 percent of the time are plotted as a function of the intensity of the noise in decibels above the threshold of hearing. Data for tones are presented for purposes of comparison. The solid line represents Eq. (2).

data obtained by Riesz[5] and by Knudsen[6] for tones. Knudsen's results do not differ markedly from those obtained for noise, but Riesz's data are quite different, especially at low intensities. Possibly Knudsen's data represent sensitivity to the "noise" introduced by the abrupt onset of his tones, or possibly Riesz's data at low intensities are suspect because of his use of beats to produce increments in intensity. Data obtained by Stevens and Volkmann[7] for a single listener at four intensities of a 1000-cycle tone seem to agree more closely with the present results than with Reisz's, but their data are not complete enough to determine a function. Churcher, King, and Davies[8] have reported data with a tone of 800 c.p.s. which compare favorably with the function of Riesz. Taken together, all these studies indicate that the difference limen for intensity is of the same order of magnitude for noise as it is for tones, at least at the higher levels of intensity.[9] At the lower intensities the discrimination for a noise stimulus may be somewhat more acute than for tones.

IMPLICATIONS FOR A QUANTAL THEORY OF DISCRIMINATION

The notion that the difference limen depends upon the activation of discrete neural units is not new. It is suggested by the discreteness of the sensory cells themselves. Only recently, however, has evidence been obtained to support the assumption that the basic neural processes mediating a discrimination are of an all-or-none character.

The principal evidence derives from the shape of the psychometric function. Stevens, Morgan, and Volkmann[10] present the argument in the following way:

[5] R. R. Riesz, "Differential intensity sensitivity of the ear for pure tones," Phys. Rev. **31**, 867–875 (1928).

[6] V. O. Knudsen, "The sensibility of the ear to small differences in intensity and frequency," Phys. Rev. **21**, 84–103 (1923).

[7] S. S. Stevens and J. Volkmann, "The quantum of sensory discrimination," Science **92**, 583–585 (1940).

[8] B. G. Churcher, A. J. King, and H. Davies, "The minimum perceptible change of intensity of a pure tone," Phil. Mag. **18**, 927–939 (1934).

[9] Of the modern investigations, only Dimmick's disagrees strikingly with the values reported here for the higher intensities. F. L. Dimmick and R. M. Olson, "The intensive difference limen in audition," J. Acous. Soc. Am. **12**, 517–525 (1941).

[10] See reference 4, p. 317.

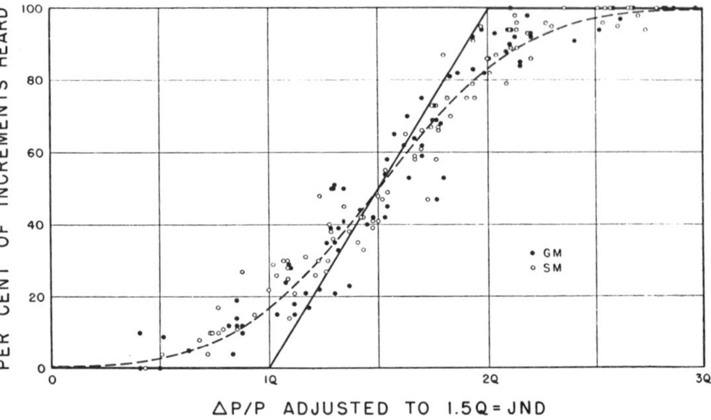

FIG. 4. The 32 psychometric functions combined in a single graph. Values of $\Delta P/P$ heard 50 percent of the time are designated as $1.5Q$, and the datum points on each function are plotted relative to this value. Each point represents 100 judgments.

> We assume that the neural structures initially involved in the perception of a sensory continuum are divided into functionally distinct units. . . . The stimulus which excites a certain number of quanta will ordinarily do so with a little to spare—it will excite these quanta and leave a small surplus insufficient to excite some additional quantum. This surplus stimulation will contribute, along with the increment, ΔI, to bring into activity the added quantum needed for discrimination . . . How much of this left-over stimulation or surplus excitation are we to expect? If [the over-all fluctuation in sensitivity] is large compared to the size of an individual quantum, it is evident that over the course of time all values of the surplus stimulation occur equally often. . . . From these considerations it follows that, if the increment is added instantaneously to the stimulus, it will be perceived a certain fraction of the time, and this fraction is directly proportional to the size of the increment itself.

When the increments are added to a continuous stimulus, however, the listener finds it difficult to distinguish one-quantum changes in the stimulus from the changes which are constantly occurring because of fluctuations in his sensitivity. In order to make reliable judgments, the listener is forced to ignore all one-quantum changes. Consequently, a stimulus increment under these conditions must activate at least two additional neural units in order that a difference will be perceived and reported. Thus, in effect, a constant error of one quantum is added to the psychometric function.

The psychometric function predicted by this line of reasoning can be described in the following way. When the stimulus increments to a steady sound are less than some value ΔI_Q, they are never reported, and over the range of increments from 0 to ΔI_Q the psychometric function remains at 0 percent. Between ΔI_Q and $2\Delta I_Q$ the proportion of the increments reported varies directly with the size of the increment, and reaches 100 percent at $2\Delta I_Q$. Such a function is illustrated by the solid line of Fig. 4.

It will be noted that the difference which is reported 50 percent of the time is equivalent to 1.5 times the quantal increment. If we take this value as defining a unit increment in the stimulus, all the psychometric functions obtained for the two listeners can be combined into a single function. In other words, we can adjust the individual intensity scales against which the functions are plotted in order to make all the functions coincide at the 50 percent point. In Fig. 4 the size of the relative increment in sound pressure, $\Delta P/P$, has been adjusted so that the increment which was heard 50 percent of the time is plotted as 1.5 times the quantal increment.

Figure 4 shows that the characteristic quantal function was not obtained in this experiment. The data are better described by the phi-function of gamma (the normal probability integral) indicated by the dashed line.

The classical argument for the application of the cumulative probability function to the difference limen assumes a number of small, indeterminate variables which are independent, and which combine according to chance. When these variables are controlled or eliminated, the step-wise, "quantal" relation is revealed.[11] If this reasoning

[11] G. A. Miller and W. R. Garner, "Effect of random presentation on the psychometric function: Implications for a quantal theory of discrimination," Am. J. Psychol. **57**, 451–467 (1944).

is correct, then the deviations of the points in Fig. 4 from the quantal hypothesis should be attributable to the introduction of random variability into the listening situation.

Is there any obvious source of randomness in the experiment? Certainly there is, for white noise is a paradigm of randomness. The statistical nature of the noise means that the calculated value of the increment is merely the most probable value, and that a certain portion of the time the increment will depart from this probable value by an amount sufficient to affect the discrimination. And in view of the fluctuating level of the stimulus, it would be surprising indeed if the rigorous experimental requirements of the quantal hypothesis were fulfilled. This situation demonstrates the practical difficulty in obtaining the rectilinear functions predicted by the quantal hypothesis. Any source of variability tends to obscure the step-wise results and to produce the S-shaped normal probability integral.

It should be noted, however, that the shape of the psychometric function is only one of the implications of the quantal argument. According to the hypothesis, the slope of the psychometric function is determined by the size of the difference limen for all values of stimulus-intensity. The present data accord with this second prediction. The standard deviations of the probability integrals which describe the data are approximately one-third the means (or $0.5\Delta I_Q$) for all the thresholds measured for both subjects. This invariance in the slope of the function is necessary but not sufficient evidence for a neural quantum, and it makes possible the representation of the results in the form shown in Fig. 4.

SYMBOLIC REPRESENTATION OF THE DATA

In order to represent the experimental results in symbolic form, the following symbols will be used:

- b numerical constant $=1.333$,
- c numerical constant $=0.066=\Delta I_Q/I$ when $I\gg I_0$,
- DL difference limen (just noticeable difference, expressed in decibels,
- f frequency in cycles per second,
- I sound intensity (energy flow),
- $I_\sim$ sound intensity per cycle,
- I_0 sound intensity which is just audible in quiet,
- I_m sound intensity which is just masked in noise,
- ΔI_Q quantal increment in sound intensity $=0.667\Delta I_{50}$,
- ΔI_{50} increment in sound intensity heard 50 percent of the time,
- L loudness in sones,
- M masking in decibels,
- N_Q number of quantal increments above threshold,
- R signal-to-noise ratio per cycle at any frequency,
- Z effective level of noise at any frequency.

An adequate description of the data in Table I can be developed from the empirical equation

$$\Delta I_Q=cI+bI_0, \quad I\geq I_0, \tag{1}$$

where the quantal increment in the stimulus-energy is assumed to have a fixed and a variable component. Since ΔI_{50}—the increment which can be heard 50 percent of the time—equals $1.5\Delta I_Q$, we can write

$$\begin{aligned} DL&=10\log_{10}(I+\Delta I_{50}/I)\\ &=10\log_{10}[1+1.5c+1.5b(I_0/I)]. \end{aligned} \tag{2}$$

From (2) it is possible to compute the just noticeable increment in decibels as a function of sensation level, although we know only the ratio between I and I_0 and not their absolute values. When the computations are carried through, the values indicated by the solid curve in Fig. 3 are obtained. The fit of this curve to the data is good enough to justify the use of Eq. (2) to obtain smoothed values of the function.

It is interesting to note that at high intensities Eq. (1) is equivalent to the well-known "Weber's Law," which states that the size of a just noticeable difference is proportional to the intensity to which it is added. Differential sensitivity characteristically departs from Weber's Law at low intensities, and Fechner long ago suggested a modification of the law to the form expressed in Eq. (1).[12] The essential feature of this equation is the rectilinear relation between ΔI and I; the obvious difficulty is the explanation of the intercept value bI_0 which appears in Eq. (1) as an additive factor. Fechner supposed that this added term is attributable to intrinsic, interfering stimulation which cannot be eliminated in the measurement of the difference limen. Body noises, the spontaneous activity of the auditory nervous system, or the thermal noise

---

[12] H. Helmholtz, *Treatise on physiological optics*, translated by P. C. Southall from 3rd German edition, "The Sensations of Vision," Vol. II (1911) (Optical Society of America, 1924), pp. 172–181.

of the air molecules have been suggested as possible sources of this background stimulation, but proof of these possibilities is still lacking. For the present, therefore, we must regard Eq. (1) as a purely empirical equation.

RELATION TO MASKING

There is an operational similarity between experiments designed to study differential sensitivity for intensity and experiments devised to measure auditory masking. This similarity is usually obscured by a practical inclination to ignore the special case where one sound is masked by another sound identical with the first.

Suppose we want to know how much a white noise masks a white noise. What experimental procedures would we adopt? Obviously, the judgment we would ask the listener to make is the same judgment made in the present experiment. In the one case, however, we present the data to show the smallest detectable increment, while in the other we use the same data to determine the shift in threshold of the masked sound. When the masked and masking sounds are identical, the difference between masking and sensitivity to changes in intensity lies only in the way the story is told.

A striking example of this similarity is to be found in the work of Reisz. In order to produce gradual changes in intensity, Reisz used tones differing in frequency by 3 cycles and instructed his listeners to report the presence or absence of beats. Although his results are generally accepted as definitive measures of sensitivity to changes in the intensity of pure tones, it is equally correct to interpret them as measures of the masking of one tone by another tone differing in frequency by 3 cycles.

Let us, therefore, reconsider the data of Table I. In this table we have presented in decibels both the sensation level of the noise and the size of the increment which can be heard 50 percent of the time. How can these data be transformed to correspond with the definition of masking?

First, consider that we are mixing two noises in order to produce the total magnitude $I+\Delta I$. Since I is analogous to the intensity of the masking sound, $I+\Delta I$ must equal the intensity of the masking sound plus the intensity of the masked sound, $I+I_m$. Thus $I_m=\Delta I$, and from

TABLE II. Masking of white noise by white noise. Quantal increments in decibels and the values of masking obtained for two listeners as a function of the sensation level of the masking noise. Computed values of masking according to Eq. (4).

Sensation level	Quantal increment in decibels		Masking obtained		Masking computed
	GM	*SM*	*GM*	*SM*	
3 db	2.37 db	2.37 db	1.61 db	1.61 db	1.66 db
5	2.21	1.51	3.26	1.18	1.88
10	0.81	0.81	3.14	3.14	3.00
12	0.67	0.61	4.22	3.80	3.76
15	0.58	0.45	6.58	5.39	5.33
20	0.33	0.37	9.00	9.54	8.99
25	0.31	0.37	13.73	14.45	13.44
32	0.27	0.27	20.06	19.97	20.25
35	0.27	0.34	23.06	24.10	23.22
45	0.29	0.30	33.33	33.53	33.20
52	0.27	0.31	40.06	40.73	40.20
55	0.27	0.34	42.97	44.10	43.20
70	0.27	0.32	57.97	58.81	58.20
82	0.22	0.32	68.32	70.81	70.20
85	0.22	0.33	72.22	73.91	73.20
100	0.19	0.27	86.43	88.06	88.20

the definition of masking M we can write

$$M=10\log_{10}(I_m/I_0)=10\log_{10}(\Delta I/I_0). \quad (3)$$

Because there appears to be some basic significance to the quantal unit, whereas the criterion of hearing 50 percent of the increments is arbitrary, we will use the quantal increment ΔI_Q in Eq. (3). ΔI_Q is defined as 0.667 times the value of the increment which is heard 50 percent of the time.

$$M=10\log_{10}(\Delta I_Q/I_0). \quad (3a)$$

Equation (3a) tells us, then, that the logarithm

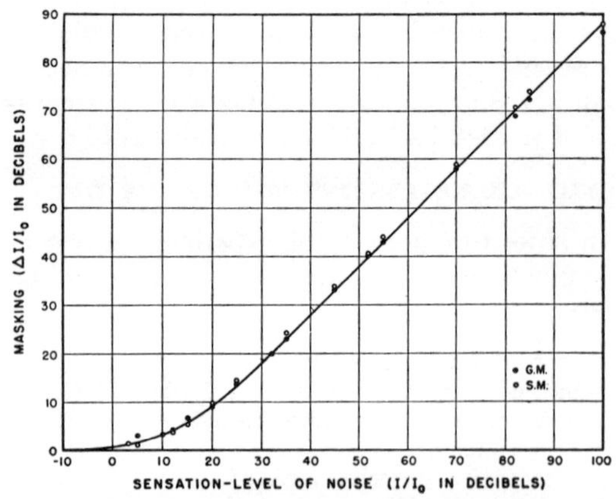

FIG. 5. Discriminable increments in intensity of white noise plotted in a manner analogous to masking experiments. Solid line represents function obtained by Hawkins for the masking of tones and speech by white noise.

of the ratio of the quantal increment to the absolute threshold is proportional to the masking of a sound by an identical sound.

It is now possible to determine the values of ΔI_Q and I_0 from the information given in Table I, and to substitute these values into Eq. (3a). The results of converting the differential thresholds into quantal increments and then into masked thresholds are given in Table II for the two listeners, and are shown in Fig. 5 where masking is plotted as a function of the sensation level of the masking noise. In addition, Table II contains values of masking which are computed when Eqs. (1) and (3a) are combined:

$$M = 10 \log_{10}[(cI/I_0) + b]. \quad (4)$$

For intensities 25 db or more above threshold, the masking noise is about 12 db more intense than the masked noise.

The obvious next step is to ask whether these results correspond to the functions obtained when noise is used to mask tones or human speech. Fortunately, we are able to answer this question. Hawkins[3] has measured the masking effects of noise on tones and speech with experimental conditions and equipment directly comparable with those used here.

Suppose, for purposes of comparison, we choose to mask a 1000-cycle tone. We find over a wide range of intensities that this particular white noise just masks a 1000-cycle tone which is 20 db less intense. Since the corresponding value is 12 db when this noise masks itself, we conclude that, for this specific noise spectrum, 8 db less energy is needed for audibility when the energy is concentrated at 1000 c.p.s. than when the energy is spread over the entire spectrum. In order to compare the forms of the two masking functions, therefore, we can subtract 8 db from the level of the noise which masks the 1000-cycle tone.

When we make this correction of 8 db in the noise level for Hawkins' data for a 1000-cycle tone and plot the masking of this tone as a function of the corrected noise intensity, we obtain the solid line shown in Fig. 5. The correspondence between this curve, taken from Hawkins' data, and the points obtained in the present experiment is remarkably close. The function computed from Eq. (4) falls too close to Hawkins' function to warrant its separate presentation in Fig. 5.

The choice of 1000 c.p.s. is not crucial to this correspondence. As Fletcher and Munson[13] have pointed out, a single function is adequate to describe the masking by noise of pure tones, if the intensity of the noise is corrected by a factor which is a function of the frequency of the masked tone. This factor is given at any frequency f by the ratio R of the intensity of the masked tone to the intensity per cycle of the noise at that frequency: $R = I_m/I_\sim$. R is experimentally determined for all frequencies at intensities well above threshold—on the rectilinear portion of the function shown in Fig. 5.

For noises with continuous spectra, the masking of a tone of frequency f can be attributed to the noise in the band of frequencies immediately adjacent to f.[14] Consequently, it is convenient to relate the masking of a tone of frequency f to the intensity per cycle of the noise at f, and to express this intensity in decibels *re* the threshold of hearing at any frequency. This procedure gives $10 \log_{10}(I_\sim/I_0)$, which can be regarded as the sensation level at f of a one-cycle band of noise. The effective level Z of the noise at that frequency is then defined as

$$Z = 10 \log_{10}(I_\sim/I_0) + 10 \log_{10} R. \quad (5)$$

When the masking of pure tones is plotted as a function of Z, the relation between M and Z is found to be independent of frequency. A single function expresses the relation between M and Z for all frequencies.

When we compare the function relating M to Z with the function obtained in the present experiment, we find that the sensation level of the noise is equivalent to $Z + 11.8$ db. Therefore,

$$I/I_0 = 15.14R(I_\sim/I_0).$$

Substituting this expression into Eq. (4) gives

$$M = 10 \log_{10}[R(I_\sim/I_0) + b]. \quad (6)$$

This equation, along with the functions relating R and I_0 to frequency, enables us to compute the masking of pure tones by any random noise

[13] H. Fletcher and W. A. Munson, "Relation between loudness and masking," J. Acous. Soc. Am. **9**, 1–10 (1937).

[14] H. Fletcher, "Auditory patterns," Rev. Mod. Phys. **12**, 47–65 (1940).

of known spectrum. When $10 \log_{10}(I\sim/I_0)$ is greater than about 15 db, b is negligible for all frequencies, and the masking can be computed more simply as $10 \log_{10}R + 10 \log_{10}(I\sim/I_0)$.

Hawkins' results show that the function of Eq. (4) can also be adapted to describe the masking of human speech by white noise.

Thus the correspondence seems complete. When the masking and the masked sounds are identical, masking and sensitivity to changes in intensity are equivalent. The results obtained with identical masking and masked noises are directly comparable to results obtained with different masked sounds. It is reasonable to conclude, therefore, that the determination of sensitivity to changes in intensity is a special case of the more general masking experiment.

It is worth noting that this interpretation of masking is also applicable to visual sensitivity to changes in the intensity of white light. Data obtained by Graham and Barlett[15] provide an excellent basis for comparison, because of the similarity of their procedure to that of the masking experiment, and because they used homogeneous, rod-free, foveal areas of the retina. When these data are substituted into Eq. (3) and plotted as measures of visual masking, the result can be described by the same general function that we have used to express the auditory masking by noise of tones, speech, and noise.

RELATION TO LOUDNESS

When Fechner adopted the just noticeable difference as the unit for sensory scales, he precipitated a controversy which is still alive today: Are equally-often-noticed differences subjectively equal? In the case of auditory loudness, the answer seems to be negative. Just noticeable differences (j.n.d.'s) at high intensities are subjectively much larger than j.n.d.'s at low intensities.

TABLE III. Loudness and the number of quanta. Sensation-level of equally loud 1000-cycle tone as a function of sensation-level of noise, with corresponding loudness in sones. Data for 12 listeners. The last column gives the corresponding number of quantal units above threshold.

Sensation-level of noise	Equally loud 1000 c.p.s. Sensation level	Stand. dev.	Loudness in sones Mean	±Stand. dev.	No. of quanta above threshold
15 db	14.2 db	4.6 db	0.036	0.015– 0.081	13
30	38.1	6.9	0.83	0.40 – 1.6	58
45	57.9	9.1	4.8	2.3 – 9.7	111
60	74.2	8.2	17.0	9 –26	163
75	86.3	7.2	37	24 –47	216
90	97.9	3.1	76	62 –88	268

In order to demonstrate that such is the case for noise as well as for pure tones, we need two kinds of information. We need to know the functions relating noise intensity to the number of distinguishable steps above threshold, and to the subjective loudness of the noise in sones. If these two functions correspond, Fechner was right and j.n.d.'s can be used as units on a subjective loudness-scale. If they do not agree, Fechner was wrong, and the picture is more complex than he imagined.

The number of differential quanta N_Q corresponding to a given sensation level of noise is readily obtained by "stepping off" the quantal increments against a scale of decibels. The pro-

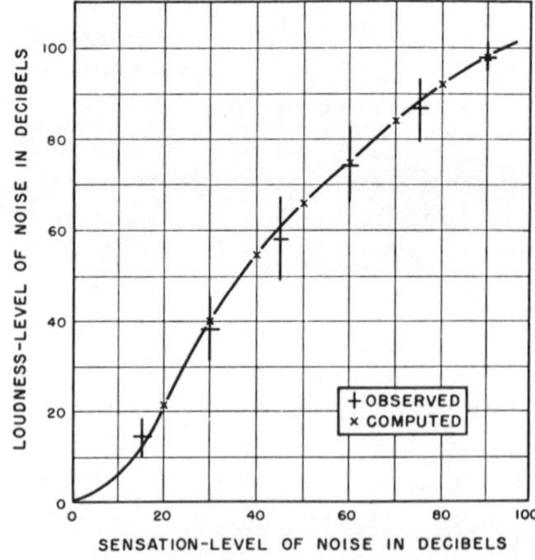

FIG. 6. Observed and computed values of the loudness level of white noise. Standard deviations of the values for 15 listeners are indicated by the lengths of the vertical bars.

[15] C. H. Graham and N. R. Bartlett, "The relation of stimulus and intensity in the human eye: III. The influence of area on foveal intensity discrimination," J. Exper. Psychol. 27, 149–159 (1940).
Crozier has used similar visual data to demonstrate that the reciprocal of the just detectable increment is related to the logarithm of the light intensity by a normal probability integral. This is deduced on the assumption that sensitivity is determined by the not-already-excited portion of the total population of potentially excitable neural effects. Crozier's equations give an excellent description of the auditory data presented here. W. J. Crozier, "On the law for minimal discrimination of intensities. IV. ΔI as a function of intensity," Proc. Nat. Acad. Sci. 26, 382–388 (1940).

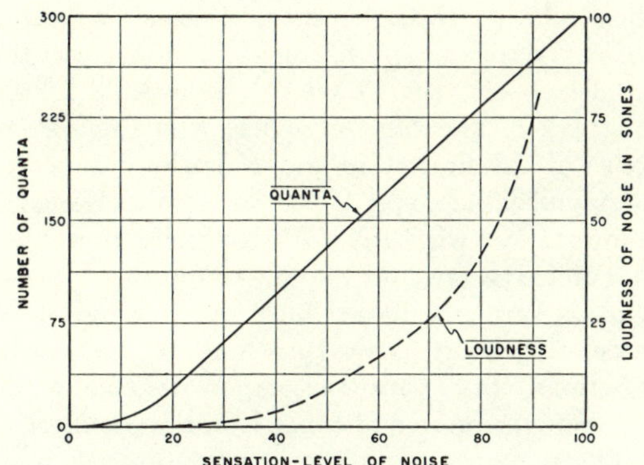

FIG. 7. Comparison of the number of discriminatory quanta with the loudness of white noise. Just noticeable increments in intensity are not subjectively equal.

cedure consists of finding the number of quantal increments per unit of intensity and then integrating:

$$N_Q = \int 1/\Delta I_Q \cdot dI. \tag{7}$$

If we substitute for the size of the quantal increment according to Eq. (1),

$$N_Q = \int \frac{1}{cI + bI_0} \cdot dI = \frac{1}{c} \ln \Delta I_Q + C. \tag{8}$$

When we convert to logarithms to the base 10, insert the values for the constants, and solve in terms of masking M, we find that

$$N_Q = 3.49M + K. \tag{9}$$

We assume that the number of quantal increments is zero when $I = I_0$, and at this point

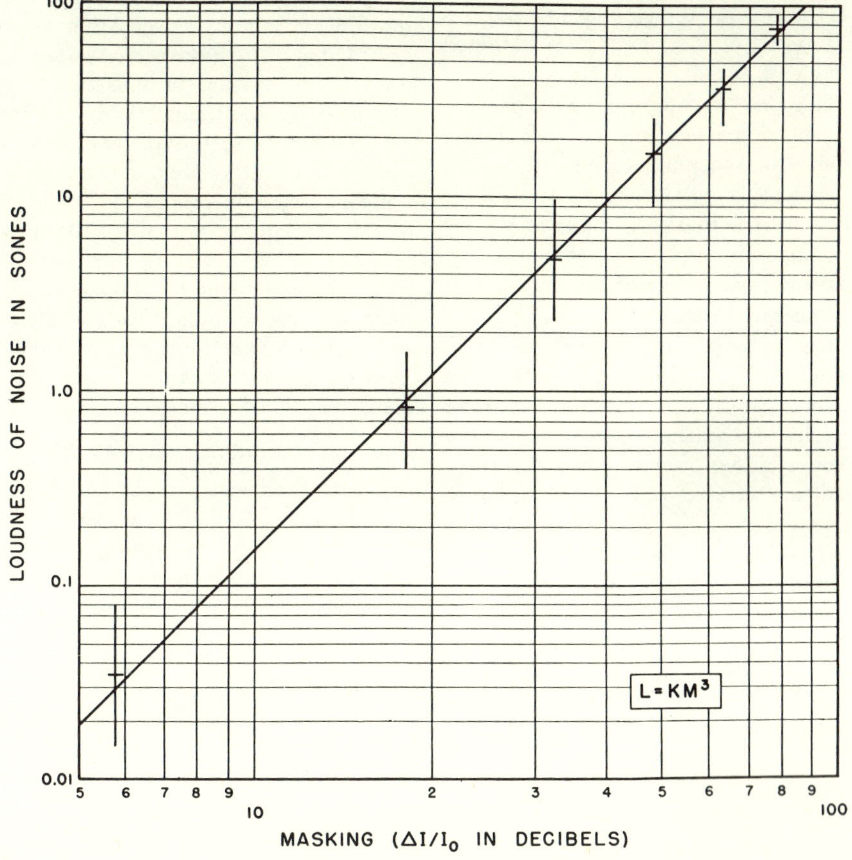

FIG. 8. Relation between loudness and masking for white noise.

Eq. (4) indicates that $M=1.46$ db. Therefore, $K=-5.1$. Values of N_Q obtained by Eq. (9) are given in Table III, and plotted in Fig. 7.

The loudness in sones was determined by requiring listeners to equate the loudness of the noise with the loudness of a 1000-cycle tone. The two sounds were presented alternately to the same ear, and the listener adjusted the intensity of the tone. Five equations were made by each of twelve listeners for the six noise-intensities studied. The result of this experiment —the level of the 1000-cycle tone which sounds equal in loudness to the noise—defines the loudness level of the noise. With these data, which are tabulated in Table III and plotted in Fig. 6, the loudness in sones is determined from the loudness-scale which has been constructed for the 1000-cycle tone. The values in sones from Stevens' loudness-scale[16] are included in Table III. Table III also gives the standard deviations of the distributions of loudness levels obtained for the 12 listeners.

Loudness can also be computed. Fletcher and Munson developed a procedure for calculating loudness from the masking which the sound produces. When this procedure is applied to Hawkins' data for the masking of pure tones by noise, we get the computed values shown in Fig. 6. The agreement between computed and experimental results is quite satisfactory.

We are now equipped to present the two functions shown in Fig. 7. The solid curve shows the number of quantal units as a function of sensation level. The dashed curve shows the loudness in sones. The discrepancy between these two curves affirms the error of Fechner's assumption. Loudness and the number of just noticeable differences are not linearly related.

When, as in the present case, two variables are both related to a third, it is possible to determine their relation to each other. Stevens[17] has used Reisz's data for pure tones to arrive at the empirical equation $L=kN^{2.2}$, where L is the loudness of the tone in sones, k is the size in sones of the first step, and N is the number of distinguishable steps. When we parallel Stevens' computation with the data for noise presented in Table III, we find that $L=kN^3$ describes the relation rather well over most of the range. It is interesting that both turn out to be power functions, but why the exponent should be different for noise and tones is not apparent.

There is an alternative way to state the relation between differential sensitivity and loudness. In the preceeding section we developed the notion that sensitivity to changes in intensity is a special case of masking, and we computed the masking of the noise on itself. Let us now examine the relation between masking, so defined, and the subjective loudness. In Fig. 5 and Table II masking is related to sensation level; in Fig. 7 and Table III loudness is related to sensation level. The relation of masking to loudness is obtained by combining these two functions. In Fig. 8 it can be seen that the expression $L=KM^3$ fits the data rather well. The loudness of a white noise increases in proportion to the third power of the masking produced by the noise on itself, i.e., the third power of the logarithm of the quantal increment in intensity. In whatever form we cast the empirical equation, however, it is obvious that faint j.n.d.'s are smaller than loud j.n.d.'s and that j.n.d.'s are not equal units along a scale of loudness.

ACKNOWLEDGMENT

The author wishes to express his gratitude to Miss Shirley Mitchell, who assisted in obtaining the experimental data, and to Professor S. S. Stevens, who contributed valuable criticism and advice during the preparation of this manuscript.

[16] S. S. Stevens and H. Davis, *Hearing* (John Wiley and Sons, Inc., New York, 1938), p. 118.

[17] S. S. Stevens, "A scale for the measurement of a psychological magnitude: loudness," Psychol. Rev. **43**, 405–416 (1936).

9

Reprinted from *Acoust. Soc. Am. J.* **19**:808-815 (1947)

The Effect of Frequency Spectrum on Temporal Integration of Energy in the Ear*

W. R. GARNER
Psychological Laboratory, The Johns Hopkins University, Baltimore, Maryland

(Received July 16, 1947)

These experiments are designed to test the following hypothesis. The rate of the temporal integration of energy in the ear (at threshold) is dependent on the width of the frequency band of the energy to be integrated. Duration is exactly equivalent to intensity only when all the energy to be integrated is in a narrow band of frequencies. The hypothesis is tested by taking advantage of the spectral distribution of energy in short tones. As a tone becomes very short, the effective band width of the energy increases. The band width of energy is essentially defined by the reciprocal of the duration of the tone. Thus as the duration of a tone decreases, not only does the total energy in that tone decrease, but the band width of energy also increases. The intensity threshold, then, has to be increased (as duration is decreased) to compensate for both effects if the hypothesis is correct. The results are in line with the predictions of the hypothesis. The width of the band necessary for maximum integration is also related to frequency and the width of critical bands.

THE MEANING OF INTEGRATION

WE speak of temporal integration of energy in the various senses when the intensive response changes as a function of duration of stimulus. Usually we speak of the change in threshold intensities, although integration does not occur only at threshold. In audition, for example, the loudness of a tone is dependent on the duration of the tone, regardless of the absolute intensity of the tone. The threshold is one limiting case of this phenomenon, and this paper is concerned only with that particular type of temporal integration.

The integrative process is never measured directly. We measure a change in threshold, and we assume that the ear has been integrating energy over a period of time if the threshold is lower for a long tone than for a short tone. If the change in threshold is exactly proportional to the change in duration, then the following equation holds.

$$I\times t=C. \qquad (1)$$

In this equation, I is threshold intensity, and t is the duration of the stimulus. With this relation, we know that for every change in the duration, there is an equivalent change in the opposite direction in the stimulus intensity. The exponent of both I and t is 1. If the exponent of t is something other than unity, then the exact equivalence between intensity and time does not hold. The more general relation is

$$I\times t^a=C. \qquad (2)$$

If, in Eq. (2) the exponent a is 0.5, then the change in threshold intensity is less than the change in duration. Intensity is proportional to the square root of duration. Such a relation still indicates the presence of integration, but time and intensity are not exactly equivalent. If, on the other hand, the exponent a is greater than unity, then threshold intensity changes faster than duration. Such cases rarely occur.

In auditory research it has become so customary to state intensities in decibels, that the logarithmic form of the above equations has been more commonly used. In its logarithmic form, Eq. (2) becomes

$$\log I+a\log t=C. \qquad (3)$$

Log$I$ is stated in decibels, so that the constant a is multiplied by a factor of 10. The value of C is determined to a large extent by the particular units of time chosen. The constant a, then, represents the number of decibels change in threshold intensity with a change of one log unit of duration.

If a in Eq. (2) is unity, then in the logarithmic form of the equation the constant is represented as 10 db. We thus have a 10-db change in

* This research was carried out under Contract N5-ori-166, Task Order I, between the Special Devices Center, Office of Naval Research, and The Johns Hopkins University. This article is Report No. 166-I-18 under that contract.

threshold for a change of one log unit in duration, and the exact equivalence between duration and intensity holds. If, on the other hand, the constant a in Eq. (2) is 0.5, then we have a change of only 5 db per log unit of duration. It is the slope of the log-log relation which determines the rate of temporal integration of energy by the ear.

NATURE OF AUDITORY INTEGRATION

Sine-wave tones

The rate of temporal integration of acoustic energy is known for several kinds of stimuli. Some of these relations have been obtained with masked thresholds, and others have been obtained with absolute thresholds. The masked threshold of pure tones as a function of duration was measured by Garner and Miller[1] who found that, between the limits of 12.5 and 200 milliseconds, the threshold changes 10 db per log unit of time. No measurements were made then with durations shorter than 12.5 milliseconds. They assumed that the same relation (within the same limits) would also be true for the absolute threshold. The extent to which this assumption is true will be shown in this paper.

Wide-band noise

Quite recently, Miller[2] obtained measures for a noise stimulus containing a wide band of frequencies at absolute threshold. He found that, under these conditions, the change in threshold is only 8 db per log unit of time, indicating a change in threshold less than the change in duration. The results of the present paper confirm this relation.

A noise is quite different from a pure tone. It contains many frequencies as compared to the single frequency of the sine-wave tone. The band width of frequencies involved in the tone is one continuum which may be used to describe a tonal stimulus. Wide-band noise and sine-wave tones are extremes on this continuum, and the slopes of integration for these two stimuli are shown in Fig. 1. These two slopes, then, indicate the two extreme slopes which should occur if only the frequency band width of the stimulus energy is varied.

Pulse-wave forms

A pulse-wave form is a stimulus which has a wide band of energy, but in which the energy is regularly spaced along the harmonics of the fundamental frequency. Measurements of the masked threshold of such tones as a function of duration were made by Garner and Mitchell,[3] and they found the slope of the curve to be 8 db per log unit of time. This is the same slope found by Miller for a wide-band noise at absolute threshold.

These same authors used a pulse-wave form with a random period between successive pulses. This stimulus is essentially a wide-band noise. The slope of the function obtained under these conditions was approximately 7 db per log unit of time, indicating even less temporal integration of energy under conditions of masked threshold than under conditions of absolute threshold for a wide-band noise. This fact may indicate some real difference between the two types of threshold in relation to the temporal integrating function.

Repeated short tones

Recent measures have been made by Garner[4] with repeated short tones. Although these ex-

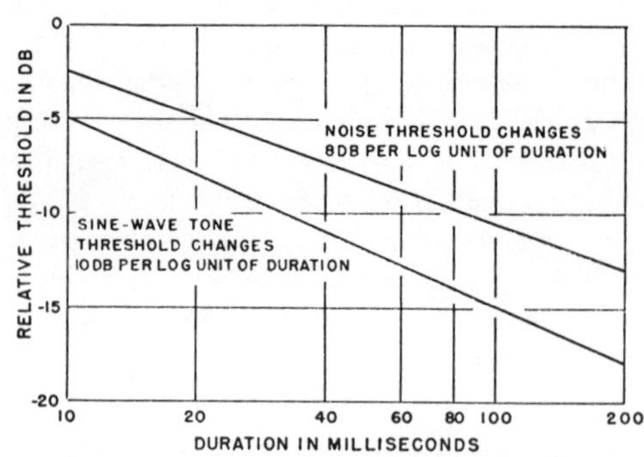

FIG. 1. The relation between threshold and duration for noise and sine-wave tones.

[1] W. R. Garner and G. A. Miller, "The masked threshold of pure tones as a function of duration," J. Exper. Psychol., in press. See also W. R. Garner and G. A. Miller, "The effect of duration on the masked threshold of tones," Part II in: "The masking of signals by noise," Psycho-Acoustic Laboratory, Harvard University (Oct. 1, 1945), OSRD Report No. 5387. (Available through the Publications Board, U. S. Department of Commerce, Washington, D. C.)

[2] Personal communication from Dr. G. A. Miller, Psycho-Acoustic Laboratory, Harvard University.

[3] W. R. Garner and S. Mitchell, Report from the Psycho-Acoustic Laboratory, OSRD Report No. 5124.

[4] W. R. Garner, "Auditory thresholds of short tones as a function of repetition rates," J. Acous. Soc. Am. **19**, 600 (1947).

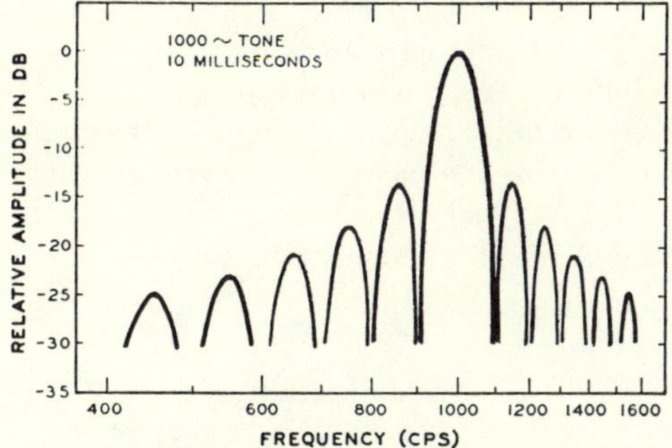

FIG. 2. Frequency spectrum of a short tone.

periments were concerned primarily with the effect of repetition rates on the threshold, duration was varied between the limits of 1 and 50 milliseconds. The results show that duration and intensity are equivalent (at masked threshold) regardless of the repetition rate. The difference in threshold between 1 and 10 milliseconds, however, was more nearly 11 db than 10 db.

Hypothesis

The nature of these many relations led to the formulation of the following hypothesis.[4] The rate of temporal integration of energy in the ear is dependent on the width of the frequency band of the energy to be integrated. Duration is exactly equivalent to intensity only when all the energy to be integrated is in a narrow band of frequencies. When the energy is in a wider band of frequencies, integration will occur, but the change in threshold will be less than the change in duration.

When that hypothesis was first stated, the further statement was made that all of the energy to be integrated must be temporally contiguous as well, but that aspect of the problem does not concern us here.

Purpose

The purpose of these experiments, then, is to test the above hypothesis. The experiments are concerned primarily with integration at the absolute threshold, but certain generalizations to the case of masked threshold are permissible. An additional purpose of these experiments is to determine to some extent the width of the frequency-band which will allow an exact equivalence between duration and intensity and to see whether this width is dependent on the general range of the band of frequencies. In other words, is the width of the band of frequencies related to the pitch function?

A great deal of equipment would be required to vary systematically the band width of frequencies about any point. Fortunately, however, such a procedure is not absolutely essential. Because of the characteristics of very short tones, this type of stimulus can be used to check the hypothesis with relatively little difficulty.

THE PHYSICS OF SHORT TONES

Any tone of a finite duration contains more than a single frequency. In the transition between zero amplitude and some finite amplitude of tone, certain frequency components are introduced other than the frequency of oscillation. These components are called transient frequencies, and the distribution of energy about any given frequency of oscillation can be determined with the aid of the Fourier integral.

Fourier analysis

A Fourier spectrum-analysis of a short tone is shown in Fig. 2. The frequency of oscillation is 1000 c.p.s. and all the energy in the short tone is distributed equally on either side of this center frequency. The energy of isolated short tones is distributed through a continuous frequency range. The individual components are not at discrete frequencies. The energy drops off from either side of the center frequency until no energy occurs at a frequency corresponding to $f_0 \pm 1/t$, where f_0 is the frequency of oscillation, and t is the duration of the tone. In the case shown, for example, no energy occurs at 900 and 1100 c.p.s. Continuous bands of energy occur above and below this main band of energy, and the width of these bands is defined by $1/t$.

The width of the main band (between frequencies of no energy) is defined by $2/t$, although $1/t$ is a good approximation of the band width defined in terms of the half-power points. With these relations, we see that the band width of energy contained in a short tone is inversely proportional to the duration of the tone. With durations as short as 1 millisecond, the band width of total energy is so great that the stimulus is essentially noise. Such stimuli sound like clicks rather than tones.

So we see that two things happen when the duration of a sine-wave tone is progressively shortened. In the first place, the total energy in the tone decreases at a rate of 10 db for a change of one log unit in duration. Thus, if the response of the ear is to total energy ($I\times t$), the threshold should change by 10 db for every change in the duration of one log unit. But at the same time the total energy is changing, the band width of the energy is changing as well. This double change enables us to test the hypothesis indirectly.

Test of hypothesis

We know that integration for a sine-wave tone is perfect down to durations as short as 12.5 milliseconds (at least for the masked threshold). The question remains: what happens with shorter durations? If the hypothesis as stated is correct, then as the duration becomes still shorter, eventually the slope of the curve in Fig. 1 should become greater than 10 db per log unit of duration. As the tone becomes shorter, the threshold intensity will have to be raised to compensate not only for the *loss* in total energy, but also for the *spread* of that energy over a greater band width. If the band width remained constant, the slope of the line should not change. But since the band width becomes greater and greater with shorter tones, the slope should change to compensate for what is essentially a loss in energy as far as the ear is concerned.

Since the frequency band width of a noise stimulus is not changed by decreasing the duration, nothing should happen to that curve as the duration is decreased. The slope should remain constant all the way down. Eventually, however, both curves should coincide, since a very short sine-wave stimulus is essentially noise.

In summary, then, the curve for noise should not change with very short durations. The sine-wave function, however, should have an increase in slope with shorter durations, followed by a flatter slope. Furthermore, both noise and tone should have the same threshold value and follow the same curve at very short durations, if the hypothesis is correct.

The specific purpose of these experiments then becomes the measurement of the change in threshold for very short durations of tone, for both noise and sine-wave stimuli. For comparison purposes, one curve is obtained in which a narrow pass band filter limits the band width of energy in the short-tone stimulus.

APPARATUS

Audio circuits

A schematic block diagram of the apparatus appears in Fig. 3. A sine-wave tone is generated by the Hewlitt-Packard oscillator, while the noise stimulus is provided by a flat-noise generator filtered with a 5000 c.p.s. low pass filter. This filter was used to prevent the earphones from being the limiting factor for the high frequencies. The duration of the tone is determined by the electronic audio-timer. The short tone is fed from the timer to attenuators and the earphones. For some measurements, the short tone was filtered by a 1000 c.p.s. band pass filter, with a pass band of 100 c.p.s. at the half-power points.

Timer operation

The electronic audio-timer has been previously described[5] in detail. The tone was always produced at a self-repeating rate of once every two seconds. The tone always started at the time axis, regardless of the duration. If the tone had been allowed to start at random in its own cycle, the transient response of the phones would have caused a considerably increased variability in the threshold measures.

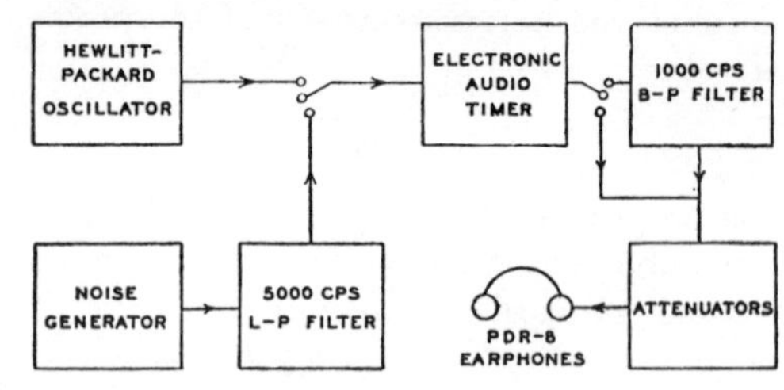

FIG. 3. Block diagram of the apparatus.

[5] R. G. Roush, "Tone burst generator," Electronics **20**, 92 (1947).

Earphones

Permoflux receivers Type PDR-8 were used. These earphones had been calibrated by the Permoflux Company, and all phones had a response essentially flat between 150 and 6000 c.p.s. The phones were mounted in Navy aviation-type headsets with doughnut cushions.

Calibrations

All reference intensities were measured on a Ballantine vacuum-tube voltmeter. The calibration curves for the phones were used to determine sound-pressure levels of the tones. All changes in intensities were obtained by means of attenuators calibrated in db.

Tone durations were calibrated by two means. Durations of 50 milliseconds and less were measured by increasing the repetition rate of the tones until the signal could be synchronized with the sweep of a Dumont Type 208 oscillograph. The actual duration was then set by counting the number of cycles of a 1000-c.p.s. tone, although for durations of 50 milliseconds, a lower frequency was used to count cycles. Durations longer than 50 milliseconds were measured with a Standard Electric Clock, Type S-1, calibrated in 1/100's of a second.

PROCEDURES

Observers

Six male college students between the ages of 18 and 25 served as observers. All observers had had previous experience as subjects in auditory experiments. The amount of this experience ranged between 50 and 125 hours of observation time, over a period of 5 months.

Methods

The data were obtained in two groups. Four men worked together in one group, and two men worked in the other group.

The men were seated comfortably in a sound-deadened room with the headsets placed on their heads. Each man had a hand-held push button with which to indicate that he heard a tone. This push button flashed a light in the experimenter's control room, so that the experimenter knew a tone had been heard. The color and arrangement of the lights identified the observer.

A method of limits was used, although tones were changed only in the direction of increasing intensity. The observer listened until he heard a tone, and then pushed his button every time he heard the tone. The experimenter increased the intensity 1 db each time the tone was presented. A threshold measure was considered obtained when an observer heard two tones in succession. After all observers had heard the tones, the intensity was decreased, and the procedure repeated.

The group of four observers listened binaurally, and made 10 observations for each condition. The group of two observers made 25 observations for each condition, and listened monaurally. This difference in procedure seemed to have little effect on the shape of the functions, and all data were averaged together for the curves presented here. Each observer's mean threshold was used to average, so that each subject, rather than each observation, received equal weighting in the final averages.

All observers listened for six to seven hours per day during the course of the experiments, with rest periods at least once an hour. The two groups were run three months apart. All conditions were completely counter-balanced for the time of day that observations were obtained. This precaution proved to be of real advantage in obtaining consistent functions at absolute threshold levels.

Conditions

Five different functions relating threshold intensity to duration were obtained. One function used a noise stimulus containing frequencies from 50–5000 c.p.s. Two functions were obtained with a 1000-c.p.s. tone. One of these stimuli was filtered with a narrow band pass filter; the other was unfiltered. Two more functions were obtained with unfiltered tones at frequencies of 250 and 4000 c.p.s.

RESULTS

Comparison of noise and 1000-c.p.s. tones

For purposes of exposition, the results are best presented in two separate sections. Figure 4 shows the results of the comparison of the noise stimulus with the two 1000-c.p.s. stimuli. The curve for noise has a slope which is almost exactly 8 db per log unit of time. The curve for the unfiltered tone has a slope of exactly 10 db per log unit of time for durations of 8 milliseconds or more. At 4 milliseconds, the slope has clearly changed, showing a rise in threshold greater than the rise which is due to a change in total energy alone. This rise continues at 2 milliseconds, but by 1 millisecond, the curve is becoming parallel with the noise curve, and the two thresholds at 1 millisecond almost coincide. It can be assumed that the two curves would coincide for even shorter durations.

The curve for the filtered tone is exactly the same as the curve for the unfiltered tone for durations of 15 milliseconds and more. As duration becomes shorter, however, the two curves deviate more and more, and the curve for the filtered tone has a slope of a little more than 17 db per log unit of duration. Theoretically, this curve should eventually have a slope of 20 db per log unit of time, since the energy in a narrow band of frequencies changes at that rate with changes in duration.

The hypothesis suggested is completely substantiated for this condition at least. The fact that the two tone curves deviate at 8 milliseconds means that the band of frequencies within which perfect integration occurs is at least greater than 125 c.p.s. The deviation of the unfiltered stimulus curve from a straight line at 4 milliseconds means that the band of frequencies must be less than 250 c.p.s. wide, at the half-power points. The best estimate from these curves is that a band of frequencies no wider than about 175 c.p.s. around 1000 c.p.s. is necessary if temporal integration of acoustic energy is to be perfect.

Relation to Critical Bands

It seems reasonable that the width of this band should be related to the frequency of the tonal stimulus. Fletcher's concept[6] of the critical band width of noise has received wide attention in recent years. The critical band width is defined as that range of noise frequencies which is equal in energy to the energy of a pure tone which is just masked by the noise. The width of this band, presumably, is determined by the minimum area of stimulation on the basilar membrane. The width of the critical band follows the same frequency function as frequency-discrimination curves and the pitch function.

[6] H. Fletcher, "Auditory patterns," Rev. Mod. Phys. 12, 47 (1940).

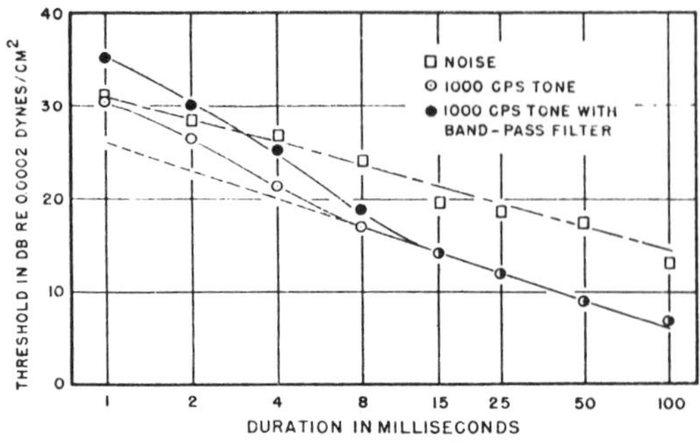

Fig. 4. The relation between absolute threshold and duration for noise and 1000-c.p.s. tones. The wide-band noise is filtered with a 5000 c.p.s. low pass filter. The filter used with the 1000-c.p.s. tone had a band width of 100 c.p.s.

The critical band at 1000 c.p.s. is approximately 50 c.p.s. The band which is necessary to insure perfect temporal integration of acoustic energy is three to four times that width. The ratio between critical bands at different frequencies, however, should be the same as the ratio of the integration bands which we are measuring. At 4000 c.p.s., then, the band within which all energy is perfectly integrated should be about 500 c.p.s. and the curve should deviate from linearity at 1 millisecond, but not at any longer duration.

Measurements at other frequencies

Figure 5 shows the results obtained at frequencies of 4000 and 250 c.p.s. The curve for 4000 c.p.s. shows practically no deviation from the straight line, with a slope of 10 db per log unit of time, and it is problematical whether deviation has begun at 1 millisecond. The curve for 4000 c.p.s. is not quite as precise as that for 1000 c.p.s., which makes it more difficult to determine exactly whether deviation from a straight line has occurred. The fact that no deviation occurs with longer durations, however, seems sufficient justification for assuming that the integration band width is related to the pitch function.

The curve for 250 c.p.s. shows quite another effect. As the duration is decreased, the threshold

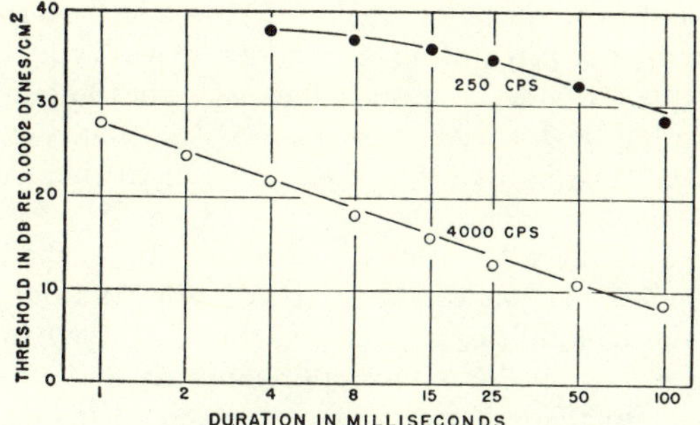

FIG. 5. The relation between absolute threshold and tonal duration for two frequencies.

rises. But the rise in threshold becomes less and less as the duration is decreased more and more. The explanation of this apparent reversal of the phenomenon becomes quite apparent after an examination of the normal audiogram shown in Fig. 6. The threshold for a 250-c.p.s. tone is very high compared to that of a 1000- or 4000-c.p.s. tone. The threshold is also changing very rapidly in that range of frequencies. When the tone becomes shorter and shorter, the increase in the band width of energy essentially throws some of the energy into a much more sensitive portion of the audiogram. The short tone has an advantage which the longer tone does not have. Eventually the 250 c.p.s. tone should have the same threshold value as a noise stimulus or a very short tone of any frequency. The only way the 250 c.p.s. tone can get to this low a threshold is for the curve to bend over as it does in Fig. 5.

DISCUSSION

Extension of the hypothesis

As the hypothesis was stated in the introductory sections, no mention was made of the extent to which the slope of the duration-threshold function would change. It was simply stated that the slope would be unity when all the energy to be integrated was in a narrow band of frequencies. The curves in Fig. 4 enable us to extend that hypothesis.

We already knew that the slope of the noise function was 8 db per log unit of duration. If the integration band to which we refer here were an all-or-none phenomenon, then whenever the band of energy was greater than this minimum band, the slope should immediately change to 8 db per log unit of time. Thus in Fig. 4, the curve for the unfiltered 1000-c.p.s. would jump immediately to coincide with the noise curve as soon as the band of frequencies was greater than that necessary for perfect integration. Since the change was gradual, however, we can assume that the slope changes gradually as the band of frequencies is increased.

In other words, we cannot make a clear distinction between a band which will provide perfect integration and bands of frequencies which are equivalent to noise. There are intermediate band widths which give integration functions with slopes between that provided by the pure-tone function and that provided by the noise function. Since the unfiltered 1000-c.p.s. tone had almost the same threshold at 1 millisecond as the noise, we can say that a band of frequencies around 1000 c.p.s. which is 1000 c.p.s. wide (as measured by the half-power points) is equivalent to a wide band noise stimulus. For bands of frequencies less than about 175 c.p.s., the integration will be perfect. For bands of frequencies between these limits, the slope of the integration function will be between 10 and 8 db per log unit of time. The narrower the band of frequencies, the more nearly will the integration be perfect.

Nature of the integration process

It is difficult to conceive of a mechanism which would account for all the phenomena mentioned in this paper. If we were concerned only with a phenomenon of integration of energy through a range of frequencies, explanations would not be so difficult. But here we are concerned with an

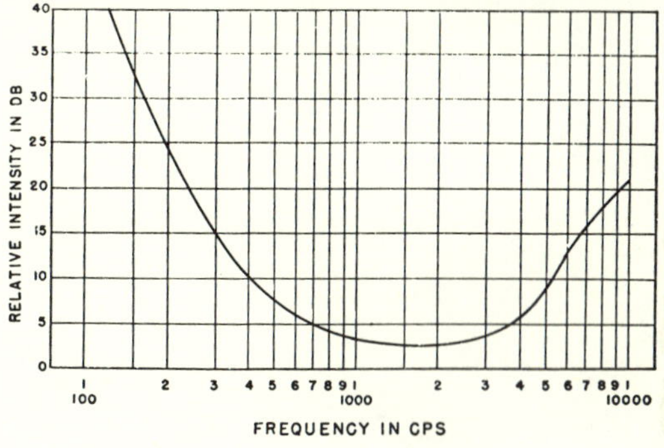

FIG. 6. The normal audiogram.

explanation of a lack of perfect *temporal* integration when the stimulus has a wide band of frequencies. We are not concerned with imperfect integration across frequencies, but rather with imperfect integration through time when many frequencies are involved.

Absolute Thresholds

If we had to explain simply the curves in Figs. 4 and 5, which involve only absolute thresholds, an explanation in terms of the normal audiogram is possible. We have evidence that the ear will integrate perfectly acoustic energy through time when all the energy is at a single frequency, or nearly so. Now when we use a wide-band stimulus, each single frequency should likewise show perfect integration with time. We have, however, the normal audiogram to consider. With the wide-band stimulus, as the duration is increased, the threshold intensity is decreased; but when the over-all intensity is decreased, the energy at very low and high frequencies falls below the threshold for those frequencies, and their energy is lost. The over-all intensity must then be increased to compensate for the loss of energy at high and low frequencies. Likewise, as the duration is increased still further, the over-all intensity could be decreased proportionately, except that some of the energy has again been lost, and the intensity must be raised to compensate for it.

We can, then, explain the lack of complete integration for wide-band noise stimuli at absolute thresholds in terms of the differential sensitivity of the ear to various frequencies. If the audiogram were flat, then the width of the band of frequencies would have no effect on the temporal integration of energy. This type of explanation is necessary to explain the shape of the curve for 250 c.p.s. The explanation, however, has disadvantages when it is used to cover all cases.

The curve for 1000 c.p.s., for example, shows deviation from the linear relationship at durations of 4 milliseconds. At this duration, the band of energy in the tone is approximately 250 c.p.s. wide at the half-power points, which means that the energy is spread between 875 and 1125 c.p.s. The change in the audiogram between these limits seems too small to account for the change in integration slope.

Masked Thresholds

The primary difficulty with this type of explanation, however, is that it cannot apply to the cases of masked threshold. When a reasonably high level of masking noise is in the listener's ear, the threshold for pure tones is almost independent of the frequency of the tone. No explanation which depends on a differential sensitivity to various frequencies can explain these curves at masked threshold—which are basically no different from the integration curves at absolute threshold. Indeed, the evidence is that there is less temporal integration for a noise stimulus at the masked level than at the absolute threshold.

ACKNOWLEDGMENT

The assistance of Mrs. Mary Hall and Mrs. Katherine Hill in recording data is gratefully acknowledged.

10

Reprinted from *Acoust. Soc. Am. J.* 8:185–190 (1937)

A Scale for the Measurement of the Psychological Magnitude Pitch*

S. S. Stevens and J. Volkmann, *Harvard University, Cambridge, Massachusetts*
and
E. B. Newman, *Swarthmore College, Swarthmore, Pennsylvania*
(Received August 4, 1936)

TWO different concepts of pitch have commonly been held. To the musician pitch has meant the aspect of tones in terms of which he arranges them on a musical scale. The musical scale divides the range of audible frequencies into octaves, which in turn are divided into tones, semi-tones, etc. Then, musically speaking, two semi-tones in different parts of the audible range are considered as equal intervals of pitch. Perceptually, however, these two semi-tones may represent unequal intervals of pitch.

To the physicist, on the other hand, pitch has generally meant frequency. "Pitch is specified scientifically by the period or frequency of vibration."[1] The error of this conception has been recently demonstrated by experiments which show that it is possible to alter the pitch of a tone without changing its frequency.[2] By increasing the intensity of tones of high frequency we raise their pitch; whereas in the case of low frequencies, an increase in intensity lowers the pitch. This change of pitch may amount to as much as half an octave[3] at certain low frequencies. Clearly, then, pitch is not frequency, nor is it correlated one-to-one with frequency.

These considerations have led to the proposal[4] that the designation of pitch should take into account the loudness of a tone. In particular, it is argued that the pitch of a given tone should be specified in terms of a reference tone at a loudness level of 40 db which is perceived as equal to the given tone in pitch. It has been proposed further that the pitch of a tone at the loudness level of 40 db should be designated by its frequency, or, alternatively, by the number of octaves that it is above a given reference frequency.

This proposal is a partial recognition of the fact that pitch, like loudness, depends upon the perceiving organism, and that the numbers used to designate values of the physical stimulus are not adequate to represent values of such a psychological magnitude. A desirable scale for the pitch of tones at the reference loudness (40-db level) would be one expressed in numbers whose values are directly proportional to the magnitude of the perceived pitch. The present experiment seeks to establish such a psychological scale of pitch.

---

* Presented at the meeting of the Acoustical Society of America, New York, October 31, 1936.

[1] E. H. Barton, *A Text-book on Sound* (Macmillan, London, 1914), p. 9.

[2] S. S. Stevens, "The Relation of Pitch to Intensity," J. Acous. Soc. Am. 6, 150–154 (1935).

[3] W. B. Snow, "Change of Pitch with Loudness at Low Frequencies," J. Acous. Soc. Am. 8, 14–19 (1936).

[4] H. Fletcher, "Loudness, Pitch and the Timbre of Musical Tones and their Relation to the Intensity, the Frequency and the Overtone Structure," J. Acous. Soc. Am. 6, 59–69 (1934).

The Problem of Sensory Scales

Controversy has for a long time centered around the proposition that it is possible to measure attributes of sensations, or to tell when one sensation is twice or three times as great as another. The truth of this proposition must depend not upon *a priori* conceptions but upon the outcome of experiment. We must first decide what we shall mean by a sensory scale (of pitch, let us say) and then determine by experiment whether or not such a scale can, in fact, be constructed. In other words, we must decide upon the criteria of the scale, and then devise operations for satisfying the criteria.

The criteria for a psychological scale were examined in a previous paper[5] in connection with the development of a scale for loudness. The following points will bear repeated emphasis.

(1) There are, in general, two types of scales, commonly referred to as *intensive* and *numerical* scales. Scales which measure intensive magnitude enable us to place the things measured in a rank-order, i.e., arrange them according to increasing magnitude. Such a scale does not, however, enable us to say how many times one magnitude is greater than another, but only that it is greater. Numerical scales, on the other hand, have numbers which express the numerical relations between things measured. Thus, when two magnitudes are measured by a numerical scale, the scale numbers can be manipulated in accordance with arithmetical laws in order to determine additional relationships such as the sum of two magnitudes, the relative separation of two pairs of magnitudes, etc.

(2) These manipulations of the numbers on numerical scales have significance only if the manipulations correspond to a set of concrete operations which can be performed on the things measured. Otherwise, the validity of the outcome of the manipulations cannot be tested empirically. The concrete operations will, in general, be different for different types of measurement. Thus, the procedure for verifying that 2 meters can be added to 2 meters to make 4 meters is very unlike that for showing that 2 henries of inductance can be added to 2 henries to give 4 henries. Similarly, in the case of sensation, we may reasonably expect to find that numerical scales are based on operations peculiar to it alone.

(3) Now, in the case of psychological measurements, most scales have been scales of intensive magnitude. What we want is a numerical scale—one whose numbers represent some aspect of the response of a living organism to a certain class of stimuli.

(4) The numbers of the numerical scale should be applied to the attribute of sensation (which is, of course, an aspect of an organism's response) in such a way that when they are manipulated according to the rules of arithmetic, one obtains a result which can be verified observationally. To the manipulations and to the result there should correspond a set of concrete operations.

(5) Although we could conceivably choose any one of several sets of operations as defining the scale,[6] that set will ultimately prove most satisfactory which leads to scale numbers bearing the most reasonable relation to the experience of the observer. A reasonable scale is one on which the number N stands for a sensation which does in fact appear to be half as great as that represented by the number $2N$, etc.

Procedure

In view of the success encountered in the construction of a numerical scale of loudness[7, 8] we employed an analogous procedure for pitch. The problem is to determine the relation between a numerical scale of perceptual pitch and the scale of frequency used to measure the stimulus. The observer was required, in our experiment, to adjust the frequency of a second tone until it sounded just half as high in pitch as a standard tone. In order to guard against the effect of intensity on pitch, tones were presented at a constant loudness level of 60 db. The fractionaation of several tones, scattered throughout the audible range, thus provides a basis for assigning numbers to the tones such that they constitute a numerical scale of perceived pitch.

[5] S. S. Stevens, "A Scale for the Measurement of a Psychological Magnitude: Loudness," Psych. Rev., 43, 405–416 (1936).

[6] C. H. Graham, "Psychophysics and Behavior," J. Gen. Psych. 10, 299–310 (1934).

[7] H. Fletcher, "Newer Concepts of the Pitch, Loudness and Timbre of Musical Tones," J. Frank. Inst. 220, 405–429 (1935).

[8] B. G. Churcher, "A Loudness Scale for Industrial Noise Measurement," J. Acous. Soc. Am. 6, 216–226 (1935).

This scale can be no more reliable than the performance of the observers. The question arises, in the first place, whether it is possible to make such a judgment about pitch. Several observers made the statement *a priori* that pitch is not something of which they could take half; yet these same observers found upon trying that the judgment is quite possible. They were not explicit as to how they made the judgment, except to say that when the second tone was set to a certain frequency, it "felt like half," whereas at other frequencies it "felt" too high or too low. Observers differed greatly in the ease with which they acquired the necessary attitude.

The following written instructions were given:

"You will be presented with two tones which differ in pitch. The pitch of one tone may be varied by turning a crank; you are to adjust this tone until its pitch is just *half* of the pitch of the fixed tone. During the course of the adjustment, take care to produce values of the variable pitch which are plainly higher than the desired half-value and other values which are plainly lower. If the fixed and the variable tones differ widely in loudness, report this fact."

Apparatus

The tones were generated by two beat-frequency oscillators. The tone from one oscillator was fixed in frequency at 125, 200, 300, 400, 700, 1000, 2000, 5000, 8000 or 12,000 cycles. The other tone could be varied continuously by the observer, who turned a small crank geared to the tuning condenser of the second oscillator (General Radio type 713-A). The observer faced the source of sound, a dynamic and a crystal speaker connected in parallel and mounted in a baffle. The experiment was conducted in a highly absorbent sound-room.

TABLE I. *Showing the geometric means of fractionations by each of five observers, and average errors for 2 observers.*

Standard Freq.	Frequency at Half-Pitch						Average Error (%)	
	Observer					Geometric Mean	Observer	
	E	*V*	*N*	*M*	*D*		*E*	*V*
125	96	84	97	87	96	90	3.4	7.5
200	131	131	123	101	107	121	7.4	6.7
300	183	205	195	118	133	171	13.0	7.8
400	237	251	237	173	253	233	13.5	9.0
700	391	407	474	256	403	384	12.3	9.8
1,000	590	640	622	391	485	558	11.0	13.9
2,000	998	979	1006	508	662	851	14.8	13.7
5,000	1930	1800	2260	1230	1590	1767	12.0	13.5
8,000	2360	2170	3110	1650	2110	2239	19.1	13.9
12,000	2970	2400	3720	2320	2980	2788	19.9	11.5

The two tones were presented alternately by a relay which switched from one to the other at two-second intervals. Care was taken to keep both tones at a loudness level of 60 db. Voltages corresponding to the 60-db level were determined beforehand in terms of the thresholds of the three of us, and then as the observer changed the frequency of the second tone, the experimenter adjusted its voltage, if necessary, to keep it at the 60-db loudness level.

Results

Five observers (two of the authors and three others) were used in the experiment. At each experimental session each observer made one fractionation of each of the 10 standard tones. Five sets of fractionations were made by 3 observers and 10 sets by 2 observers. These 10 sets were made in order to get an indication of the reliability with which an observer is able to set one pitch to half of the value of another pitch. The averaged results for each observer are presented in Table I. In averaging it appeared reasonable to take the geometric mean of the individual adjustments rather than the arithmetic mean, in order to compensate for the fact that the differential sensitivity of the ear (measured in cycles per second) is less for high than for low frequencies. In taking the final

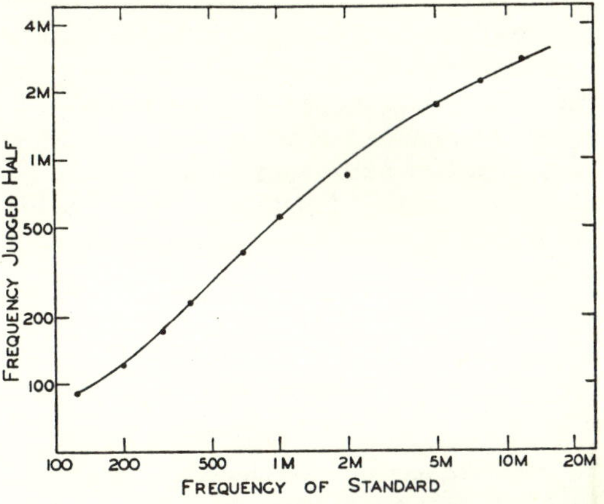

FIG. 1. The ordinate represents the frequency of the tone whose pitch was judged half as high as the pitch of the standard tone (abscissa). The smooth curve was fitted visually to the geometric mean of the adjustments of five observers. The point at 2000 cycles deviates from the general trend, due to the tendency of observer M to select values an octave below the other observers at this frequency.

average for the 5 observers their individual averages were weighted according to the number of judgments made by each.

These observers show good agreement, considering the supposed difficulty of fractionating pitch. Only one of them (M) departs significantly from the average of the group. He is a trained musician, and reported an inability to disregard octaves and other musical intervals when setting the second tone at half the pitch of the first. The other observers were apparently not confused by the recognition of these musical relationships. Observer M, however, tended to come more into line with the other observers as the experiment proceeded. His earlier settings were also upset by his conscious effort to imagine what "zero pitch" might be. It appears that a somewhat non-analytical attitude is necessary on the part of the observer if he is to maintain a consistent criterion for his judgment.

In order to construct a pitch scale the averaged results were plotted as in Fig. 1, and a smooth curve was fitted visually to the points. Then, from this smooth curve we proceeded to construct the *pitch function* in Fig. 2. We assigned the number 1000 to the pitch of a 1000-cycle tone and determined from Fig. 1 the frequency of the tone which sounds half as high and which should have, therefore, the number 500 assigned to it. Similarly for the pitch number 250, etc. The result is a function (Fig. 2) which has, within the limitations of our particular procedure, the numerical significance which we set out to give it; namely, the numbers on the pitch scale are related to each other as the subjective magnitudes of the pitches. A pitch of 1000 units (mels[9]) is subjectively twice as high as a pitch of 500 units. "Twice as high" is, of course, defined by the operations of this experiment.

Relation of the Pitch Function to Other Data

Having established a pitch scale, we can use it to measure certain psychological magnitudes, and by comparing it with physiological data, we can obtain a suggestion as to the probable basis of the judgment of pitch magnitudes.

[9] The name *mel* was chosen as a name for the subjective pitch unit. It was taken from the root of the word *melody*.

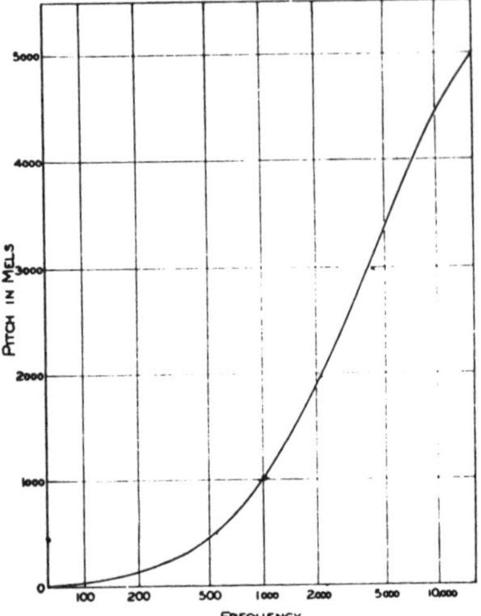

Fig. 2. The pitch function, showing the relation of perceived pitch (in mels) to the frequency of the stimulus. The values in mels are derived from the curve of Fig. 1; the 1000-cycle tone is arbitrarily assigned the value of 1000 mels.

Relation of pitch to DL's

Psychologists have long debated the proposition that all just-detectable increments in frequency (difference limens or DL's) are subjectively equal in magnitude. Now, if each DL increases the pitch of a tone by a constant amount, the summated DL's should give a pitch scale which agrees with the scale in Fig. 2. In order to test this hypothesis we integrated graphically the DL's determined by Shower and Biddulph[10] and obtained the values shown in Fig. 3. The integration was made of the data for the loudness level of 60 db. Several assumptions are possible as to the best limits of integration. For the lower limit we chose 60 cycles, because at lower frequencies Shower and Biddulph found an anomalous decrease in the size of the relative DL's. The number of DL's below 60 cycles is so small, however (about 10 or 20) that their effect on the total integration is negligible for our purpose. At the upper end we integrated as far as available data would permit (about 12,000 cycles). This coincides with the highest tone we actually used in determining the pitch function in Fig. 2.

[10] E. G. Shower and R. Biddulph, "Differential Pitch Sensitivity of the Ear," J. Acous. Soc. Am. 3, 275–287 (1931).

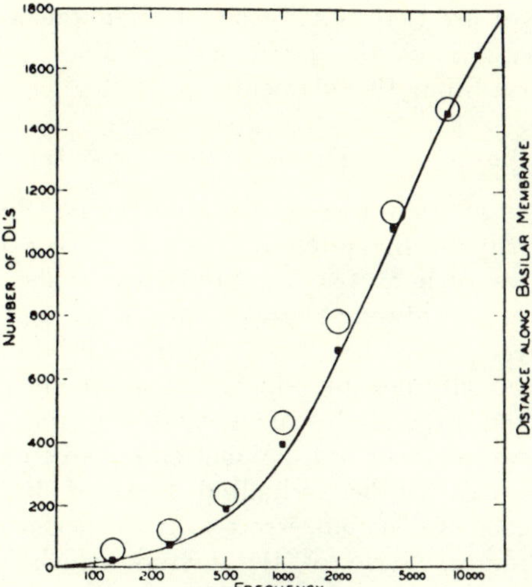

FIG. 3. The relation of the pitch function (solid curve) to the integrated DL's (solid squares) and to the experimental location of resonant positions on the basilar membrane (circles). The ordinate scale (on left) shows the number of DL's for pitch as a function of frequency when the integration is made at the 60 db loudness level. The pitch scale in mels can be obtained by multiplying the ordinate values by the factor 2.83. The relative locations of resonant areas on the basilar membrane are obtained by laying the linear extent of the membrane along the ordinate scale. Thus the ordinate on the right represents the relative linear extent of the membrane both in man and guinea pig.

The close agreement of the integrated DL's and the pitch function (Fig. 3) shows clearly that, within the limits of accuracy of present measurements, all DL's for pitch, at a constant loudness level, are of equal subjective magnitude. This conclusion is unlike that reached in the case of loudness[11] where DL's increase rapidly in size with increasing intensity of the stimulus. The fact that the size of DL's for pitch is constant, whereas the size of DL's for loudness varies, testifies to the fact that pitch and loudness are based on quite dissimilar physiological mechanisms. Perhaps the two judgments of loudness, magnitude and DL, involve different types of physiological mechanisms, whereas the judgments of magnitude and DL for pitch are based upon the same type of physiological mechanism. Both magnitudes and DL's for pitch depend upon discrimination of the *location* of stimulation on the basilar membrane. Loudness appears to depend upon the total *number* of fibers stimulated in the auditory nerve. The mechanism underlying the judgment of DL's for loudness is as yet undetermined.

Relation of the pitch scale to basilar mechanics

Experiments designed to determine the location of the region of the basilar membrane which is resonant to different frequencies have been conducted by means of the electrical recording of potentials generated in the ears of guinea pigs.[12, 13] Surgical damage to the basilar membrane at a particular location results in a decreased sensitivity to tones of a certain frequency. The "map" of the basilar membrane obtained by correlating locations of lesions with abnormalities in the corresponding audiograms is almost precisely the same "map" as that resulting from an integration of DL's for pitch. The latter is based on the assumption that for each DL the two tones being discriminated must stimulate parts of the basilar membrane separated by a constant distance.

Now, if we let the ordinate of Fig. 3 represent the linear extent of the basilar membrane, and plot the resonant positions as a function of frequency, we obtain the function suggested by the circles in Fig. 3. The size of these circles represents approximately the probable error of the measurements made in the work with guinea pigs. The obvious correspondence between the locations of the resonant regions determined by experiment and by integration of DL's, and their correspondence in turn to the pitch function suggests an interesting hypothesis. Apparently, when an observer is asked to set a second tone to half the pitch of a given tone, he changes its frequency until it stimulates a position on the basilar membrane midway between the position stimulated by the given tone and the apical end of the membrane. He is, of course, not aware of these locations as such, but the underlying physiological process which makes comparison of pitches possible seems to be characterized chiefly by spatial differentiation. Although there are subsequent central nervous processes, the form of certain discriminatory functions is evidently imposed by the receptor mechanism.

[11] S. S. Stevens and H. Davis, "Psychophysiological Acoustics: Pitch and Loudness," J. Acous. Soc. Am. **8**, 1–13 (1936).

[12] S. S. Stevens, H. Davis and M. H. Lurie, "The Localization of Pitch Perception on the Basilar Membrane," J. Gen. Psych. **13**, 297–315 (1935).

[13] E. Culler, Ann. Otol. Rhin. Laryn. **44**, 808–814 (1935).

Relation of the pitch scale to musical intervals

An interesting application of the pitch scale is the measurement of the size of musical intervals. We can measure the subjective size of the various octaves by determining from Fig. 2 how much the pitch changes in going from one octave to the next. In a similar way we can measure the size of other musical intervals. In general, the subjective size of any musical interval is approximately proportional to the slope of the pitch function (Fig. 2) at the frequency which falls in the middle of the interval.

In order to illustrate these relationships, the subjective size of successive octaves and fifths, as measured in mels, is plotted in Fig. 4. The plot for other intervals would be similar in form but different in ordinate value.

Quite definitely, musical intervals become subjectively larger as frequency increases up to the fourth octave above middle C (up to 4096 cycles). In other words, throughout the useful musical range, intervals increase in subjective magnitude with increasing frequency of the stimulus. This conclusion is not entirely novel. The eminent psychologist-musician, Stumpf,[14] decided that in spite of the great difficulty of making these subjective comparisons, the upper octaves are perceptually larger than the lower octaves. Thus the pitch scale enables us to confirm Stumpf's judgment.

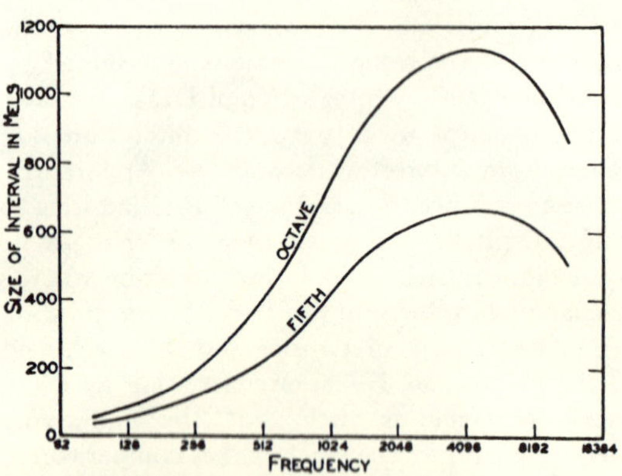

FIG. 4. The size of musical intervals in terms of mels. The upper curve shows the perceived size of octaves as a function of the geometric mean of the limiting frequencies. The lower curve shows in a corresponding manner the perceived size of fifths.

[14] C. Stumpf, Tonpsychologie I, 250 (1883).

DISCUSSION

The question arises concerning the possibility of verifying the pitch function by other procedures such as bisecting tonal intervals, i.e., setting a third tone to a value half-way, in pitch, between two other tones. Such verification is theoretically possible—in fact it is theoretically required if the pitch scale is valid. The ability of any two methods of fractionation or bisection to confirm each other is limited, however, by the existence of constant errors in the experimental procedures. Some of the factors which may introduce constant errors are the size of the interval, the position of the interval on the frequency scale, the order of presentation of the stimuli, the rate of presentation, the position of the variable tone before the observer begins the adjustment, and the effect of what is known as "absolute judgment," namely, a tendency to adjust the variable tone to a value which is to some extent independent of the two limiting tones, but dependent upon preceding judgments. The choice of a function to be used as a pitch scale will, therefore, be subject to revision whenever the sources of constant errors in the experimental procedures can be detected and eliminated.

The method of bisection has been applied to tonal intervals. The results of different investigators, however, have thus far been contradictory.[15] Some workers have insisted that the bisection is made at the arithmetic mean and some claim evidence for bisection at the geometric mean. A famous historical controversy was waged about this point.[16] From the form of the present pitch function it is evident that the bisection of an interval should depend upon the position of the interval on the frequency scale. Hence, both parties to the controversy may be correct.

[15] C. C. Pratt, "Comparison of Tonal Distance," J. Exper. Psych. 11, 77–87 (1928).
[16] E. B. Titchener, Experimental Psychology 2, part 2, 232–248 (1905).

11

Reprinted from *Psychol. Rev.* 43:405-416 (1936)

A SCALE FOR THE MEASUREMENT OF A PSYCHOLOGICAL MAGNITUDE: LOUDNESS

BY S. S. STEVENS

Harvard University

A scale adequate to the measurement of the subjective magnitude of sensation has long been sought by psychophysicists. Scales, such as those obtained by summating difference limens, have been proposed, but they have turned out to be scales of intensive magnitude, *i.e.*, scales which enable us to tell whether one sensation is greater than another without, however, permitting us to say *how much* greater.[1] In other words, it has not been possible to apply to these scales numbers for which the usual laws of mathematics could be shown to hold when the numbers were given operational meaning, *i.e.*, identified with concrete operations performed upon the organism.

I

The Problem of the Scale

We devise scales for the purpose of facilitating the description of natural phenomena in terms of functional relationships expressed, if possible, by the symbols of conventional mathematics. Consequently, it is desirable to assign numbers in each scale which not only denote the order within the scale (for which the letters of the alphabet would serve well enough), but also designate the relative magnitudes of the phenomena to which the scale is applied. When this is done, the scale numbers can be manipulated in accordance with arithmetical laws in order to determine additional relationships such as the sum of two magnitudes, the relative separation of two pairs of magnitudes, etc. However, the outcome of the purely

[1] The operational basis of psychological measurement has been treated by D. McGregor, Scientific measurement and psychology, Psychol. Rev., 1935, 42, 246–266.

formal[2] (mathematical) manipulation of the scale numbers has no empirical significance unless the manipulations and their results can be identified with some concrete operations. Thus, in the case of a scale of length, 3 cm. plus 3 cm. equal 6 cm. both formally and empirically, because the operation of adding lengths can be carried out and the formal result verified empirically. In the case of electrical inductances 3 henries plus 3 henries equal 6 henries, but here the physical process of adding the two inductances in order to verify the relationship is very different from that of adding two lengths. A coil of wire whose inductance is 3 henries does not become one of 6 henries when we simply double the length of the wire. Other criteria have to be chosen to define the scale used in the measurement of inductance. Similarly, for every scale obeying the laws of addition, the physical process represented consists of a different set of operations.

Now, in the case of sensation what we want is a scale for the measurement of some aspect of the response of a living organism to a certain class of stimuli. Two conditions should be satisfied. First, the scale numbers should be applied to the attribute of sensation in such a way as to make the scale one of true numerical magnitude, which means simply that if the numbers are manipulated according to the rules of arithmetic, the result (and the manipulations) correspond to a set of physical operations. Secondly, although at the outset we could conceivably choose any one of several sets of operations as defining the scale,[3] that set will ultimately prove to be most satisfactory for a subjective scale when it leads to scale numbers bearing a reasonable relationship to the experience of the observer. Thus, the scale would be satisfactory if the magnitude of the attribute of sensation to which the number 10 is assigned should appear to be half as great to the experiencing individual as that to which the number 20 is given, and twice as great as the magnitude to which the number 5

[2] For the distinction between what is here meant by formal and empirical statements see S. S. Stevens, Psychology, the propaedeutic science, *Philos. Sci.*, 1936, 3, 90-103.

[3] For a recent discussion of three of these sets of operations see C. H. Graham, Psychophysics and behavior, *J. Gen. Psychol.*, 1934, 10, 299-310.

is given. With such a scale the operation of addition consists of changing the stimulus until the observer gives a particular response which indicates that a given relation of magnitudes has been achieved. In other words, a subjective scale is a scale of response, and the response of the observer who says "this is half as loud as that" is one which, for the purpose of erecting a subjective scale, can be accepted at its face value.

A scale, then, which would enable us to designate the *numerical* as well as the *intensive* magnitude of an attribute of sensation can be constructed according to the criterion that, having assigned a particular number N to a given magnitude, the number $N/2$ shall be assigned to the magnitude which appears half as great to the experiencing individual. Obviously, in the application of this criterion we are limited by our ability to devise operations for the determination of fractional magnitudes of sensation.

We do not measure the magnitude of a sensation, but only of a particular dimension or aspect of sensation within a single sensory modality. Thus a scale for each of the four attributes [4] of auditory sensation could conceivably be devised, and the experience attendant upon stimulation by a pure tone could be described by four numbers, one for its position on each of the four subjective scales. Any two numbers will, of course, uniquely determine the tone.

In proceeding to the construction of a scale for an auditory attribute, loudness let us say, we are confronted with the possibility of measuring the attribute as a function of either one of the two dimensions of the stimulus, frequency and intensity, since each attribute is a function of both dimensions.[5] However, in the case of loudness it is obviously more satisfactory to hold frequency constant and determine loudness as a function of intensity, since this function is single valued, and variation is possible over the entire range of the attribute. (At a fixed level of intensity loudness is not a single valued function of frequency.)

[4] For a discussion of the criteria of auditory attributes see S. S. Stevens, The operational definition of psychological concepts, PSYCHOL. REV., 1935, **42**, 517-527.

[5] S. S. Stevens, The attributes of tones, *Proc. Nat. Acad. Sci.*, 1934, **20**, 457–459.

Having decided, then, upon the function which we wish to establish, it remains for us to devise procedures that will yield results satisfying the criteria which define the scale. Loudness is a name which we give to a class of discriminatory responses on the part of an organism under certain restricted conditions of 'set' and stimulation, and it is these responses which must provide the basic operations that we seek. In other words, the subjective judgments (responses) of the observer must provide the ultimate test of the validity of the numbers on the scale as representative of degrees of loudness. The utilization of the observer's discriminations in this way presupposes, of course, that he is capable of making valid judgments of the numerical ratio of one impression to another. How he acquired this ability is irrelevant to the present problem, providing he *has* the ability.

If the observer is able to make what we can accept as valid judgments of the ratio of two loudnesses, the problem becomes simply one of finding the particular ratio and the experimental conditions which will make the judgments most reliable. In the case of loudness the simple ratio 1 to 2 has been determined with good consistency by several investigators, and four general methods have been used to establish it.[6]

1. The observer is required to make a direct estimate by varying the intensity of one tone until it sounds half as loud as another. Several variations of this procedure are possible. This method is necessarily the most basic (although not necessarily the most reliable) one in view of the criteria previously laid down regarding the nature of the loudness scale, and the other methods are valid only in so far as they offer alternative ways of getting the same results.

2. The second method makes use of the fact that the two ears are connected in such a way that a tone introduced into one ear sounds half as loud as the same tone introduced into both ears. (The ears are apparently connected in a manner analogous to voltaic cells in series in that summation occurs, whereas the eyes suggest somewhat a parallel connection.)

[6] B. G. Churcher, A loudness scale for industrial noise measurements, *J. Acoust. Soc. Amer.*, 1935, **6**, 216–226.

The procedure then is to have the observer adjust the intensity of a tone in one ear until it sounds as loud as a given tone in both ears. The validity of the results of this method are checked by their agreement with those of the first method.

3. Since differential sensitivity to intensity is a function of the intensity level, the loudness of a tone, heard binaurally and yielding the same difference limen as a tone heard monaurally, might be considered half as loud as the latter provided again that these results agree with those gotten by the first method.

4. Two tones of equal loudness which are sufficiently separated in frequency so as not to stimulate overlapping areas on the basilar membrane ought to yield, when presented together, a loudness twice as great as either one alone. By equating a third tone first to one and then to both, the desired ratio of loudnesses should be obtained.

II

The Loudness Scale

The results of recent studies which utilized these methods have been reviewed and summarized by Churcher,[7] who concludes that sufficiently good agreement is shown to warrant the construction of a loudness scale based upon the weighted average of the results of several experiments. Thus the curve labeled '*loudness*' in Fig. 1 he constructed by assigning arbitrarily the number 100 to the loudness of a tone (1000 cycles) 100 db above the standard reference threshold of 0.0002 bars. Consequently the number 50 means an intensity which sounds half as loud as 100 and the number 10 an intensity which sounds one tenth as loud, etc. This curve expresses completely, therefore, the relation between a dimension of the stimulus and an attribute of auditory sensation.

On the physiological side, H. Davis and the author have measured the magnitude of the electrical potentials generated in the cochleas of guinea pigs in response to stimulation by a 1000-cycle tone at various intensity levels. These potentials (obtained from three animals) are plotted as circles in Fig. 1.

[7] B. G. Churcher, *op. cit.*

The values were multiplied by a factor to make the value at 80 db above threshold correspond to the loudness curve at

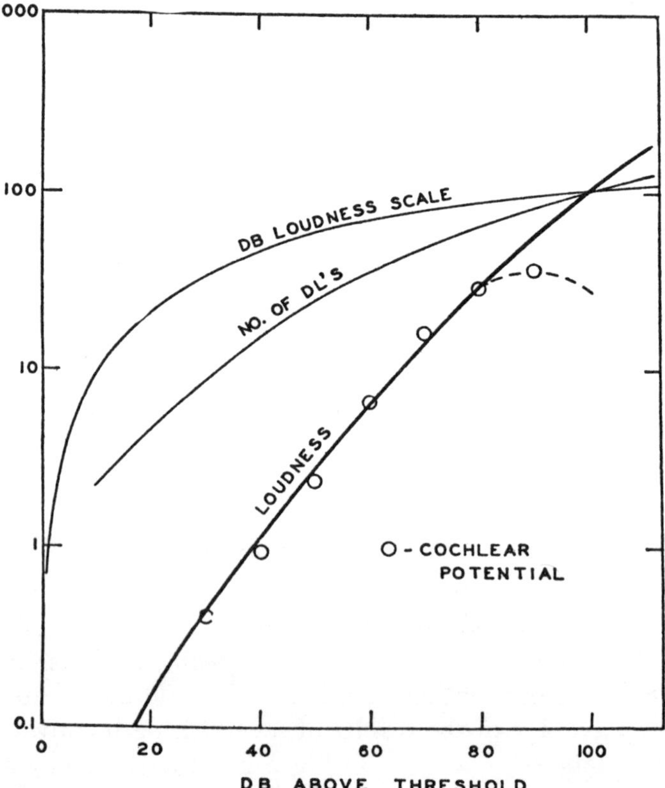

Fig. 1. The relation of loudness and number of DL's to the intensity of the stimulus at 1000 cycles. The curve for loudness was obtained from a consideration of the results of several experiments reviewed by Churcher. The circles represent the magnitude of the electrical response generated in the cochleas of guinea pigs and recorded on a cathode-ray oscillograph. The values were multiplied by a constant to make them coincide with the loudness curve at 80 db above threshold. Above that intensity the potentials decrease with intensity due to an overload effect. The curve for the number of DL's above threshold was adjusted to correspond to the loudness curve at 100 db and therefore the ordinates for this curve are relative values only. The db loudness scale, which is simply tne locus of points for which the ordinate value is equal to the abscissa value, is to illustrate the divergence between the true loudness scale and the decibel scale by which we usually measure the stimulus.

that intensity in order to facilitate the comparison of the two functions. The close agreement suggests not only that it is possible to establish a valid scale for loudness, but also that there exists in the sense-organ a directly measurable process whose magnitude, to a first approximation, is the same function of intensity as is the loudness scale.[8] It should be noted in this connection that, since the loudness curve of Fig. 1 represents averaged data from several individuals, it has the 'properties of an average.' Consequently it may not be as useful for deducing the nature of the mechanism of the response to loudness as would be the case if it represented homogeneous data from a single ear, for which the properties (variability, etc.) were known.

Since the loudness scale will probably be utilized extensively by psychophysiologists and acoustical engineers, it seems appropriate to select and name a fundamental unit of loudness. The loudness of a 1000-cycle tone 40 db above threshold, listened to with both ears, recommends itself as the logical unit, because 1000 cycles has been selected as the reference-frequency for loudness comparisons leading to the determination of *loudness level*, and the loudness level of 40 db above threshold has been proposed as the reference-level for determining the *pitch* of a tone.[9] Incidently, on Churcher's scale (Fig. 1) the value 1 corresponds almost exactly to an intensity of 40 db above threshold. Such a unit should prove to be of the right order of magnitude for general usefulness, since it is only about one-third of one per cent of the maximal loudness the ear can support. As we shall see later this unit corresponds in order of magnitude to the differential thresholds of moderately intense tones of the musical scale. As a name [10] for the unit the word *sone* is proposed.

The Measurement of Difference Limens

Armed with a scale for the measurement of subjective magnitudes, it now becomes possible to answer the question

[8] A more complete discussion of the physiological correlates of loudness is scheduled to appear in the *J. Acoust. Soc. Amer.*, July, 1936.

[9] H. Fletcher, Loudness, pitch and the timbre of musical tones and their relation to the intensity, the frequency and the overtone structure, *J. Acoust. Soc. Amer.*, 1934, **6**, 59–69.

[10] The name *phone* was proposed by the author at the meeting of the Acoustical Society of America, Harvard University, December, 1935, but was found to be objectionable because in Germany *phon* is used to designate the equivalent of a decibel. There appear to be no such objections to the word *sone*, however.

which has agitated psychologists since the days of Fechner regarding the subjective size of a just noticeable difference (DL). Fechner assumed that all DL's are subjectively equal and proceeded forthwith to integrate them in an effort to determine the magnitude of sensation. However, it has been found that summating the same number of DL's for two tones of different frequency does not yield equal loudnesses.[11] Work on equal sense-distances also failed to confirm Fechner's assumption, but suggested that the DL's at high intensities are subjectively larger than those at low intensities, although it could not be said how much larger.[12] It should be noted that we are not here concerned with the constancy of the Weber-fraction, which was *another* of Fechner's assumptions, but only with the problem of subjective magnitude, *i.e.*, the ability of an added just noticeable difference to contribute an increment to the total subjective effect of the stimulus.

If Fechner's first assumption were correct, the summated DL's would yield a function proportional to the loudness function shown in Fig. 1. However, a determination of the number of DL's contained in a 1000 cycle tone as a function of intensity gives the relationship labeled 'No. of DL's' in Fig. 1. This curve was obtained from an integration of Riesz's [13] measurements of differential sensitivity. Riesz's values were multiplied by a constant in order to make the two curves correspond at 100 db and thereby reveal the wide divergence between the two functions. The curve marked 'db loudness scale' has been inserted in an effort to correct the impression that the decibel scale is a fair measure of loudness. If it were, this curve would correspond to the loudness curve.

[11] E. B. Newman, The validity of the just noticeable difference as a unit of psychological magnitude, *Trans. Kansas Acad. Sci.*, 1933, 36, 172–175.

[12] E. B. Titchener, A text-book of psychology, New York, 1910, p. 218. Titchener, however, rejected the implication that the DL's are not equal. He argued that the stimulus-error might have invalidated the measurements of equal sense-distances. A final answer to the question of the relation of summated equal sense-distances to the loudness scale obtained by the procedure outlined in the present paper cannot be given until more adequate measurements have been made.

[13] R. R. Riesz, Loudness and the minimum perceptible increment in intensity, *J. Acoust. Soc. Amer.*, 1933, 4, 211–216.

Now, Fig. 1 shows the relationship between loudness and intensity, and between the number of DL's and intensity. We can proceed, therefore, to determine the relation between the number of DL's and loudness and thereby to measure the one in terms of the other, just as we measure the ratio of one distance to another by determining the relation of each separately to a third scale. The relation turns out to be very nearly exponential as is shown by the fact that, by plotting the two functions in logarithmic coördinates, straight lines are obtained (see Fig. 2). In order to plot these functions for frequencies other than 1000 cycles it was necessary to put the data through the following series of transformations. From the data of Fletcher and Munson [14] the loudness level of the tone was determined as a function of intensity level, and the loudness corresponding to each loudness level was obtained from the loudness curve of Fig. 1. Thence the relation of loudness to intensity level was obtainable. Next the relation of number of DL's to sensation level (db above threshold) was obtained from Riesz's data, and then, by adding the threshold intensity level, the number of DL's as a function of intensity level was found. Hence, knowing the relation of both loudness and number of DL's to the scale of intensity level, we could determine their relation to each other. This computation was made for tones of 200, 4000 and 7000 cycles—the tones for which complete data were available.

In fitting lines to the data in Fig. 2 the best fitting straight line (visually determined) was passed through the points for 200 cycles, and then lines parallel to it were drawn through the other sets. Then, if the lines are taken as defining the relationship between loudness and the number of DL's above threshold, the equation shown in Fig. 2 can be written. The constant K can be determined from the intercepts of the lines with the loudness axis. The exponent is the same for all frequencies because the slopes of the lines are the same. Of course, since the data for the higher frequencies could best be

[14] H. Fletcher and W. A. Munson, Loudness, its definition, measurement and calculation, *J. Acoust. Soc. Amer.*, 1933, 5, 82-108.

fitted by curves slightly concave downward, the exponent is not strictly constant, but the data probably do not warrant

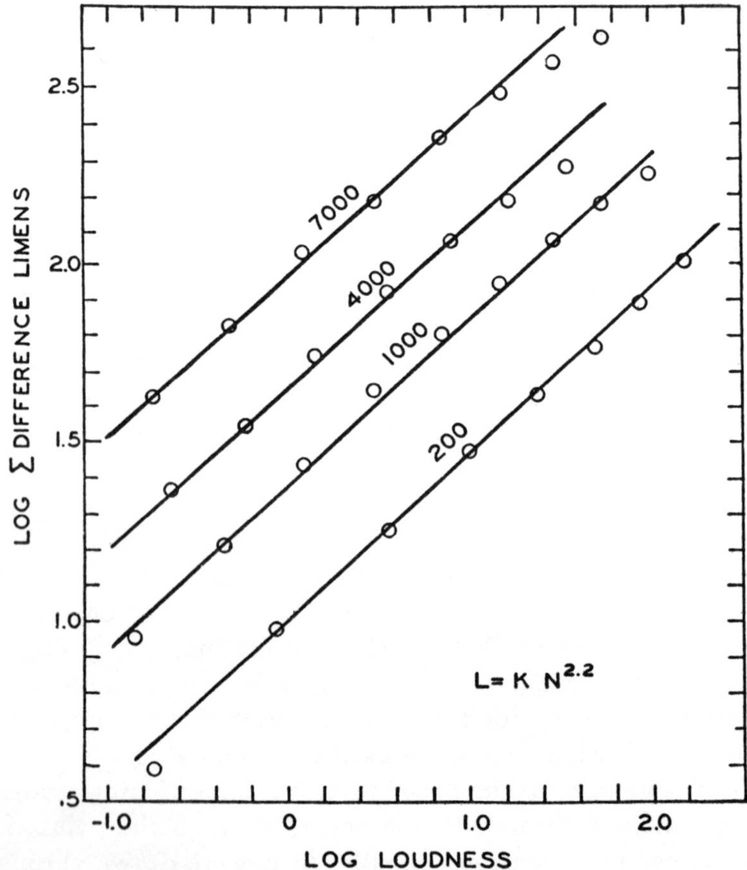

FIG. 2. The relation of loudness to number of DL's for tones of four different frequencies. The points for 7000 cycles have been shifted 0.5 logarithmic units upward on the ordinate scale in order to facilitate plotting, since the function for 7000 cycles lies between those for 1000 and 4000 cycles. L represents loudness, N the number of DL's above threshold and K is a constant determined by the intercepts of the lines on the axis of log loudness at zero value of the ordinate. The values for K are: .0070, .00112, .00028, .00070 for 200, 1000, 4000, and 7000 cycles respectively.

more precision in the determination of the exponent than has been used here. On Fechner's assumption the exponent would be unity.

Now, to measure the size in sones of the first DL above threshold we may set $N = 1$, so that the size becomes equal to the value of K. In Fig. 3 the magnitude of the first DL is plotted as function of the frequency of the tone. The general relationship would be the same for the Nth DL. The DL's for tones at about 3000 cycles are all subjectively smaller than those at other frequencies.

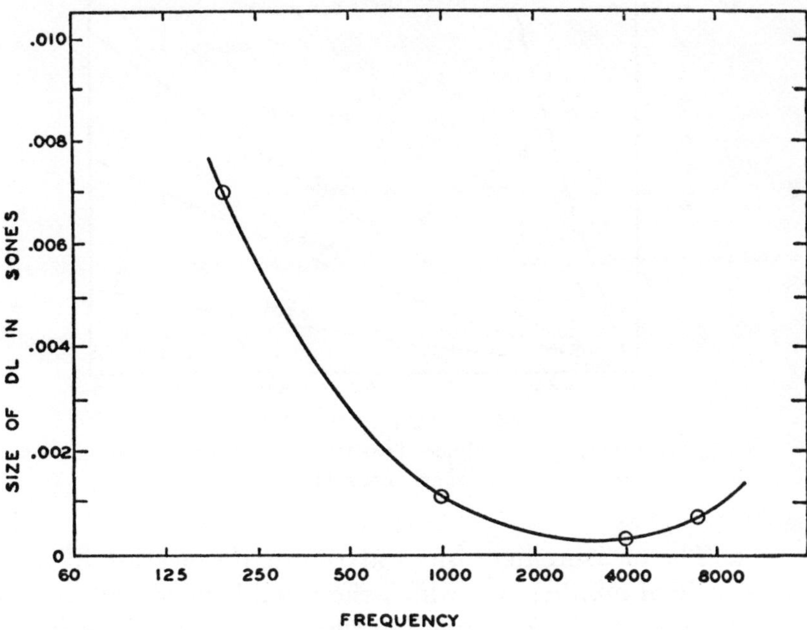

FIG. 3. The variation of the subjective magnitude of the first DL above threshold as a function of frequency. The circles are for the four frequencies for which values were computed. The curve was fitted visually.

Not only does the subjective magnitude of a DL depend upon the frequency of a tone, but it varies also as a function of the number of the DL above threshold. This relationship is shown in Fig. 4. The equation in Fig. 4 relating the size of a DL to its number is obtained by differentiating the equation in Fig. 2. The vast disparity between the subjective magnitudes of different DL's for a tone of given frequency is astonishing in view of the original assumption by which they were considered equal. Their integration for the purpose of obtaining a reasonable numerical scale for the measurement of the magnitude of 'sensation' is obviously not valid.

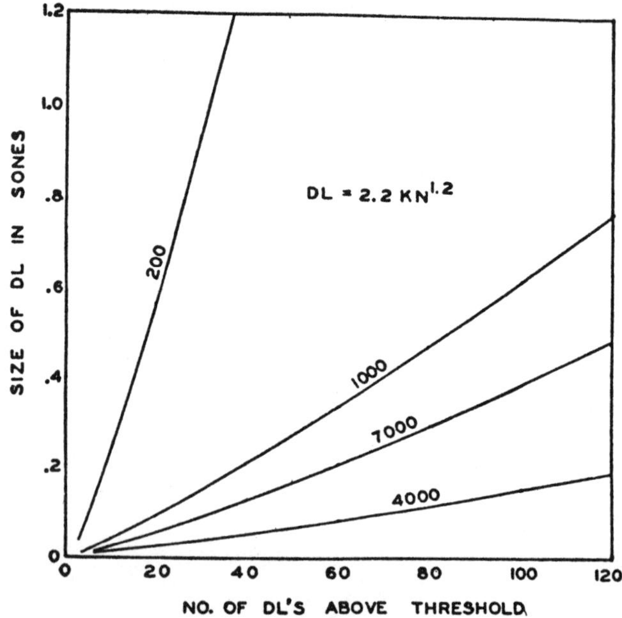

FIG. 4. The subjective magnitude of the DL's as a function of their number above threshold.

SUMMARY

1. The measurement of an attribute of sensation in terms of a scale of numbers for which the usual laws of addition are valid can be achieved providing there exist operations for the determination of fractional values of the attribute.

2. Four methods are available for determining the half value in the case of the attribute loudness.

3. A loudness scale has been erected on the basis of the results of several experiments. It is proposed that the unit of the scale be the loudness of a 1000 cycle tone 40 db above threshold heard with both ears, and that it be called a *sone*.

4. In terms of this scale the subjective magnitude of the just noticeable difference has been measured. The size of DL's is different at different frequencies, and at a fixed frequency it is proportional to the 1.2 power of the number that the DL is above threshold.

Part III

PITCH MECHANISMS AND PITCH PERCEPTION

Editor's Comments on Papers 12 Through 18

12 FLETCHER
The Physical Criterion for Determining the Pitch of a Musical Tone

13 SCHOUTEN
The Perception of Subjective Tones

14 LICKLIDER
A Duplex Theory of Pitch Perception

15 MILLER and TAYLOR
Excerpt from *The Perception of Repeated Bursts of Noise*

16 DAVIS, SILVERMAN, and McAULIFFE
Some Observations on Pitch and Frequency

17 DOUGHTY and GARNER
Excerpt from *Pitch Characteristics of Short Tones. I. Two Kinds of Pitch Threshold*

18 CHIH-AN and CHISTOVICH
Frequency-Difference Limens as a Function of Tonal Duration

Considering that the history of music begins long before that of psychological acoustics, it is scarcely surprising that pitch has occupied the central role from the very beginning of the study of audition. But as experimentation replaced introspection and conjecture, musical considerations exerted progressively less influence on the study of pitch. This state of affairs must be at least partly attributed to the fact that musical listeners find it especially difficult to extend credibility to any simple theory of auditory analysis. For such listeners, the ability to listen to (for example) a vocalist being accompanied by a piano playing the melody in unison, and to hear these two spectrally interwoven signals as two separate, easily distinguished sounds, admits of no simple form of analysis; yet this is one of the very simplest of musical listening tasks. For those who discern effortlessly that it is the clarinet rather than the oboe that produces a particular supporting harmony in a full orchestra passage, the physics of the auditory operation ought to seem even more impressive.

But whatever the approach, it takes but a moment's reflection to convince even the beginning student of psychological acoustics that the primary auditory dimension is pitch. Musical listening aside for the moment, our responses to changes in frequency tell us, for example, whether things are accelerating or decelerating, whether an impact involved a large or a small body, whether a moving source is approaching or receding, whether an incompletely identified source (such as a barking dog) is apt to be large or small, whether wind velocity is increasing or decreasing, and often whether a question is being asked or a positive statement made.

In our discussion of classical psychoacoustics, the development of a laboratory scale of pitch and the exploration of the fineness of frequency resolution was discussed. As we noted, that work was almost solely confined to responses to steady-state pure tone signals. One practical meaning of the statement that pitch occupies a central position in audition is that we make pitch judgments about an extremely wide variety of waveforms. Though individuals vary widely in the nature of their pitch responses and in their pitch discrimination ability, most normal hearers can recognize and reproduce melodic pitch sequences with reasonable accuracy, and for some listeners nearly every sound has pitch as one of its salient attributes. The story of the musician and his friend wandering through the forest may be apocryphal, but it well illustrates how ubiquitous the pitch response may be for some auditors. When a sudden sound occurs and the friend asks "What was that?" the musician immediately replies "B-flat, I think."

Perhaps the most cogent implication of the incident is that pitch responses range themselves along an impressively varied continuum—not only because of the great disparity in the predilection of different listeners for automatically assigning pitch to various sounds but in their widely differing ability to do so even under instruction. If we hold this in mind as we peruse the history of experimentation on pitch, it may help to explain some otherwise puzzling disagreements about pitch behavior. Not always recognized either is the fact that subjects differ also in the *number* of pitches they hear in a complex sound, particularly in those with poorly established fundamentals. Such unwonted sources of variability leave the pitch theorist to face the problem of whether pitch models should encompass what the auditory system *can* do, as exemplified by the unusual—not necessarily musical—listener, or what the average system *does* do in the pitch domain.

However rare the pitch-dominated listener may be, from the earliest recorded history of interest in audition, pitch has occupied a central—one might say the central—role. Undoubtedly one reason this comes about, in addition to the almost universal appeal of music, is the fact that frequency is relatively invariant under the vagaries of sound transmission; this does not hold for intensity or spectrum. Thus on the relevant subjective dimensions, pitch remains invariant in various acoustic environments to a much greater degree than does loudness or timbre.

This preoccupation with pitch concepts in audition has persisted in one form or another since the time of Pythagoras. Long before the development of psychophysics in the experimental sense, the pitch response of listeners was the aspect of audition that interested physicists and philosophers. Quite obviously this was directly related to participation in musical activity. But human powers of frequency discrimination were more a source of wonderment than a potential subject for scientific study.

According to Wever's excellent account (Wever, 1949), the first proposal that mechanical resonance in the ear separated high and low tones for the listener was made by DuVerney in 1683. From this point on, the model of the sympathetically vibrating strings contained in the peripheral auditory mechanism developed, confidently at first and then haltingly in the face of some criticism, until Helmholtz (1863) established it more firmly. From the start, since the impetus came from musical discussion and argument, interest in the functioning of the ear focused on concepts of frequency patterns and frequency discrimination. Almost all of Helmholtz's theorizing about the operation of the auditory system centers on the ability of the human auditory system to analyze complex sounds in the fourier sense and to make both fine distinctions and accurate interval (ratio) judgments in the frequency domain.

Delezenne (1826–1827) evidently was one of the earliest to advance the psychophysically oriented notion that measurements of the pitch-discrimination capabilities of musical listeners should weigh heavily in arguments about the appropriateness of small-frequency distinctions in assigning musical scale values. Though earlier workers disputed the relevance of certain frequency distinctions between musical scales, Delezenne evidently was the first to report some reasonable semblance of a psychophysical approach to a problem dealing with pitch.

The practical problem is the one eventually solved by equal-tempered tuning. For many years before Delezenne, argument arose about the auditory efficacy of the comma—the discrepancy in the tuning of the same note if one arrives at that tuning by successive simple ratios. Beginning with a standard tone and moving up by four successive musical fifths (3:2) one arrives at the same note as by moving up two octaves and a major third (5:4). The numerical discrepancy between these two notes, which on a keyboard instrument must be identical, is 81/80. This is a musical (syntonic) comma. Delezenne desired to show that listeners, both musical and untrained, could distinguish less than this difference.

His test instrument was a single-string sonometer with a string length (between fixed bridges) of 1147mm and marked in millimeter gradations. Its half-length frequency, for checking responses to departures from unison tuning, was 240Hz. Tones for the other intervals in the Delezenne experiment were determined by the ratio required, but they all lay within an octave of middle C.

Delezenne acted as his own experimenter, presenting a pair of tones and asking his subjects to judge whether the interval was sharp or flat as he moved the sonometer bridge (presumably randomly) from the position specified for the mathematically defined position for the given interval. He extracted several judgments from each subject at each position and was very careful not to allow his subjects to be influenced by seeing the changes he made in the position of the movable bridge.

Delezenne reported that at a frequency of 240Hz, his musical listeners could detect a deviation from unison of approximately a quarter of a comma—that is, the ratio of the two notes that could be discriminated was $(81/80)^{0.2807}$. This he characterized as "the extreme limit of sensitivity of the human ear." The outcome for "persons who had never tried to compare sounds" was detection of a departure from unison of $(81/80)^{0.561}$, approximately half a comma.

Delezenne gives only one figure for detectable mistuning of the octave: $2(81/80)^{0.31}$, nearly a third of a comma. This was the change occasioned by moving the bridge of the sonometer 1mm, apparently the smallest change attempted for the octave. Presumably this is for the expert ear. It seems unexpectedly small for that interval in view of the now-well-established fact that the subjectively satisfactory octave is greater than the precise 2:1 ratio.

For the musical interval of the fifth (3:2), Delezenne gives a figure of only about one-sixth of a comma for musical persons to detect mistuning and nearly twice that—about a third of a comma—for other persons. For the major third, the only figure given appears to be for skilled listening and is close to a fourth of a comma: $(81/80)^{0.284}$.

For those who think of pitch-discrimination skills in terms of

$\Delta f/f$, Delezenne's measurements give the following values in percentages:

	Musician	Unskilled
Unison	0.36	0.73
Octave	0.40	
Fifth	0.21	0.43
Major third	0.36	

Delezenne's work is of special interest in psychological acoustics because he used a number of listeners, both trained and untrained, he carefully kept extraneous clues from intruding, he tried to control loudness, and he reported his results in log units of his basic interval, the comma.

Thus his effort is well worth noting since it occurred prior to the rise of experimental sensory psychology, yet in principle and in rough outline, it resembles the experiments of several decades later. It was nearly coincident with the very beginnings of quantification of sensory magnitudes in Germany. Fechner's *Elemente der Psychophysik* did not appear until more than thirty years later.

A better grasp of the nature of pitch developed during the ensuing decades. Seebeck (1841), with his siren experiments, raised the question of the relative importance of having energy at the fundamental versus responding to waveform pulsing rate. Ohm (1843), supported by Helmholtz, insisted on the importance of spectral definition: energy at the fundamental frequency. This whole discussion was coincident with the search for anatomically identifiable resonant elements in the auditory system, and such nonresonance hypotheses as Seebeck's created but little stir. Rutherford's telephone theory (1886) never was juxtaposed with Seebeck's suggestion that periodicity itself might be the primary factor mediating the pitch sensation.

With the advent of the electronic transmission of sound, the problem arose in a different guise: Why did apparent pitch remain the same over a telephone system that did not transmit low frequencies? The phenomenon could be verified with other kinds of filters. Fletcher approached the problem with the equipment available at the Bell Laboratories in the manner, and with the results, shown in Paper 12. He concluded that the nonlinear response of the middle ear reintroduced energy at the fundamental frequency and thus maintained the original pitch of the complex tone in spite of filtering. The rationale for this conclusion drew heavily on the use of an exploring tone to locate tones attributable to nonlinearity in the mechanical auditory system. Fletcher's example of the effects of nonlinear distortion on the low end of the spectrum is particularly intriguing. Considering that each of the ten equally strong partials of the complex tone used as 114dB SPL (100 dynes/cm^2) and from ten different oscillators, the overall sound pressure level impressed on the middle ear was 124dB. One hopes the implied inner ear spectrum in his figure 3c was calculated rather than actually measured by the exploring tone method.

Fletcher's concepts of the restoration of fundamental pitch coincided with the Helmholtz version. But by the time of his 1929 book, *Speech and Hearing,* Fletcher specifically stated that these perceptions could also be accounted for by the timing pattern of nerves responding to the higher potentials of the complex tone. Stevens and Davis (1938) subscribed explicitly to the Fletcher version without even a mention of Seebeck's experiments. It is fascinating, from the superior vantage point of four decades later, to contrast the treatment by Stevens and Davis of what was later to emerge as periodicity pitch with that by Wever. Wever and Bray (1937) unequivocally subscribed to the concept of a pitch mediated by rate of nerve impulses. They asserted:

> As the discharge from the segment of the basilar membrane common to the two beating tones approaches a smooth wave, it gives in perception a rough low tone, of a pitch corresponding to the rate of beats (beat-tone or difference tone). An increase in the beat frequency gives a tone of higher pitch and smoother quality, as the volleys of nerve discharges become more rapid and more continuous. The point of this theory is that a series of nervous discharges, with a rate of, say, 30 per second, will give rise to a tone of the same pitch, regardless of the place of origin in the cochlea: regardless of whether the discharge arises in the action of the basilar membrane as a whole (or a large section of it), or in the action of some limited region of that membrane under the influence of two adjacent, interacting frequencies. [P. 113]

Later in the same article they made a still more adventuresome statement:

> We do not deny the existence of middle-ear distortion; no doubt it appears for stimuli that are sufficiently strong. Thus it may happen that under particular circumstances the same low tone is doubly represented in the action of the ear: directly in the response of the cochlea through distortion in the middle ear, and also in the interaction of two adjacent frequencies in the membrane. [P. 114]

But these views on pitch from interacting adjacent frequencies were definitely not endorsed by Stevens and Davis. Their book, published a year later than the article just quoted, was easily the most influential work in audition for the next few decades. Whereas Wever believed, as we have seen, that a beating complex becomes tonal as beats increase beyond about thirty per second and that the perceptual result is a pitch, Stevens and Davis, in their rather complete discussion of beating phenomena and roughness, studiously avoid the pitch label, using it only once in reference to Wever's work on beats.

One should not imply that any of these workers was unaware, even during this early period, of the efficacy of neural time patterns in auditory processing. In his "Space Time Pattern Theory of Hearing," Fletcher (1930) incorporated the time pattern of neural firings as part of the message from the ear to the brain and specifically noted that at least up to 500Hz, and probably further, this should afford a cue for the pitch of pure tones. Stevens and Davis (1936) were among the first to be acquainted with the frequency-following properties of the auditory nerves but thought they saw problems with postulating neural periodicity as the physiological correlate of pitch.

In the same year of the Stevens and Davis publication, Schouten began a series of highly useful reports. The first of them appears here as Paper 13. One incidental and long-unrecognized service he performed was to point out the untenable nature of the use of the beats of exploring tones ("best beats") to measure subjective harmonics. But more immediately relevant to our scanning of the history of pitch, he separated the two kinds of of pitches that occur when the lower partials are missing from a complex tone. In a later paper (Schouten, 1940), he named the second kind of pitch—the one not attributable to energy at the fundamental—the *residue,* the pitch that remains if one cancels out the difference-tone distortion that appears at the frequency of the fundamental, and which has a different perceptual quality than the fundamental sinusoid of the same pitch. This is precisely the pitch postulated by Wever and Bray (1937). Thus nearly a century had gone by before Seebeck's idea that periodicity rather than spectral location could be the basis for pitch was revived independently by Wever and Bray and by Schouten and was soon theoretically supported by Licklider's duplex theory of pitch (Paper 14). Licklider acknowledged the influence of the work of Schouten, of Miller and Taylor (Paper 15) on interrupted noise, and of Davis, Silverman, and McAuliffe (Paper 16) on filtered click trains. And, of course, Wever had espoused the notion of time-pattern pitches long before, but there was by no means complete agreement on the interpretation of these data. Garner (1952) attacked the idea of a time-oriented pitch mechanism on the grounds of parsimony. He definitely discredited the idea that the work of Miller and Taylor and of Davis et al. required a new mechanism of pitch perception. Apparently the earlier Schouten work had little influence before 1950.

Over the two decades following the Licklider exposition, there were a number of investigations of pitches that appeared to be time-pattern mediated—notably the work of Thurlow and Small (1955) on sweep pitch, Cramer and Huggins (1958) on binaurally created pitch, McClellan and Small (1967) on time separation pitch, and Fourcin (1965) and Bilsen (1966) on repetition pitch. Plomp (1966) did perhaps the most complete marshalling of experimental evidence for the effect, both from his own work and previous investigators. Later, however, he became persuaded that spectral cues are likely to be the predominant ones (Plomp, 1975, 1976).

The demonstration by Miller and Taylor in 1948 (Paper 15) that subjects could match the pitch of a sinusoid or a square wave to the interruption rate of a white noise was welcomed by some as proof positive that time pattern alone can mediate a pitch response. It is the forerunner of a whole series of experiments on the possibility of pitch sensation in the absence of spectral clues that is worth tracing separately. Over the three decades since that experiment, experts have remained about evenly divided on whether periodically interrupted noise contributed anything useful to the understanding of the pitch response. Actually three camps can be identified: The "unbelievers" are persuaded that a bona fide match cannot be made—that all results can be explained by the presence of a not-completely-masked train of switching transients making audible a conventional pulse train of the appropriate period. (See Pollack, 1969, for a précis of this view.) Of a similar persuasion are those who point out that, in spite of retaining a long-term flat spectrum, interruption of a given rate yields an increased variance in the spectrum at points related to the interruption rate. This offers the possibility of a spectral clue for those not comfortable with time-oriented pitch.

The second group embraces those who believe the match is indeed made to the interruption rate, but that labeling it a pitch match is erroneous because listeners report no feeling of tonality. Garner (1952) asked that we retain the distinction between "intermittency" and pitch, implying that the former was involved in the matches of interrupted noise to tonal signals. Plomp (1976) expresses this view very carefully when he says, "Using the word 'pitch' in the instructions, the author assumed that his subjects 'matched some property of the stimulus that, by their own admission, may or may not be related to pitch'" (p. 130). Measurements by Harris (1963), Campbell (1963), and Ritsma and Hoekstra (1974) seem to agree that the jnd for both interrupted noise and other periodicity pitch is close to 2 percent and thus suspiciously larger than the jnd for tonal pitch in the same range.

The third group finds interrupted noise sufficiently tonal that melodies "played" by changing interruption rates can be recognized (Viemeister and Burns, 1975) and musical intervals identified, though not as confidently as those produced with conventional tones (Burns and Viemeister, 1976; Wicke and Houtsma, 1975). Burns and Viemeister employed a sinusoidal (100 percent) modulation and took admirable precautions to minimize unwanted spectral cues. We are left with considerable puzzlement about the failure of some previous experimenters to achieve a tonal experience or, worse still, to effect even a suitable match. Bilsen (1977) recently reported that in an experiment in his laboratory using experienced observers, "for an on-time fraction of, for example, 50%, all observers were unable to hear a periodicity pitch, not even a sensation of tonality." Perhaps the naturally wide range of pitch skill and behavior and the small subject samples conspire to create these disturbing discrepancies.

For many years the investigation of pitch perception in the laboratory has been narrower in scope than one might predict from the prevalence of pitch-related responses in everyday listening. Much of the usefulness of the pitch response as sensory information deals with recognition of fairly rapid frequency changes. Even in much of music listening, this principle holds. Yet only a modest proportion of experimental work on pitch deals with temporal patterns of pitch or with pitch of impulsive sounds. Part of this lack should be attributed to the absence of suitable transducers for such experiments. In fact, one must consider that early experimenters exploring the pitch of transient signals worked with formidable limitations.

One early study that was highly regarded was an effort by Bürck, Kotowski, and Lichte (1935), who presented their subjects with two very short, immediately adjacent tone bursts. They changed the length of the two bursts and asked their subjects to report at what duration the bursts became tonal. The criterion for tonality was the hearing of two pitches rather than a single short burst of sound. They found that with a separation of about a full musical tone between the two frequencies, each of the tones had to last about 10msec to lead to two discriminable pitches.

A little earlier Kucharski (1930) had taken a quite different approach to the same problem. He used widely separated frequencies but very short durations. When he had his subjects compare 750Hz and 1000Hz at durations of only about 0.5msec, he found they could distinguish the two pitches and that his musical listeners recognized the interval as a fourth. Similarly for single-cycle presentations of 100Hz and 150Hz, he reported that his five listeners could hear the pitch difference and that four of them identified the musical interval as a fifth.

The modern counterpart of these studies is found in a report by Wier and Green (1975). They presented their subjects with two short contiguous tonal bursts, or rather they presented a single tone burst of two equal segments that changed frequency after the first segment. These two-frequency bursts were always presented in pairs with the order of frequency reversed for the second member of the pair. The subjects indicated which member of the pair proceeded from high to low. With large frequency separation—from 1kHz to 2kHz—subjects could perform close to 90 percent correct down to durations of 2msec for a single segment. When the frequency separation was smaller, discernment of the direction of frequency change was more difficult, but for the same 2msec duration performance was still about 75 percent for a frequency separation of 25 percent (a musical major third).

The two earlier studies seem to arise from the view that there is a certain minimum duration at which periodic signals achieve tonality. This they have in common with the approach taken by Doughty and Garner about a dozen years later in 1947. Since this is a study often cited by American authors as the basis for believing there is a definite duration threshold for tone pitch, the experimental part of that paper is reproduced here (Paper 17). Even though these same authors did a companion study on pitch as a function of duration (Doughty and Garner, 1948), they concerned themselves there with only the question of a pitch change with duration. They were not concerned with the relevance of the $\Delta f \Delta t$ question to pitch perception.

If one believes, as I do, that the pitch response to short signals is the most useful area for the study of pitch, then the orientation proposed by Doughty and Garner in 1947 is a step in the wrong direction. Doughty and Garner chose to dichotomize the pitch response into "tone pitch" and "click pitch," and they explored the "threshold" for these two types of pitch response. The report is included here because it has frequently been cited—and still is—as the basis for the clean separation between tonal pitch and nontonal pitch. One of its historical antecedents has been the conviction that it takes a specific minimal number of cycles of a driving frequency to elicit a pitch response. Kucharski's results should have dispelled this notion, but subsequent history indicates it did not do so. As recently as 1967, Pollack was interested in establishing the "tonal threshold" for pulse trains.

Békésy (1929) held a much more defensible view of the way one should establish the lower limit of duration for signals to possess the pitch attribute. How confidently a signal can be said to possess pitch depends on the precision with which it can be matched. Békésy showed that at 800Hz, the difference limen for frequency, $\Delta f/f$, changed from about 0.003 to nearly 0.01 as duration was decreased from 375msec to about 15msec.

Békésy's suggestion that the jnd in frequency is a function of the signal's duration for any short tones was developed further by Turnbull (1944), who plotted for three widely spaced frequencies (128Hz, 1024Hz, and 8192Hz) the increase in frequency difference necessary to maintain a 75 percent correct pitch discrimination performance. One noteworthy aspect of Turnbull's report is his recognition that performance of the transducer is crucial for short signals. Turnbull viewed his output waveforms on an oscilloscope and made the visual judgment that at 128Hz, for example, the first three cycles were primarily "transients." Noting that one of his subjects still achieved 75 percent correct when the driving signal was applied to the transducer for less than three cycles, Turnbull wisely concluded that there could have been "a characteristic difference between the transients produced by the two frequencies distinguished." This point is developed further later on.

The conviction that neural processing improves on the frequency resolution of the cochlea motivated Liang and Chistovich (Paper 18) to repeat and extend Turnbull's work on the dependence of pitch discrimination on tonal duration. These authors were interested in imposing some physiological lawfulness on the form of the function, though considering the small number of listeners, the limitations of equipment and the post hoc nature of the rationale offered, it must be considered only a beginning.

Cardozo (1962) pursued the notion of a time-frequency uncertainty principle in interpreting his data on the pitch of short tonal pulses. His measurements at 1kHz indicate that the jnd for tone-burst durations greater than 50msec is 0.001f and that for durations less than this, the data fit the expression, $\Delta f \cdot \Delta t = 5 \times 10^{-2}$. Liang and Chistovich preferred a different expression to fit their data over this same range of duration, but Cardozo's formulation could easily fit their results. Ronken (1971), making measurements at a single frequency, used the signal envelope to control effective bandwidth and measured the jnd (Δf_{75}) over a comparable range of durations. Ronken's data seem to indicate that effective duration of signal is more important than the spectrum shape imposed by the envelope in determining pitch-discrimination ability in the range of durations below about 50msec. Ronken's gaussian-envelope data actually fit Cardozo's $\Delta f \Delta t$ constant of 0.05 much better than Cardozo's own data.

There are good reasons for proceeding as Ronken did by selecting the envelope that represents the desired correspondence between spectrum spread and effective duration before attempting to explain the short-duration limits of tonal signals. A number of independent experiments have shown that pitch can be reliably assigned to the period between two transients. Jenkins-Lee (1971) took great pains to produce acoustic signals that, measured in the ear canal, departed negligibly from single-cycle sinusoids. He found that the direction of a change of 10 percent in frequency (period) could be detected with a probability of 75 percent. However, if even those "ideal" signals generate a period-related onset and offset transient—perhaps in the cochlea—then an unwanted aspect of the signal is affording a rewarding clue (to the subject), and the wrong conclusions can be drawn.

There has been a gradually increasing recognition of a strong dependence of pitch precision—and probably also of pitch quality—on signal duration, for short signals. But it was not until over forty years after Stewart (1931) pointed out the relevance of the uncertainty principle that Moore (1973) used the $\Delta f \cdot \Delta t$ model at a sufficient number of frequencies and durations to test its adequacy. Moore's conclusion is that time pattern appears to mediate the pitch response to short tonal signals up to a frequency around 5000Hz, above which place, or spectrum, takes over. We have noted earlier the evidence that around this same frequency pitch discrimination deteriorates rapidly for long tonal signals. Siebert (1970) had already pointed out that in theory either periodicity or place clues could yield enough precision to account for the auditory discrimination data available.

Even considering the variability of results from different experiments, these analyses indicate a most impressive frequency analyzer for short tonal signals. Oddly, many experts (see for example Pollack, 1969; Gulick, 1971, p. 142) appear to prefer the dichotomy promulgated (perhaps unintentionally) by Doughty and Garner's 1947 report. Perhaps the psychologist's predilection for categorical perception contexts underlies the preference.

BINAURAL PITCH

Occasionally evidence has been presented that the pitch response can be elicited with cues that exist only in signal relations between the two ears—that is, that a particular pitch will be heard solely as the result of the manner in which the two signals are combined through binaural processing. The interaural signal configurations that have been used are most unlikely to occur in ordinary listening, but the results indicate that pitch processing can—not necessarily does—take place centrally. These reports have had a rather dramatic influence on theories of pitch perception. When Cramer and Huggins (1958) demonstrated the creating of a pitch through a particular interaural phase relation over one segment of the spectrum of a noise with no spectral or temporal clues in either monaural signal, Licklider's duplex theory of pitch perception became a triplex theory (Licklider, 1959) to accommodate the phenomenon. Similarly when Houtsma and Goldstein (1971) created a "missing fundamental" pitch from one harmonic partial in each ear, extant models for pitch processing felt obliged to accommodate this new phenomenon. Bilsen (1977), noting that there are a number of interaural phase configurations for which pairs of harmonically spaced narrow bands of noise can produce the equivalent of Schouten's residue pitch, reasoned that for both monaural and dichotic* signals, pitch processing is best described by the creation of a central spectrum. This is then scanned for spectral peaks, followed by "calculation" of the best-fitting harmonic spectrum.

*The term *dichotic* is used for signals delivered to the two ears through phones with one or more interaural parameters controlled more extensively than is possible when only distance and the presence of the head determine the difference between the two ears.

Presumably distinctly binaural melodies can be created as Schroeder (1959) did monaurally, by sequential interaural phase shifts of appropriately chosen harmonics, much as Kubovy and Cutting (1974) did with interaural time delay of selected tones from a tone cluster. Even the controversial pitch of periodically interrupted noise could probably be created exclusively binaurally by an extension of the technique used by Nieder and Creelman (1965), who created the appearance of a central pitch by having in the opposite ear a continuous (uninterrupted) version of the interrupted noise. Had they filled the silent periods in the interrupted ear with an uncorrelated noise, the pitch should appear only when signal is present at both ears.

For such reasons, pitch still continues to be the area of psychological acoustics that generates much interest and some controversy. Rather than funnelling toward a single model of pitch perception, we have several competing ones, and these still fail to encompass a large proportion of recognized pitch phenomena.

REFERENCES

Békésy, G. V. 1929. Zur theorie des hörens: Über die eben merkbare amplituden- und frequenz-änderung eines tones; die theorie des schwebungen physik. *Zeitschrift* **30**:721–745.

Bilsen, F. A. 1966. Repetition pitch: Monaural interaction of a sound with the same, but phase shifted sound. *Acustica* **17**:295–300.

Bilsen, F. A. 1977. Pitch of noise signals: Evidence for a "central" spectrum. *Acoust. Soc. Am. J.* **61**:150–161.

Bürck, W., P. Kotowski, and H. Lichte. 1935. Die hörbarkeit von laufzeitdifferenzen. *Elektr. Nachr. Tec.* **12**:355–367.

Burns, E. M., and N. F. Viemeister. 1976. Nonspectral pitch. *Acoust. Soc. Am. J.* **60**:863–869.

Campbell, R. A. 1963. Frequency discrimination of pulsed tones. *Acoust Soc. Am. J.* **35**:1193–1200.

Cardozo, B. L. 1962. Frequency discrimination of the human ear. *Fourth Int. Cong. Acoust., Copenhagen, Paper H16.*

Cramer, E. M., and W. H. Huggins. 1958. Creation of pitch through binaural interaction. *Acoust. Soc. Am. J.* **30**:413–417.

Delezenne, M. 1826–1827. Sur les valeurs numèriques des notes de la gamme. *Recl. Trav. Soc. Sci. Agric., Arts de Lille.* **8**:1–57.

Doughty, J. M., and W. R. Garner. 1948. Pitch characteristics of short tones. II. Pitch as a function of tonal duration. *J. Exp. Psychol.* **38**:478–494.

DuVerney, J. G. 1683. *Traité de l'organe de l'ouie.* Paris.

Fletcher, H. 1930. A space time pattern theory of hearing. *Acoust. Soc. Am. J.* **1**: 311–343.

Fourcin, A. J. 1965. The pitch of noise with periodic spectral peaks. *Fourth Int. Congr. Acoust., Copenhagen, Paper B42.*

Garner, W. R. 1952. Hearing. *Annl. Rev. Psychol.* **3**:85–104.

Gulick, W. A. 1971. *Hearing: physiology and psychophysics.* New York: Oxford University Press.

Harris, G. G. 1963. Periodicity perception using gated noise. *Acoust. Soc. Am. J.* **35**:1229–1233.

Helmholtz, H. L. F. von. 1863. *Sensations of tone.* New York: Dover (reprint ed., 1954).

Houtsma, A. J. M., and J. Goldstein. 1971. Perception of musical intervals: Evidence for the central origin of the pitch of complex tones. *MIT Res. Lab. Elec. Tech. Rep. 484.*

Jenkins-Lee, J. E. 1971. Pitch perception for minimum tone bursts: Single periods. Ph.D. diss. Stanford University.

Kubovy, M., and J. E. Cutting. 1974. Hearing with the third ear: Dichotic perception of a melody without monaural familiarity cues. *Science* **186**:272–275.

Kucharski, P. 1930. Nouvelles expériences sur les facteurs determinants de la sensation tonale. *C. R. Soc. Biol.* **104**:1249–1252.

Licklider, J. C. R. 1959. Three auditory theories. In *Psychology: A study of a science,* ed. S. Koch, pp. 141–144. New York: McGraw-Hill.

McClellan, M. E., and A. M. Small, Jr. 1967. Pitch perception of pulse pairs with random repetition rate. *Acoust. Soc. Am. J.* **41**:690–699.

Moore, B. C. J. 1973. Frequency difference limens for short-duration tones. *Acoust. Soc. Am. J.* **54**:610–619.

Nieder, P. L., and C. D. Creelman. 1965. Central periodicity pitch. *Acoust. Soc. Am. J.* **37**:136–138.

Ohm, G. S. 1843. Über die definition des tones, nebst daran geknüpfter theorie de Sirene und ähnlicher tonbildender vorrichtungen. *Annu. Phys. Chem.* **59**: 513–565.

Plomp, R. 1966. *Experiments on tone perception.* Soesterberg, Netherlands: Institute for Perception RVO-TNO.

Plomp, R. 1975. Auditory psychophysics. *Annu. Rev. Psychol.* **26**:207–232.

Plomp, R. 1976. *Aspects of Tone Sensation.* New York: Academic Press.

Pollack, I. 1967. Number of pulses required for minimal pitch. *Acoust. Soc. Am. J.* **42**:895 (L).

Pollack, I. 1969. Periodicity pitch for interrupted white noise—fact or artifact? *Acoust. Soc. Am. J.* **45**:237–238 (L).

Ritsma, R. J., and A. Hoekstra. 1974. Frequency selectivity and the tonal residue. In *Facts and models in hearing,* ed. E. Zwicker and E. Terhardt, pp. 156–163. Berlin: Springer-Verlag.

Ronken, D. A. 1971. Some effects of bandwidth-duration constraints on frequency discrimination. *Acoust. Soc. Am. J.* **49**:1232–1242.

Rutherford, W. A. 1886. A new theory of hearing. *J. Anat. Physiol.* **21**:166–168.

Schouten, J. F. 1940. The residue, a new component in subjective sound analysis. *K. ned. Akad. Wet. Proc.* **43**:356–365.

Schroeder, M. R. 1959. New results concerning monaural phase sensitivity. *Acoust. Soc. Am. J.* **31**:1579 (A).

Seebeck, A. 1941. Beobachtungen über einige bedingungen der entstehung von tönen. *Ann. Phys. Chem.* **53**:417–436.

Siebert, W. M. 1970. Frequency discrimination in the auditory system: Place or periodicity mechanisms. *IEEE Proc.* **58**:723–730.

Stevens, S. S. and H. Davis. 1936. Psychophysiological acoustics: Pitch and loudness. *Acoust. Soc. Am. J.* **8**:1–13.

Stevens, S. S., and H. Davis. 1938. *Hearing: Its psychology and physiology.* New York: Wiley.

Stewart, G. W. 1931. Problems suggested by an uncertainty principle in acoustics. *Acoust. Soc. Am. J.* **2**:325–329.

Thurlow, W. R., and A. Small, 1955. Pitch perception for certain periodic auditory stimuli. *Acoust. Soc. Am. J.* **27**:132–137.

Turnbull, W. W. 1944. Pitch discrimination as a function of tonal duration. *J. Exp. Psychol.* **34**:302–316.

Viemeister, N. F., and E. M. Burns. 1975. Nonspectral pitch. *Acoust. Soc. Am. J.* **58**:S83 (A).

Wever, E. G. 1949. *Theory of hearing.* New York: Wiley.

Wever, E. G., and C. W. Bray. 1937. The perception of low tones and the resonance-volley theory. *J. Psychol.,* **3**:101–114.

Wicke, R. W., and A. J. M. Houtsma. 1975. Musical pitch of interrupted white noise. *Acoust. Soc. Am. J.* **58**:S83 (A).

Wier, C. C., and D. M. Green. 1975. Temporal acuity as a function of frequency difference. *Acoust. Soc. Am. J.* **57**:1512–1515.

12

Reprinted from *Phys. Rev.* 23:427–437 (1924)

THE PHYSICAL CRITERION FOR DETERMINING THE PITCH OF A MUSICAL TONE

By Harvey Fletcher

Abstract

Effects upon pitch and quality of musical sounds of eliminating certain component frequencies.—A high quality telephone system was used to reproduce musical sounds from the voice, the piano, the violin, the clarinet and the organ without any appreciable distortion. Into this telephone system electrical filters were introduced which made it possible to eliminate any desired frequency range. Results with this system show that only the quality and not the pitch of such musical sounds changes when a group of either the low or high frequency components is eliminated. Even when the fundamental and first seven overtones were eliminated from the vowel *ah* sung at an ordinary pitch for a baritone, the pitch remained the same. These results were checked by a study of synthesized musical tones produced by ten vacuum tube oscillators, with frequencies from 100 to 1000 at intervals of 100. It was found that three consecutive component frequencies were sufficient to give a clear musical tone of definite pitch corresponding to 100, and that in general when the adjacent components had a constant difference which was a common factor to all components, a single musical tone of pitch equal to this common difference was obtained, but not otherwise. *Explanation of the results in terms of mechanism of the ear.* Recent work on hearing has shown that the transmission mechanism between the air and the inner ear has a non-linear response which accounts for the so-called subjective tones. When the components of low frequency are eliminated from the externally impressed musical tone, they are again introduced as subjective tones before the sound reaches the nerve terminals. Calculation of the magnitude of these subjective tones from the non-linear constants of the ear shows that the results on pitch are what might be expected.

Sound spectra of ten typical musical sounds, obtained with an electrical automatic harmonic analyser to be described by Wegel and Moore, are given for *ah* sung at pitch d, $\bar{a}$ sung at a, piano c_1, piano c', violin g', clarinet c, organ pipe c_1 for three pressures, and organ pipe c'.

THIS paper describes some experiments which show that the fundamental and a large number of harmonics from a compound tone may be eliminated without changing the pitch of the tone. This is contrary to the general belief that the pitch of a musical tone is determined by the vibration frequency of the fundamental. Although the idea of producing a musical tone which has a lower pitch than that corresponding to any single component frequency is not entirely new, the extent to which this method of producing low pitched tones can be carried has not been appreciated.

Composition of Musical Tones

A musical tone is usually composed of a large number of component frequencies. In the voice and in most musical instruments, it is well known that these components are harmonics, i.e. the component frequencies stand in the ratios of the integers 1, 2, 3, etc.; the characteristic quality of the tone is determined by their relative magnitudes.

Sound spectra for various types of musical sounds are shown in Fig. 1. In the charts shown in this figure the abscissas give the frequency in

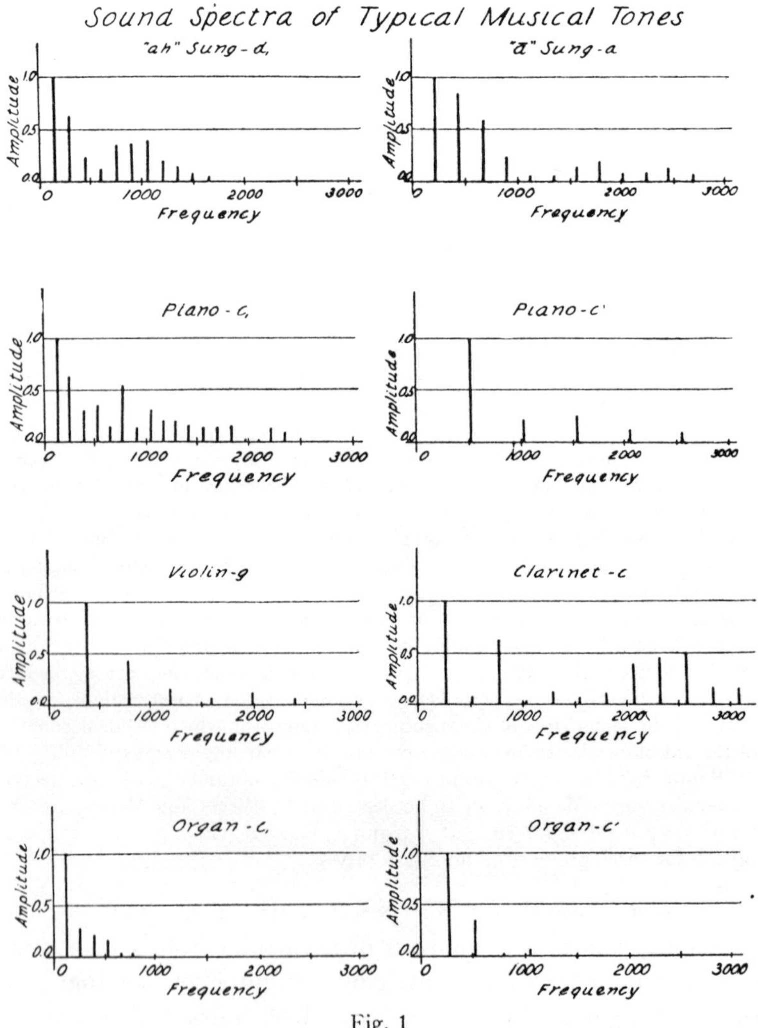

Fig. 1

double vibrations, or cycles per second. The ordinates give the relative amplitude of the harmonics, plotting the fundamental as unity. The spectra for the piano represent the average values of the components during the first few seconds after the strings are struck. The sound spectra for organ pipes change very markedly when the blowing pressure changes. Those shown represent a typical case.

The analyses of these tones were made by the electrical harmonic analyzer which has been recently developed in the Bell System Research Laboratories. A full report covering the design and operation of this analyzer will soon be published by Wegel and Moore,[1] who are responsible for its development. The sounds to be analyzed are picked up by a condenser transmitter[2] which converts the sound wave into a faithful electrical copy. This electrical copy of the sound wave is ther amplified and sent into the electrical harmonic analyzer for analysis. The analyzer consists essentially of a resonant circuit for which the frequency of resonance may be varied from 80 to 6,000 in steps of only a few cycles. Consecutive readings of the current transmitted through this circuit for each value of the resonant frequency are recorded photographically. The operations are entirely automatic, so that it requires only about five minutes from the time the machine is started until a completed picture of the sound spectrum comes out of the camera-box.

Measurement of the Pitch of a Musical Tone

The pitch of a tone as usually understood is the place on the musical scale to which the tone is referred. A pure tone,—that is, one consisting of a single component or frequency—has a definite pitch which anyone experienced in music will correlate with that frequency. By changing the frequency of such a pure tone its pitch can be made the same as that of any compound musical tone. Consequently a vibration frequency number can be associated with each pitch although, as will be seen presently, a component having such a frequency may not be present in the musical tone. The pitches as used in this paper are expressed on the International Tempered Scale, $a=435$ cycles per second.

The pitch of the musical tones used in this investigation were determined by comparison with a standard, giving a fairly pure tone. This standard tone was produced by a telephone receiver, which was connected to a vacuum tube oscillator. Its pitch was adjusted to any desired value by making the proper setting on the oscillator.

The question might be asked, What happens to a tone if some of the upper harmonics are eliminated? Its is well known that the pitch is

[1] Wegel and Moore, presented before A.I.E.E. at Philadelphia, Feb. 8, 1924
[2] Wente, Phys. Rev. (2) **10**, 39, 1917

TABLE 1

Effect of the Elimination of Various Components on the Pitch and Quality of Various Musical Sounds

Source	Pitch	Eliminated components	Eliminated frequencies	Pitch change	Quality
Voice–*ah*	*d*(145)	F	0–250	No change	Inappreciable change
		F & 1–2	0–500	" "	Small change
		F & 1–4	0–750	" "	Large change
		F & 1–7	0–1250	" "	Very large change
		F & 1–9	0–1500	Uncertain	Noise
		6–∞	1000–∞	No change	Small change
		3–∞	500–∞	" "	Large change
		F & 1–2 & 6–∞	0–500 & 1000–∞	" "	Very large change
Voice–*ā*	*a*(218)	F	0–250	No change	Slight change
		F & 1–2	0–750	" "	Sounds like *ah*
		F & 1–4	0–1250	" "	Small change
		F & 1–5	0–1500	" "	Between *ah* & *ō*
		6–∞	1500–∞	" "	"
		3–∞	750–∞	" "	Sounds like *ō*
		F & 1–2 & 8–∞	0–750 & 2000–∞	" "	Very weak *ah*
Piano	*c*(129)	F	0–250	No change	Small change
		F & 1–2	0–500	" "	Metallic
		F & 1–5	0–750	" "	Clanging
		For more harmonics eliminated the tone lost all musical character			
		6–∞	750–∞	No change	No brilliance
Piano	*c''*(517)	F'	0–750	No change	Small change
		F & 1	0–1250	" "	Metallic
		All harmonics	750–∞	" "	Pure tone; Musical brilliance lacking
Violin	*g'*(388)	F	0–500	No change	Large change
		F & 1	0–1000	" "	Very large change
		F & 1–2	0–1500	Uncertain	Non-musical
		2–∞	1000–∞	No change	Violin quality gone
Clarinet	*c'*(259)	F	0–500	No change	Large change
		F & 1–2	0–1000	" "	Very large change
		F & 1–4	0–1500	" "	Non-musical
		7–∞	2000–∞	" "	Large change
		2–∞	750–∞	" "	Pure tone (no clarinet quality)
Organ pipe	*c*(129)	F	0–250	No change	Small change
		F & 1–2	0–500	" "	Large change
		F & 1–4	0–750	Uncertain	Noise
		15–∞	2000–∞	No change	Very small change
		6–∞	750–∞	" "	Small change
Organ pipe	*c'*(259)	F	0–500	No change	Large change
		F & 1–2	0–1000	Uncertain	Non-musical
			2000–∞	No change	Small change
			750–∞	" "	Sounds dull

unaltered, but the quality of the tone is changed. An equally interesting question is, What happens to a tone if the fundamental and some of the lower harmonics are eliminated? The answer to this question is the same as to the first one, namely, the pitch remains the same but the quality is altered.

Results

For the purpose of obtaining quantitative data relating to this question, use was made of the high-quality telephone system which has been described in previous papers.[3] The efficiency of this telephone system is approximately constant for the various frequencies throughout the range used in this investigation. Also, for the range of intensities which were used, the system has a linear response, so that no frequencies other than those in driving force were introduced. Consequently, the sound coming out of the receiver is a faithful copy of that which goes into the transmitter. Electrical filters[4] were introduced into this system, so that any portion of the spectrum could be eliminated. The characteristics of these filters were such that the amplitudes of the eliminated harmonics were reduced to values between .001 and .0001 of those obtained without the filter.

The results of the tests with the musical sounds indicated in Fig. 1 are shown in tabular form in Table 1. The judgments of pitch and quality were made by three persons familiar with music. In every case they agreed unanimously in the statements made in the 4th and 5th columns. The musical tones were produced at loudness[5] values between 70 and 80 units. These loudness values correspond approximately to intensities of 10^7 and 10^8 times the minimum audible intensity. In the second column of this table, the letter F refers to the fundamental and the numbers refer to the overtones, thus (F & 1-6) means that the fundamental and the first six overtones were eliminated. It is seen that the vowel *ah* sung at a pitch *d* is affected only slightly in pitch or quality when the fundamental and first two overtones are eliminated. Even with the fundamental and first six overtones eliminated, the pitch still very definitely corresponds to the pitch of a pure tone with the frequency of the fundamental, namely, 145 cycles per second. The harmonic analysis of this filtered tone shows no frequencies below 1000 cycles per second. Eliminating all of the overtones above the sixth changes the quality by about the same amount as eliminating the fundamental and first and second overtones. The data also indicate that if the fundamental and all of the upper and lower harmonics except the third, fourth and fifth

[3] R. L. Wegel, Journal A.I.E.E., October, 1921

[4] H. Fletcher, Jour. Franklin Inst. June 1922; also Phys. Rev. **15**, 513, 1920

[5] For the meaning of the term loudness as used here see article by H. Fletcher, Jour. Franklin Inst., Sept. 1923

are eliminated, the remaining compound tone has the same pitch as the fundamental, although the quality of the sound is very different from that of the sound *ah*.

As indicated in the table, similar results were obtained for the vowel *ā*, sung at the pitch *a*. Still other vowels were tried with similar results. In general, neither the quality nor the pitch of notes from a rich baritone or contralto voice is appreciably affected by eliminating the fundamental and the first two to three overtones. If, however, higher overtones are eliminated, the musical quality (in particular the richness) is noticeably affected and this is true even though the omitted overtones are all above the fifteenth. The high harmonics do not seem to be so essential for good quality in a soprano voice. Experimental tests showed the rather unexpected result that the elimination of all the harmonic frequencies above 2000 cycles affects the musical quality of a bass, a baritone or a contralto voice to a greater extent than the quality of a high soprano voice.

The table shows that the quality of the principal musical instruments is much more seriously affected by the elimination of the lower parts of their characteristic sound spectra than the quality of the sung vowels by a similar elimination. In any case such eliminations do not change the pitch, for this remains constant as long as the filtered sound can be recognized as a musical tone.

These results were confirmed in a very striking manner by using ten separate vacuum tube generators for producing the component frequencies. These generators were adjusted to give the frequencies 100 to 1000 at intervals of 100. They were all connected to a special telephone receiver and the currents regulated so that the pressure amplitude of the components of the sound emitted by the receiver were equal. By suitable switching arrangement any one of the components could be eliminated. When they were all impressed upon the receiver a full tone resulted which had a definite pitch corresponding to 100 cycles per second. The elimination of the 100-cycle component produced no noticeable effect. The elimination of any other single component had no effect upon the pitch and almost none upon the tone quality, although by careful listening, its introduction and withdrawal could be detected in most cases. Even with the first seven components eliminated, leaving only 800, 900 and 1,000, the pitch corresponded to a frequency of 100. When only two components were left, they were heard as separate tones, the fundamental subjective tone at 100 being still plainly audible but much weaker than either component. Any three consecutive components were sufficient to give the tone a pitch corresponding to 100, as, for example, 200, 300, 400 or 600,

700, 800 etc. When four consecutive components were sounded, the fundamental subjective tone was very prominent. When all of the components were sounded this fundamental seemed to be louder than the other components and dominated the tone.

The tests just described were made when the loudness[5] of the 700-cycle tone was at 90. When only three components, 700, 800, 900 were used and the loudness of the combination greatly decreased, it was found that the 100-cycle subjective tone disappeared when the loudness of the combination was approximately 45 units. At this loudness, the three tones were heard as separate tones, the 900 cycle one being the last to disappear as the loudness approached zero. When five or more consecutive components were used, the pitch seemed to remain the same for low values of the loudness even down to zero, although for these very low values, it was very difficult to judge pitch.

If the components 200, 400, 600, 800 and 1,000 were used, the pitch corresponded to 200 cycles, i.e. to the octave of the compound tone discussed above. This tone still had the same pitch when the 200 and 400 cycle components were eliminated. Any two consecutive pairs gave the subjective tone 200 but only very weakly. Combination 300, 600 and 900 gave a harmonious sound, the listener having the tendency to hear the combination as separate musical tones.

From the results which have been described, one might conclude that the pitch of a musical tone was determined by the common difference in the frequencies of the harmonics, rather than by the frequency of the lowest component. This conclusion suggested trying a combination of frequencies which are separated by a common difference, but which are not necessarily multiples of this common difference. The combination 100, 300, 500, 700 and 900 was tried and it was found to have no definite pitch, but sounded like a noise. However, one could distinctly hear the subjective tone at 200 cycles. Similarly, the combinations 100, 400, 700, 1,000 and 100, 500, 900 and 200, 500, 800 were tried and found to have no definite pitch and to be entirely lacking in musical quality.

Further evidence of the above phenomenon was made possible by means of a carrier telephone system which was available in the laboratory. The technique of carrier telephony makes it possible to displace all the frequencies constituting a compound tone by the same absolute amount upward or downward. Thus, if the compound tone of ten components which has been described were transmitted through such a system when the carrier at the transmitting end differed from the carrier at the receiving end by 30 cycles, the frequencies received would be 130, 230, etc. up to 1030. It is found that such a shift destroys the musical quality which the original tone possessed. If the fundamental is very predominant this shift raises the pitch, but the inharmonic tones produce a harshness and the tone loses its musical character.

Structure of "Harmonic" Tones from Such Wind Instruments as the Bugle

In this connection it is interesting to examine the structure of those tones produced on wind instruments by changes in the blowing intensity rather than by changes in the length of the vibrating air column. When

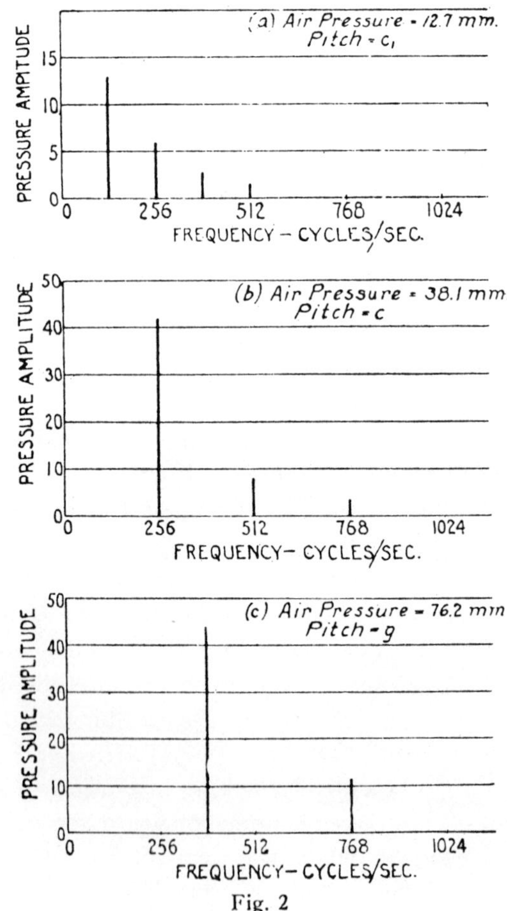

Fig. 2

the air pressure blowing an organ pipe or horn is continuously increased, the pitch of the emitted tone corresponds first to the fundamental and then it suddenly jumps to that corresponding to the first overtone and then to that corresponding to the second overtone, etc. As is well known, it is this effect that makes it possible to produce the different notes on a bugle. One might expect to find all the harmonics of the fundamental in each of these notes. However, this would be contrary to the observations we have just described. In fact, we find from a few experiments upon organ pipes that the overtones are all present in appreciable amount when and only when the pitch of the tone is that corresponding to the fundamental but when the pitch corresponds to the first overtone, only those components which are multiples of the first overtone are perceptible. This is clearly shown in the sound spectra given in Fig. 2, obtained by means of the harmonic analyzer which has been described. They represent the sound emitted by an organ pipe when it was blown with the various pressures indicated on the charts.

Explanation of the Results

It is possible to explain these experimental facts concerning pitch from our conception of the mechanism of the ear. The recent work[6] on this subject which has been carried on in the Bell System Laboratories, has shown that the ear displays a non-linear response to external applied forces. This non-linearity produces subjective tones; all the summation, the difference, and the harmonic frequencies as well as the impressed frequencies produce nerve stimulation. When the fundamental and first few overtones are eliminated from the external tone, they are again introduced by the ear mechanism as subjective tones although of course with different intensities. The changes in the relative intensities of the components impressed upon the nerve endings produce the observed changes in quality.

For example, in Fig. 3, the top chart (a) shows that sound spectrum described above, which was produced by 10 oscillators working into a single telephone receiver. The currents from the oscillators were adjusted so that the pressure amplitudes produced in the outer ear canal were all equal to approximately 100 dynes per square centimeter. When these component tones are transmitted through the ear mechanism the relative amplitudes of the elements producing nerve stimulation are quite different from those shown in Chart (a). If the component tones are impressed separately upon the ear as single tones then the relative amplitudes of these elements which stimulate the inner ear would be represented by chart (b). The ordinates represent the relative sensitivity of the ear to the various frequencies.[7] If the ear had a linear response this same chart would represent the relative amplitudes when all the components were sounding simultaneously.

[6] See Wegel and Lane, Phys. Rev. **21,** 705, 1923; also Fletcher[4]

[7] See Fletcher and Wegel, Phys. Rev. **19,** 553, June 1922

The third chart (c) shows the redistribution brought about by the non-linearity of the ear, that is, it represents the actual spectrum produced in the average inner ear that is excited by the tone represented in chart

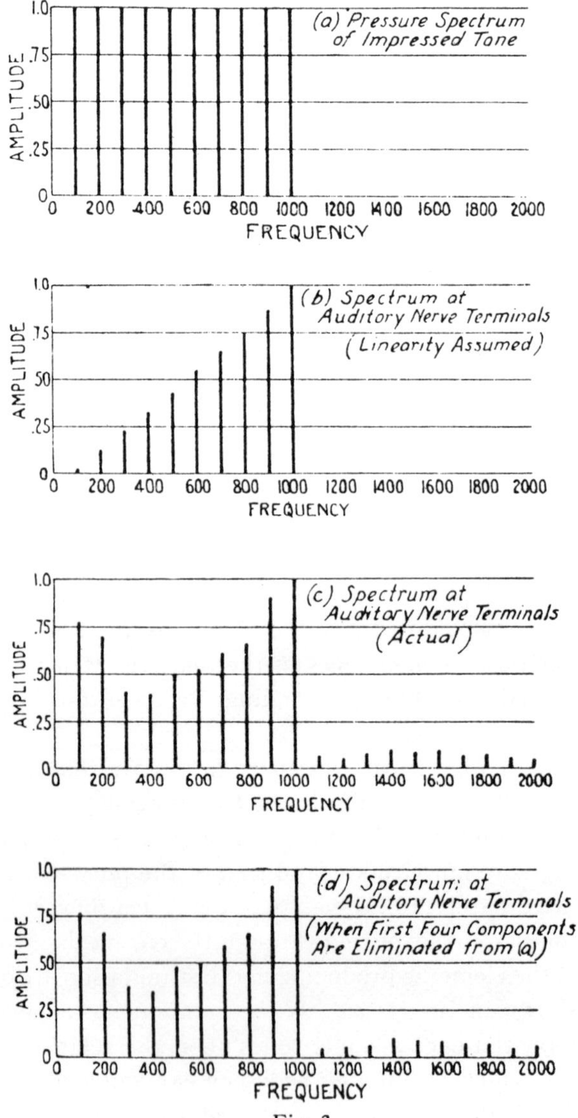

Fig. 3

(a). The fundamental is greatly increased due to the nine difference tones from adjacent components uniting to reinforce the fundamental.

The fourth chart (d) shows the spectrum in the inner ear when the first four components are eliminated from the impressed tone. That is, it represents the condition when the oscillators which are sending out 100, 200, 300 and 400 vibrations per second are switched off. Since the lower components in the inner ear spectrum are principally due to the higher frequency components of the pressure spectrum, the elimination of the first few components of the latter spectrum produces very little effect upon the former.

The constants used in computing these redistributions were obtained from experimental measurements by Wegel and Lane[6] of the magnitudes of the subjective tones. A comparison of the last two charts shows very clearly why one should expect the pitch of the two tones to be the same. If the impressed tones are all decreased without changing their relative magnitudes the resulting inner ear spectra will be different from that shown in these charts. Consequently the quality of the musical tone as well as its intensity will change as the loudness of the musical tone approaches zero. For these low intensities the inner ear spectrum approaches that shown in chart (b).

13

Reprinted from *K. ned. Akad. Wet. Proc.* **41**:1086–1093 (1938)

THE PERCEPTION OF SUBJECTIVE TONES

J. F. Schouten

It is a well-known fact that the ear sometimes perceives tones which do not correspond with any of the Fourier-components of the objective sound. Of these "subjective" tones the difference tones and the summation tones are the best perceptible. When a pure tone of increasing intensity is presented to the ear, the tone quality gradually changes from a pure one into a harsh or rough one. This change of quality is generally ascribed to a generation of higher harmonics in the ear, which is most probably due to non-linear distorsion in either the middle or the inner ear.

The existence of these subjective [1]) harmonics was demonstrated independently by FLETCHER [2]) and by VON BÉKÉSY [3]) with the aid of the method of beats. If a tone of say 200 cycles of high intensity is sounded together with an "exploring" tone of 406 cycles of low intensity, the ear perceives 6 beats per second. These beats are interpreted as an interference between the objective tone of 406 cycles and the subjective tone of 400 cycles (the second harmonic) which is generated within the ear.

At a certain intensity of the exploring tone the beats are reported to be most pronounced. This intensity is taken as the intensity of the subjective second harmonic. In the same way the best beat obtained with an exploring tone of 606 cycles gives the intensity of the subjective third harmonic, etc. FLETCHER and VON BÉKÉSY give data of 8 and 5 harmonics resp., obtained by means of this method.

A peculiarity of their results is that the percentaged intensity of the harmonics is almost constant over a wide range of intensities of the fundamental tone. Practically all known non-linear mechanisms, however, produce harmonics, the percentaged intensity of which is strongly dependent upon the intensity of the fundamental tone.

CHAPIN and FIRESTONE [4]) and TRIMMER and FIRESTONE [5]) investigated the influence of the phase of an objective harmonic on the tone quality,

---

[1]) We shall, throughout this paper, use the term "objective" when referring to the actual sound pressure and the term "subiective" when referring to the sound heard by the ear.

[2]) H. FLETCHER, J. Acoust. Soc. Am., **1**, 311—343 (1929).

[3]) G. VON BÉKÉSY, Ann. Phys., **20**, 809—827 (1934).

[4]) E. K. CHAPIN and F. A. FIRESTONE, J. Acoust. Soc. Am., **5**, 173—180 (1933).

[5]) J. D. TRIMMER and F. A. FIRESTONE, J. Acoust. Soc. Am., **9**, 24—29 (1937).

when added to the fundamental tone. The fundamental tone and its next five harmonics were generated by means of 6 electrostatic inductor alternators. In this way it was possible to add a certain harmonic of known intensity and phase to the fundamental tone.

If the second harmonic is generated in the ear, one might expect that, by addition of an appropriate amount of second harmonic to the objective sound, the tone quality as well as the intensity of the sound perceived would become dependent upon the phase of this objective second harmonic. In one phase (phase A) the objective and the subjective harmonic would just counterbalance, in the opposite phase (phase C) the two would reinforce one another.

This phase effect was found, according to expectation, at an intensity level of 104 db and about 10 % second harmonic. In phase A the addition of the objective harmonic produced a sound perception of smoother tone quality and of less intensity than that produced by the objectively pure tone. In phase C the tone obtained a rough or dissonant element and became of greater loudness.

The same authors [5]) severely criticize the use of the method of beats as a quantitative method of measuring the subjective harmonics, especially so because the presentation of the exploring tone might change the amount of harmonics generated in the ear and might give rise to disturbing overtones and combination tones. Below we shall describe a phenomenon which seems to justify this criticism.

Optical arrangement for the production of synthetic sound.

We constructed an optical apparatus for the production of sound of any prescribed waveform. One period of the desired waveform (in this case the fundamental tone) is drawn in polar coordinates on stiff paper in such a way that one period corresponds with forty degrees.

The paper enclosed between the drawn waveform and the circle passing through the largest negative value of the waveform is then cut out. The paper, which can be shoved into a holder H_1 (Figs. 1 and 2), is illuminated homogeneously by a point source of light P. A revolving wheel W containing 9 narrow slits S is placed immediately behind a holder H_1 and is driven by motor M.

By means of a lens L an image of the light source P is formed in the photo-electric cell C. The light transmitted by the slit wheel, which is linearly proportional to the prescribed waveform, is finally transformed into sound by means of the photo-electric cell C, an amplifier and a loud-speaker. A cathode ray oscillograph O permits to visualize the waveform actually obtained. The fundamental frequency is 200 cycles.

Measurements of the intensity level of the fundamental tone and of the higher harmonics were carried out by means of an electrostatically calibrated condenser microphone and a wave analyzer. If a pure sine is cut out, the amount of higher harmonics introduced by faults in the optical system and by non-linearity in the electrical and the acoustical system is measured to be limited to 1 %.

For studying the phase effect use was made of a second holder H_2

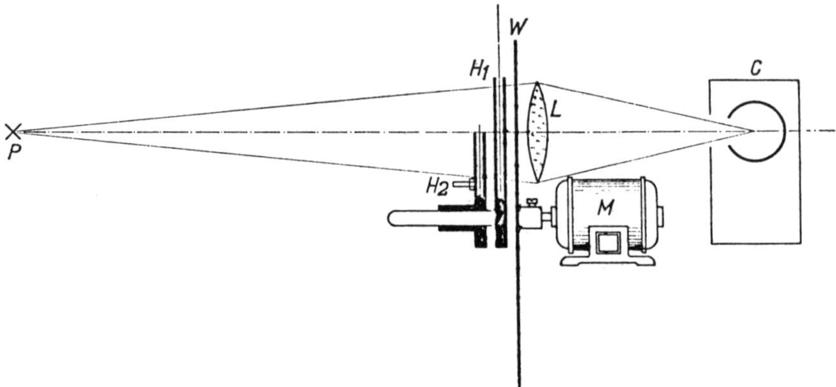

Fig. 2. *Sketch of the apparatus used for obtaining synthetic sound.* The holders H_1 and H_2, holding the desired waveform, are illuminated homogeneously by the point source of light *P*. The light transmitted by the slits of the rotating wheel *W* is concentrated by means of lens *L* into the photoelectric cell *C*.

which could be turned round the axis of symmetry. In this way a harmonic of continuously varying phase could be added to the fundamental tone.

At an intensity level of 105 db and an objective second harmonic of 4—8 %, a very marked phase effect upon the tone quality is heard. At this level the second harmonic can even be heard separately to vanish (phase *A*) or to reappear. If the phase is adjusted in such a way that the second harmonic is no longer perceptible and the objective second harmonic is then removed, the subjective harmonic can actually be heard to be present in the objectively pure sound. After a few seconds this subjective harmonic seems to blend with the fundamental tone and cannot be heard separately again until after comparison with the sound of phase *A*.

At higher intensity levels the phase effect on the tone quality still exists, although the second harmonic is no longer separately perceptible. The tone acquires a strongly increasing rough quality.

The phase effect on the intensity confirmed the findings of previous investigators [4, 5]).

That indeed in phase *A* the effect of the objective second harmonic consists in suppressing the subjective harmonic generated in the ear, can be beautifully demonstrated by combining the phase method with the method of beats.

For this purpose a tone of 406 cycles was produced by a second loudspeaker. It should be expected that in phase *C*, where the subjective harmonic is reinforced, strong beats occur, whereas in phase *A*, where the subjective second harmonic is suppressed, the beats should vanish. A strong phase effect for beats was indeed found, which confirmed the above hypothesis.

A disturbing effect, however, was noticed. Although at phase A the beats of the second harmonic practically vanish, other beats, which probably can be best described as beats of the fundamental tone, remain audible. These beats have the same frequency as those of the second harmonic. The only explanation presenting itself seems to be that these beats are due to the fundamental tone of 200 cycles and the difference tone of the fundamental and the exploring tone of 206 cycles. This effect confirms the criticism of TRIMMER and FIRESTONE [5]) in sofar that one should be very cautious before interpreting beats heard between the tones 200 and 406 as being due to the second harmonic and the exploring tone alone. As neither FLETCHER nor VON BÉKÉSY explicitly mention that the beats heard were beats of the second harmonic and not of any other tone, the possibility remains that this effect affected their measurements, which give values so greatly differing from those obtained by other methods.

In figure 3 values are represented of the percentage second harmonic and the intensity level of the fundamental tone at which the phase effect

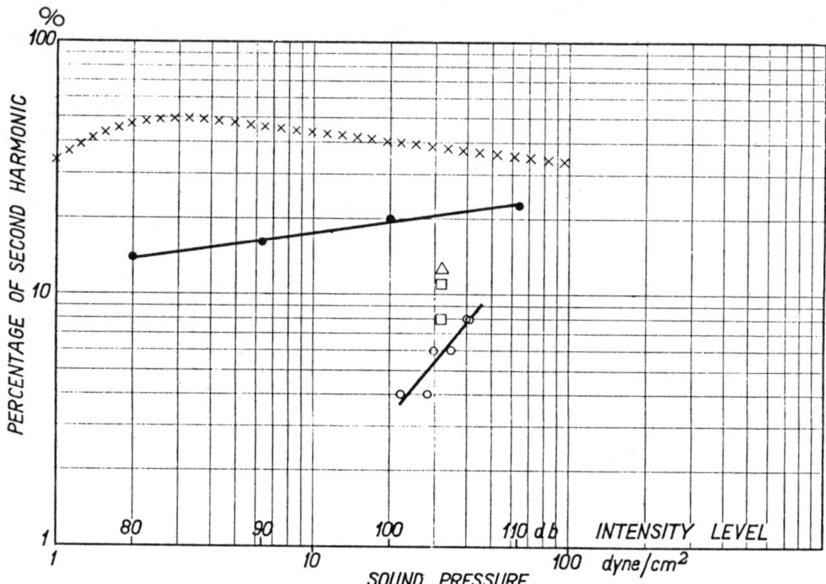

Fig. 3. *The percentaged intensity of the second harmonic generated in the ear as a function of the intensity level.*

● ● ● ●	FLETCHER	best beat method
× × × ×	VON BÉKÉSY	best beat method
△ △ △ △	CHAPIN and FIRESTONE	phase method: minimum loudness
□ □ □ □	TRIMMER and FIRESTONE	phase method: minimum loudness and minimum roughness
○ ○ ○ ○	Our measurements	phase method: minimum roughness and minimum beats

on tone quality and beats was best pronounced. These values may give a fair impression of the intensity of the subjective second harmonic. For comparison the values obtained by other observers are also given.

Subjective tones and the perception of pitch.

Some sounds exhibit the peculiarity that the fundamental tone is missing or of very low intensity compared to the higher harmonics. As an example we reproduce (Figs. 4 and 5) photographs of the sound spectra obtained from strips of sound film on which the lowest *g* of the violin and the vowel "a" in "father" are recorded [6]).

The pitch ascribed to these tones, however, is that of the missing fundamental. Similar results were obtained by FLETCHER [8]) with sounds from which the lower harmonics were artificially removed.

The customary and attractive hypothesis [8]) to account for this effect is to assume that the fundamental tone, although not present in the objective sound, is generated as a subjective tone in the ear. Because of the non-linear distorsion in the ear this fundamental tone would occur as the difference tone of all adjoining harmonics and would thus be of great strength.

It should be stated that the tacit assumption underlying this hypothesis is that the perception of pitch is determined by the lowest harmonic actually present in the ear.

There is one objection which might be raised beforehand against this hypothesis, namely that even at lowest intensities no one was yet reported to judge the pitch of these tones an octave higher. Subjective tones, however, do not become noticeable until above a certain intensity level.

In order to study this effect, we used the waveform *A* reproduced in figure 6. This waveform can be described as a periodic impulse of finite width (one twentieth of the fundamental period). A periodic true impulse contains all harmonics in equal strength. The periodic impulse of finite width contains the lower harmonics in gradually decreasing strength. The tone quality is very sharp.

By using the procedure described in the above paragraph, the fundamental tone could be exactly cancelled. The intensity of the fundamental in the actual sound field was ½ % of the second harmonic. The waveform is represented in fig. 6, *B*.

After that the same setting was made but now subjectively. It was found that these adjustments are very critical and therefore easy to make. For

---

[6]) It can be shown [7]) that the diffraction pattern of variable-width sound film provides a visual Fourier-analysis of the registered sound. This rule only holds true on the horizontal axis of symmetry of the spectrum. The intensity of the lines, is proportional to the square of the amplitudes of the harmonics.

[7]) J. F. SCHOUTEN, Nature, **141**, 914 (1938).

[8]) H. FLETCHER, Phys. Rev., **23**, 427—437 (1924).

very slight alterations of the phase or the amplitude of the periodic impulse the fundamental could be heard separately in the sound again.

Contrary to expectation the objective and the subjective settings practically coincided, which means that no subjective fundamental of

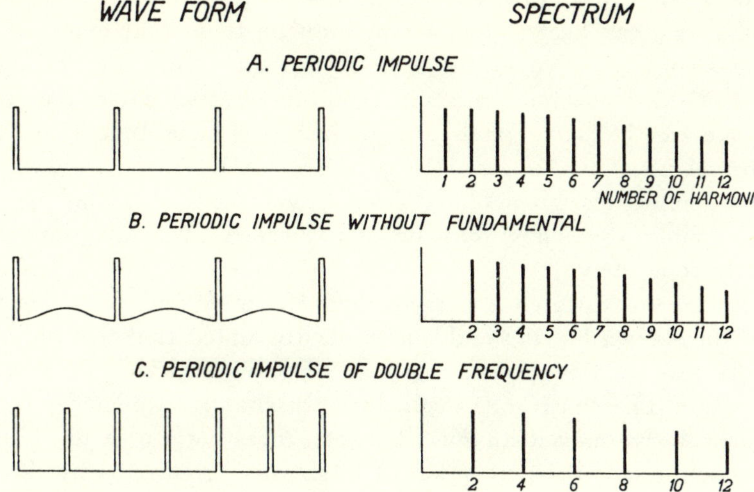

Fig. 6. *Various periodic impulses and their Fourier spectra.*
Waveform *A*: periodic impulse of finite width. Frequency 200 cycles. The spectrum contains all harmonics in gradually increasing intensity.
Waveform *B*: same as *A*. The fundamental tone is suppressed.
Waveform *C*: periodic impulse of double frequency (400 cycles).

appreciable intensity is formed in the ear. The amount of the subjective fundamental for pressure amplitudes of the same order as those used in the experiments with a pure tone is certainly less than 3 %.

We shall, however, leave this part of the matter aside for the present and turn to another surprising phenomenon. No matter whether the fundamental is generated in the ear or not, the subjective fundamental can be made to vanish completely. This can be corroborated by means of the method of beats. If an additional tone of 206 periods is presented to the ear, 6 beats per second are distinctly heard at random settings. These beats, however, disappear completely at the setting obtained above. We are, therefore, justified in concluding that indeed no fundamental tone is present in the ear at that setting.

The pitch ascribed to this tone (waveform B), however, is the same as the pitch of the periodic impulse with fundamental tone (waveform A) and is an octave lower than the pitch of a periodic impulse of frequency 400 (waveform C).

It is not without interest to analyse the sound impressions obtained from the three waveforms somewhat further. By concentrating the attention (the difficulty of which has been so adequately formulated by

HELMHOLTZ [9])) on the fundamental, the second and the third harmonic, each of these can be heard separately in waveform *A*. We might say that, as to the actual perception, this sound consists of four entities: a sharp tone of pitch 200 and the pure tones of pitch 200, 400 and 600. The relative prominence of these four entities is so strongly dependent upon the concentration of the attention that it is scarcely an exaggeration to say that one can hear at will a tune built on these four tones.

In the sound with waveform *B* there are three separate entities. The second and third harmonic are still separately recognizable, the rest is a sharp tone of the *same* pitch and almost the same timbre as that of waveform *A*.

The sound impression obtained from waveform *C* was that of a sharp tone of double frequency; we did not succeed in hearing any of the harmonics separately.

Sometimes the difference between waveform *A* and *B* is heard as a jump of an octave, but it should be explicitly stated that this only occurs when the attention is concentrated on the lowest harmonic perceptible in the sound. The sharp tone itself does not change in pitch.

Historically we may distinguish between three stages. In the first stage it was thought that the perception of pitch was determined by the lowest harmonic present in the objective sound. It was then found that tones which either naturally or artificially miss the fundamental tone and even some of the lower harmonics still have a pitch equal to that of the fundamental tone.

In the second stage it was assumed that the fundamental tone, although not present in the objective sound, is generated in the ear as a subjective tone. It is now found that tones which miss the fundamental, even as a subjective tone, still may have the pitch of the fundamental tone.

Therefore the perception of pitch is not determined by the lowest harmonic present in the ear, although the ear is sometimes capable of ascertaining whether the fundamental tone is (subjectively) present in the sound or not.

One might ask now whether there is any sense in this behaviour of the ear. There is scarcely any sense in it, if we look at the Fourier spectrum. Why should the pitch of a pure tone be the tone itself and that of a sharp tone be the frequency difference of its harmonics? There is very much sense in it, if we look at the oscillogram, because, as in figure 6 *B*, although the fundamental tone is missing, the oscillogram is still periodic with the frequency of the fundamental tone.

There must be some way in which the ear, when perceiving pitch, is able to become aware of this fundamental period of the oscillogram.

Eindhoven, 29th November 1938.

---

[9]) H. V. HELMHOLTZ, Lehre von den Tonempfindungen.

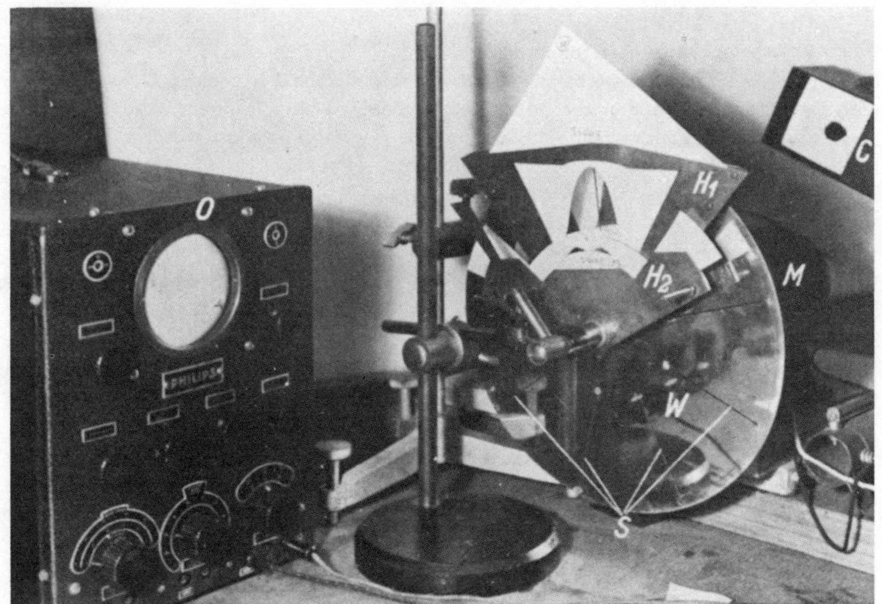

Fig. 1.

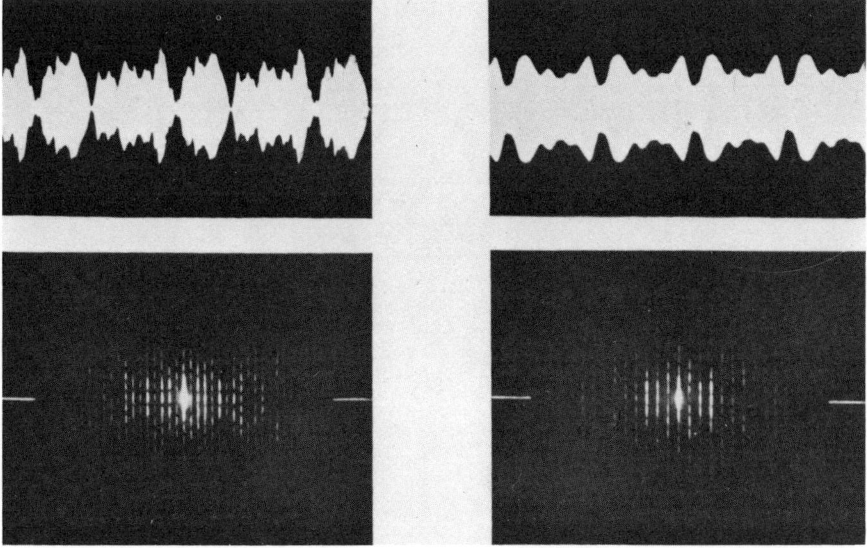

Fig. 4.

Fig. 5.

LEGENDS TO FIGURES:

Fig. 1. *Photograph of the apparatus used for obtaining sound of any prescribed waveform.* The fundamental tone is cut out in the paper held by holder H_1, whereas the second harmonic is cut out in the paper held by holder H_2. The papers are illuminated homogeneously. The light transmitted by the slits S of the rotating wheel W driven by motor M is proportional to the desired waveform. The light is concentrated into the photo-electric cell C. The cathode ray oscillograph O serves to visualize the waveform actually obtained.

Fig. 4. *Above*: tenfold enlargement of a strip of sound film on which the lowest *g* of the violin is recorded (193 cycles).
Below: photograph of the pattern obtained from this strip by diffraction of light. The intensity of the lines on the horizontal axis of symmetry provides a visual Fourier analysis of the sound recorded on the film. Note the very low intensity of the fundamental tone.

Fig. 5. *Above*: tenfold enlargement of a strip of sound film on which the vowel "a" in "father" is recorded (290 cycles).
Below: photograph of the diffraction pattern obtained from this strip. Note the very low intensity of the fundamental tone.

14

Reprinted from *Experientia* 7:128-133 (1951)

A Duplex Theory of Pitch Perception[1]

By J. C. R. LICKLIDER[2], Cambridge, Mass.

Theories of pitch perception have shared the presupposition that pitch is a unitary attribute of auditory experience. It is by no means entirely clear, however, that such is the case. In some musical circles, in the older psychological literature[3], and in recent papers on absolute pitch[4], pitch is held to be duplex in nature. Two pitch-like qualities are distinguished. They are given various pairs of names by various authors: tone height and tone chroma, ordinary pitch and chroma, pitch and quality, pitch and tonality, etc. If such a distinction is warranted—and several considerations suggest that it is—the part of auditory theory that concerns the perception of pitch is in need of modification.

The stimulus basis for pitch is also duplex: On the one hand we have frequency, on the other hand, periodicity. That frequency and period are reciprocally related is not sufficient reason for throwing one away and examining only the other, for with each one is associated a method of analysis. Of the two methods, one—frequency analysis performed by an array of band-pass filters—has been incorporated into auditory theory. The cochlea is almost universally regarded as being an extended wave filter that distributes oscillations of different frequencies to different places. The possibility that the other method, autocorrelational analysis, plays a role in the auditory process has been neglected[5].

Autocorrelational analysis is an analysis, carried out entirely within the time domain, that yields the same information as the power spectrum which is obtained through analysis in the frequency domain. WIENER's famous theorum[6] shows that the autocorrelation function and the power spectrum of a wave are a FOURIER transform pair. The attractiveness of autocorrelational analysis *per se* therefore lies not in revealing anything that cannot be found through frequency analysis; it lies in the fact that the operations involved in carrying out the autocorrelational analysis are quite different from those involved in making the frequency analysis.

The essence of the duplex theory of pitch perception is that the auditory system employs both frequency analysis and autocorrelational analysis. The frequency analysis is performed by the cochlea, the autocorrelational analysis by the neural part of the system. The latter is therefore an analysis not of the acoustic stimulus itself but of the trains of nerve impulses into which the action of the cochlea transforms the stimulus. This point is important because the highly nonlinear process of neural excitation intervenes between the two analyses.

The neural mechanism of analysis

In so far as the frequency analysis is concerned, the duplex theory follows the resonance-place theory of HELMHOLTZ[1] and the space-time pattern theory of FLETCHER[2]. If we designate the lengthwise dimension of the uncoiled cochlea as the x-dimension, we can describe the cochlear frequency analysis by saying that the cochlea transforms the stimulus time function $f(t)$ into a running spectrum $F(t, x)$, position x being the neural correlate of stimulus frequency. Thus the cochlea does, in a rather different way and perhaps with less resolution in frequency, essentially the same thing as the Sound Spectrograph developed by the Bell Telephone Laboratories[3]. The running spectrum, a spatial array of time functions, is transmitted brainward by neurons of the auditory nerve. Neurons terminating at x_b near the base of the cochlea act as a group to carry $F(t, x_b)$, while those terminating at x_a near the apex carry $F(t, x_a)$, and the others in between handle other parts. Each $F(t, x_i)$ is an integral over the behaviors of many neurons. The contribution of an individual neuron, say tha jth neuron in group i, is $N_{ij}(t)$, a function that has either the value 0 (quiescent) or 1 (firing).

It will facilitate the description of the autocorrelational analysis if we think of it, at first, as being performed upon the individual functions $N_{ij}(t)$. The running autocorrelation function of $N_{ij}(t)$ is defined[4] (see appendix) as

[1] The preparation of this paper was supported by a contract between Massachusetts Institute of Technology and the Air Force Research Laboratories, Cambridge, Mass.

[2] Acoustics Laboratory, Massachusetts Institute of Technology Cambridge, Massachusetts.

[3] G. RÉVÉSZ, *Zur Grundlegung der Tonpsychologie* (Viet & Co., Leipzig 1913). – MAX F. MEYER, Psychol. Bull. *11*, 349 (1914).

[4] A. BACHEM, J. Acoust. Soc. Amer. *9*, 146 (1937).

[5] The suggestion has been made by R. M. FANO of the Research Laboratory of Electronics and by L. A. DE ROSA of the Federal Telecommunication Laboratories, Inc., that the cochlea may operate more nearly as an autocorrelator than as a filter. This suggestion is quite different from, and in fact quite contrary to the hypothesis proposed in the present paper.

[6] N. WIENER, Acta math. *55*, 117 (1930).

[1] H. VON HELMHOLTZ, *Sensations of tone* (English translation by A. J. ELLIS, London, 1895, of *Die Lehre von den Tonempfindungen*, 2nd English ed., Longmans, Green, & Co., London, 1885).

[2] H. FLETCHER, J. Acoust. Soc. Amer. *1*, 311 (1930).

[3] J. C. STEINBERG and N. R. FRENCH, J. Acoust. Soc. Amer. *9*, 146 (1946); and a series of articles by members of the Bell Telephone Laboratories in the same issue. Also R. K. POTTER, G. A. KOPP, and HARRIET C. GREEN, *Visible speech* (D. Van Nostrand Co., Inc., New York, 1947).

[4] R. M. FANO, J. Acoust. Soc. Amer. (in press). Also K. N. STEVENS, J. Acoust. Soc. Amer. (in press). These papers are, respectively, on the mathematical relations between running autocorrelation functions and power spectra and on autocorrelation functions of speech sounds.

$$\varphi_{ij}(t, \tau) = \overline{N_{ij}(t)\, N_{ij}\,(t-\tau)} \qquad (1)$$

in which τ is the variable interval by which $N_{ij}(t)$ is delayed to produce $N_{ij}\,(t-\tau)$ and the overline designates a running integral over the more or less recent past of t. Therefore $\varphi_{ij}(t, \tau)$ is simply a running accumulation of recent values of the product of $N_{ij}(t)$ and the same function delayed by τ. It provides a progressive description of the periodicity of the discharges of neuron ij.

The nervous system is nicely set up to perform running autocorrelational analysis. The operations specified by expression (1) are to delay the input function $N_{ij}(t)$ by a variable interval τ, to multiply the delayed function $N_{ij}\,(t-\tau)$ by the original function $N_{ij}(t)$, and to determine the running integral $\varphi_{ij}(t, \tau)$ of the product. A chain of neurons makes an excellent delay line. The spatial aspect of synaptic summation provides approximate multiplication. And the temporal aspect of synaptic summation gives us running integration. The theory postulates, therefore, that the lower centers of the auditory system perform the three operations.

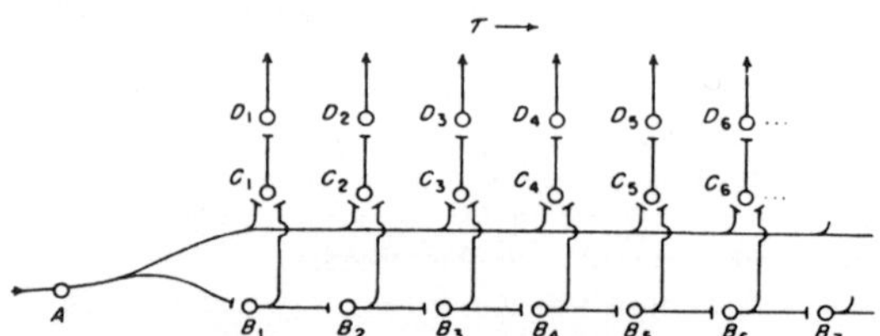

Fig. 1. – *Basic schema of neuronal autocorrelator.* A is the input neuron, B_1, B_2, B_3, ... is a delay chain. The original signal and the delayed signal are multiplied when A and B_k feed C_k, and a running integral of the product is obtained at the synapse between C_k and D_k, where excitation accumulates whenever C_k discharges and dissipates itself at a rate proportional to the amount accumulated. Since these operations correspond to the definition of running autocorrelation, the excitatory states at D_1, D_2, D_3, ... provide a display of the running autocorrelation function of the input time function, the temporal course of the discharges of A.

The basic neuronal connections are shown in Fig. 1. The state of neuron A is $N_A(t)$. If each synaptic delay in the chain B is $\Delta\tau$, the chain gives us $N_A(t)$ under various delays. The state of neuron B_k, for example, is $N_A\,(t-k\Delta\tau)$. Assuming, with McCulloch and Pitts[1], that both A and B_k must fire almost simultaneously to make C_k fire, we have

$$N_{C_k}\,(t) = N_A(t)\, N_A\,(t-k\Delta\tau). \qquad (2)$$

Neuron C_k impinges upon neuron D_k. Excitation is built up at D_k by the discharges of C_k and dissipates itself spontaneously, perhaps at a rate proportional to the amount accumulated. The excitation at D_k at a particular instant t is therefore

[1] W. S. McCulloch and W. Pitts, Bull. Math. Biophys. *5*, 115 (1943).

$$E_{D_k}(t) = \overline{N_{C_k}\,(t)}. \qquad (3)$$

Substituting in (3) the value of $N_{C_k}\,(t)$ from (2), we obtain

$$E_{D_k}(t) = E(t, k\Delta\tau) = N_A(t)\, \overline{N_A\,(t-k\Delta\tau)}. \qquad (4)$$

Since expression (4) is equivalent to the definition (1) in every respect save for the substitution of $k\Delta\tau$ for τ, $E(t, k\Delta\tau)$ is an approximation of the running autocorrelation function of $N_A(t)$. Viewing the arrangement of Fig. 1 as a neuronal autocorrelator, we therefore identify the lengthwise dimension of the delay chain with τ, and we regard the time-varying excitation at D_1, D_2, .., D_k., as a spatial display of successive cross-sections of the autocorrelation function[1].

We must now take into account the facts that sensory systems have many neurons roughly in parallel and that the important physiological quantities appear to be averages or integrals over sets of neurons. We therefore think of neuron A as but one of many neighbors; it is, let us say, the jth neuron in the ith group terminating along the basilar membrane of the cochlea. It is the behavior $F(t, x_i)$ of the group, not $N_{ij}(t) = N_A(t)$ of the individual neuron, that is subjected to autocorrelational analysis. The arrangement of Fig. 1 must be modified by introducing many neurons in parallel with A. Each has its own delay chain, but the outputs of several delay chains are fed to C_1, C_2, .., C_k.. Finally, many sets like C_1, C_2, .., C_k. impinge upon D_1, D_2, .., D_k.. We substitute for the assumption that both A and B_k must discharge to fire C_k the more plausible assumption that the accumulation of excitation at C_k must reach a certain level, which may vary secularly. Other neurons in parallel with C_k have other thresholds. These are distributed in such a way that the behavior of the group of neurons in parallel with C_k is related nonlinearly to the input, which is approximately $F(t, x_i)$ plus $F\,(t-k\Delta\tau,\ x_i)$. The nonlinearity gives rise to an output that is a rough approximation of the arithmetic product of the two components of the input.

In order to obtain the running integral of the product, we follow in principle the description given in the preceding paragraphs. However, as soon as we substitute groups of neurons for individuals, we may redefine the output of the neuronal autocorrelator in terms of the actual behavior of groups of neurons, which is more directly observable than the excitatory state defined as the output in expression (4). To do this, we need only assume that the behavior of the

[1] For the sake of simplicity, we assume here that delay in time is proportional to distance traversed in the neural tissue. If the tissue should prove to be non-homogeneous, we should designate the lengthwise dimension of the delay chain as $y = y(\tau)$. This would parallel our procedure in handling frequency, which is not transformed linearly into the x-dimension: we labeled the spatial dimension $x = x(\omega)$ instead of ω itself.

group of neurons in parallel with D_k is roughly proportional to E_{D_k}. As soon as we take that step, however, we see that the chain of neurons $D_1, D_2, .., D_k$. (introduced in the first place only to facilitate the description by separating the operations) can be eliminated. We can give the synapses at $C_1, C_2, .., C_k$. responsibility for both multiplication and integration. The former depends upon the nonlinearity of the synaptic relay, the latter upon its sluggishness. Let us therefore amend the notation and call the behavior of the group of C-neurons (i.e. the output of the system) $\varphi(t, \tau)$.

We have thus far an arrangement of neurons that determines approximately the running autocorrelation function of $F(t, x_i)$. The arrangement has a simple network of neurons as its basic schema. However, it is not in essence a digital machine. Since the basic operations involve integrations over sets of neurons, the discontinuity of the discharges of the individual neurons is smoothed over and does not appear in $\varphi(t, \tau)$. For the same reason, exact replication of the neuronal arrangement shown in Fig. 1 is not required. In fact, a certain amount of statistical variation of microstructure is quite as desirable for the functioning of the mechanism as it is bound to occur in neural tissue.

Bringing together the cochlear frequency analysis and the neuronal autocorrelation, we note that our discussion of the latter has given us the autocorrelation function of a single channel of the cochlear output. The cochlear frequency analysis transforms $f(t)$ into $F(t, x)$, of which $F(t, x_i)$ is but one part, separated spatially from the others. Our $\varphi(t, \tau)$ describes only the signal in the ith channel; it is $\varphi(t, \tau, x_i)$. We must think of the neural arrangement, therefore, as extended in two spatial dimensions. The one corresponding to frequency is the x-dimension, or the dimension of the nervous tissue into which the lengthwise dimension of the cochlea projects. The whole arrangement for determining autocorrelation functions is replicated in the x-dimension. The τ-dimension is functionally orthogonal to the x-dimension, and we can think of it, at least for convenience of graphical representation, as being spatially orthogonal, also. The over-all system, then, yields a representation of the stimulus $f(t)$ in two spatial dimensions and time, a running autocorrelation $\varphi(t,\tau,x)$ of the components in each of many frequency bands. The arrangement is shown schematically in Fig. 2.

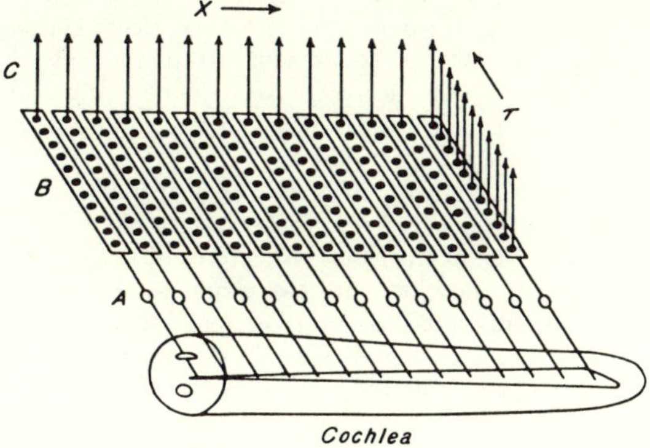

Fig. 2. – *Schematic diagram of overall analyzer.* At the bottom is the uncoiled cochlea. Its lengthwise dimension and the corresponding dimension in the neural tissue above it is designated the x-dimension. The cochlea performs a crude frequency analysis of the stimulus time function, distributing different frequency bands to different x-positions. In the process of exciting the neurons of the auditory nerve, the outputs of the cochlear filters are rectified and smoothed. The resulting signals are carried by the groups of neurons A to the autocorrelators B, whose delay- or τ-dimension is orthogonal to x. The outputs of the autocorrelators are fed to higher centers over the matrix of channels C, a cross-section through which is called the (x, τ)-plane. (Output arrows arise from all the dots; some are omitted in the diagram to avoid confusion.) The time-varying distribution of activity in the (x, τ)-plane provides a progressive analysis of the acoustic stimulus, first in frequency and then in periodicity.

Relations between theory and observation

The duplex theory accounts immediately for two observations that cause ordinary place theories great difficulty. These are the observations of MILLER and TAYLOR[1] on the pitch of interrupted white noise and of SCHOUTEN[2] on the residue phenomenon. MILLER and TAYLOR found that their listeners could match with an oscillator tone the pitch of random fluctuation noise that was chopped into segments (on half the time, off half the time) at rates between about 40 and 250 per second. According to the duplex theory, both the tone and the interrupted noise produce activity in the same stria of the (x, τ)-plane. The distributions of activity set up by a 100-c.p.s. sinusoid and white noise interrupted 100 times per second are shown schematically in Fig. 3, A and B (see Fig. 3).

The basis for the pitch match is evident.

The acoustic stimulus that gives rise to SCHOUTEN's effect consists of the high-frequency harmonics of a frequency in the interval 30 to 300 c.p.s. SCHOUTEN's listeners reported that the high-frequency sound had about the same pitch as a (low-frequency) sinusoid of the same fundamental period. Repeating SCHOUTEN's work with a spectrum consisting of lines at 4,000, 4,100, 4,200, ..., ROSENBLITH[3] found that many of his listeners made the same judgment: they matched the high-frequency sound in pitch with a sinusoid of about 100 c.p.s. However, some insisted that the pitch of the sound was quite high[4]. The distribution of activity in the (x, τ)-plane, shown in Fig. 3C, shows that both reports are reasonable. There is simply a disagreement among the listeners about which of the attributes—the one based on periodicity in τ or the one based on position in x—is meant by "pitch".

[1] G. A. MILLER and W. G. TAYLOR, J. Acoust. Soc. Amer. *20*, 171 (1948).

[2] J. F. SCHOUTEN, Philips Tech. Rev. *5*, 226 (1940).

[3] W. A. ROSENBLITH, Progress Report II (PNM–6) of the Psycho-Acoustic Laboratory, Harvard University (1947).

[4] A similar division of judgment of pitch was reported by H. DAVIS at the June, 1950, meeting of the Acoustical Society of America. DAVIS' acoustic stimulus was a carrier of about 2000 c.p.s. modulated at 123 c.p.s.

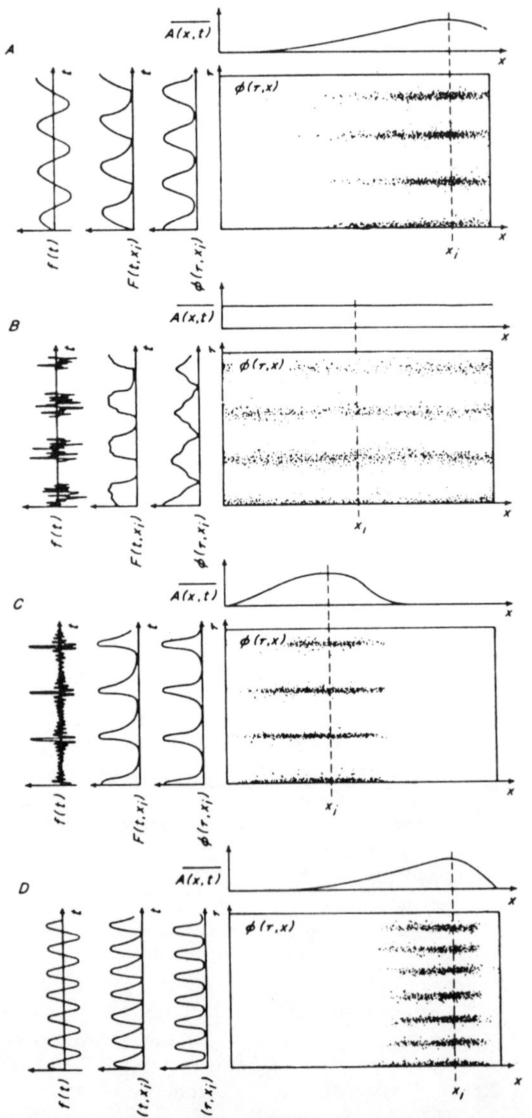

Fig. 3. – *Schematic illustrations of duplex analysis. A* represents the analysis of a 100-c.p.s. sinusoid, *B* of white noise interrupted 100 times per second, *C* of a set of high-frequency harmonics of 100 c.p.s., and *D* of a 200-c.p.s. sinusoid. At the left in each plot are shown the stimulus waveform $f(t)$, the waveform $F(t, x_i)$ of the signal carried by the first-order neurons (acting as a group) at x_i, and the autocorrelation function $\varphi(\tau, x_i)$ of $F(t, x_i)$. At the top of each plot is the distribution of activity along the length of the cochlea: $\overline{A(x, t)}$ is the root-mean-square of the instantaneous amplitudes of oscillation $A(x, t)$ at various positions along the cochlear partition[15]. $F(t, x,$ results from the rectification and smoothing of $A(x, t)$. The density of stippling in the rectangle represents $\varphi(\tau, x)$, the autocorrelation functions of the signals in the various x-channels. (Since the signals are in steady state, the t-dimension is omitted here.) Note that the first three (x, τ)-plots are similar in the τ- but not in the x-dimension. This corresponds to the fact that they are subjectively similar in one pitch-like attribute but not in another. *D* is somewhat similar to *A* in the τ-dimension: the odd-numbered maxima of $\varphi(\tau, x)$ in *D* coincide with the maxima in *A*. This corresponds to the subjective uniqueness of the octave relation.

The octave relation, the musical third, fourth, and other consonant intervals are understandable on essentially the same basis. When the frequencies of two sounds, either sinusoidal or complex, bear to each other the ratio of two small integers, their autocorrelation functions have common peaks. The 200-c.p.s. sinusoid in Fig. 3*D* gives rise to maximal activity wherever the 100 c.p.s. sinusoid of Fig. 3*A* does, and also in the strips that are half-way between. Furthermore, making use of the phenomenon illustrated in Fig. 3*C*, we note that the fundamental components of complex sounds need not be energetically present in the acoustic stimulus. The non-linearity of the neural excitation process introduces a component at the fundamental frequency before the autocorrelational analysis occurs. This fact explains the "case of the missing fundamental"[1].

The duplex theory also accounts for the subjective difference between the difference tone, heard when two moderately strong primary tones are presented to the ear, and a sinusoid of the difference frequency. It may account for the distinction between the two pitch-like attributes made by the listeners with "absolute pitch" who place a tone in the right region of the scale on the basis of ordinary pitch and then fix the note precisely with the aid of chroma. And it may account for some of the differences that have been noted between low-frequency and high-frequency hearing. The autocorrelational analysis must operate only for frequencies (frequencies of modulation *or* frequencies energetically present in the stimulus) that can be represented by volleys in the first-order neurons. Although there is evidence[2] that the volley principle operates up to 3,000 or 4,000 c.p.s., the effect at those frequencies is very weak, and it is safer to restrict the autocorrelational analysis to 1,000 c.p.s. or less. (It is unlikely that synapses provide delays of less than a millisecond, though of course axonal delays of almost any smaller duration may be postulated.)

A final comment concerns the plausibility of the autocorrelational schema from the neurological point of view. One of the essential features of the schema is division of the input into two channels, one with and one without built-in delay. In his histological investigation of the cochlear nucleus, Lorente de Nó[3] found that the first-order auditory fibers branch, one division taking a one-synapse route to the next relay station, the other passing into a region of dense ramifications and thicket-like synaptic connections. Furthermore, recent work of Galambos, Rosenblith, and Rosenzweig[4] shows that it is entirely reasonable to postulate

[1] S. S. Stevens and H. Davis, *Hearing, its psychology and physiology* (John Wiley and Sons, Inc., New York, 1938). – J. F. Schouten, Proc. K. Ned. Akad. Wet. *43*, 356 (1940).

[2] E. G. Wever, *Theories of hearing* (John Wiley and Sons, Inc., New York, 1949).

[3] R. Lorente de Nó, Laryngoscope *43*, 1 (1933).

[4] R. Galambos, W. A. Rosenblith, and M. R. Rosenzweig, Periodic Status Report IX (PNM-18) of the Psycho-Acoustic Laboratory, Harvard University (1949).

for the cochlear nucleus the delay of 1/30 sec. that is required if the autocorrelator is to operate as low as 30 cps. These considerations, together with the fact that the autocorrelator should be as near the cochlea as possible so that it may operate upon the signal before temporal resolution is lost, suggest that the cochlear nucleus may be the site. It is perhaps best, however, not to commit the theory at the present time to a definite statement about the location of the mechanism.

APPENDIX

Autocorrelation

The running autocorrelation function defined roughly by expression (1) in the text is a generalization of the function known to mathematicians[1] as the unnormalized autocorrelation function

$$\varphi(\tau) = \lim_{\mu \to \infty} \frac{1}{\mu} \int_{-\mu/2}^{\mu/2} f(t)\, f(t + \tau)\, dt. \qquad (5)$$

$\varphi(\tau)$ is the average over all time of the product of the original time function $f(t)$ and the same function advanced by τ. The generalization is achieved by relaxing the requirement, which of course cannot be met in practice, that the average extend over all time. In general, we know nothing about the futures of the messages we receive. Certainly, the auditory system operates only upon the present and the not-extremely-far-distant past of the acoustic stimulus. We therefore take a running average (or, what amounts to the same thing, a running integral) instead of the average over all time. We also reverse the sign of the τ, so that we delay the signal instead of advancing it. This, again, avoids operating upon the future. The reversal of sign makes no difference to $\varphi(\tau)$ because, as defined in (5), it is an even function, symmetrical about $\tau = 0$. However, the substitution of the running integral for the all-time average requires explication.

As shown in Fig. 4, the first two operations in the determination of the running autocorrelation may be thought of as the same (except for the reversal of the sign of τ) as the first two operations in the determination of the function defined in (5). The function to be analyzed, $f(t)$, is shown as the heavy line in A. The first step is to delay $f(t)$ by a variable interval τ. In the figure, delaying $f(t)$ by τ_j (i.e. by one particular value of the variable τ) yields $f(t - \tau_j)$, which is shown as a dashed line. The second step is to multiply the original function by the delayed function. The product $\Pi(t, \tau_j) = f(t)\, f(t - \tau_j)$ is shown in B. We should of course have a set of such product functions, one for each value of the variable τ, instead of the single one shown in the figure.

[1] N. WIENER, *Extrapolation, interpolation, and smoothing of stationary time series* (John Wiley and Sons, Inc., New York, 1949).

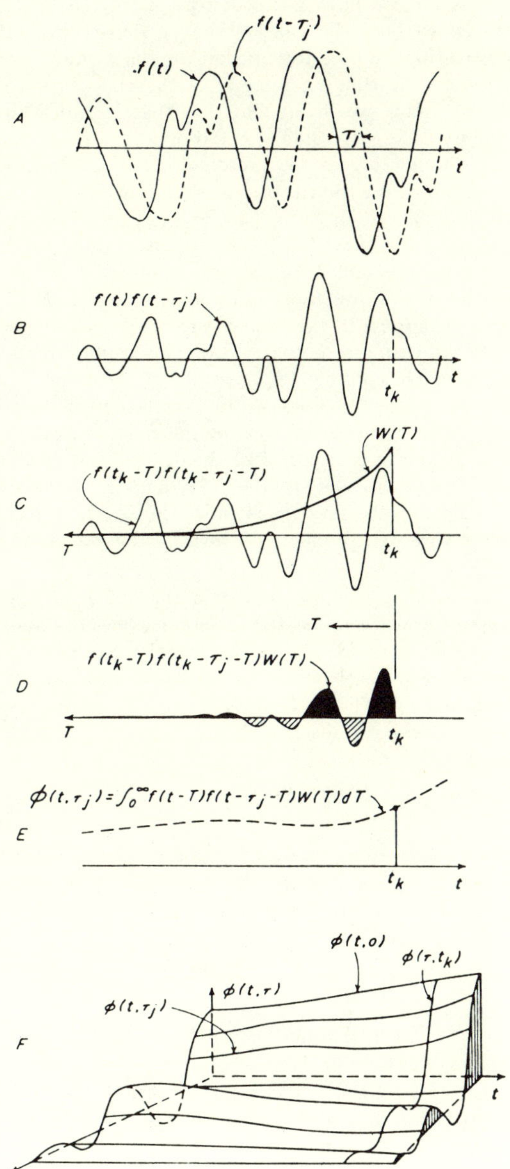

Fig. 4. – *Steps in the determination of the running autocorrelation function.* A shows the original function $f(t)$ and the delayed function $f(t - \tau_j)$. Their product is shown in B. In C, the instant t_k is taken as the present, and the product is re-expressed as a function of T, the distance into the past of t_k. The weighting function $W(T)$ determines the strength of the contribution of each past ordinate of the product to the autocorrelation coefficient. In order to let time t flow from left to right, the scale of T is oriented in the reverse direction as indicated by the arrows in C and D. The curve of D is the weighted product. It is integrated, the solid areas being considered positive and the cross-hatched areas negative, and the integral is plotted above t_k in E. Letting the present flow along in time and repeating the process for other values of time than t_k, we obtain the dashed curve in E. And, finally, we replicate the whole analysis for other values of the delay than τ_j. This generates the surface $\varphi(t, \tau)$ shown in F. The surface is the running autocorrelation function.

Thus far, we have proceeded as instructed by (5), but as we take the third step, we depart from it, substituting running integration for the average over all time. The running integral is the convolution of $\Pi(t, \tau_j)$ and a weighting function that specifies how strongly each past value of the product contributes to the accumulation at the present instant t_k. As in C, therefore, we rewrite the product as a function, not of t, but of distance T into the past of t_k. The choice of the weighting function $W(T)$ is to a considerable extent arbitrary: we might define any number of running autocorrelation functions, one for each possible $W(T)$. For the purpose of the duplex theory, a declining exponential with a time constant of 2 or 3 milliseconds is a reasonable choice. [$W(T)$ need not be defined for negative values of T.] The autocorrelation coefficient $\varphi(t_k, \tau_j)$ is then the integral of the weighted product over the entire past of t_k, but the distant past receives so little weight that it is effectively ignored. The result of weighting the product is shown in D. The integral of the weighted product is shown by the dot above t_k in E.

The procedure illustrated in A through E of Fig. 4 must of course be repeated for other values of t and τ. Repeating it for all t yields the function $\varphi(t, \tau_j)$ represented by the dashed line in E and shown again as a contour in F. Then repeating it for other values of τ generates the surface

$$\varphi(t, \tau) = \int_0^\infty f(t - T)\, f(t - \tau - T)\, W(T)\, dT. \qquad (6)$$

This is the running autocorrelation function for which expression (1) is a short-hand definition. The overline in (1) specifies that the operation

$$\int_0^\infty [\qquad\qquad]\, W(T)\, dT \qquad (7)$$

is applied to the product $f(t)\, f(t - \tau)$ after $t - T$ has been substituted for t.

Interpretation of the autocorrelation function is often facilitated, especially in cases in which we either naturally or through force of habit think in terms of frequency, by use of the WIENER theorem:

$$\left.\begin{aligned} \Phi(\omega) &= \frac{1}{2\pi}\int_{-\infty}^{\infty} \varphi(\tau)\cos\omega\tau\, d\tau \\ \varphi(\tau) &= \int_{-\infty}^{\infty} \Phi(\omega)\cos\omega\tau\, d\omega \end{aligned}\right\} \qquad (8)$$

Expression (8) tells us, for example, that the autocorrelation function of any sinusoid is a cosine function, the period in τ being the same as the period in t. Taking advantage of the fact that, if signals are superposed, the autocorrelation function of the sum may be found by superposing the autocorrelation functions of the individual signals, we can obtain the autocorrelation function of any signal that has a line spectrum by superposing cosine functions. Other aids to intuition are useful if the signal to be analyzed has a continuous spectrum. It is by no means necessary, however, to make the mental detour through the frequency domain. Some signals lend themselves more naturally to autocorrelational than to spectral analysis. The easiest way to find the spectra of telegraph and teletype messages, for example, is to determine the autocorrelation function first and then to take its Fourier transform.

The foregoing comments about the relation between the autocorrelation function and the power spectrum refer to $\varphi(\tau)$ and $\Phi(\omega)$, both of which involve integration over all time. Fortunately, analogous statements can be made about the running autocorrelation function, defined in (6), and the running power spectrum, measured with band-pass filters. FANO[1] has shown that, if the weighting function $W(T)$ in (6) is a declining exponential, and if the filters employ certain simple arrangements of resistances, capacitances, and inductances, the FOURIER transform relation extends to the running autocorrelation function and the running power density spectrum.

A final comment concerns the distinction between normalized and unnormalized autocorrelation functions. Often, the distinction is not made explicit. In communication engineering, the function defined in expression (5) is usually called "the autocorrelation function" without qualification. The signal $f(t)$ may have any average power; it may include a d-c component. "Autocorrelations" greater than unity may therefore arise. In other fields, especially those in which "correlation" means PEARSON product-moment correlation, it is natural to normalize $f(t)$ before operating upon it. The normalization eliminates the d-c component (sets the mean at 0) and adjusts the average power to unity (sets the variance at 1). The magnitude of the coefficient of autocorrelation is restricted to the interval $-1 \leqq \varphi \leqq 1$ by the normalization. For the autocorrelation function based on the average over all time [expression (5)], the normalization changes only the zero point and the scale factor; it leaves the shape unaltered. For the running autocorrelation function [expression (6)], however, the distinction is fundamental. In Fig. 4F, for example, the contour $\varphi(t, 0)$ would be a straight line at $\varphi = 1$ if the function were normalized. As the figure stands, unnormalized, $\varphi(t, 0)$ is the running average power (or squared amplitude) of $f(t)$.

[1] R. M. FANO, *op. cit.*

15

Reprinted from pages 171–177 and 181–182 of *Acoust. Soc. Am. J.* 20:171–182 (1948)

The Perception of Repeated Bursts of Noise[1]

GEORGE A. MILLER AND WALTER G. TAYLOR
Psycho-Acoustic Laboratory, Harvard University, Cambridge, Massachusetts
(Received December 1, 1947)

WHEN we measure the sound pressure at various frequencies in a continuous white noise, we find all the audible frequencies are present in approximately equal magnitude. Suppose we interrupt this noise at regular intervals. These interruptions can be regarded as a modulation of the amplitude of the noise by a square wave. Amplitude modulation produces sidebands around the carrier frequency. But with noise, the carrier is itself a band of frequencies, and sidebands are produced around all the frequencies in the band. Consequently, the interruption of a noise 200 times a second scatters energy outside the original band of noise frequencies, but over the audible frequency range no radical change is made in the uniformity of the noise spectrum. So long as the system is linear and detection does not occur, the frequency of 200 c.p.s.—representing the rate of modulation—is not intensified in the spectrum. Over the audible range, a wave analyzer reveals no difference in the shapes of the spectra of an interrupted and of a continuous white noise.

The interesting fact is that the ear discerns what the wave analyzer does not. A noise interrupted 200 times per second does not sound like a continuous noise. If Ohm's acoustic law—and Helmholtz's resonance theory of hearing which was built upon Ohm's law—applied strictly, the two noises would sound alike, which they do not. There is the possibility, of course, that the mechanical non-linearity of the middle ear acts to detect the modulation. When the two noises are reduced to 20 or 30 db above threshold, where the auditory mechanism presumably operates in a linear manner, the perceived differences should disappear. Since the difference does not disappear at these low intensities, mechanical non-linearity cannot be used as an explanation.

From an experimental point of view, the advantage of interrupted noise is that interruptions do not produce significant changes in the spectrum transduced by the earphones. If the listener notices changes in the sound, therefore, he is noticing them on the basis of the wave form and not on the basis of a frequency analysis of the various components in the sound. Consequently, an interrupted random noise can be used to explore the conditions under which changes in the wave form can be reported. We have found that some listeners have considerable success in matching the frequency of a pure tone to the rate of interruption of the noise up to 200 or 300 interruptions per second. Above this frequency the differential sensitivity to the rate of interruption becomes very poor, although qualitative differences between interrupted and continuous noises remain detectable, under some conditions, up to much higher rates of interruption.

For convenience in discussing these experiments we would like to introduce terminology

[1] This research was carried out under contract with the U. S. Navy, Office of Naval Research (Contract N5ori-76, Report PNR-43).

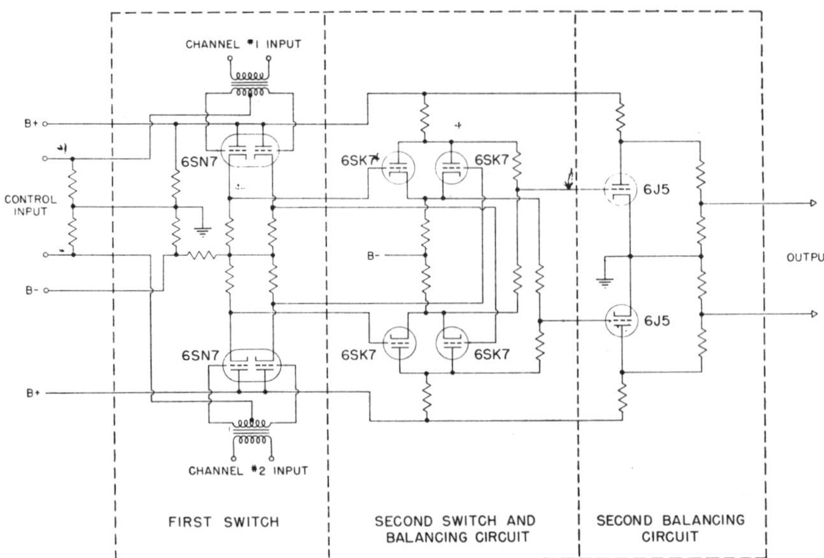

Fig. 1. Schematic diagram of the circuit used to interrupt the noise.

which parallels that used for the flicker experiments in vision. An interrupted noise whose intermittency can be perceived by a listener will be said to *flutter*. The rate of interruption will be called the *flutter frequency*, and the highest flutter frequency at which the interruption can be detected will be called the *critical flutter frequency*. The noise between two successive interruptions is a *burst*, and the portion of the total time occupied by noise bursts is the *sound-time fraction*.

CRITICAL FLUTTER FREQUENCIES AND AUDITORY FUSION

Under what conditions can auditory flutter be detected? The variables are, basically, those made familiar by experiments on visual flicker: intensity, rate, and sound-time fraction. Any two of these variables can be held constant while the third is varied until the listener reports that the interrupted stimulus is perceptually continuous.

In the present experiment it was convenient to establish a given rate of interruption and a given sound-time fraction and to permit the listener to adjust the intensity until the critical value (the point at which fusion occurs) was determined. A constant criterion for continuousness was provided the listener by alternating between interrupted and continuous noise. The listener then varied the intensity to the point at which he could not detect the alternation between the two noises. Thus fusion is here defined as the inability to discriminate interrupted from continuous sound.

The equipment for producing these stimuli began with a single noise generator. The noise voltage was led through two channels, one channel containing an electronic switch. The electronic switch chopped the noise into bursts at rates which could be varied between 0.1 and 5000 times a second for variable portions of the total on-off cycle. The two noises were then equated in apparent loudness, and a timing device alternated the two sounds in the listener's earphone (Permoflux PDR-10) every 1.5 seconds. A motor-driven attenuator was inserted in the line to the earphone, and the listener was able to vary the intensity of the noises over a range of 120 db. The listener was located in a separate, sound-deadened room along with the earphone and the manual switch which controlled the motor driving the attenuator. All other equipment was outside the listener's room.

A schematic diagram of the electronic switch, developed by P. W. Dippolito, is shown in Fig. 1. It consists of two switches in series, the first providing a differential of about 35 db between the on and off conditions, the second providing about 45 db. With this arrangement it is possible to present stimuli at relatively high levels without danger of a background signal leaking through when the channel is turned off. When only one channel is used, the signal is interrupted in accordance with the switching voltage applied to the control input. When both channels are used, the two signals are alternated. With the auxiliary equipment used in the present experiment, where an effectively instantaneous transition from on to off was employed, the balancing circuits operated to reduce the peak voltage of the switching 'spike' more than 20 db below the peak voltage of the signal passed without distortion. The train of pulses so introduced into the signal was inaudible under the conditions of these experiments. For longer transition times between on and off, the spike can be reduced more than 40 db below the peak amplitude of the signal.

The experimenter set up a given flutter rate and sound-time fraction. The listener then heard the continuous noise alternating every 1.5 seconds with the interrupted noise. The listener decreased the intensity of these sounds until he could no longer discriminate between them. At this point he announced his plight to the experimenter, who recorded the amount of attenuation and proceeded to change the interrupted noise for the next presentation. The attenuator readings were expressed as the equivalent sound pressure levels (db above 0.0002 dyne/cm^2) which the earphone would generate in a rigid cavity of 6 cc. The sensation level (db above threshold for hearing the noise) is obtained by subtracting 10 db from the sound pressure level. The level of the interrupted noise is given in terms of the level of the burst alone and not as an average over a longer period of time.

The results for two listeners, who made from two to ten judgments for each point, are shown in Fig. 2, where the burst intensity is plotted as a function of rate of interruption with the sound-time fraction as the parameter. The complete functions were obtained for sound-time fractions of 0.90 and 0.75. A sound-time fraction of 0.50 produced a detectable flutter well above 1000 interruptions per second, but we were not confident that the earphone would transduce the interrupted wave in a meaningful form at these higher rates. The frequency response of the earphone cuts off rather sharply above 7000 c.p.s., and the standard deviation of the energy in successive bursts of noise increases rapidly at high rates of interruption. By using Rice's formula for the standard deviation of the energy as a function of duration and pass band,[2] we calculated that an ideal pass band between 0 and 6500 c.p.s. yields a standard deviation 72 percent as large as the mean energy for a burst of noise lasting 0.25 msec. In other words, if a band of noise containing frequencies up to 6500 c.p.s. is interrupted 2000 times each second for a sound-time fraction of 0.50, almost a third of the bursts will fall more than 2.4 db above or more than 5.6 db below the mean value of the energy in the bursts. Similar computations for other rates of interruption show that such a noise is not a satisfactory stimulus when the duration of the

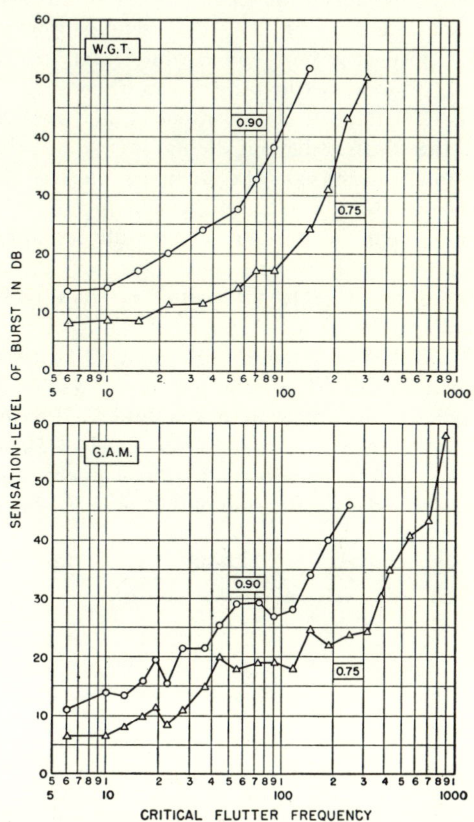

FIG. 2. The sensation level at which an interrupted noise could not be distinguished from a continuous noise is plotted as a function of the flutter frequency for two listeners and two noise-time fractions, 0.90 and 0.75. For more intense noises the flutter could be perceived.

[2] S. O. Rice, J. Acous. Soc. Am. 14, 216–227 (1943).

bursts gets much below a millisecond. After working against these technical difficulties, we obtained the impression that the upper limit for the detection of the flutter of noise interrupted half the time is in the neighborhood of 2000 interruptions per second, but the psychophysical data were too variable to be conclusive. With an electroacoustic transducer capable of transducing a uniform noise spectrum up to 20,000 c.p.s., however, this upper limit for the 0.50 sound-time fraction should be determinable.

The two contours obtained for sound-time fractions of 0.90 and 0.75 are similar in form to the functions obtained for visual flicker. With a fixed on-off fraction and a fixed rate of interruption, the flutter disappears as the intensity of the sound is lowered toward threshold. For any given intensity and sound-time fraction, the flutter disappears when the rate of interruption is great enough. And if the intensity and rate are set, the flutter disappears as the sound-time fraction is increased. The striking difference between auditory flutter and visual flicker is, of course, the higher rates at which auditory flutter can be detected. Apparently the auditory system is more sensitive to interruptions than is the visual system.

When the two listeners are compared, it will be noted that G.A.M. was better able to detect the presence of the flutter than was W.G.T. If we cut across the curves at a sensation level of 50 db, W.G.T. was able to detect 135 bursts per second with a sound-time fraction of 0.90 and 300 bursts

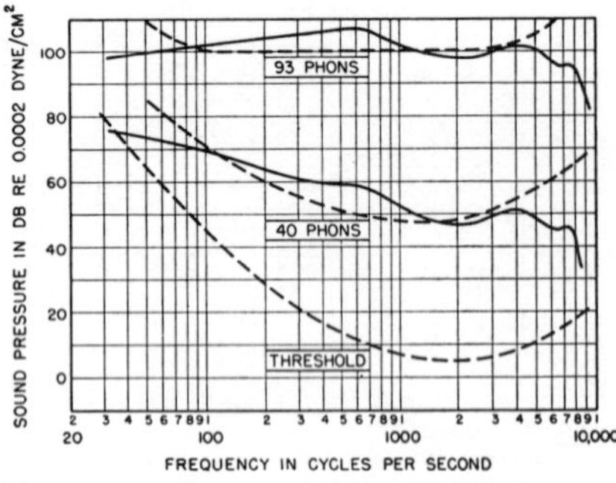

FIG. 3. Solid curves represent the sound pressure level at the listener's ear as a function of frequency. The dashed functions represent equal loudness contours at equivalent intensities. For the two intensities used in the pitch-matching experiments, the loudness of the tones was approximately constant at all frequencies.

with a fraction of 0.75. The corresponding values for G.A.M. are 270 and 750 bursts per second, about twice as large. Since the process of interruption produces no change in the spectrum of the noise, we assume that the listener perceives directly the modulation in the amplitude of the sound.

The shape of the functions in Fig. 2 can be predicted on the basis of the sensitivity of the ear to changes in the intensity of noise and the rate at which the auditory system recovers from stimulation. At 50 db a change of about 0.4 db in the level of a white noise can be detected, and so the rate of decay during the silent interval can be computed. The ear must recover from stimulation at a rate of at least 0.4 db per silent interval. When the computation is carried out for W.G.T., we find that his ear must have recovered from stimulation at a rate of about 0.51 db per msec., while G.A.M.'s ear recovered at a rate of 1.14 db per msec. If we extrapolate from these values to estimate the time it would take to recover 50 db to the quiet threshold, it amounts to 98 and 44 msec., respectively. These values are in fair agreement with the critical duration of 65 msec. to decay to threshold which was determined by previous experiments.[3] Indeed, a satisfactory description of the data of Fig. 2 is obtained if we assume that the perception would decay to threshold over a period of 98 msec. for W.G.T. and 44 msec. for G.A.M. at all intensities, and that the silent interval is just long enough to permit a sensory decay of one detectable step. Thus the results from this experiment are in essential agreement with the hypothesis that the decay time from any level of stimulation to threshold is a constant value for each listener.

THE PITCH OF INTERRUPTED NOISE

Some listeners reported that repeated bursts of random noise have a pitch corresponding to the rate of interruption. The pitch is vague, rough, and diffuse, but no other term than pitch seems to describe how 100 interruptions per second differ perceptually from 200 per second. According to a resonance theory of hearing, pitch depends upon the acoustic spectrum and the place on the basilar membrane where the com-

[3] G. A. Miller, "The perception of short bursts of noise," J. Acous. Soc. Am. 20, (1948).

ponent frequencies have their maximum effects. With repeated bursts of noise, however, the entire membrane is stimulated periodically, and the nature of the stimulus would seem to preclude any resonant localization of the disturbance at a particular point corresponding to the rate of interruption. That a perception of pitch can be produced by such a stimulus is, therefore, a matter worth looking into.

The pitch of a complex sound is usually considered to be that pitch of a pure tone which sounds equal in pitch to the complex sound. This definition suggests a simple experiment. To determine the pitch of a complex sound we ask some "average normal ears" to select a pure tone whose pitch sounds equivalent. The simplest procedure is to allow the listener to adjust the frequency of an oscillator until he is satisfied with the match. The fact is, however, that a complex sound does not have a single pitch, but has many pitches. A listener will give a variety of responses when tested over a period of time. Most of his responses are related by some simple multiple to the fundamental frequency of the complex sound, but a few represent original ideas of the listener. Confronted with such data it is no simple matter to decide what "the" pitch is, and the best we can do is to speak of the accuracy with which the frequencies are matched.

These considerations dictated the design of the following experiment. Listeners were asked to adjust the frequency of a pure tone to the same pitch as that of an interrupted noise. In order to minimize changes in loudness, equalizing networks were used in the oscillator circuit in an attempt to approximate the equal loudness contours as frequency was varied. Figure 3 shows the comparison of the response characteristic actually used with the equal loudness contours at the two levels investigated. Flutter frequencies from 30 to 2000 per second were employed at both 50 and 100 db over-all sound pressure levels of the noise. As an experimental control, the listeners were also asked to match the pure tone to a square wave and to a series of rectangular pulses (duration of pulse = 40 μsec). A final check was provided by having them match the frequency of the square wave to the rate of interruption of the noise. In all four experimental conditions care was taken to have the two sounds to be compared

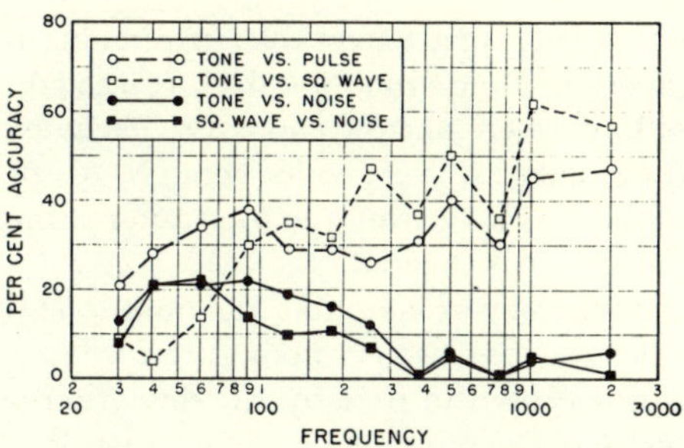

FIG. 4. The percentage of the judgments which fell within a narrow range on either side of the basic period of the standard is plotted as a function of the standard frequency. Open circles represent the accuracy in matching the pure tone to pulses; open squares, to square waves. The filled circles represent the accuracy in matching a pure tone to the flutter frequency of the noise; filled squares, the accuracy in matching a square wave to the flutter frequency.

at very nearly the same loudness: the effect of loudness upon pitch should not influence the experimental results.

A timer alternated the two sounds in the listener's earphone. The listeners were instructed to make their setting without looking at the dial of the oscillator. Once the setting was made, they recorded the frequency and the experimenter proceeded to set up the next experimental condition. Ten listeners with normal hearing were used. They were instructed in the concepts of pitch and timbre by a short discussion of musical instruments which play the same pitch, but do not sound alike. Since the subjects were well above normal intelligence, they quickly grasped the nature of the problem set for them. Five judgments were made by the ten listeners for each condition, and thus 50 judgments are available for each comparison.

The results showed that, for the two intensities studied, there was a very slight improvement in the accuracy of the match at the higher intensity. The magnitude of this effect was about the same for all the signals which were matched, and thus does not discriminate between the pitch character of the tonal and atonal sounds. The data for all 10 listeners at both levels have been pooled in the functions of Fig. 4, where the accuracy in matching the two frequencies is plotted as a function of frequency. Accuracy was defined as the percentage of the judgments which fell within a specified range on either side of the fundamental frequency of the complex sound. This range was taken as ±(1 just detectable increment in the frequency of a pure tone +0.02f). It was felt that these limits were narrow enough to exclude most random guesses, yet wide enough to permit normal errors in hearing the tone and reading the frequency from the dial.

The accuracy of matching the pure tone to the complex sounds was very poor at low frequencies. This was caused in part by the deviation of the intensity of the pure tone from an equal loudness contour at low frequencies, and in part by the insensitivity of the ear for the low fundamental as opposed to the harmonics of the complex waves.

At low frequencies, pure tones were matched more accurately to the frequency of the pulses than they were to the square waves. This difference is related to a phenomenon sometimes called "the case of the missing fundamental." A train of pulses at low pulse repetition frequencies has a very stable pitch which persists unchanged even when the lowest components of the sound are eliminated. The square wave, on the other hand, is much less stable in pitch when the fundamental is attenuated. In the present experiment, the ear acted as a filter to attenuate the intensity of the low frequency components, and this filtering affected the pitch of the pulses less than it affected the pitch of the square waves. At the high frequencies, on the other hand, the square wave is more similar to the sinusoidal wave than is the train of pulses, and hence the difference in accuracy is reversed. The large increase in accuracy for both pulses and square waves at high frequencies may reflect the elimination from these high tones of the harmonics above the cut-off frequency of the earphone.

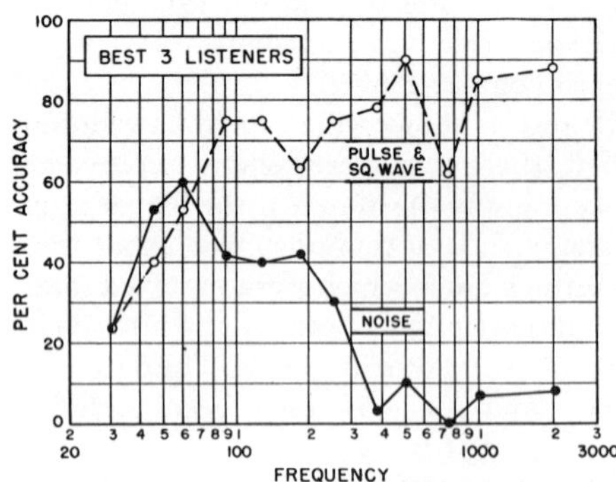

FIG. 5. Only the three most accurate listeners are presented. Judgments of the pitch of pulses are combined with those for square waves to give the single function shown by the open circles. Closed circles represent the accuracy in matching the flutter frequency of the noise with both pure tones and square waves.

The present interest in Fig. 4, however, is in the fact that our listeners had considerable success in matching a tone to an interrupted noise for rates of interruption up to 200 or 250 per second. At flutter frequencies below about 100 per second the accuracy is as high in matching the rate of interruption as it is in matching the frequency of pulses or square waves. When the rate of interruption is raised, however, the accuracy for the noise decreases and the accuracy for the complex tonal signals increases. The distribution of judgments at the higher rates of interruption of the noise are not greatly different from the distribution we might get if the listeners turned the oscillator dial completely at random. The fact that the distributions for high flutter frequencies were not completely random can be attributed to a "salient number tendency" in some of the listeners. Judgments of 500 or 1000 c.p.s., for example, occurred more frequently than would be expected by chance alone. Apparently some listeners intended a report of 500 c.p.s. to mean "in the neighborhood of 500 c.p.s." rather than "exactly 500 c.p.s." The tendency for the judgments to pile up at certain salient numbers, therefore, is not attributable to a real discrimination of pitch above 375 interruptions per second. It seems safe to conclude that, for a sound-time fraction of 0.5, the pitch character of interrupted noise disappears when the rate of interruption is increased above about 300 per second.

The data suggest that the characteristic of the sound which determines its pitch changes as a function of frequency, intermittency being a predominant feature at low frequencies, spectral composition at high. The transition is apparently a gradual one with considerable overlap from about 100 to 300 c.p.s. This conclusion agrees with the picture of the mechanics of the human cochlea developed by Békésy. Some degree of mechanical frequency analysis is obtained in the cochlea down to about 30 c.p.s., but the mechanical resolution (as indicated by the breadth of the resonance curves) is especially poor be-

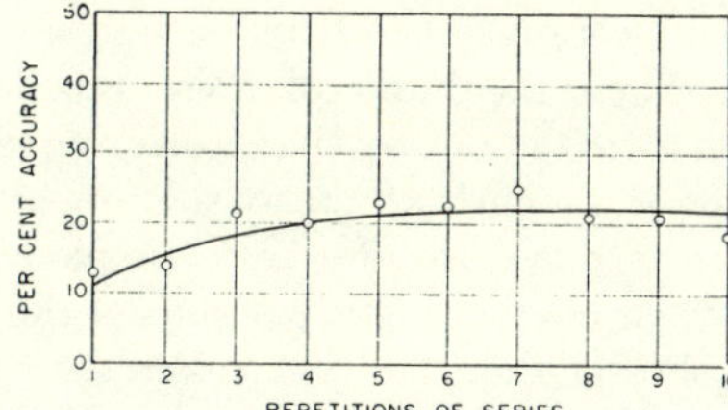

FIG. 6. Showing the slight improvement in accuracy as a function of successive trials when the listener was informed of the accuracy of his response.

tween 30 and 200 c.p.s.[4] Above 200 c.p.s. the resolution improves until a maximum is reached between 1000 and 3000 c.p.s. "Below 200 c.p.s. there is a continuously increasing broadening of the resonance curve."[5] The poor mechanical resolution over the range of frequencies below 200 c.p.s. is presumably supplemented by a neural mechanism capable of reporting the intermittent nature of the stimulation. The ability of listeners to match tones to the rates of interruption of a noise is direct evidence for the existence of such a neural mechanism.

The individual differences among the subjects' ability to match pitches were quite striking. After the experiment was completed the listeners were given the pitch and tonal memory portions of the Seashore Musical Aptitude Test. The listeners were ranked in order by their scores on this test, and again by the percentage of the "correct" judgments they made during the pitch-matching experiments. These two rank orders correlated positively with a correlation coefficient of 0.75. Apparently some of the listeners, though possessing normal audiograms, were low in general musical aptitude. One listener, for example, failed consistently to make accurate matches under any of the experimental conditions. In order to give a better picture of what some listeners are able to do in the way of matching frequencies, we have selected the three most accurate of the ten listeners and presented their results in Fig. 5. For convenience, the two conditions under which tonal sounds (pulses and square waves) were judged are combined, and the two conditions using interrupted noise are combined. The general picture is much the same as for the entire group, but it is more obvious that

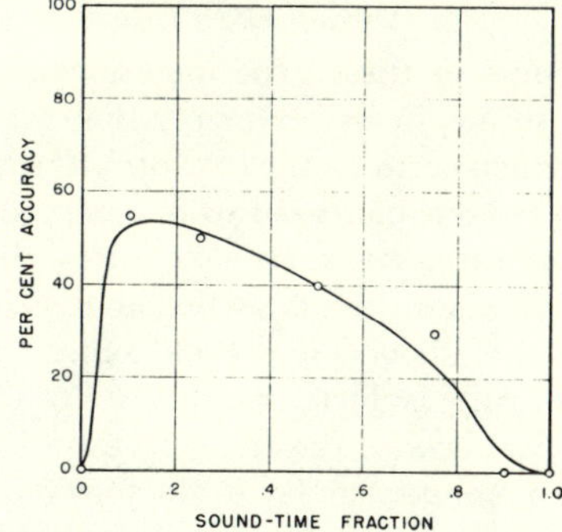

FIG. 7. The accuracy in matching the frequency of a tone to the rate of interruption of a noise varies with the noise-time fraction.

these three listeners were matching the slower rates of interruption with considerably better than chance success.

In view of the poor performance of many of the subjects we felt that a period of training might increase their accuracy. This training was given for the pure tone *vs.* interrupted noise conditions. Twenty-five frequencies of interruption between 30 and 1920 per second were used, and the listener made his response as before. After each judgment, however, the experimenter told the listener his judgment was "correct," or, if it was not correct, the listener was told what the correct setting was. He then changed his oscillator to the correct frequency and listened to the two sounds. The series of 25 frequencies was repeated 10 times with each of five listeners, and the accuracy is plotted in Fig. 6 as a function of successive repetitions. This situation resulted in little learning, as the curve in Fig. 6 shows. Apparently the large individual differences in the accuracy of matching a tone to the rate of interruption of a noise depend upon fundamental differences in perceptual ability and not upon any failure to grasp the nature of the judgment which they were called upon to make.

All the experiments described above employed a sound-time fraction of 0.5. In order to estimate the importance of this variable for the pitch of interrupted noise, two listeners matched a pure tone to noise (100-db sound pressure level) interrupted between 55 and 180 times a second for different fractions of the total time. The results are shown in Fig. 7. The greatest accuracy was achieved for sound-time fractions less than 0.5.

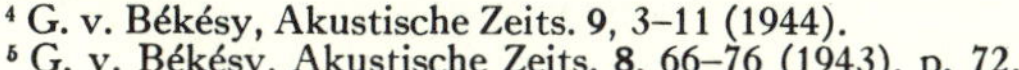

[4] G. v. Békésy, Akustische Zeits. 9, 3–11 (1944).
[5] G. v. Békésy, Akustische Zeits. 8, 66–76 (1943), p. 72.

[*Editor's Note:* Material has been omitted at this point.]

DISCUSSION

The results of these experiments can be summarized by a description of the perceptual changes which occur as the rate of interruption of a random noise is increased from a very slow to a very rapid rate. At very slow rates the noise comes on, persists, decays to threshold, is followed by a period of silence, and then comes on again. When the rate is increased to 10 to 15 interruptions per second, the successive bursts begin to fuse in a manner similar to the fusion obtained with sinusoidal waves. The pitch character of the noise begins to emerge and is quite distinct for most listeners at interruption rates of 40 per second. Over the range from about 40 to 250 interruptions per second the impression of a definite pitch persists, and differential sensitivity to rate is comparable in accuracy to differential sensitivity for the frequency of sinusoidal waves. From about 250 to 2000 interruptions (assuming a sound-time fraction of 0.5) a qualitative difference between the interrupted noise and a steady noise can be detected, but no pitch seems to accompany the changes in rate of interruption. For more rapid rates the interrupted noise is indistinguishable from the continuous noise. Thus four phases can be distinguished: (1) successive bursts, (2) a train of bursts having a pitch character, (3) a noise differing slightly in quality from continuous noise, and (4) a continuous noise.

If we look to the auditory system to find phases in its operation corresponding to these four perceptual phases, we arrive at the following description. Below about 10 per second the bursts can probably be regarded as separate events with little interaction upon one another. Miller[3] has presented evidence supporting the notion that the perceptual decay of a noise is complete in about 60–65 msec. for most listeners. Thus at 10 bursts per second, with a sound-time fraction of 0.5, the perceptual decay of one burst would not be completed before the next burst occurs, and the neural processes representing the successive bursts should begin to tread upon each other's heels and to fuse into a steady train.

From about 20 to 250 bursts per second, therefore, the level of neural activity is presumably fluctuating in synchronism with the bursts of noise. This synchronism might continue to higher frequencies were it not for the mechanism of the cochlea. When the burst of noise reaches the cochlea it is spread out by that analyzing mechanism over the length of the basilar membrane. The time it takes for the high frequencies to activate their characteristic portions of the membrane is shorter than the time taken for the low frequencies, since the low frequencies must travel the entire length of the membrane to the helicotrema. Békésy[5] has shown that approximately 5 msec. are necessary for a pulse to travel the length of the cochlear duct. A second burst of noise separated from the first by less than 5 msec. would activate the high frequency portion of the membrane before the first burst had stopped stimulating the end near the helicotrema. A silent interval of 5 msec. corresponds to a duration of 10 msec. for the total on-off cycle, and 10 msec. corresponds to an interruption rate of 100 per second. Since the pitch character and the ability to detect changes in the frequency of the flutter begin to deteriorate above 100 bursts per second, it is reasonable to associate this perceptual change with the occurrence of two successive patterns of activity on the basilar membrane. At 250 bursts per second the temporal separation between bursts is 2 msec., and the last 5 mm of the membrane are active at the moment the next burst begins to travel down the cochlear duct. Neural impulses from the two bursts start up the auditory nerve at the same time, and the discrimination of pitch deteriorates greatly.

Although the nervous discharges representing successive bursts of noise must begin to overlap seriously when the bursts are separated by less than 2 msec., the last of the preceding discharge comes from a different group of receptor cells than the first of the following discharge. A small group of cells located at a single point along the membrane will continue to discharge intermittently even though their activity overlaps that of other cells at a distant point. Thus, qualitative differences between the interrupted noise and a continuous noise can be detected, even though pitch discrimination is gone. The intermittent character of the activity is apparently an effective cue for the detection of interruptions up to the point where successive bursts occur so rapidly that the neural process does not have time to decay by a just detectable step before the next burst arrives. Assuming that upon termination of a noise 100 db above threshold the neural process decays over a period of 65 msec. and that 0.4 db is necessary to detect a difference in intensity, it turns out that 0.25 msec. would be necessary for a just detectable decrement. This duration is equivalent to a flutter frequency of 2000 bursts per second, a figure which corresponds to the highest rate at which the presence of interruptions can be detected with a sound-time fraction of 0.5.

16

Reprinted from *Acoust. Soc. Am. J.* **23**:40–42 (1951)

Some Observations on Pitch and Frequency*

H. DAVIS, S. R. SILVERMAN, AND D. R. MCAULIFFE
Central Institute for the Deaf, St. Louis, Missouri

(Received October 2, 1950)

"Tone-pips" were produced by brief rectangular electrical pulses being delivered through two sound-effects filters in cascade with both high and low cut-offs set at 2000 cps. Nearly all of the acoustic energy of the final signal was found to be concentrated in a band about an octave wide and centering at 2000 cps. The pulsing frequency was varied independently between 90 and 150 pips per second.

Listeners describe the resulting sound as a "metallic buzz." Listeners vary greatly in their ability to identify the two "pitches" present in this sound and in the accuracy with which they match with a pure tone either the pulsing frequency (about 130 per second) or the band-pass frequency (2000 cps in the present series). Errors of exactly one octave are particularly common.

In the theoretical discussion we argue that the "pitch" of a pure tone is a double attribute compounded of "buzz" (correlated with frequency of volleys of nerve impulses) and "body" (correlated with position of maximum stimulation on the basilar membrane).

INTRODUCTION

THIS study was initiated to test the theory that the pitch of tones below 1000 cps is uniquely determined by the frequency of successive volleys of nerve impulses in the auditory nerve.[1] In our program abstract[2] we emphasized some of our present observations that are contrary to the frequency theory of pitch perception, but experiments done since the abstract was written have led us to incorporate much of the frequency theory into our own thinking. The present paper is still only a preliminary report, however, of some psycho-physical studies that we have carried out with "tone-pips," and an outline of our present views on the problems of pitch.

TONE-PIPS

"Tone-pips" are brief trains of waves at a constant frequency, say 2000 or 4000 per second, modulated rapidly to a maximum amplitude in about three waves and then back to a low level in 3 to 10 waves. Singly they sound like ticks, knocks, or thuds, depending on the frequency. We developed these simple acoustic stimuli for use in our animal experiments. They are produced by passing a rectangular electrical pulse of appropriate duration through two filter sections in cascade. We employ two sound-effects filters, each with attenuation of 18 db per octave and each with high pass and low pass both set to the nominal frequency desired. The tone-pip can sometimes be further purified or modified by acoustic filtering of the output of the electro-acoustic transducer or by taking advantage of a mechanical resonance. Figure 1 shows oscillograms illustrating the various steps in the production of typical tone-pips.

We deliver the tone-pips to our listeners through a PDR-10 receiver or, in our experiments on guinea pigs, through an Atlas PM-25 loudspeaker coupled to 5 feet of garden hose.

Figure 2 shows the acoustic spectrum of a series of 2000 cps tone-pips obtained with a General Radio Wave Analyzer 736-A set for 4-cycle band width. The line spectrum was obtained when the pips were delivered to the filter at a frequency of 150 pips per second. The continuous spectrum was obtained by observing the swing of the meter needle to individual pips at 1 per second as the analyzer frequency was slowly altered. A similar spectrum was shown by a Panoramic Sonic Analyzer.[3] Notice that the energy is nearly all concentrated in a band about an octave wide and particularly

* This work was carried out under Contract N6onr-272 between the ONR and Central Institute for the Deaf.

[1] E. G. Wever, *Theory of Hearing* (John Wiley and Sons, Inc., New York, 1949).

[2] H. Davis, S. R. Silverman, and D. R. McAuliffe, J. Acoust. Soc. Am. 22, 674 (1950).

[3] Kindly loaned by Dr. George Kreezer, Department of Psychology, Washington University.

that no energy within 60 decibels of the maximum appears at 150 per second, which is the pulsing frequency.

Most of our present observations were made with 2000-cps pips at 90 to 150 pips per second and at the 30- or 40-db sensation level. These frequencies were chosen to get complete dissociation of the two frequencies, i.e., *cycles* per second and *pips* per second, without getting too close to the limits of the auditory range.

Physiological observations on guinea pigs reported elsewhere[4] indicate that, with 2000-cps pips 40 db above threshold, (a) a particular area about the middle of the cochlea is stimulated, (b) each fiber that responds gives only 1 impulse per pip because of its refractory period, (c) the volley principle is at work: two or perhaps three groups of fibers are excited at intervals of 0.5 msec. We conclude that the frequency of impulses in each of the active fibers is at the pulsing rate, say 150 per second. The group of fibers that carries this frequency corresponds broadly, however, to the 2000-cps position on the basilar membrane. A definite frequency of impulses is set up in the "wrong" set of fibers.

PSYCHO-ACOUSTIC OBSERVATIONS

The subjective sensation on listening to 2000-cps pips at 90 to 150 pips per second, 40 db SL, has been reported by all nine of our listeners as a "buzz."

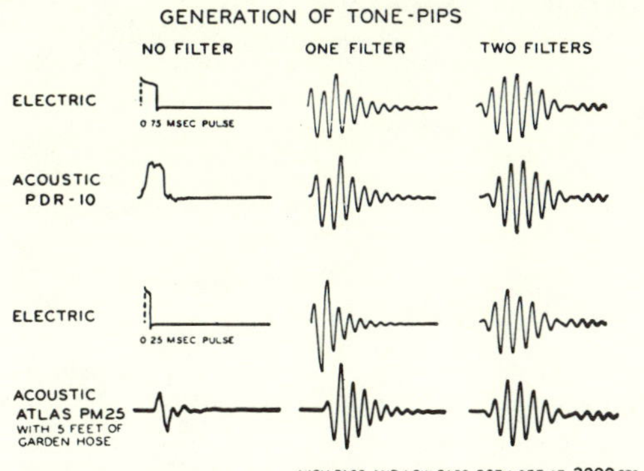

FIG. 1. Our electric pulse is actually rectangular. The distortion in this figure is due to the frequency characteristics of the recording amplifiers. The distortion of the filtered patterns and acoustic pulses is negligible, however. The choice of duration of pulse is critical for obtaining the simple patterns shown. These patterns, produced with pulses one-half and one-and-a-half times the basic wavelength passed by the band-pass filters, are among the simplest and most symmetrical. The pip employed in the present experiments is the second from the top in the third column. Note the close correspondence between electric and acoustic patterns when two filter sections are used. The production of a strong 2000-cps component by the Atlas PM 25 when no filter is used depends largely on the use of a piece of garden hose instead of the intended horn. A loose pack of pipe-cleaners in the hose nearly suppresses a strong component at 8000 cps.

Acoustic oscillograms were obtained with a 640AA condenser microphone. The PDR-10 is coupled to it with a 6-cc coupler. With the Atlas PM 25 the microphone is set in the "free field" 3 cm from the end of the hose at the position usually occupied by the ear of the experimental animal (guinea pig).

[4] H. Davis, C. Fernández, and D. R. McAuliffe, Proc. Nat. Acad. Sci., U. S. **36**, 580–587 (1950).

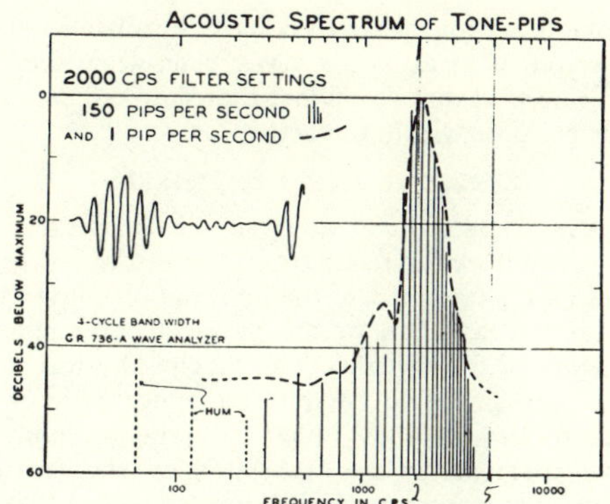

FIG. 2. The wave form of the pips is indicated as well as the acoustic analysis. With 1 pip per second the hum is stronger relative to the signal and makes readings uncertain below 200 cps.

Adjectives commonly used are "rough" and "metallic." No listener has been able to hear a low tone, like that aroused by a sine wave at the pulsing frequency, even when specifically directed to listen for it. Many observers deny that the "buzz" has *any* pitch, until either the basic frequency or the pulsing frequency is altered. A few, apparently those who do the most listening to music, recognize one or the other pitch: either the one corresponding to *cycles* per second or else the one corresponding to *pips* per second. No unsophisticated listener has yet spontaneously reported the presence of both pitches. All listeners, however, agree that the sound has a pitch as soon as either of the physical frequencies is varied. They say that the sound becomes lower and more "wooden" when the cycles per second are reduced to 1000 and that it becomes higher, smaller, and sharper when the frequency is increased to 4000 cps. They also say that it "sounds like a siren getting up speed" when the pips are increased gradually from 60 to 150 per second.

Our listeners vary greatly in their ability to make pitch-matches to the "buzz." A pure tone is presented to them alternately with the buzz and at equal loudness for 1-sec periods. All our listeners agree that "the matching is difficult because the sounds are so unlike." Some of them match the 2000-cps frequency quite well, sometimes with great precision. Others find the 130 per second frequency easier to match and *may* be very precise with few errors of more than 3 cycles per second. At other times the same subjects may make consistent systematic errors.

The commonest error, which most listeners mention spontaneously, is choice of the wrong octave, i.e., a frequency double or half of the basic frequency or of the pulsing frequency. It is interesting that the difficulty of identifying the octave correctly seems equally great for both of the actual frequencies involved. Other simple harmonic ratios are often chosen as well as the octaves, sometimes with precision and confidence, particularly by the more "musical" listeners. (This finding was completely unexpected.) Some of our listeners have made errors as great as 2 octaves, even when they did match, and were quite confident that they had matched, the correct note within the octave.

COMMENT AND HYPOTHESES

We may expect the greatest simplicity of theory in the long run if we can relate subjective sensations to the *physiological* parameters of the information delivered to the brain rather than to the physical parameters or dimensions of the stimulus. The psycho-physical correlations may prove to be quite complicated. For example: *frequencies* above 4000 cps (and probably all audible frequencies) are translated in the ear into *positions*, i.e., to *choice of channel*; but below 800 cps (and perhaps, by the volley principle, up to 4000 cps) information as to frequency is *also* carried in the form of *time-intervals between impulses*. Pure tones set up a *particular* relation between these two types of information; but a series of tone-pips gives a very different relation. The tone-pips are heard as "a very different sound."

We may safely postulate that all of the information that is actually delivered to the brain will appear in some attribute of sensation. The problem is to relate the attributes correctly to the classes of information which are conveyed by different physiological processes.

The usual operational definition of pitch seems to be "that attribute which allows us to match frequencies of sounds." It now seems clear that either place or frequency or both may be the physiological correlate(s) of physical frequency. We therefore do not regard pitch as a single attribute, but as a composite of "buzz" (the correlate of physiological frequency) and "body" (the correlate of physiological place or channel). "Buzz" probably also contributes to or determines "rate," "successiveness," and perhaps "roughness." It is what Schouten's "residue"[5] contributes to hearing, but it may be contributed by lower harmonics or by the fundamental as well. "Body" is closer to what we ourselves have formerly thought of as "pitch," and it probably contributes strongly to both the "volume" (size) and "density" of sounds. We regard musical chroma or key as a higher order attribute that may be based on either "buzz" or "body" or both.

Our observations, analysis, and theorizing are in close agreement with those of Miller and Taylor.[6] The theory that emerges incorporates much of the frequency theory as stated by Wever,[7] but more observations are needed.

---

[5] J. F. Schouten, Philips tech. Rev. **5**, 286–294 (1940).

[6] G. A. Miller, and W. G. Taylor, J. Acoust. Soc. Am. **20**, 171–182 (1948).

[7] E. G. Wever, reference 1, p. 1.

17

Reprinted from pages 351, 354-356, and 365 of *J. Exp. Psychol.* 37:351-365 (1947)

PITCH CHARACTERISTICS OF SHORT TONES. I. TWO KINDS OF PITCH THRESHOLD *

BY J. M. DOUGHTY AND W. R. GARNER

The Johns Hopkins University

[*Editor's Note:* Material has been omitted at this point.]

Results

Preceding the experiment proper, approximately 500 judgments, over a period of two weeks, were made by each of the two *S*s on these thresholds. The criteria for the thresholds were constantly emphasized during this training period.

Training periods.—The time to make a single judgment decreased steadily during the training period. In the early stages of training, an *S* would take as long as five min. to make a single judgment. In the final stages, the average length of time was cut to about 30 sec. Judgments at the low frequencies of 125 cps and 250 cps remained the most difficult to make throughout the entire experiment, and invariably took the longest to make. This was probably due to the phase differences in the onset of the sound—a crucial factor at low frequencies. Phase at the onset of the tone was not controlled during the running of the experiment, but a post-experimental investigation of its effect indicated that the effect was non-existent at frequencies of 250 cycles and above.

By the end of the training period, the *S*s reported that judgments of both click-pitch and tone-pitch were relatively easy to make at all frequencies higher than 250 cycles, with the click-pitch threshold being the more clear-cut of the two.

Preceding the second part of the experiment, another training period was given during which the *S*s made approximately 250 judgments for the two types of pitch throughout the intensity range stated and over the three frequencies used. This training was only for the purpose of giving the *S*s practice at recognizing click-pitch and tone-pitch at low intensity levels.

Results: Effect of Frequency

Table I shows the relation between frequency and duration of a tone in msec. for the click-pitch and tone-pitch thresholds. The thresholds for each frequency are based on the average of 40 observations obtained from the two *S*s over four experimental periods.

* This research was carried out under Contract N5ori-166, Task Order I, between the Special Devices Center, Office of Naval Research, and The Johns Hopkins University. This article is Report No. 166-I-14 under that contract.

TABLE I

THE RELATION BETWEEN FREQUENCY AND DURATION OF A TONE IN MSEC. FOR TWO KINDS OF PITCH THRESHOLDS

The intensity is 110 db *re* 0.0002 dynes/cm.[2]

	Frequency (cps)						
	125	250	500	1000	2000	4000	8000
Click-pitch	17.9	10.5	5.8	4.4	4.6	4.1	4.0
Tone-pitch	24.2	16.8	12.9	10.2	10.2	8.8	9.6

For all observations the intensity level remained constant at 110 db *re* 0.0002 dynes/cm.[2]

Fig. 3 is a graphical representation of the data from Table I, and it can be seen from this figure that click-pitch and tone-pitch follow

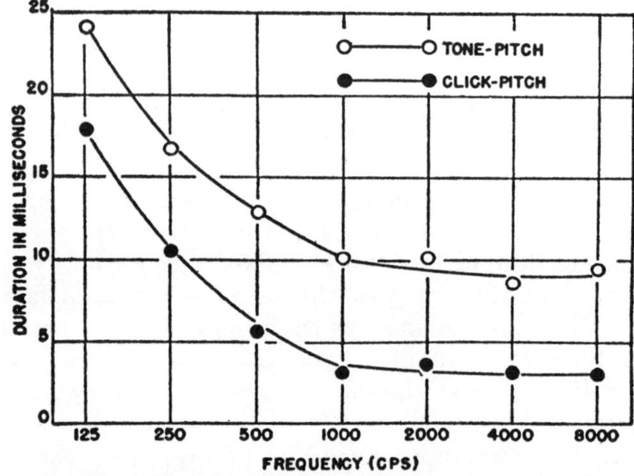

FIG. 3. The relation between frequency and the tonal duration required for two types of pitch The data for these two curves are obtained from Table I, and each plotted point represents the average of 40 observations obtained from two *Ss*. The intensity of the tone is 110 db *re* 0.0002 dynes/cm.[2]

two very distinct curves throughout the frequency range from 125 cps to 8000 cps. The duration threshold for the perception of *click-pitch* is shorter at all frequencies than that for perception of *tone-pitch*, which is, of course, to be expected.

The thresholds for both types of pitch are longest at the low frequencies of 125 cps and 250 cps. They become shorter in the range of frequencies to which the ear is most sensitive, i.e., 1000 cps to 4000 cps, and remain fairly constant throughout this range of frequencies and up to 8000 cps.

Difference between thresholds.—Two facts are evident from these curves. In the first place, the difference in duration required for the click-pitch and the tone-pitch thresholds is not a relative matter, but rather is a constant. For example, it does not take twice as great a duration to go from click-pitch to tone-pitch regardless of the duration required for click-pitch, but it appears to require about six msec. more duration, for any frequency and any duration. The maximum difference in duration between any two thresholds is 7.1 msec., and the minimum difference is 4.7 msec. While there is some tendency for the time difference to become less as the frequency is increased (and as the duration for click-pitch is decreased), still that trend is very small compared to the relative constancy of the difference. Thus, it would seem that only increased duration, and not number of cycles, is responsible for the change from click-pitch to tone-pitch.

In the second place, as the frequency is changed, it requires neither a constant duration nor a constant number of cycles to obtain either of the thresholds. For frequencies above 1000 cps, duration is relatively constant. For frequencies below 500 cps, there is a tendency for the number of cycles to remain constant (more true for click-pitch than tone-pitch), although this tendency is far from exact. In other words, as long as the minimum duration required for click-pitch involves at least two to three cycles, that duration will be constant. When the frequency is so low, however, that an insufficient number of cycles would be involved, the duration must be increased so that at least two complete cycles are encompassed in the tone. For example, for frequencies of 125, 250, and 500 cps, the duration is not constant, although in each case the duration is equivalent to between two and three complete cycles (click-pitch). For frequencies above that, however, the duration is constant, indicating that the number of complete cycles increases proportionate to the frequency.

[*Editor's Note:* Material has been omitted at this point.]

References

1. Bürck, W., Kotowski, P., & Lichte, H. Der Aufbau des Tonhöhenbewusstseins. *Elek. Nachr.-Techn.*, 1935, **12**, 326–333.
2. Bürck, W., Kotowski, P., & Lichte, H. Die Hörbarkeit von Laufzeitdifferenzen. *Elek. Nachr.-Techn.*, 1935, **12**, 355–362.
3. Roush, R. G. Tone burst generator. *Electronics*, 1947, **20**, No. 7, 92–96.
4. Stevens, S. S., & Davis, H. *Hearing: Its Psychology and Physiology*. New York: John Wiley, 1938.
5. Turnbull, W. W. Pitch discrimination as a function of tonal duration. *J. exp. Psychol.*, 1944, **34**, 302–316.

18

Reprinted from *Sov. Phys. Acoust.* **6**:75-80 (1960)

FREQUENCY-DIFFERENCE LIMENS AS A FUNCTION OF TONAL DURATION

Liang Chih-an and L. A. Chistovich

I. P. Pavlov Physiological Institute, Academy of Sciences, USSR, Leningrad

(Translated from: Akusticheskii Zhurnal Vol. 6, No. 1, pp. 81-86, January-March, 1960)

Original article submitted June 2, 1959

The dependence of frequency-difference limens on tonal duration is investigated. The results reveal different forms of the relationship in the regions of short ($t < T_1$), medium ($T_1 < t < T_2$), and long ($T_2 < t$) durations. The change in T_1 and T_2 with a change in the signal frequency is studied. The authors discuss the possible physiological interpretation of the constants T_1 and T_2.

One of the most astonishing peculiarities of hearing is the possibility of distinguishing very small frequency differences between tones in the very coarse frequency analysis of sound executed by the cochlea. This contradistinction between the imperfection of sound analysis by the colchlea and the precision of the end-resultant distribution has been widely discussed in the literature, and many hypotheses have been put forth regarding the mechanisms of the auditory system that make the resolving power sharper. Much less attention has been drawn to the fact that the time required for the build-up process in the cochlea has been computed as a few msec [1], whereas the frequency-difference limens continue to be reduced with increasing signal duration up to 0.1-0.3 sec [2]. Comparing these two groups of factors, it is reasonable to assume that one of the reasons for the refinement is the ability of the nerve branches of the auditory system to accumulate information relevant to the signal frequency from the process already established in the cochlea.

It is evident that an investigation of the dependence of the difference limen on the tonal duration should yield some information on the behavior of the summation of information by the nerve branches of the auditory system. A dependence of this type was determined by Turnbull [2], but the procedure that he used for the measurement fosters certain objections. In Turnbull's experiments the short tone used was always compared with a standard tone of constant duration (0.5 sec). It is known that when the tonal duration is shortened it begins more and more to turn into a click, so that the increase observed by Turnbull in the discrimination threshold with shortening of the tone to be compared could be connected not only with the frequency discrimination of the short sinusoidal signals becoming worse, but with difficulties in comparing short signals with a long one. It is possible that this very circumstance must be explained by the fact that for signals shorter than 17-37 msec Turnbull could not in general measure the difference limens. In view of this, it seemed necessary to us that Turnbull's experiments be repeated, but using signals of identical duration for both the variable signal and standard.

The tests were conducted on two human subjects, the authors of the present paper (hereafter denoted in the figures and text by A and B). Both of the auditors had normal hearing and were trained in auditory measurements. The measurement of threshold was performed by the method of frequency matching. A schematic of the experimental setup is shown in Fig. 1. The tone sources were two audio oscillators. One of the oscillators 1, which was the source of the standard signal, was placed outside the dead room 2 and its frequency was controlled by the experimenter. The other oscillator 3 was placed in the room, its frequency controlled by the auditor. The outputs of the oscillators were fed in turns by means of the relay 4, controlled by a mechanical interrupter, to the input of the electronic key 5, which ensured the necessary signal duration. The key was triggered by the same relay, connected with the mechanical interrupter. The signals were delivered from the output of the key (segments of a sinusoid, switched on and off with random phase) through the attenuators 6 and 7 to the TD-6 electrodynamic earpiece 8.

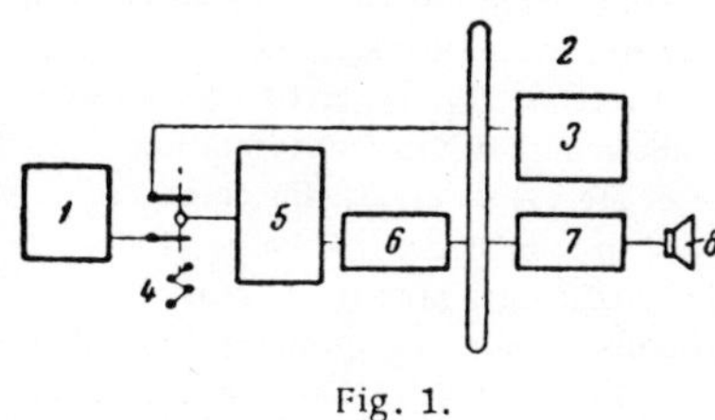

Fig. 1.

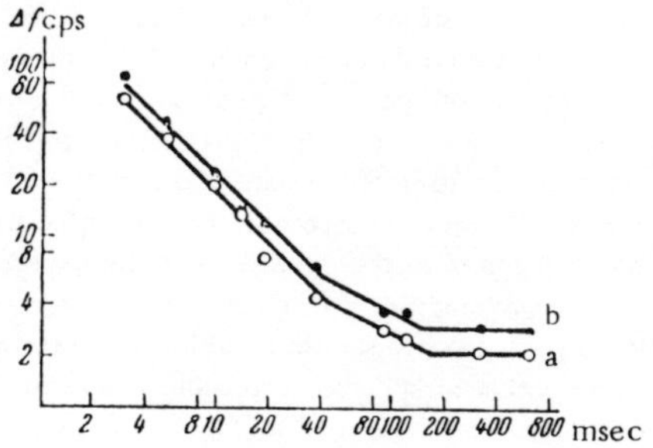

Fig. 2.

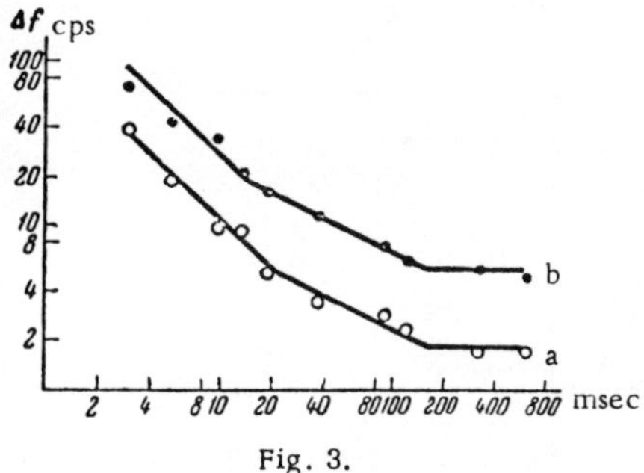

Fig. 3.

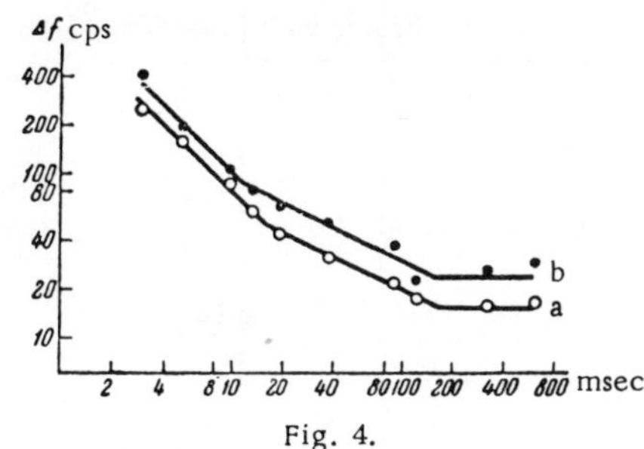

Fig. 4.

The signals were delivered in pairs. The interval between the variable and standard signals was 2.5 sec. The variable signal was the first of the pair. At the beginning of the determination the frequency of the variable signal was always made considerably different from the frequency of the standard (above and below it in an equal number of cases), then the auditor gradually varied the frequency of the variable signal until both signals were perceived as the same. After the frequency of the variable signal had been matched by the auditor the experimenter measured the deviation of the adjusted frequency from the frequency of the standard. For this both oscillators fed the same earpiece and the frequency of the standard-signal generator 2 was changed until the beats between tones disappeared. On the basis of 20-40 deviations for individual determinations the standard deviation was computed and taken as the threshold for the given tonal duration.

The dependence of the difference limens (Δf) on the signal duration (t) so obtained for three different values of the signal frequency is shown in Figs. 2, 3, 4, which refer to experiments with tonal frequencies of 250, 1000, and 4000 cps, respectively. It can be seen that the auditors differed in the absolute values of Δf, but the form of the dependence for the two auditors was similar. In comparing the curves obtained for the different frequencies, it is notable that, although the range of durations within which the dependence of Δf on $\underline{t}$ was observed was approximately the same in all three cases, the curves differ considerably in form.

In order to exhibit these differences in the curve forms distinctly, we tried to approximate the curves by three straight-line segments. It turned out that a satisfactory approximation to the experimental relations could be obtained with the description of these by the following expressions:

$$\Delta f = k\,(T_1/t) \quad \text{for} \quad t < T_1, \tag{1}$$

$$\Delta f = k\,(T_1/t)^{1/2} \quad \text{for} \quad T_1 < t < T_2 \tag{2}$$

$$\Delta f = k\,(T_1/T_2)^{1/2} = c \quad \text{for} \quad T_2 < t, \tag{3}$$

where Δf is the difference limen, t is the signal duration, T_1 is the first critical duration, T_2 is the second critical duration, k is a constant depending on the frequency.

From these expressions it follows that on the segments of the curves corresponding to very small signal duration ($t < T_1$) the difference limen decreases in direct proportion to the increase in signal duration. As evident from the curves in Figs. 2, 3, 4, the duration of this interval is shortened with increasing signal frequency, i.e., T_1 is a diminishing function of the signal frequency.

On the second interval of the curves ($T_1 < t < T_2$) the difference limen continues to decrease with increasing duration, but the rate of this decrease is lessened, the threshold is proportional to the square root of the signal duration. Finally, when the signal duration reaches T_2, further reduction in the threshold ceases, i.e., its magnitude becomes no longer dependent on the signal duration. In order to calculate the constants of interest, T_1, T_2, and k, the following procedure was used: from Eq. (1) it follows that for small signal durations the product of the discrimination threshold and the duration is constant and equal to kT_1. Therefore, making use of the values of Δf for duration known to be small, we should be able to determine the series of values of Δft and to take as the true value of kT_1 that for which the sum of the deviations in the experimental values of Δft is the smallest (in practice it proved to be very near the average of the Δft series). Further, making use of the points on the middle part of the curve, which is described by Eq. (2), we should be able to determine the series of values of $\Delta f(t)^{1/2} = k(T_1)^{1/2}$ and also to find the most probable value of $k(T_1)^{1/2}$. From the values of kT_1 and $k(T_1)^{1/2}$ we determined k and T_1. For determining T_2 the values of Δf from the third segment of the curve was used. From Eq. (3) it follows that $T_2 = (k\sqrt{T_1}/\Delta f)^2$.

TABLE 1

f, cps		T_1, msec	T_2, msec	*k*, cps
250	A	40.9	163.8	4.2
	B	38.4	148.8	5.9
1000	A	19.9	187.9	5.2
	B	14.4	185.0	18.3
4000	A	16.0	144.0	49.6
	B	11.6	123.2	91.0

TABLE 2

f, cps		T_1, msec	*k*, cps
125	A	117.0	1.7
	B	91.6	2.3
500	A	28.0	3.9
	B	19.8	9.8
800	A	11.7	504
	B	6.8	283

The values of T_1, T_2, and k thus determined for three signal frequencies are shown in Table 1.

From the table it follows that T_1 changes substantially with a change in the signal frequency, where this variation behaves regularly: T_1 increases with increasing frequency. The variations in T_2 are considerably less and do not follow so simple a pattern. According to our data, T_2 is greatest at a frequency of 1000 cps; according to Turnbull's data, the limiting duration for which the difference limen depends on the duration is the smallest at 1000 cps. This contradiction with Turnbull's data, plus the fact that the differences in T_2 at different frequencies are comparatively small, forces us to assume these differences to be nonexistent, being connected instead with measurement errors. Therefore, in constructing the curves in the graphs of Figs. 2, 3, 4 we adopted the same constant value of T_2 for all frequencies, and this value was defined as the average of the values of T_2 cited in Table 1. It was 165.2 msec for A and 152.3 msec for B.

Having constructed the curves of Figs. 2, 3, 4 on the basis of the constants given above, we then had to determine how much they corresponded to the experimental points. Since the difference limens determined in our experiments represented nothing more than the standard deviation of the frequency adjusted by the auditor from the frequency of the standard, we could compare the two dispersions [3]. In doing this it was assumed that the calculated values of Δf represented the true values of the standard deviation, determined for an infinite number of measurements. The calculations were made for all 60 points. It turned out that only for one point was the difference from the theoretically calculated value significant (at the 0.1% level). For 49 points z was less than the corresponding 5% level, for 10 points z was less than the corresponding 1% level. Consequently, we could conclude that the approximation adopted for the empirical relations was fully admissible.

Assuming further that the dependence of Δf on t differed at different frequencies only because of the different values of k and T_1, we could determine these constants at other frequencies, by conducting measurements for just a few durations. The measurements were performed at frequencies of 125, 500, and 8000 cps. Two durations in the region $t < T_1$ and one very large duration were used. On the basis of the values of Δf determined for a large duration, $k(T_1)^{1/2} = \Delta f(T_2)^{1/2}$ was computed. From the experimental data for the small durations $kT_1 = \Delta ft$ was determined. Then from this the values of the constants T_1 and k were calculated. They are listed in Table 2.

Let us analyze the results obtained. It is obvious that in considering the dependence of the difference limen on the signal duration a spectral approach can be used. It is well known that the width of the spectrum of a segment of a sinusoid is inversely proportional to the duration of the segment. Consequently, the relation $\Delta f = kT_1/t$ (for $t < T_1$) determined above can be interpreted in another way, such that for sufficiently wide spectra of the signal the difference limen is proportional to the width of the spectrum. This fact is found in correspondence with Stevens' data [4] for an investigation of the difference limens for damped oscillations with varying time constants, and with the data of Michaels [5], who studied the difference limens for noise bands with different bandwidths. However, as shown by these authors, a linear dependence between the width of the spectrum and the difference limen is maintained only for sufficiently wide signal spectra. It must, of course, be violated when the width of the signal spectrum becomes comparable with the bandwidth of the frequency-selective elements of the ear. It is evident that the minimum signal spectrum width, above which a linear dependence is maintained between signal spectrum and the difference limen, can serve as an index of the bandwidth of the frequency-selective elements of the ear. Defining the minimum signal spectrum width (W) as $1/T_1$, we can find the dependence of W on the signal frequency from our data. This dependence is shown in Fig. 5, where the values of W calculated from the values of Q and the values of the critical bands defined by various authors ($W = f/Q$, $W = {}^1/_3\ W_{cr}$) are also shown. It can be seen that the dependence so determined is nearly the same as that given by certain other authors (the crosses denote the data of Schafer and others [6], the vertical marks denote the data of Stevens [4], the triangles denote the data of Hamilton [7], and the squares the data of Makita and Miyatani [8]) and, in addition, differs considerably from the well-known dependence for the critical bands [9, 10]. Proceeding from the values of the critical bands, considerably smaller values of T_1 should be anticipated at high frequencies.

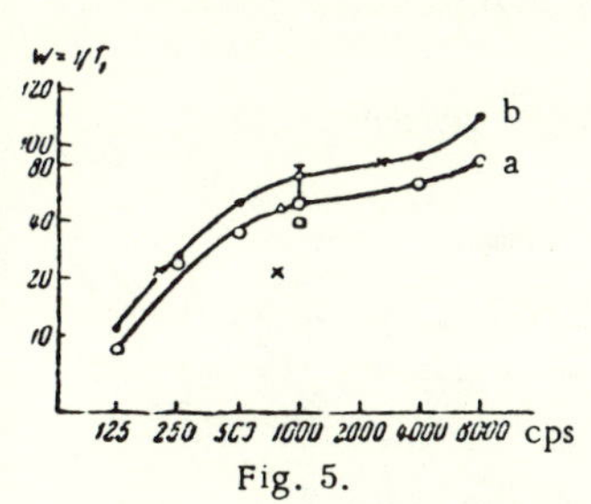

Fig. 5.

However, if the change in Δf over the range of durations below T_1 yet can be attributed to the build-up process in the cochlea, then the further lowering of the threshold to T_2 can in no way be considered from this point of view. The fact that T_2 is very large (152- and 165-msec for our auditors) and obviously does not depend on the signal frequency prompts the assumption that it reflects a certain time constant for the functioning of the nerve section of the auditory system.

Papers on the investigation of the dependence of sound-detection threshold on its duration [11, 12] have shown that 100-200 msec is the critical time during which the auditory system integrates the signal. The same values of the critical time were found in an investigation of the dependence of sound loudness on its duration [13] and in an investigation of the loudness discrimination of two short signals in rapid succession [14]. It is natural that we should pose the question: is our observed improvement in the differential threshold over the tonal duration interval from T_1 to T_2 then not a manifestation of the same effect of summation, or time-averaging of the signal? For the consideration of this problem it is necessary to recall that in psychological experimentation some measure of the fluctuations in the perceptible values of signal frequency is adopted as the difference limen [15]. Thus, in our experiments the standard deviation in a sound frequency, perceived as coinciding with a standard, from the frequency of the standard was adopted as the difference limen.

To whosoever happened to be perceiving the signal frequency (point of maximum in the excitation distribution in the cochlea or any other chosen point) it became obvious that the information concerning it is repeatedly, throughout the on-time of the sound, transmitted from the cochlea to the central branches of the auditory system. If the nerve system is capable of taking the time average of the transmitted signal, then it is reasonable to expect that with an increase in the time of transmittal (signal duration) the fluctuations in the mean values will be reduced. If n is the number of transmitted values of the frequency, then the standard deviation of the average value of the frequency will be diminished in proportion to the square root of n. In other words, if the improvement in the threshold with increasing tonal duration occurs simply as the result of a time-averaging of the frequency values transmitted from the cochlea, then the decrease in difference limen has to proceed in proportion to the square root of the tonal duration. It can be seen that this exactly corresponds to the dependence that was determined experimentally.

Consequently, both the values of T_2 and the nature of the dependence of the difference limen on tonal duration foster the opinion that the improvement over the interval from T_1 to T_2 is attributable to the occurrence of the averaging mechanism of the nerve branches of the auditory system.

Hence,we can make the following conclusions:

1. The frequency-difference limen for a tone varies as a function of the tonal duration.

2. For small durations ($t < T_1$) the frequency-difference limen is reduced in direct proportion to the increasing duration.

3. For medium durations ($T_1 < t < T_2$) the frequency-difference limen is reduced in direct proportion to the square root of the increase in duration.

4. For sufficiently large durations ($t > T_2$) the frequency-difference limen becomes constant and independent of duration.

5. The critical duration T_1 follows a regular diminution with increasing tonal frequency (for Subject A from 117.0 msec at 125 cps to 11.7 msec at 8000 cps, for B from 91.6 msec at 125 cps to 6.8 msec at 8000 cps). The critical duration T_2 is more or less the same for all frequencies (for A it was equal, on the average, to 165.2 msec, for B it was 151.3 msec).

6. It appears likely that the values of T_1 are determined by the width of the frequency-selective elements of the ear, while T_2 represents the time of summation (averaging) of information on the signal by the nerve branches of the auditory system.

LITERATURE CITED

[1] G. Békésy, "Resonance curve and decay period at various points on the cochlear partition," J. Acoust. Soc. Am. 21, 245-254 (1949).

[2] W. W. Turnbull, "Pitch discrimination as a function of tonal duration," J. Exp. Psychol. 34, 302-316 (1944).

[3] R. A. Fisher, Statistical Methods for Researchers [in Russian] (Gosstatizdat, Moscow, 1958).

[4] K. N. Stevens, "Frequency discrimination for damped waves," J. Acoust. Soc. Am. 24, 76-79 (1952).

[5] R. M. Michaels, "Frequency-difference limens for narrow bands of noise," J. Acoust. Soc. Am. 29, 520-522 (1957).

[6] T. H. Schafer, R. S. Gales, A. C. Shewmaker and P. O. Thompson, J. Acoust. Soc. Am. 22, 490-496 (1950).

[7] P. M. Hamilton, "Noise-masked thresholds as a function of tonal duration and masking-noise bandwidth," J. Acoust. Soc. Am. 29, 506-511 (1957).

[8] Y. Makita and S. Miyatani, "The time in which equilibrium state of audition is established. Part 3," J. Phys. Soc. Japan 5, 241-243 (1950).

[9] H. Fletcher, Speech and Hearing in Communication (N. U., 1953).

[10] E. Zwicker, G. Frottorp and S. S. Stevens, "Critical bandwidth in loudness summation," J. Acoust. Soc. Am. 29, 548-557 (1957).

[11] W. R. Garner and C. A. Miller, "The masked threshold of pure tones as a function of duration," J. Exp. Psychol. 37, 293-303 (1947).

[12] D. M. Green, T. G. Birdsall and W. P. Tanner, "Signal detection as a function of signal intensity and duration," J. Acoust. Soc. Am. 29, 523-531 (1957).

[13] I. Pollack, "Loudness of periodically interrupted white noise," J. Acoust. Soc. Am. 30, 181-185 (1958).

[14] L. A. Chistovich and V. A. Ivanova, "Critical time for the determination of loudness," Fiziol. Zhur. SSSR 46, 1, 20-25 (1960).

[15] J. R. Pierce and E. N. Gilbert," On AX and ABX limens," J. Acoust. Soc. Am. 30, 593-595 (1958).

Part IV

SEPARATION OF SIMULTANEOUS SIGNALS

Editor's Comments on Papers 19 Through 24

19 MAYER
Researches in Acoustics

20 WEGEL and LANE
Excerpt from *The Auditory Masking of One Pure Tone by Another and Its Probable Relation to the Dynamics of the Inner Ear*

21 EGAN and HAKE
On the Masking Pattern of a Simple Auditory Stimulus

22 FLETCHER
Excerpt from *Auditory Patterns*

23 ZWICKER, FLOTTORP, and STEVENS
Critical Band Width in Loudness Summation

24 GREEN
Application of Detection Theory in Psychophysics

One of the most useful properties of the auditory system—and certainly to the scholar in audition one of the most impressive—is its ability to separate simultaneously present signals or, on occasion, to process two independent signals concurrently. So admirably is this performed in our daily listening that beginning students in audition find it difficult to recognize that all these signals arrive at the ear as a linear addition of the sound pressure variations from all sources.

But there is no way for a system to be perfect in this regard. If the auditory system deserves admiration for its simultaneous processing, it is because it arrives at a suitable compromise between extremely fine frequency resolution and optimum time-pattern tracing. In a way it is unfortunate that the focus of study of this aspect of auditory processing has been its failure to separate concurrent signals. Fortuitously this is the facet most amenable to experimental analysis and quantification. Yet the principle that ought to filter through all this study of the masking of one signal by another is the remarkable accomplishment of the system as a sensory input in keeping the organism apprised of the varied acoustical events transpiring at any given moment in our noisy, yet multisignal-dependent, environment.

What ought to remain uppermost, then, as one gets embroiled in the details of masking experiments, is the fact that the principle of primary interest is the inverse of masking: frequency analysis by the auditory system. For this reason, even though this part will deal with the papers that have made important contributions to our knowledge of masking in psychological acoustics, I have chosen a title that will remind the reader of the preferred orientation.

As we saw with the concept of pitch, frequency analysis by the auditory system has a longer history than psychoacoustics itself. In fact, the ear is the oldest frequency analyzer known. Long before Helmholtz began his experiments to sharpen and confirm the frequency-separating properties of the ear—experiments that combined with the formulation of Ohm's psychoacoustic law to solidify Helmholtz's promulgation of the resonance principle of the cochlea—expert musical listeners were aware of the relation of the partials (overtones) to the fundamental of the complex tone. Mersenne (1636), for instance, knew the ratios of partials to the fundamental and apparently could hear out at least the first seven partials.

Practitioners of solfeggio, knowing since Pythagoras of the integral ratios of the modes of vibration of strings, could readily "auditorize" where the note of a given partial should be and could employ the auditory analyzer to ascertain whether that note was present in a particular complex sound. Particularly following Helmholtz's endorsement of Ohm's principle of auditory analysis, many expert listeners reported instances of the "hearing out" of partials—in one case as high as the twenty-seventh. (See Plomp, 1966, for a review of this activity.)

Quantification of the results of such experiments had to await development of better analyzers. In Paper 13, primarily concerned with pitch, Schouten measured the first twelve partials of a complex tone by matching each in loudness to a sinusoid. Similarly Wegel and Lane, in their masking paper reproduced in Paper 20, estimated the strength of the harmonics generated in the ear during stimulation by strong tones by recording the amplitude of an exploring tone that produced the most prominent beat with the harmonic in question. This one widely used method, however, turns out to be of questionable accuracy. But mostly, simply because of the difficulty and the imprecision of making that type of measurement of auditory frequency resolution, the earliest formal specification of the ear's ability to separate signals took the form of designating the degree to which it failed to do so: the study of masking.

The early history of masking is well portrayed by the first two papers reproduced here. Mayer (Paper 19) discussed his experiments from a direct interference or "obliteration" point of view, and one must admire his ingenious attempts at quantification. He was not content with simply reporting his demonstration that "high sounds cannot obliterate low sounds" but suggested that this finding would "introduce profound modifications into the hypotheses heretofore framed respecting the mechanism and functions of the ear." This has indeed been the case.

By the time of the appearance of the Wegel and Lane paper in 1924 (Paper 20), psychoacoustics was beginning to benefit from electronic control and measurement of acoustic signals. Scarcely any serious student of audition will be unaware of the content of this paper, but it is well worth reading for didactic purposes in addition to its historical interest. The definition of masking in the Acoustical Terminology of the American Standards Association (1961) reads like a paraphrase of the Wegel and Lane definition. The concept of the masking audiogram of a signal is introduced in this 1924 paper. It portrays dramatically the fact first noted by Mayer that high tones are obliterated by low tones. We now know that when we record the response from any eighth nerve fiber, its frequency response expands primarily toward lower frequencies as the level of the stimulating signal increases; thus it follows that strong low tones will usurp the neural channels normally carrying information about higher frequencies. Exceptions to this masking pattern are rare, but Tobias (1977) has recently presented data showing that for tones 250Hz and below, the asymmetry is not so marked. Perhaps, as he suggests, this indicates the frequency range where the cochlear amplitude pattern no longer exhibits a maximum, and the steep slope of the mechanical low-pass filter is missing.

A rather prominent feature of the Wegel and Lane masking curves is the nonmonotonic nature of the masking function at multiples of the frequency of the masking tone. (See p. 271 of the paper.) This rise in interference, along with the sensation of beats, led to the conviction that the phenomenon is attributable to distortion products at these frequencies. Several years after the appearance of the Wegel and Lane paper, Fletcher (1930) introduced some data gathered using the method of best beats to estimate the level of the harmonic distortion components generated in the auditory system.* These data, and the method itself, were accepted by most theorists as evidence of the degree of nonlinearity of the ear.

Békésy (1934) made the most extensive, or at least the most completely reported, set of measurements by the best-beat method, varying

*This is essentially the same procedure as that described on p. 272 of Wegel and Lane for estimating the strength of the subjective harmonics.

the primary tone over a wide range and noting that "the magnitudes of the harmonics are unexpectedly large" and that "at the larger intensities the overtones vary almost in proportion to the fundamental, though at low intensities they change more rapidly" (p. 334 of Wever translation).

Trimmer and Firestone (1937), speaking of the American work on measurement by best beats, voiced some skepticism about the method, noting that the listeners could not be certain the beats they listened to were actually changes in the harmonic being measured. Lewis, who had been using an electrostatic complex tone generator with phase-locked partials, pointed out (1940) that if one changes the phase of an externally introduced tone of the same frequency, the cochlear resultant changes amplitude in the fashion predicted by the presence of a "subjective harmonic." He therefore appeared to be endorsing both the steady tone (same frequency) and the beating tone method of measuring auditory distortion.

But it was Schouten (Paper 13), in the Netherlands, who performed the definitive experiment in 1938. He also had a complex tone generator (optical) with a provision for controlling phase relations of the partials. First of all, he measured the second harmonic with essentially a cancellation method and showed that—at least over the narrow range that he measured—the energy in the harmonic increased nearly as the square of the increase in the primary, as it should. Schouten pointed out that this was not true for the best-beat measurements of Fletcher or Békésy.

Schouten's brilliant maneuver, however, was the direct combination of the cancellation method and the beating method. Having found the phase of his externally produced harmonic that cancelled the subjective harmonic, he then reintroduced the beating tone and noted that beats were still heard. These are now known as "beats of mistuned consonance" (Plomp, 1966). Unfortunately Schouten's report, perhaps because of the loss of communication during the war, had little immediate effect on the use of the best-beat method to estimate aural distortion products. American workers continued to endorse best beats as the method for measuring harmonic distortion and ascribed the irregularities in the pure-tone masking curves to the presence of these products at the levels indicated in the Fletcher graph.

Egan and Hake (Paper 21) noted this difficulty with the measurement of pure-tone masking, along with other irregularities attributable to the interaction of the several frequencies present and generated instead the masking pattern for a band of noise narrow enough to preserve the general shape of the tonal masking pattern but broad enough to minimize the effects of beats and difference tones. As the authors note, Fletcher and Munson (1937) had already made such measurements for the same reasons. Fletcher and Munson, however, reported these measurements only sketchily, whereas Egan and Hake very carefully contrast the patterns resulting from the two kinds of measurement.

Bilger and Hirsh (1956) did a more complete job of investigating the masking of tones by bands of noise. They used noise bands an equal number of pitch units in width (250 mels) and spaced by that same distance from about 400Hz to 5kHz. Masking audiograms for these bands behaved very much as the Egan and Hake measures would predict, except for a surprising departure below the band for high levels of noise. Here there appeared to be low-frequency energy in the cochlea, later shown (Deatherage et al., 1957a, b) to be related to the regularity (or lack of it) with which the amplitude envelope of the signal exceeded the limits of linear operation. The effect of this translated energy on the audibility of low-frequency signals was labeled *remote masking.*

Masking of tones by other tones has proved to have both other problems and other uses than masking by noises (see, for example, Greenwood, 1972), and the masking of harmonic partials by the fundamental presents even more special difficulties (Lamoré, 1977).

A more complete view of the principles involved in the separation of signals by the ear was offered by Fletcher (Paper 22) in his work on auditory patterns. The first few pages of the paper present a brief general view of hearing as it was understood in 1938, but it is particularly the concept of "critical bands" in hearing—the ubiquitous filter-like mechanism that characterizes peripheral frequency resolution—that owes its genesis to the Fletcher paper. Fletcher's assumption that a signal in noise is perceived half the time when the energy of the signal is equal to that of the masking noise led to specific estimates of the effective width of the band actually contributing to the masking (see p. 55 of the paper).

Hawkins and Stevens (1950) measured the detectability of tones in broad-band random noise and show excellent agreement with Fletcher in the ratio of the sound pressure level of the tone to the pressure spectrum level of the noise at the frequency of the tone. They were properly a little more prudent in stating that this relation is "usually interpreted as defining the width of the band of frequencies that actually contributes to the masking of a tone located at the center of the band" (p. 10).

The logical sequel to the effort to determine a prototypical masking pattern has been the use of noise bands to deduce the form of the auditory filter. Filter terminology, though it increases the risk of oversimplification, has been highly useful in describing general aspects of rudimentary auditory analysis, particularly since the Fletcher paper.

Ideally Fletcher's data points, as he gradually narrowed a broad-band noise and plotted the level of the tone just masked by the remaining noise (see p. 55 of Paper 22), would delineate the shape of the filter. By drawing only the straight lines of his figure 17, Fletcher seems to restrict his interest to the effective (equivalent flat-topped, steep-skirt) width. Schafer and his coworkers (Schafer et al., 1950) tried the complementary maneuver of beginning with a very narrow band and plotting the detectable level of the tone as the noise band increased. Their data fit about equally well to a simple resonance curve or a flat-topped, sharp-cornered shape.

Much wider applicability of this filter-like concept to auditory behavior was established by the report of Zwicker, Flottorp, and Stevens (Paper 23) on a number of experiments that indicated about the same degree of frequency resolution for a variety of responses. The paper gives an excellent view of the early empirical establishment of the critical band, includes detection experiments encompassing a greater variety of signals than the Fletcher study, and also presents evidence from signal behavior above threshold.

Shortly following, Greenwood (1961) presented a greatly improved and extended version of the Fletcher experiment on the change in the level of a tone just masked by a band of noise as a function of the noise-bandwidth. He began with narrow bands and gradually increased the width until the center frequencies no longer showed an increase in just-detectable level with further increase in bandwidth. Greenwood fitted triangular-shaped functions to his masked audiograms, much influenced, apparently, by Fletcher's reasoning. But Greenwood's estimate of the critical band width was based on that noise-bandwidth that first showed a flat portion in the masked audiogram and did not require an assumption about the relative energy in the two signals when the tone was just audible. His bandwidths, thus estimated, agree with those by Zwicker et al.

Since the bandwidths estimated by these other experiments differ from the Fletcher calculation for pure tones in noise by a factor of about 2.5, one might conclude that further processing of this output of the critical-band filter is such that the system is able to detect the presence of the signal half the time when the signal to noise ratio at the filter output is -4dB. Actually, in 1937, when Fletcher and Munson reported their method of calculating loudness from masked audiograms, they noted: "It is found that a better agreement between calculated and observed results for single frequency tones is obtained if the masking at the frequency of the masking tone is taken as about 4dB below the level of the masking tone." If Fletcher had concluded from this that a tone is just masked by a noise when the level of the tone is 4dB less than the noise that is masking it, rather than when the energy of tone and noise are equal, his critical band would have been the same width as those of Zwicker et al.

Recently Patterson (1976) added a still more sophisticated measure to this series of attempts to portray the shape of the auditory filter that separates tonal signals from masking noises. In contrast to the technique of Fletcher and Greenwood, Patterson began with a masking noise that had a wide gap at the location of the tone to be masked, ideally wide enough that the tone would be detectable at the same level whether his noise was present or not. He then plotted the level of the tone necessary to keep it just detectable as the gap was gradually narrowed—that is, as he filled the filter from both sides. The plot of these tone levels as a function of noise-gap width should be the integral of the filter shape as it operates in the detection of tones in interfering noise. Patterson fitted an analytic function to these values of just-detectable tones and emerged with a filter whose equivalent square width agrees well with the critical bandwidths estimated by other methods.

Particularly germane to the problem of frequency resolution in the cochlea is the experiment by Goldstein (1967) showing that when two tones f_1 and f_2 are closely spaced in the cochlea ($f_2/f_1<1.1$), a third appears at the output with frequency $2f_1-f_2$. Actually a series described by $(n+1)f_1-nf_2$ can be shown to be present, but the level decays rapidly with increasing n so that only $2f_1-f_2$ has been of interest. This evidence of nonlinearity in the ear actually touched off more activity in auditory neurophysiology than in psychological acoustics. Goldstein pointed out, however, that canceling two tones of the series led to a sharp reduction in the "musicality" of the sound, so that one might conjecture that for sounds that contain a high proportion of energy in their upper partials (>10), the quality of the sound is definitely influenced by this nonlinear aspect of the ear's behavior. Greenwood (1971, 1972) showed that the effect can also be seen in measurements of the masking of one tone by another, or the masking of tones by narrow bands of noise.

Since the Fletcher experiment, but increasingly following the Zwicker, Flottorp, and Stevens report, the analog of the filter has been invoked to describe the frequency-analysis aspect of auditory processing. But, as frequently occurs, the simplicity that makes the model attractive carries an attendant risk. We may be highly conversant with the principles of filter operation, but we do not often work with filters closely resembling the implied auditory models. In the laboratory, filters do not center appropriately and simultaneously on salient points in the spectrum as we must suppose they do in auditory analysis of changing complex signals. Perhaps if we are continually cognizant of the versatility of the entire processing network and of how much further analysis apparently takes place following the initial filtering, we can be less occupied with arguments about whether the filter width changes as a function of level or duration of the signal. No matter how simple the task may seem to the experimenter, the complex adaptive processor (sensory system) utilizes whatever it has available to optimize performance.

The significant papers included in this section and the work noted in the brief review of masking experiments make it clear that the detection of one signal in the presence of another has been for a long time a very useful tool in the attempt to understand and quantify the behavior of the auditory analyzer. But in the late 1950s workers in auditory psychophysics were forced to take a critical look at their methods and their terminology. The precipitating event was the promulgation by Tanner and his colleagues at the University of Michigan of a mathematical model for the detection of a signal in an interfering noise. Green's paper reproduced here (Paper 24) is not the original work that spawned a critical reappraisal of past and current work on detection of weak signals (signals of nearly the same level as the interfering noise). Until specially tailored expositions for auditory psychophysicists appeared (and they were numerous), a monograph by Tanner, Swets, and Green (1956) was the document most likely to be open on the desk of any auditory researcher. But Green's synopsis is briefer, somewhat broader in coverage, and written by one of the most able proponents of the relevance of the theory to audition.

As for the more lasting influence of this reform, one need only note the rather profound change in terminology alone to note that the effect was more than transitory. Though it is true that much of the ear's performance goes beyond the detection of signals in noise, so has the influence of the theory; and it has made a profound difference in the thinking and the training of a generation of scholars in audition.

REFERENCES

Békésy, G. V. 1934. Über die nichtlinearen Verzerrungen des Ohres. *Ann. Phys.* **20**: 809-827. Translated in E. G. Wever, *Experiments in hearing.* New York: McGraw-Hill, 1960.

Bilger, R. C., and I. J. Hirsh. 1956. Masking of tones by bands of noise. *Acoust. Soc. Am. J.* **28**:623-630.

Deatherage, B., R. C. Bilger, and D. H. Eldredge. 1957a. Remote masking in selected frequency regions. *Acoust. Soc. Am. J.* **29**:512-514.

Deatherage, B., H. Davis, and D. H. Eldredge. 1957b. Physiological evidence for the masking of low frequencies by high. *Acoust. Soc. Am. J.* **29**:132-137.

Fletcher, H. 1930. A space time pattern theory of hearing. *Acoust. Soc. Am. J.* **1**: 311-343.

Fletcher, H., and W. A. Munson. 1937. Relation between loudness and masking. *Acoust. Soc. Am. J.* **9**:1-10.

Goldstein, J. L. 1967. Auditory nonlinearity. *Acoust. Soc. Am. J.* **41**:676-689.

Greenwood, D. D. 1961. Auditory masking and the critical band. *Acoust. Soc. Am. J.* **33**:484–502.

Greenwood, D. D. 1971. Aural combination tones and auditory masking. *Acoust. Soc. Am. J.* **50**:502–543.

Greenwood, D. D. 1972. Masking by narrow bands of noise in proximity to more intense pure tones of higher frrquency: Application to measurement of combination band levels and some comparisons with masking by combination noise. *Acoust. Soc. Am. J.* **52**:1137–1143.

Hawkins, T. E., Jr., and S. S. Stevens. 1950. Masking of pure tones and speech by white noise. *Acoust. Soc. Am. J.* **22**:6–13.

Lamoré, P. 1977. Pitch and masked threshold in octave complexes in relation to interaction phenomena in two-tone stimuli in general. *Acustica* **37**:249–257.

Lewis, D. 1940. Support for the exploring tone method of measuring aural harmonics. *Psychol. Rev.* **47**:169–183.

Mersenne, M. 1636. *Harmonie universelle.* Trans R. Chapman. The Hague: Nijhoff, 1957.

Patterson, R. D. 1976. Auditory filter shapes derived with noise stimuli. *Acoust. Soc. Am. J.* **59**:640–654.

Plomp, R. 1966. *Experiments on tone perception.* Soesterberg, Netherlands: Institute for Perception RVO-TNO.

Schafer, T. H., R. S., Gales, C. A. Shewmaker, and P. O. Thompson. 1950. The frequency selectivity of the ear as determined by masking experiments. *Acoust. Soc. Am. J.* **22**:490–496.

Tobias, J. V. 1977. Low-frequency masking patterns. *Acoust. Soc. Am. J.* **61**: 571–575.

Trimmer, J. D., and F. A. Firestone. 1937. An investigation of subjective tones by means of the steady tone phase effect. *Acoust. Soc. Am. J.* **9**:23–29.

Tanner, W. P., Jr., J. A. Swets, and D. M. Green. 1956. Some general properties of the hearing mechanism. *Univ. Of Michigan Elec. Defense Grp., Tech. Rep. No. 30.*

19

Reprinted from *Philos. Mag.* 2:500–507 (1876)

RESEARCHES IN ACOUSTICS

Alfred M. Mayer*

CONTENTS.

1. On the Obliteration of the Sensation of one Sound by the simultaneous action on the ear of another more intense and lower sound.
2. On the Discovery of the Fact that a Sound, even when intense, cannot obliterate the Sensation of another Sound lower than it in pitch.
3. On a proposed Change in the usual Method of conducting Orchestral Music, indicated by the above discoveries.
4. Applications of the Interferences of Sonorous Sensations to Determinations of the Relative Intensities of Sounds.

THIS communication is preliminary to an elaborate paper on the above subjects. For conciseness and clearness I present the few facts I have now to offer in the form of notes of experiments.

1. *On the Obliteration of the Sensation of one Sound by the simultaneous action on the ear of another more intense and lower sound.*

Experimental Observations on the Obliteration of one Sound by another.—Several feet from the ear I placed one of those loud-ticking spring-balance American clocks which make four beats in a second. Then I brought quite close to my ear a watch (made by Lange, of Dresden) ticking five times in the second. In this position I heard all the ticks of the watch, even those which coincided with every fourth tick of the clock. Let us call the fifth tick of the watch which coincided with one of the ticks of the clock, its fifth tick. I now gradually removed the watch from the ear and perceived that the fifth tick became fainter and fainter, till at a certain distance it entirely vanished and was, so to speak, "stamped out" of the watch†.

Similar and more striking experiments were made with an

* Communicated by the Author.

† In the publication of this paper in 'Nature,' Aug. 10, 1876, my friend Mr. Alexander J. Ellis, F.R.S., appends the following note to the above experiment:—"The precise numbers of ticks in a second here mentioned are not necessary for roughly observing and understanding these phenomena. I observed them by a common American pendulum-clock placed on a table (which increased the power of its half-second ticks), and a watch beating five times in two seconds. The Rev. Mr. Haweis informs me that he has often noticed a similar effect at night with ordinary watches. The sensation produced by the obliteration of the tick when the proper distance of the watch from the ear has been attained, and the consequent sudden division of the ticks into periods separated by silences, is very peculiar. It is difficult not to believe that some accident has suddenly interfered with the action of the watch instead of merely with our own sensations."—A. J. E.

old silver watch, beating four times to the second, by causing this watch to gain about thirty seconds an hour on the clock, so that at every two minutes the ticks of the watch and clock exactly coincided. When the watch was held near the ear, every one of its ticks was heard distinctly ; but on gradually removing it from the ear the ticks of the watch became fainter and fainter at the coincidences, and when the watch had been removed to a distance of nine inches from the ear the ticks of the watch were utterly obliterated during *three* whole seconds of its ticks about the time of coincidence. On removing the watch to a distance of twenty-four inches I found that I lost its ticks during *nine* seconds about the time of coincidence. It is here important to remark that the ticks of the clock are *longer* in duration, as well as *lower* in pitch, than those of the watch. With the watch remaining at a distance of twenty-four inches from the ear, I listened with all my attention as tick by tick the watch approached the time of coincidence. Since the ticks of the watch are shorter in duration than those of the clock, they are *overlapped* by the others about the time of coincidence. Hence as, so to speak, the short ticks of the watch glided tick after tick under the long ticks of the clock, I perceived that more and more of the duration of each successive watch-tick became extinguished by the tick of the clock, until only the *tail* end of the short tick of the watch was left audible ; and at last even this also crept under the long tick of the clock, and the whole of the ticks of the watch were rendered inaudible for *nine* seconds, at the end of which time the front or *head* of the watch-tick, as we may call it, protruded beyond the clock-tick, and then slowly grew up into a complete watch-tick as before. In this succession of events the tick of the old silver watch (made by Tobias) disappears with a sharp *chirp* like a cricket's, and reappears with a sound like that made by a boy's marble falling upon others in his pocket. By this experiment, therefore, a gradual analysis is made of the effect of the tick of the clock on the tick of the watch, affording a beautiful illustration of the fact that one sonorous sensation may overcome and obliterate another.

Experiments to determine the relative Intensity of the Clock-ticks which obliterate the Watch-ticks.—The clock was placed on a post in the middle of an open level field in the country on nights when the air was calm and noiseless. The ticks of the clock became just inaudible when my ear was removed to a distance of 350 feet. The ticks of the watch became just inaudible at a distance of twenty feet. The ratio of the squares of these numbers makes the ticks of the clock about 300 times as intense as those of the watch. On the same nights that I made the above determinations I also put the clock on the post, and placing against my zygomatic process a slender stick graduated to inches and tenths, I stood with my ear at distances from the clock of from eight to sixteen feet, and then slid the watch above and along the stick (taking care that it did not touch it) until it reached such a distance from the ear that its fifth tick just disappeared. Knowing the relative intensities of the ticks of clock and watch when placed at the same distance from the ear, the law of the reciprocals of the squares gives the relative intensities when the clock and watch are at the several distances obtained in the above experiments. Large numbers of such experiments have been made; and the results agree perfectly well when we take into consideration, first, the difficulty thrown in the path of the determinations by the *gradual* fading away of the watch-ticks as they approach coincidence with the clock-ticks, and secondly, the impossibility of arriving at *any* result at all if the slightest noise (the rustle of a gentle breeze, the piping of frogs, the bark of a distant dog) should fall on the ear of the observer when engaged in making an experiment. The general result of the numerous experiments thus made shows that the sensation of the watch-tick is obliterated by a coincident tick of the clock when the intensity of the clock-tick is *three times* that of the watch-tick. This result, however, must be regarded as merely approximative, not only from the manner in which it was obtained, but from the *complexity* of the sounds on which the experiments were made. It is interesting, however, both as being, I believe, the first determination of this kind that has ever been made, and as having opened out a new and important field of research in physiological acoustics.

Experiments on the Interference of the Sensations of Musical Sounds.—Reserving the further development of my discoveries for future papers, I will now briefly describe some of the more prominent and simple phenomena which I discovered in experimenting with *musical sounds.* At the outset I will remove an objection always made by those versed in acoustics but unacquainted with these new phenomena. It is as follows:—"You say that one sound may obliterate the sensation of another; but are you sure that the real fact is not an alteration of the *quality* of the more intense sound by the action of the concurrent feebler vibration?" I exclude this objection by experimenting as follows:—An open or closed organ-pipe is sounded forcibly; and at a few feet from it is placed the instrument emitting the sound to be obliterated, which may be either a tuning-fork on its resonance-box or a closed organ-pipe communicating with a separate bellows. Suppose that in the following experiment both tuning-fork and closed organ-pipe produce a note higher in pitch than the more intense or extinguishing sound of the open organ-pipe. Now sound the fork alone strongly, and alternately shut and open its resonance box with the hand. We can thus obtain the sound of the fork in a *regular measure of time*. When the ear has well apprehended the intervals of silence and of sound thus produced, begin the experiment by sounding the open pipe and tuning-fork simultaneously. Now if any change is thus effected in the quality of sound emitted by the open pipe, this change cannot occur except when the fork is sounded, and hence, if it occurs at all, it must occur in the regular measure in which the fork is sounded. The following are the facts really observed. At first every time that the mouth of the box is open the sound of the fork is distinctly heard and changes the quality of the note of the open pipe. But as the vibrations of the fork run down in amplitude the sensations of its effect become less and less till they soon entirely vanish, and not the slightest change can be observed in the quality or intensity of the note of the open organ-pipe, whether the resonance box of the fork be open or closed. Indeed at this stage of the experiment the vibrations of the fork may be suddenly and totally stopped without the ear being able to detect the fact. But if instead of stopping the fork when it becomes inaudible we stop the sound of the open organ pipe, it is impossible not to feel surprised at the strong sound of the fork which the open pipe had smothered and had rendered powerless to affect the ear. If we replace the tuning-fork by a closed organ-pipe of the same pitch, the results will be the same ; but in this case I adjust the intensity of the higher closed pipe to the point of extinction by regulating the flow of air from the bellows by a valve worked with a screw. The alternation of sound and silence is obtained by closing and opening the mouth of the closed pipe by the hand.

2. *On the Discovery of the Fact that a Sound, even when intense, cannot obliterate the sensation of another Sound lower than it in pitch.*

High Sounds cannot obliterate Low Sounds.—A new and remarkable fact was now discovered. No sound, even when very intense, can diminish or obliterate the sensation of a concurrent sound which is lower in pitch. This was proved by experiments similar to the last, but differing in having the more intense sound higher (instead of lower) in pitch. In this case, when the ear decides that the sound of the (lower and feebler) tuning-fork is just extinguished, it is generally discovered on stopping the higher sound that *the fork,* which should produce the lower sound, *has ceased to vibrate.* This surprising experiment must be made in order to be appreciated. I will only remark that very many similar experiments, ranging through four octaves, have been made, with consonant and dissonant intervals, and that scores of different hearers have confirmed this discovery. It is important to understand that this phenomenon depends solely on *difference* of pitch, and not at all on the absolute pitch of the notes. Thus a feeble c''' (1024 double vibrations) is heard as distinctly through an intense e''' (1280 double vibrations) as a feeble c (128 double vibrations) is heard through an intense g (192 double vibrations) or an intense c' (256 double vibrations).

The development of the applications and of the further illustrations of these discoveries would occupy too much space; I must therefore restrict myself to mentioning some of the most interesting. Let a man read a sentence over and over again with the same tone and modulation of voice, and while he is so doing forcibly sound a c' pipe (256 double vibrations). A remarkable effect is produced, which varies somewhat with the voice experimented on; but the ordinary result is as follows. It appears as though two persons were reading together, one with a grave voice (which is found by the combination of all the reader's real vocal sounds below c in pitch, or having less than 256 double vibrations), the other with a high-pitched voice, generally squeaky and nasal, and, I need not add, very disagreeable. Of course the aspirates come out with a distressing prominence. I have observed many curious illustrations of this change in the quality of the tone of the voice, caused by the entire or partial obliteration of certain vocal components, while listening to persons talking during the sound of a steam whistle, or in one of our long, resonant American railway carriages. Experiments similar to those on the human voice can be made, with endless modifications, on other composite sounds, as those of reed-pipes, of stringed instruments, of running water, &c. With one of my c (128 double vibrations) free Grenié reeds, I get very marked results. Using as a concurrent sound an intense c' (256 double vibrations), I perceive the prime or fundamental simple tone c to be unaffected in intensity, while all the other partial tones (higher harmonics or overtones, as they are sometimes called) are almost obliterated, except the fifth partial (or fourth upper partial e'', of 640 double vibrations, and the sixth partial (or fifth upper partial) g'' (of 768 double vibrations), which come out with wonderful distinctness. The fact that the lowest, or prime partial tone in the majority of ordinary compound musical tones is strongest, is due (among other reasons) to the fact that the sensation of each partial tone of which the whole musical tone is composed, is diminished by the action on the ear of all the components or partial tones *below* it in pitch. Thus the higher the pitch of any component or partial tone the greater the number of lower components which tend to obliterate it. But the prime, or lowest, component partial tone is not affected by any other. Another illustration I cannot resist giving. At the end of the street in New York in which I resided, there is a large fire-alarm bell, the residual sound of which, after its higher components have disappeared, is a deep simple tone. This bass sound holds its own with total indifference to the clatter of horses, or to any sounds *above* it in pitch. It dies out with a smooth gradient, generally without the slighest indentation or break produced by the other sounds of the street. Indeed, in this case, as in all others where one sound remains unaffected by intense higher notes, the observer feels as though he had a special sense for the perception of the graver sound—an organ entirely distinct from that which receives the impress of the higher tones.

That one sonorous sensation cannot interfere with another which is lower in pitch is a remarkable physiological discovery, and, next after the demonstration of the fact that the ear is capable of analyzing compound musical sounds into their constituent or partial simple tones, is probably the most important addition yet made to our knowledge of the nature of hearing. It cannot fail to introduce profound modifications into the hypotheses heretofore framed respecting the mechanism and functions of the ear.

3. *On a proposed Change in the usual Method of conducting Orchestral Music, indicated by the above discoveries.*

We have seen how an intense sound may obliterate, entirely or in part, the sensations of certain partial tones or components of any musical tone, and thus produce a profound change in its quality. In a large orchestra I have repeatedly witnessed the entire obliteration of all sounds from violins by the deeper and more intense sounds of the wind instruments, the double-bases alone holding their own. I have also observed the sounds of the clarinets lose their peculiar quality of tone and consequent charm from the same cause. No doubt the conductor of the orchestra heard all his violins, ranged as they always are close around him, and did not perceive that his clarinets had lost that quality of tone on which *the composer* had relied for producing a special character of expression.

The function of the conductor of an orchestra seems to be threefold. First, to regulate and fix the time. Secondly, to regulate the intensity of the sounds produced by the individual instruments, for the purpose of expression. Thirdly, to give the proper quality of tone or *feeling* to the whole sound of his orchestra, considered as a single instrument, by regulating *the relative intensities* of the sounds produced by the various classes of instruments employed. Now this third function, the regulation of relative intensities, has hitherto been discharged through the judgment of the ears of a conductor who is placed in the most disadvantageous position for judging by his ears. Surely he is not conducting for his own personal gratification, but for the gratification of his audience, whose ears stand in very different relations from his own in respect of their distance from the various instruments in action. Is it not time that he should pay more attention to his third function, and place himself in the position occupied by an average hearer? This position would be elevated, and somewhere in the midst of the audience. The exact determination of its place would depend on various conditions which cannot now be considered. That the position at present occupied by the conductor of an orchestra has often allowed him to deprive his audience of some of the most delicate and touching qualities of orchestral and concerted vocal music I have no doubt, and I firmly believe that when he changes his position in the manner now proposed, the audience will have some of that enjoyment which he has too long kept to himself. During the past winter, in the Academy of Music at New York, and this spring at Offenbach's concerts, I fully confirmed all the foregoing surmises, by placing myself in different parts of the house to observe the different results; and my opinions were fully shared by others who have a more delicate musical organization than I can lay claim to.

In large orchestras these interferences of sonorous sensations are so multiplied and various as to be beyond our mental conception. By taking them up in detail, however, some general laws may be evolved. But it will be impossible to formulate such laws until, first, we are in possession of a *quantitative* analysis of the compound tones of all musical instruments (that is, until we know the relative loudness of the partial tones of which they are composed at all parts of their compass), and, secondly, we have determined throughout the musical scale the relative intensities of the sounds (of simple tones) when obliteration of the sensations of higher (simple) tones supervenes. The powerlessness of one sound to affect the sensation due to another sound lower than itself in pitch greatly simplifies this problem.

4. *Applications of the Interferences of Sonorous Sensations to Determinations of the Relative Intensities of Sounds.*

Quantitative analysis of the compound tones of musical instruments is now the great desideratum of the composer. It is only after we know the relative intensities of the components of typical musical tones used in orchestral performances that we can so regulate their intensities as to give those qualities of sound which the composer desires to be heard. Thus it at once becomes evident that the instruments used in orchestral music should be very differently constructed from those used for solos or quartets. In orchestral instruments certain *characteristic* upper partials (overtones, harmonics) should predominate in order to find expression in the midst of other and graver sounds. Such orchestral instruments will therefore have exaggerated peculiarities in their qualities of tone which will render them unfit to be played on alone and uninfluenced by other orchestral notes. It is surely not hopeless to anticipate that empirical rules may be attained, which will guide the musical-instrument-maker to the production of those special qualities of tone required in orchestral instruments. It is fortunate that the very phenomena of the interferences of sonorous sensations will assist in the much-desired solution of the problem of measuring the intensity of a sound (simple tone), either when existing alone or as component of an ordinary musical (compound) tone. On this subject I am now engaged. It is evident (by way of illustration) that, so far as concerns the measure of the relative intensities of sounds *of the same pitch*, this problem has already received the simplest solution by merely placing these sounds at various distances and obliterating the sensations they excite by means of a constant and standard sound of a lower pitch. But I reserve a description of this work for a more formal publication.

20

Reprinted from pages 266-276 of *Phys. Rev.* **23**:266-285 (1924)

THE AUDITORY MASKING OF ONE PURE TONE BY ANOTHER AND ITS PROBABLE RELATION TO THE DYNAMICS OF THE INNER EAR

By R. L. Wegel and C. E. Lane

Abstract

Auditory masking of one pure tone by another.—Using an air damped telephone receiver supplied with current with a proper combination of two frequencies, as source, the amount of masking by tones of frequency 200 to 3500 was determined for frequencies from 150 to 5000 per sec. The magnitude of a tone is taken as the logarithm of the ratio of its pressure to the threshold value, and masking is taken as the logarithm of its threshold value with masking to that without. The curves of masking as function of magnitude are approximated straight lines as a rule except for rounded feet, of slope s intersecting the magnitude axis at minimum masking magnitude m. For a given masking frequency n the slope increases from zero through nearly 1.0 for a frequency near n, then more slowly, approaching about 3 to 4 for the highest frequencies measured. The intercept is small or zero below n, then increases rapidly, approaching the value 3 for high frequencies. Except when the frequencies are so close together as to produce beats, the masking is greatest for tones nearly alike. When the masking tone is loud it masks tones of higher frequency better than those of frequency lower than itself. When the masking tone is weak, there is little difference. If the masking tone is introduced into the opposite ear, no appreciable masking occurs until the intensity is sufficient to reach the listening ear through the bones of the head. At intensities considerably above minimum audibility, there is no longer a linear relation between the sound pressure and the response of the ear. Data are given showing *combinational tones* resulting from this non-linearity when two tones are simultaneously introduced in the ear. The presence also of *subjective overtones* in a loud tone accounts for the large amount of masking of tones higher than itself by a loud masking tone.

Dynamics of inner ear.—The data on masking together with Knudson's data on frequency sensibility are interpreted in terms of the *dynamical theory of the cochlea* which ascribes its frequency selectivity to a passing of vibrations along the basilar membrane and a shunting through narrow regions of the membrane at points depending on the frequency. Conjectured curves are given for a few single frequencies of the amplitude of vibration of this membrane as a function of the distance along it.

Part I. Auditory Masking of One Pure Tone by Another

1. INTRODUCTION

In past work on audition very little attention has been given to the phenomenon of masking. A. M. Mayer[1] has left a more complete record of observations on masking than any one else. He concludes that

[1] Mayer, Phil. Mag. **11**, 500, 1876

low frequency sounds may completely "obliterate" higher frequencies of considerable intensity but higher frequencies do not "obliterate" lower ones. In his experiments he used organ pipes for low frequencies and tuning forks for the high ones. With the organ pipe sounding, the action of the fork could be made intermittent by moving the hand to and fro over the mouth of a resonance box with which it was used. He describes his results in part as follows: "As the vibrations of the fork run down in amplitude, the sensations of its effect become less and less until they soon entirely vanish. Indeed the vibrations of the forks may be suddenly and totally stopped without the ear being able to detect the fact. But if instead of stopping the fork when it becomes inaudible, we stop the sound of the organ-pipe, it is impossible not to feel surprised at the strong sound of the fork which the open pipe had smothered and had rendered powerless to affect the ear. No sound, even when very intense, can diminish or obliterate the sensation of a concurrent sound which is lower in pitch. This was proved by experiments similar to the last, but differing in having the more intense sound higher (instead of lower) in pitch."

The experiments of Mayer are of course only qualitative. The work described in this paper was undertaken to obtain quantitative data and to find an explanation for the phenomena observed.

2. *Definition of masking.* Unless otherwise specified, whenever the term masking is used, it is intended to mean the masking of one tone by another when both are introduced in the same ear. For convenience in presenting data, the magnitude of a tone is defined as the ratio of its pressure to that of its minimum audible value. A logarithmic scale is used in plotting. If a minimum audible pressure of one tone is p_1 and the introduction of a second tone changes its minimum detectable value to p_2, the ratio p_2/p_1 is taken as the magnitude of the masking of the first tone by the second and is likewise plotted on a logarithmic scale. In this paper the term pressure is used to signify the root mean square value of the sound pressure in the external ear passage.

3. *Range of intensities and frequencies of the tones used.* Fig. 1 is a diagram of the auditory sensation area.[2] This figure practically describes itself. It shows that the region of sensation covered by these experiments includes the most important range of frequencies and intensities. The higher levels in this region near the threshold of feeling are generally impracticable for extended experimentation because they induce tinnitus. The very low and very high frequencies are not covered in this work because they are of lesser importance, and furthermore, intense and

[2] See Wegel, Proc. Nat. Acad. Sci., July, 1922 and Bell System Tech. J., Nov. 1922.

pure tones at low frequencies and intense tones at high frequencies are produced with difficulty.

4. *Masking as a function of intensity.* Fig. 2 shows the amount of masking of various frequencies from 250 to 4,000 cycles produced by an 800 cycle tone, plotted as a function of the magnitude of this masking tone. For example, the first curve shows the amount of masking, as already defined, of 250 cycles plotted as a function of the magnitude of an 800 cycle masking tone. Each plotted point represents the average of

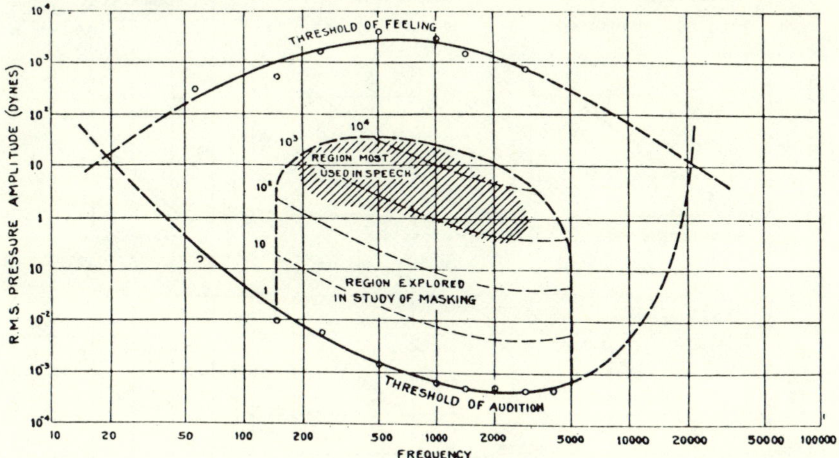

Fig. 1. Auditory sensation area.

four observations taken in succession at one time. In all figures the masking tone is designated by F_1 and the masked by F_2. These curves were all obtained for one observer except the dash-dot ones, which are included here to show the small amount of variation usually found when taking masking data for different observers of normal hearing.

The curves do not all pass through the origin as they evidently should except, as will be explained later, when the tones produce beats. The minimum audible reference value used was the average taken over a period of several days. Plotted in this way it was found that such curves varied from day to day near minimum audibility but for the higher intensities checked within the experimental error. The general magnitude of the deviation of the lower end of the curve from the origin will be seen from the variations shown by the curves. This shows that the ear is quite variable in its behavior near minimum audibility, but comparatively constant for louder tones. The curves as corrected by the dotted lines represent a close approximation, in each case, to the average curve which would have been obtained if the observations had extended over a long period of time. This correction does not apply when the tones produce beats.

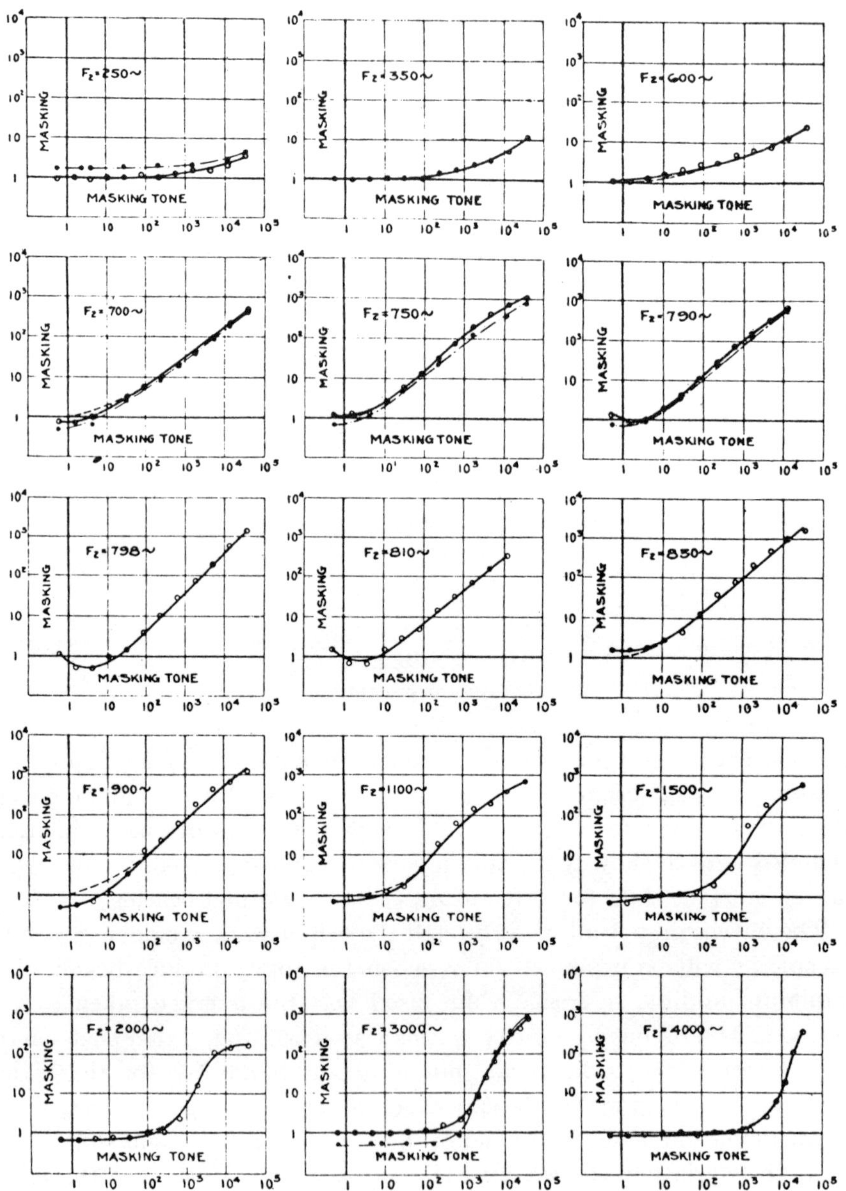

Fig. 2. Data for masking tone of 800 cycles.

Fig. 3 shows some of the corrected curves from Fig. 2 reproduced on common axes. Curves for masking tones of 200, 300, 400, 600, 1200,

1800, 2400 and 3500 cycles are also included in this figure. The frequency of the masked tone is indicated on each curve.

From the figures certain general facts are evident. A tone of a frequency much below the masking tone is not perceptibly masked for the lower range of intensities and hardly more than perceptibly so when the tones are very loud. A tone of much higher frequency than the masking

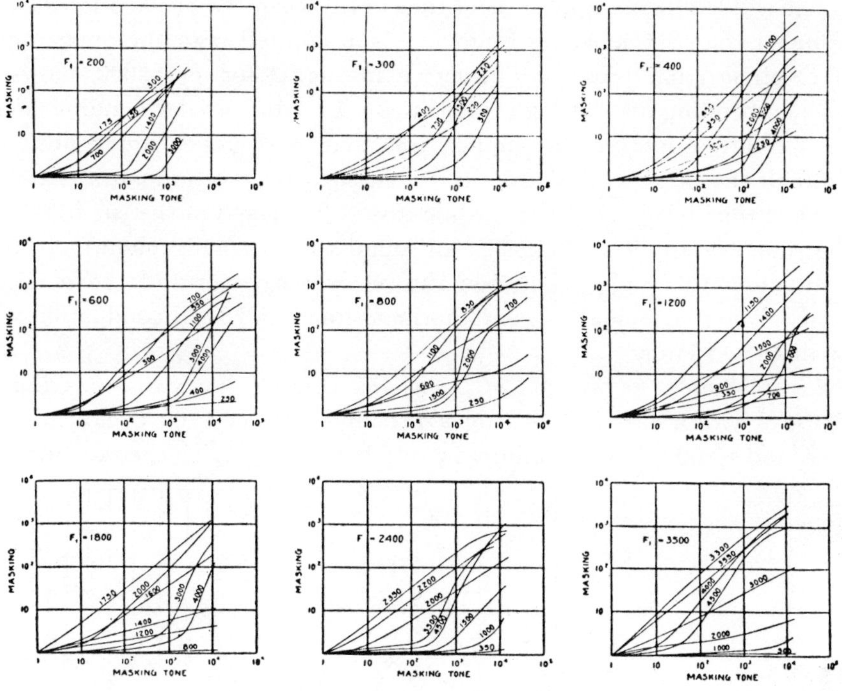

Fig. 3. Masking for tones in same ear.

tone is not perceptibly masked for the lower range of intensities, but at a rather definite high intensity masking occurs perceptibly and quickly becomes very great as the masking tone is increased. In general, masking is greater when the tones lie close together, the curves approaching straight lines with 45° slopes, intercepting the axis of abscissas at about ten times the minimum audible pressure of the masking tone.

When the tones are close enough together in frequency to beat, they do not give masking curves in the same sense as when farther apart. They represent measurements of the minimum perceptible fluctuation of the beating tone. Two such tones, separately inaudible, but each not lower than one-half the minimum audible pressure, will obviously beat when introduced together in such a way as to be alternately audible and inaudible. This effect accounts for the depression in the curve at low intensities in Fig. 2 for $F_2=790$, 789 and 810. At higher intensities the magnitude of the minimum perceptible beating fluctuation may be obtained from the difference between abscissas and ordinates. The minimum detectable amount of this fluctuation has been found to decrease as the beat frequency decreases, approaching a value which would be expected from ear sensibility data.

The sudden increase in slope of the curves when the masked frequency is higher than the masking frequency is associated with the appearance of combinational tones. The curve in Fig. 2 for $F_2=2000$ shows a decided bending over at high intensities. This and similar bendings may be accounted for on the supposition that both tones are conducted through the head to the opposite ear in such relative amounts that the masked tone is detected there while it is still masked in the ear to which the sound is applied. It has been found that a small amount of bone conduction takes place between the receiver ear cap and the mastoid bone. The phenomena of combinational tones and head conduction will be discussed later.

5. *Masking as a function of frequency.* Fig. 4 shows the masking of tones of various frequencies by a masking tone of 1200 cycles at 160, 1000 and 10,000 times its minimum audible value. With the exception of

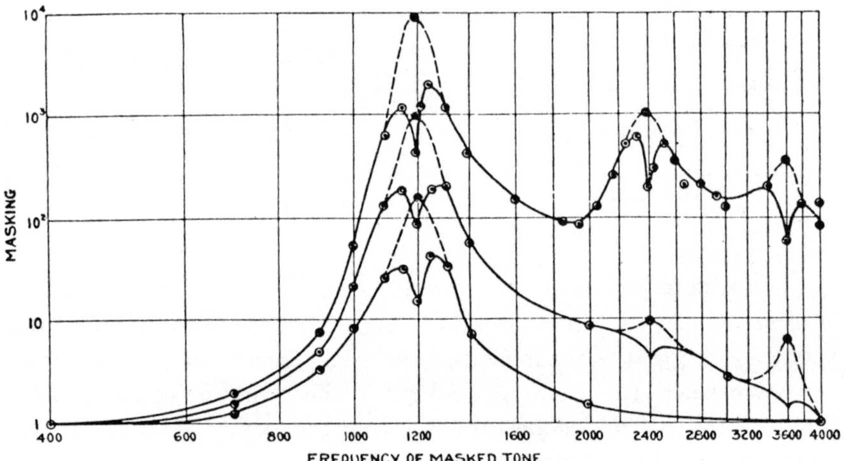

Fig. 4. Masking of various frequencies by 1200 cycles.

the region near the masking frequency where beats occur, the lowest curve shows a gradual falling off of masking as the masked frequency departs on either side from the masking frequency. Within the region of beats, the amount of masking decreases as the masking frequency is approached. The intersection of the curves at the masking frequency may be interpreted to give intensity sensibility. The highest curve differs in that its characteristics in the region of the first and second overtones of the masking frequency are much like those in the neighborhood of the masking frequency. It resembles such a curve as might be expected from a knowledge of the lowest curve if three masking frequencies, 1200, 2400 and 3600 cycles were present, with relative magnitudes of 1:0.1:0.025. An harmonic analysis of the sound as picked up by a condenser transmitter, showed that these tones were not appreciably present in the air. These and other tests were made, in fact, in all measurements recorded in this paper, and in no case was the distortion in the receiver detectable. Since beats are obtained at the frequencies of overtones, it is concluded that these harmonics are introduced subjectively in the ear due to some non-linear characteristic of its response. The magnitude of these overtones may be obtained experimentally by increasing the intensity of a secondary tone of such a frequency as to beat with the harmonic, to a point where beats are most prominent and taking the intensity of this

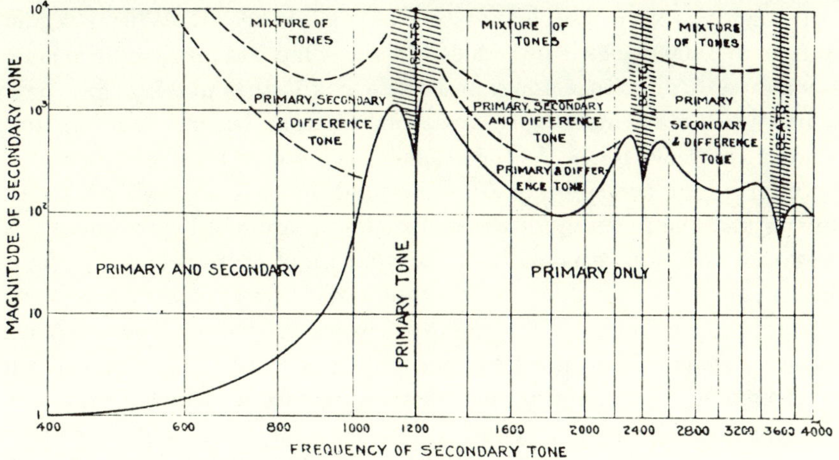

Fig. 5. Sensation caused by two pure tones.

tone to be equal to the intensity of the overtone. The dots represent the magnitudes of the harmonics so determined. This method is not very accurate because the intensity of the variable tone at which the most prominent beats are heard tends to be somewhat higher than the fixed overtone. The middle curve represents a transition between the other two. It indicates harmonic components of relative magnitudes 1:.01:.006. These curves show that a tone masks frequencies higher than itself better than lower frequencies only when it is loud.

6. *Non-linearity of response of the ear.* The character of the sensation, when two tones are acting together on the ear, varies considerably with the relative frequency and intensity values. Fig. 5 represents the sensa-

tion caused by a tone of fixed frequency, 1200 cycles, and magnitude 10^4, in combination with various secondary tones of which the frequencies are represented by the abscissas and the magnitudes by the ordinates. The continuous curve is the same as the top curve in Fig. 11. The various areas represent ranges of magnitude and frequency of the secondary tone in which combinational tones of various kinds, as indicated, appear. As any secondary tone of a frequency below about 1000 cycles, for example 800, is gradually brought up in intensity from a sub-audible value to a point at which it is just detectable, it is first heard as a separate tone along with the primary tone. In the lower part of this range, the intensity of the secondary tone may be increased to very large values and still be perceived independently of the primary. When, however, the intensity of the secondary tone is increased to a point indicated by the dotted line, the difference tone is distinguishable and increases gradually in relative intensity as the area above this line is crossed. At the high intensities in this region, a very complex mixture of tones is heard. When a secondary tone of 1900 cycles is introduced in the same way, its presence is first detected by a difference tone, and the secondary is not heard. As the intensity is further increased, the secondary tone becomes audible along with the difference tone. As the intensity is increased to the higher levels, the mixture of tones becomes more and more complex. With this explanation, the meaning of the rest of the figure will be obvious.

A careful analysis was made of the mixture of tones present in the ear when a primary of 1200 at a magnitude 6×10^4 was present along with a secondary of frequency 700, of about the same intensity. The component frequencies were determined by introducing a third tone of known variable frequency and determining the frequencies at which beats occur. If f_1 represents the primary, and f_2, the secondary, the frequencies found in the mixture were f_1, 1200 cycles; f_2, 700; f_1+f_2, 1900; f_1-f_2, 500; $2f_1$, 2400; $2f_2$, 1400; $3f_1$, 3600; $3f_2$, 2100; $2f_1+f_2$, 3100; $2f_1-f_2$, 1700; $2f_2+f_1$, 2600; $2f_2-f_1$, 200 (?); $4f_2$, 2800; $2f_1+2f_2$, 3800; $2f_1-2f_2$, 1000; $3f_1+f_2$, 4300; $3f_1-f_2$, 2900; $3f_2+f_1$, 3300; $3f_2-f_1$, 900. No attempt was made to determine their magnitudes although this can probably be done approximately by measuring the intensity of the exploring tone at which the beats at each frequency are most prominent. With the exception of the frequency $4f_1$, this series is all that would be expected if the response of the ear were non-linear and represented by the equation:

$$x=a_0+a_1p+a_2p^2+a_3p^3+a_4p^4.$$

In this equation, x is the response of the mechanism of the middle ear; a_0, a_1, a_2, etc., are constants, and p is the pressure in the ear canal. While frequencies introduced by higher powers of the pressure were probably present, they were very faint and no careful search was made for them. No careful investigation has yet been made of this phase of audition. Results of further work may call for modifications of the interpretation

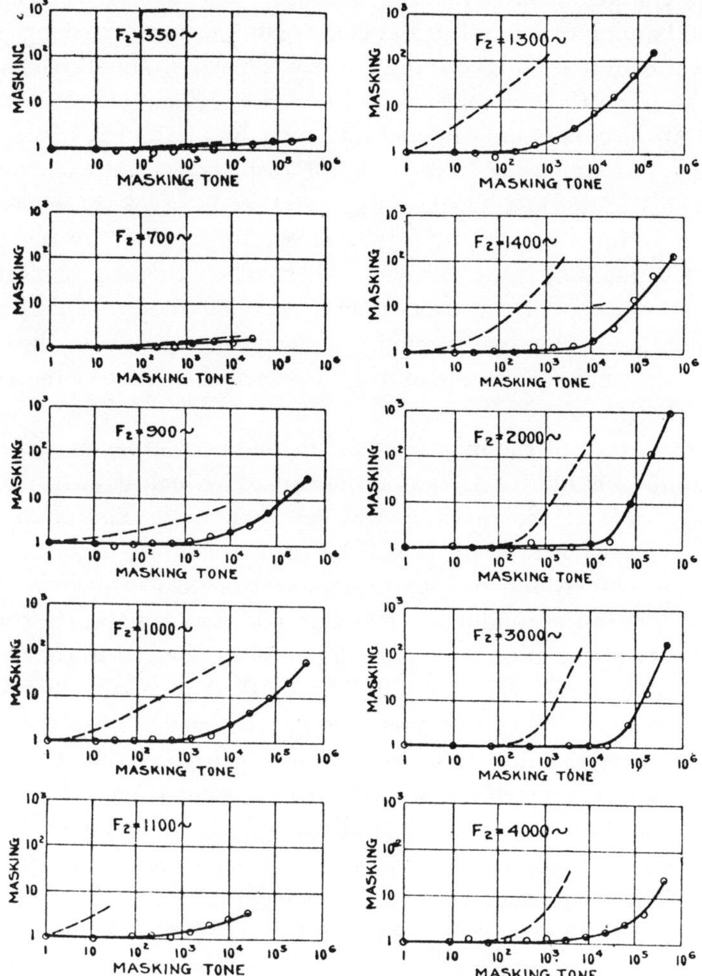

Fig. 6. Masking data for tones in opposite ears, masking tone 1200 cycles.

given here. It may be interesting to note in this connection that one of the striking characteristics of some kinds of abnormal hearing has been found[2] to be an exaggerated departure from linearity.

7. *Masking with tones in opposite ears.* Fig. 6 gives the masking when the masked and masking tones are introduced in opposite ears. The dotted curves show the corresponding data for tones in the same ear. The two sets of curves are nearly alike except for displacement in the

ratio of $1:10^2$ to $1:10^3$ along the horizontal axis. These curves may be explained by assuming that there are two kinds of masking, central and peripheral, the former being generally relatively small and resulting from the conflict of sensations in the brain and the latter originating from overlapping of stimuli in the end organ. Central masking is probably always present to a certain extent whereas peripheral masking can only occur when the two tones excite the same region on the basilar membrane. All large amounts of masking may be attributed to peripheral masking. The similarity, except for the displacement already noted, of the two sets of masking curves indicates that most of the masking for loud tones in opposite ears is peripheral masking, caused by the conduction of the masking tone through the head to the opposite ear with sufficient intensity to cause peripheral masking there. This presumes an attenuation of the tone through the head from one ear to the other of the same order of magnitude as the displacement between the two sets of masking curves.

The magnitude of the masking tone in these experiments was referred to the minimum audible value for the ear into which it was introduced. The magnitude of the masking was referred to the minimum audible value for the opposite ear. It will be seen, therefore, according to the explanation offered above, that the amount of displacement of a curve gives the sum of the conduction loss through the head and the difference in sensitivity of the two ears. If both had been referred to the minimum audible value of the ear receiving the masked tone, the displacement would have given the attenuation through the head. Since the two ears of the observer did not differ greatly in sensitivity, this displacement gives the proper order of magnitude for the attenuation.

There is still further evidence that when a tone is introduced into one ear by a telephone receiver, the opposite ear is also excited but to a lesser degree. Cases of persons very deaf in one ear have been noted for which 10^2 to 10^3 times the current is required for audition with the receiver on the deaf ear over that for the receiver on the good ear. Also, when the sound for the receiver on the deaf ear is audible, it may be greatly enhanced by placing the finger in the good ear, indicating that the sound is not only heard first in the good ear but that it arrives there by bone conduction. Furthermore when two tones of the proper frequencies to beat are introduced in opposite ears the best beats[3] are always heard when one of the tones is over 100 times the amplitude of the other and the relative intensities for hearing these best beats are nearly indepen-

[3] In this connection, see G. W. Stewart, Phys. Rev. **9**, 514, 1917. Stewart's conclusions are somewhat at variance with those arrived at here.

dent of the sensitivity of the ear to which the louder tone is applied. In fact this ear may be entirely deaf, or, if normal, its sensitivity may be lowered by plugging, and best beats will still be heard at the same relative currents through the receivers.

In view of the approximate agreement of all the evidence of head conduction, it seems safe to conclude that this phenomenon actually exists and that it accounts for the resemblance of the two sets of masking curves in Fig. 6. This attenuation through the head, of course, applies only when telephone receivers are used in the ordinary manner as the sound source. When other sources were used, different values of attenuation were found.

[*Editor's Note:* Part II is a discussion of the dynamics of the inner ear and has been omitted since it is not pertinent to the topic of this volume.]

21

Reprinted from *Acoust. Soc. Am. J.* **22**:622–630 (1950)

On the Masking Pattern of a Simple Auditory Stimulus*

James P. Egan and Harold W. Hake
University of Wisconsin, Madison, Wisconsin
(Received April 15, 1950)

MEASUREMENTS of the masking effects of an auditory stimulus provide data from which the excitation pattern of the masking stimulus may be derived. In 1924 Wegel and Lane[1] published the first quantitative results showing the masking of pure tones by pure tones. The masking audiograms which these investigators obtained showed how marked is the spread of action produced by a simple auditory stimulus.

The masking pattern of a pure tone is complicated, however, by various phenomena not directly related to the degree of excitation as it is measured by the masked stimulus. In the first place, when the masked stimulus, f_s, is nearly the same in frequency as the masking stimulus, f_p, beats occur, and the amount of masking is much less than at more distant points. Furthermore, the production of a difference tone, $f_s - f_p$, by the distortion of the masking and masked stimuli, makes it possible to detect the presence of the masked stimulus long before its intensity is sufficient to provide its characteristic pitch. When the difference tone is detected, the amount of masking measured at f_s depends upon the amount of distortion in the ear under test and upon the amount of masking at the frequency $(f_s - f_p)$ of the difference tone. Clearly, under these conditions, the degree of excitation at the frequency f_s is not adequately measured by the amount of masking at f_s. Fletcher and Munson[2] were fairly successful in avoiding these difficulties by using bands of noise as the masking stimulus. With this stimulus the effects on masking due to beats and to difference tones are largely, but not entirely, obviated. The measurements reported below provide further support for the use of narrow bands of noise in the determination of the masking pattern of a simple auditory stimulus.[3]

EXPERIMENTAL PROCEDURE

The masking audiograms of two stimuli were determined. One masking stimulus was a pure tone of 400 c.p.s., generated by a beat frequency oscillator (General Radio Co., Type 1304-A). To ensure the purity of this tone it was passed through the same narrow band-pass filters used for the other masking stimulus. The second masking stimulus was a narrow band of noise obtained by passing a noise (gas tube) with uniform spectrum level through narrow band-pass filters (two wave filters, General Radio Co., Type 530-A). The resulting band of noise was about 90 c.p.s. wide, measured three decibels down from the broad peak, and had a center frequency of 410 c.p.s. The over-all voltage level of this band of noise was measured directly and also checked by calculation from the over-all voltage measurements of a wider band of noise (0–1000 c.p.s.) and the measured filter characteristics. Since the noise had a uniform spectrum level, the level-per-cycle was taken to be $-10 \log_{10}\Delta f$ decibels relative to the over-all level, where Δf is the band width of the noise whose over-all level is known. The voltage levels measured at the earphone were converted to sound-pressure levels (S.P.L. or decibels re 0.0002 dyne/cm^2) by means of the calibration curve of the earphone.

All measurements were monaural, and the masking and masked stimuli were presented by means of a dy-

* This research was supported in part by the Research Committee of the Graduate School of the University of Wisconsin from special funds voted by the State Legislature.

[1] R. L. Wegel and C. E. Lane, "The auditory masking of one pure tone by another and its probable relation to the dynamics of the inner ear," Phys. Rev. **23**, 266–285 (1924).

[2] H. Fletcher and W. A. Munson, "Relation between loudness and masking," J. Acous. Soc. Am. **9**, 1–10 (1937).

[3] A recent article by W. A. Munson and M. B. Gardner, "Loudness patterns—a new approach," J. Acous. Soc. Am. **22**, 177–190 (1950), points out the difficulties encountered in the determination of the excitation or loudness pattern of a pure tone. These investigators employed a novel technique in which a test tone of brief duration is presented a short time after the masking stimulus is turned off. By this method they obtained measures of residual masking which are evidently free of the complications due to beats, difference tones, and aural harmonics. Their important new findings are not related to the amount of simultaneous masking in a simple manner, however.

namic earphone (Permoflux Corp., Type PDR-10) held in a headband and coupled to the ear by means of a small rubber cushion. Under these conditions the sound pressure at 400 c.p.s. near the entrance to the auditory canal does not differ appreciably from that obtained with the artificial ear (6 cc coupler) used for calibration of the earphone.[4] The contralateral ear was also covered by means of a PDR-10 earphone held in the headband and sealed against the external ear by means of a small rubber cushion. The internal consistency of the results obtained with low and high intensities of the masking stimulus as well as independent checks (the masking of the contralateral ear by white noise and the auditory localization of the masked tone near its masked threshold) indicate that any cross-stimulation of the contralateral ear did not appreciably affect the results.

Once the sound-pressure level of the masking stimulus is correctly measured, discrepancies between the actual pressure of the masked stimulus and that found with the artificial ear do not affect the determination of masking, since a difference between two intensities at the same frequency is the required datum. Consequently, the marked low frequency leak (below 300 c.p.s.), which is present when the earphone is worn, does not introduce errors in the masking results.

The masking audiograms for each of these masking stimuli were determined at various sound-pressure levels. The number of intensities used varied somewhat from listener to listener, and the particular intensities will be indicated along with the results.

In all, seven subjects served in the experiment. Two of these *Ss* had marked hearing losses at low frequencies, and their results are not included in the present report. Each of the other five *Ss* had normal hearing. The curve showing the average absolute threshold as a function of frequency for these five *Ss* agrees remarkably well with that published by Sivian and White[5] for minimum audible pressures with monaural listening. At 100 c.p.s. the deviation from Sivian and White is 4 db. From 200 to 5000 c.p.s. the deviation at any frequency is less than 2 db.

The amount of masking was measured in the usual way. The absolute threshold in quiet for pure tones was first determined as a function of frequency. Four-

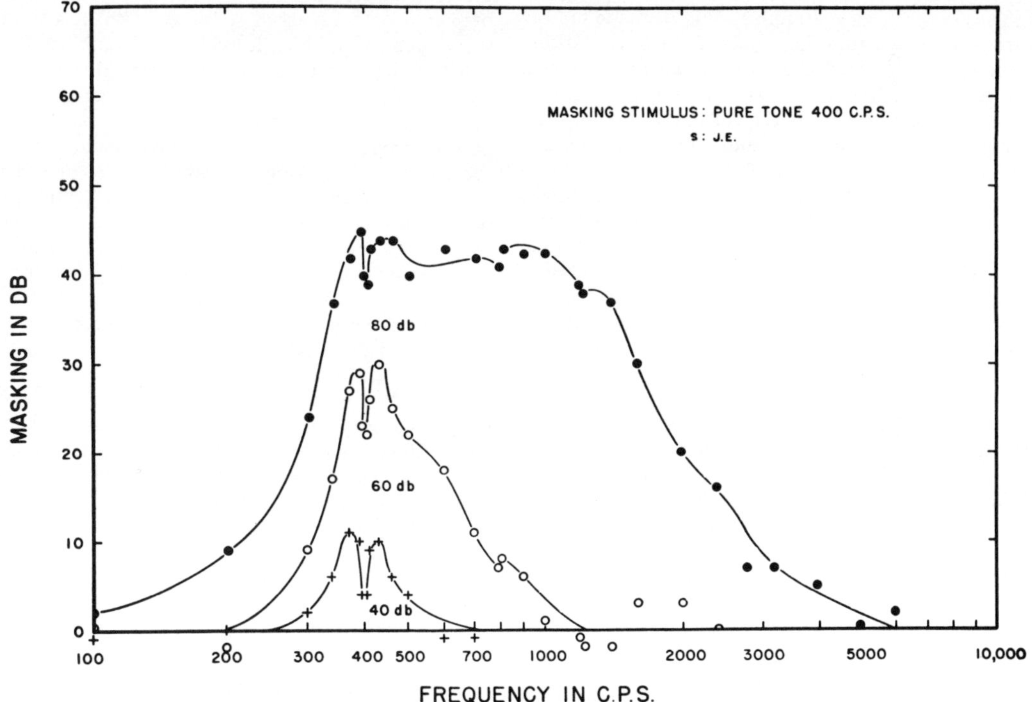

FIG. 1. The curves are masking audiograms of a pure tone of 400 c.p.s. The number under each curve is the sound-pressure level (decibels re 0.0002 dyne/cm²) of the masking tone (0 db sensation level corresponds to 15 db S.P.L. at 400 c.p.s.). The abscissa represents the frequency of the masked tone and the ordinate represents the shift in decibels of its absolute threshold. Note how asymmetrical the curves become as the intensity of the masking stimulus is increased.

[4] F. M. Wiener and A. S. Filler, "The response of certain earphones on the ear and on closed couplers," in a report of research issued by the Psycho-Acoustic Laboratory Harvard University, under a contract with the U. S. Navy, Office of Naval Research, Contract. N5ori-76, Project order II, Report PNR-2, December 1, 1945.

[5] L. J. Sivian and S. D. White, "On minimum audible sound fields," J. Acous. Soc. Am. 4, 288–321 (1933).

teen tones ranging from 100 to 8000 c.p.s. were used for this purpose. At least two measurements were made at each frequency by each subject. Then the thresholds were redetermined in the presence of the masking stimulus. The 29 pure tones used as the masked stimuli, f_s, were: 100, 200, 300, 340, 370, 390, 397, 403, 410, 430, 460, 500, 600, 700, 797, 803, 900, 1000, 1197, 1203, 1400, 1597, 2000, 2400, 2800, 3200, 4000, 5000, and 6000 c.p.s. Another oscillator (General Radio Company, Type 1304-A) was used to generate the masked stimulus, f_s. When the masking stimulus was a 400 c.p.s. pure tone, special care was exercised to ensure that the relative calibration of the two oscillators, one for the masking and one for the masked stimulus, was correct. Thus, when the masked stimulus was near 400 c.p.s., the experimenter first adjusted the frequency of the oscillator used for the masked stimulus until it gave zero beat against the oscillator used for the masking stimulus (400 c.p.s.). Then the incremental tuning dial, calibrated in one-cycle steps, was set to give the appropriate frequency for the masked stimulus. The same procedure was followed when the frequency of the masked stimulus differed from an aural harmonic by 3 c.p.s. In this case the masked stimulus could be made to beat clearly against the aural harmonic of the pure masking stimulus, and zero beat was easily obtained. Because a large number of frequencies were tested, and because the repeated calibration of the oscillators held up the masking tests, only one determination of the masked threshold by each subject was feasible.

For the determination of both quiet and masked absolute thresholds the test tone, f_s, was presented automatically by means of an electronic switch which turned the tone on and off at regular intervals. The duration of the test tone was 0.7 sec. After an interval of 0.7 sec. the test tone sounded again. The effects of transients were minimized by turning the tone on or off over a period of about 0.1 sec.

In all tests the subject adjusted an attenuation network, calibrated in one decibel steps, until he found his own threshold. He was carefully instructed in the procedure of "bracketing" his threshold. When such a method is carefully employed, the datum from a single trial is actually the result of a series of judgments made by the subject before he selects the final setting. When the test tone was at or near threshold, the subject could effectively turn off the masked tone by throwing 10 db additional attenuation in the pad, an aid which some subjects find useful.

In determining his masked threshold the subject used the criterion "detection of anything." Thus, with a masking stimulus of 400 c.p.s. and a masked stimulus of 300 c.p.s., he would hear, in addition to the masking tone, the characteristic pitch of a 300 c.p.s. tone. At 397, however, he would hear nearly two beats while the test tone was on and then a short interval during which the masking stimulus sounded without waver. Under these conditions his task was to adjust the attenuator dial until he could just detect the presence of the beat. Again, when a tone of 600 c.p.s. was near the threshold of detection (masked threshold) in the presence of a loud tone of 400 c.p.s., he would typically hear a tone whose pitch corresponded to a tone of 200 c.p.s. ($f_s - f_p$). For all masked thresholds, he adjusted the attenuator until he could just detect that something happened at the regular intervals during which the test tone f_s was on.

RESULTS AND DISCUSSION

Typical masking audiograms of a pure tone of 400 c.p.s. are shown in Fig. 1. The number under each curve designates the sound-pressure level of the masking stimulus. As was found by Wegel and Lane,[1] the masking audiogram of a stimulus of low intensity is nearly symmetrical when frequency is plotted on a logarithmic scale. However, at the higher intensities of the masking stimulus, the aural harmonics of the pure masking tone help to spread the action of the primary stimulus up the frequency scale. The curves also show the well-known "dips" due to beats between the masked stimulus and the masking stimulus or its aural harmonics. When the frequency of the masked stimulus is 397 or 403 c.p.s., the amount of masking is evidently determined by the value of the differential threshold for intensity at 400 c.p.s. As the frequency of the masked stimulus increases up to 430 c.p.s., the amount of masking increases and passes through a maximum. Above about 430 c.p.s. the amount of masking decreases because presumably the ear is now successfully analyzing the complex tone into its two components. The masked tone is then heard as a separate component. At the higher intensities of the masking stimulus, the masking curve passes through a minimum between 400 and 800 c.p.s. The curve drops as much as it does because the difference tone, $f_s - f_p$, is detectable before the masked stimulus is heard with its characteristic pitch.

Figure 2 shows the masking audiograms for the same subject when the masking stimulus is a narrow band of noise. It is evident that the masking pattern is not nearly as complicated by beats, harmonics, and difference tones as is the masking pattern of a pure tone. The "beat" heard in the immediate vicinity of 410 c.p.s. is no longer prominent, and the test tone, f_s, is heard as a "buzz" or "rattle." Furthermore, when the over-all S.P.L. of the band of noise is 80 db, the test tones of 797 and 803 c.p.s. appear with only a slight "flutter" or "roughness." Careful listening tests also indicate that a masked tone of 500 or 600 c.p.s. is detected in terms of that tone and not by means of a difference tone.

A comparison of Figs. 1 and 2 shows that, at the lower intensities of the masking stimulus, the masking audiogram of the pure tone lies wholly under the corresponding masking audiogram of the band of noise. With the masking stimulus at an over-all S.P.L. of 80 db, however, the pure tone of 400 c.p.s. masks the high frequencies better than the band of noise.

The relation between the amount of masking at a certain frequency and the intensity of the masking stimulus is better illustrated by Figs. 3 and 4. Figure 3 shows the amount of masking at a given frequency as a function of the intensity of the masking tone of 400 c.p.s. The curve which shows the amount of masking at 430 c.p.s. has a slope of one only at intermediate intensities of the masking stimulus; at higher intensities the curve departs more and more from linearity. The curves for 1000 and 1400 c.p.s. show how great is the increase of masking at frequencies just above the second and third aural harmonics of the pure masking stimulus. These curves ultimately cross the curve for 430 c.p.s., a fact which verifies the result obtained by Wegel and Lane.[1]

In Fig. 4 are shown the corresponding curves of masking produced by the narrow band of noise. For this masking stimulus the curve that shows the amount of masking at 430 c.p.s. is a linear function with a slope of one over most of its course. The equation of this curve over its linear portion is: $M=10\log_{10}(I_m\Delta f_k/I_0\Delta f_m)$, where M is the amount of masking in decibels, I_m is the over-all intensity of the masking noise, Δf_m is the band width of the masking noise in c.p.s., Δf_k is the width of a critical band in c.p.s., and I_0 is the threshold intensity of the masked tone measured in the quiet. Now, $10\log_{10}\Delta f_m$ is 19.5 db; $10\log_{10}\Delta f_k$ obtained by using the narrow band of noise is 14.5 db for this subject; and his absolute threshold is 14 db S.P.L. at 430 c.p.s. Therefore, the simplified equation of the curve is $M=\beta-19$, where β is the band pressure level (decibels re 0.0002 dyne/cm²) of the masking stimulus. (The fact that k is only 14.5 db is discussed below.)

Figures 5 and 6 show for a different subject the same set of relations as those of Figs. 1 and 2. This subject (HH) was also used to obtain data comparable to those of Figs. 3 and 4, but they are not included because they are so similar to the data presented.

Figure 7 shows the average data for five subjects (JE, LG, HH, LS, and MS). The individual data of two of the *Ss* (JE and HH) have been presented. The other three *Ss* show essentially the same relations between the two masking audiograms as those shown by the average curves. With a masking stimulus at an over-all sound-pressure level of 80 db, four of the five *Ss* show that tones above about 1000 c.p.s. are masked more by a pure tone of 400 c.p.s. than by the narrow band of noise. The intensity of the masking stimulus at which an individual's masking audiogram for a pure tone of 400 c.p.s. crosses the audiogram for a band of noise

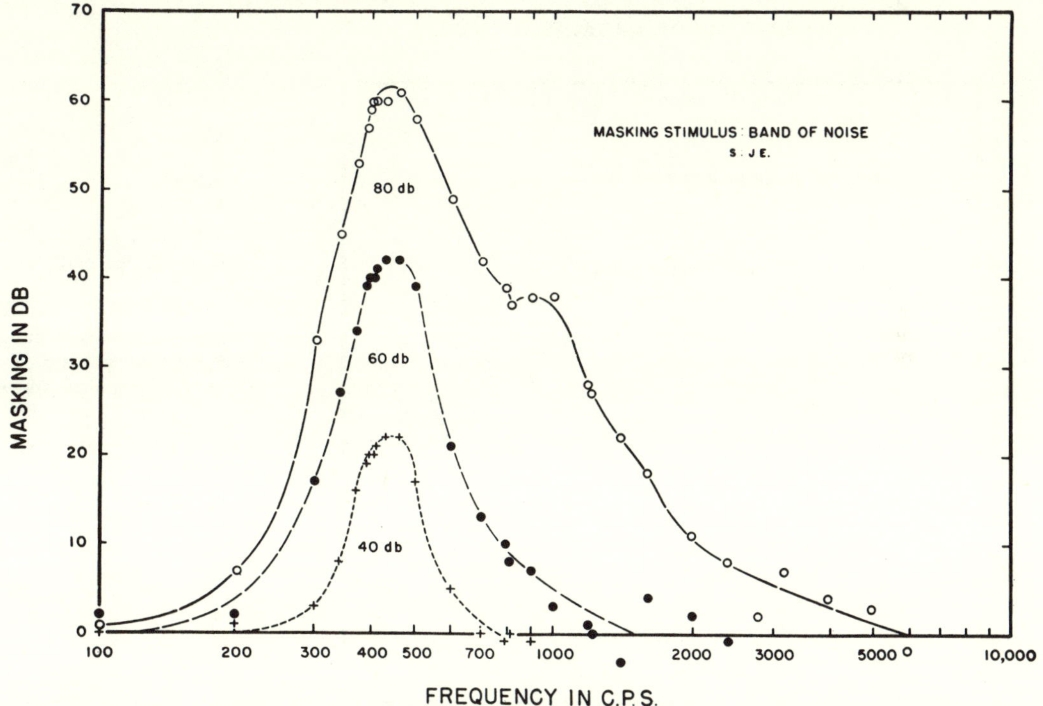

FIG. 2. These curves are masking audiograms of a band of noise (90 c.p.s. wide, centered at 410 c.p.s.). The parameter is the over-all sound-pressure level of the masking noise. These curves represent better than those for a pure tone the masking patterns of an auditory stimulus whose energy is confined to a narrow frequency region; but the masking at 410 c.p.s. still does not have the same meaning as the masking at more distant points, because the masked tone at about 410 c.p.s. is detected as a "buzz" or "rattle"

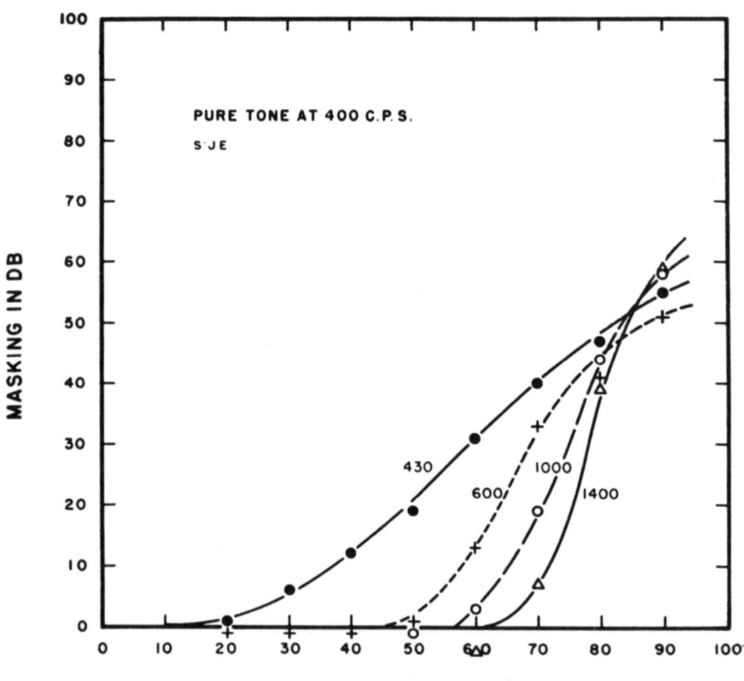

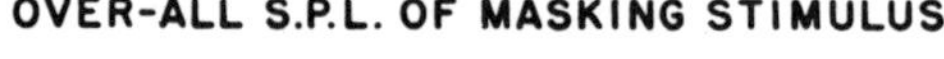

FIG. 3. Each curve shows the amount of masking at a given frequency as a function of the intensity of the masking tone of 400 c.p.s. Note how the curve for the masked tone of 430 c.p.s. departs from linearity at the higher intensities of the masking stimulus, and how the curves for 1000 and 1400 c.p.s. cross the curve for 430 c.p.s. at high intensities.

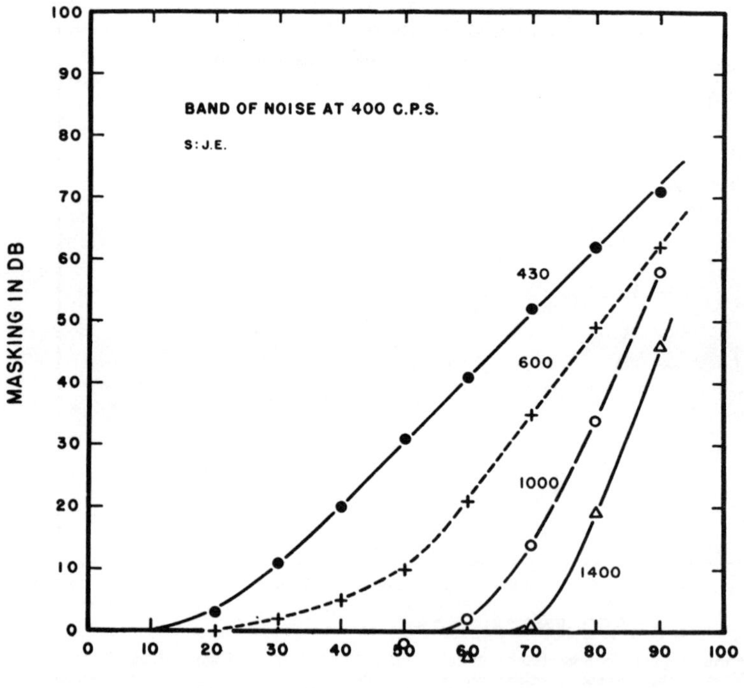

FIG. 4. Each curve shows the amount of masking at a given frequency as a function of the intensity of the narrow band of masking noise (90 c.p.s. wide, centered at 410 c.p.s.). The curve that shows the amount of masking at 430 c.p.s. is a linear function with unit slope over most of its course.

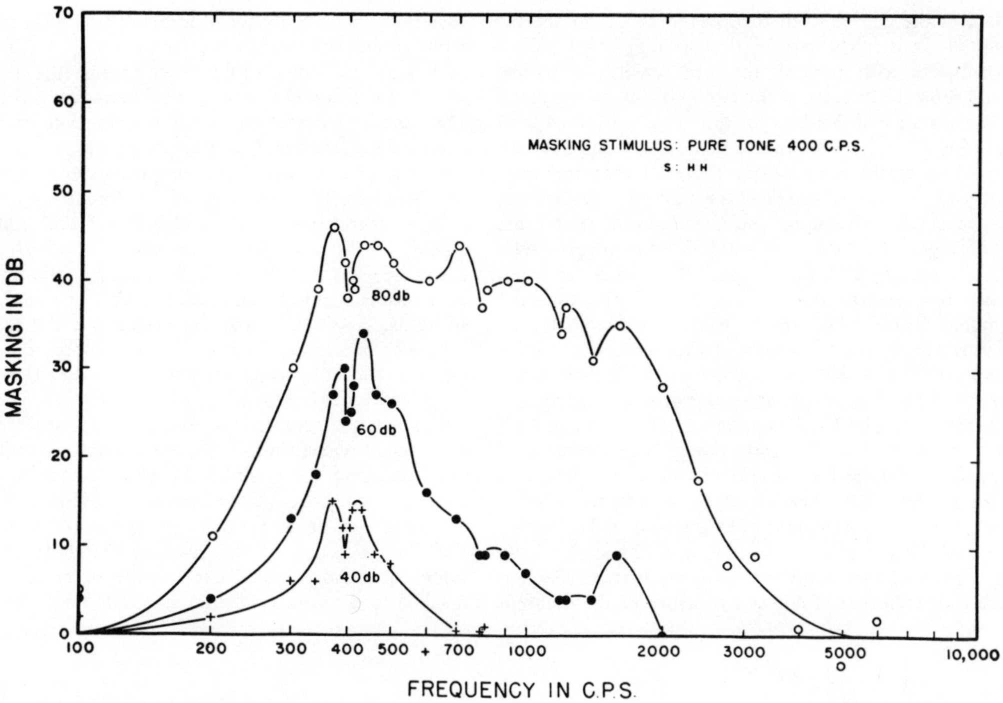

FIG. 5. Masking audiograms of a pure tone of 400 c.p.s. These curves show for a different subject the same relations as those of Fig. 1.

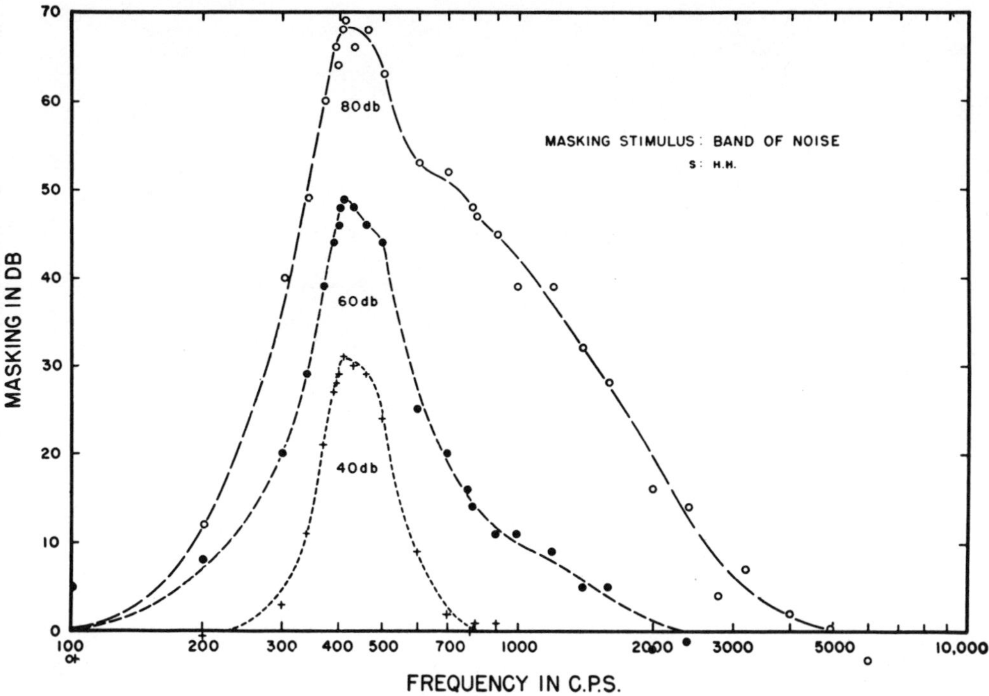

FIG. 6. Masking audiograms of a narrow band of noise (90 c.p.s. wide, centered at 410 c.p.s.). These curves show for a different subject the same relations as those of Fig. 2.

indicates the degree of distortion in the ear of the individual. It is fairly certain that at higher intensities all subjects with normal absolute sensitivity curves would show the crossing of the two masking audiograms.

The variance of the data for the five *Ss* obtained with the band of noise was analyzed into various sources. Inspection of the data clearly revealed that the variability of the *masked threshold* for a given tone depends to a marked degree upon the frequency of that tone. Accordingly, the data were subdivided into three sets. One set consisted of the masked thresholds for tones whose frequencies were below that of the masking stimulus. Those tones whose frequencies were in the same region as the frequency of the masking stimulus comprised the second set, and the tones higher in frequency than that of the masking stimulus composed the third set. The total number of judgments in each set was 20, 35, and 35, respectively. The measures of variability obtained by these analyses are shown in Table I. The column headed "*S.D.* of judgments by an average *S*" may be thought of as the standard deviation of a distribution of a large number of thresholds for a single masked tone measured with an average listener. Such a distribution provides a measure of the inherent variability or of the error of measurement that remains after differences due to the frequency of the masked tone and individual differences among the listeners have been removed from the total variance of the data. The standard deviation of the distribution of means, one for each listener, is a measure of differences among listeners. (The differences among the listeners were not significant for the four tones of low frequency.)

It is clear from the data of Table I that the variability of the masked thresholds is relatively small when the energy of the masked stimulus is concentrated in the same band of frequencies as that of the masking stimulus. However, when the masking is the result of "spread" of action of the masking stimulus, the variability is relatively large, particularly so when the spread is up the frequency scale.

It was not considered meaningful to perform a similar analysis of variance for the data obtained with the pure masking tone, since the assumption of homogeneity of variance for the frequencies grouped into one set could not be met. Although the criterion used in the determination of the masked threshold was the same throughout, the basis for the detection of the masked tone varies markedly as pointed out above.

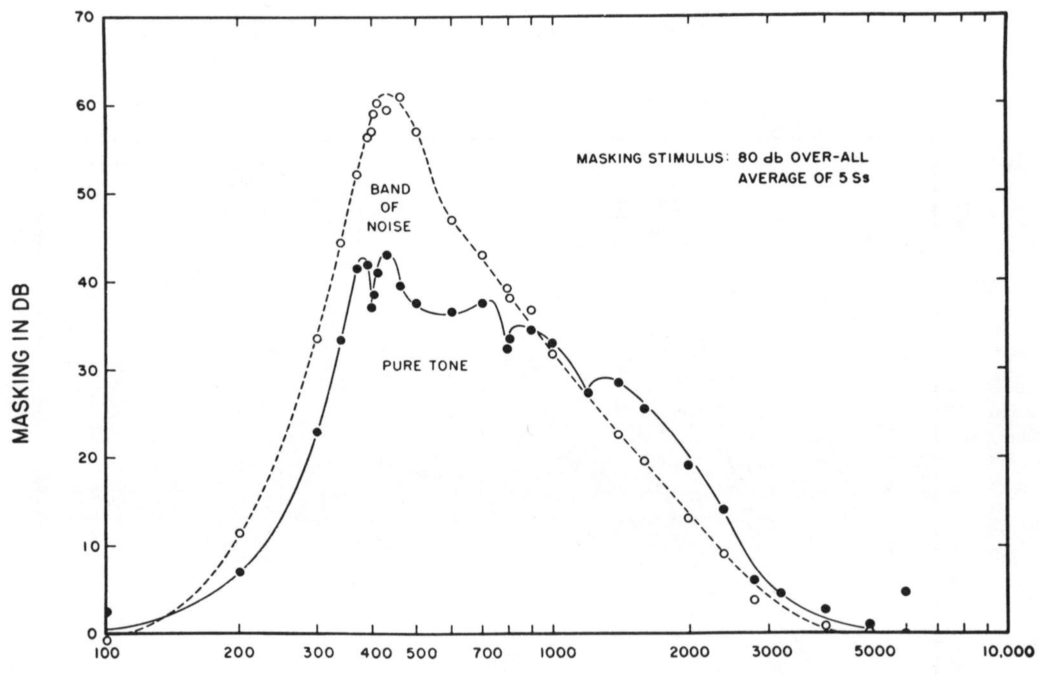

FIG. 7. These two curves show the difference between the masking audiograms of a pure tone of 400 c.p.s. and of a narrow band of noise (90 c.p.s. wide, centered at 410 c.p.s.) with each presented at an over-all sound-pressure level of 80 db (decibels re 0.0002 dyne/cm²). Comparison of the two curves shows how much the masking pattern of a pure tone is complicated by beats, aural harmonics, and difference tones. The dips are due to beats, and the broad minimum between 400 and 800 c.p.s. is due in part to the detection of the masked tone by means of the difference tone and in part to the additional masking produced by the aural harmonic of 800 c.p.s. These masking audiograms are based upon the average of 5 *Ss* with normal hearing.

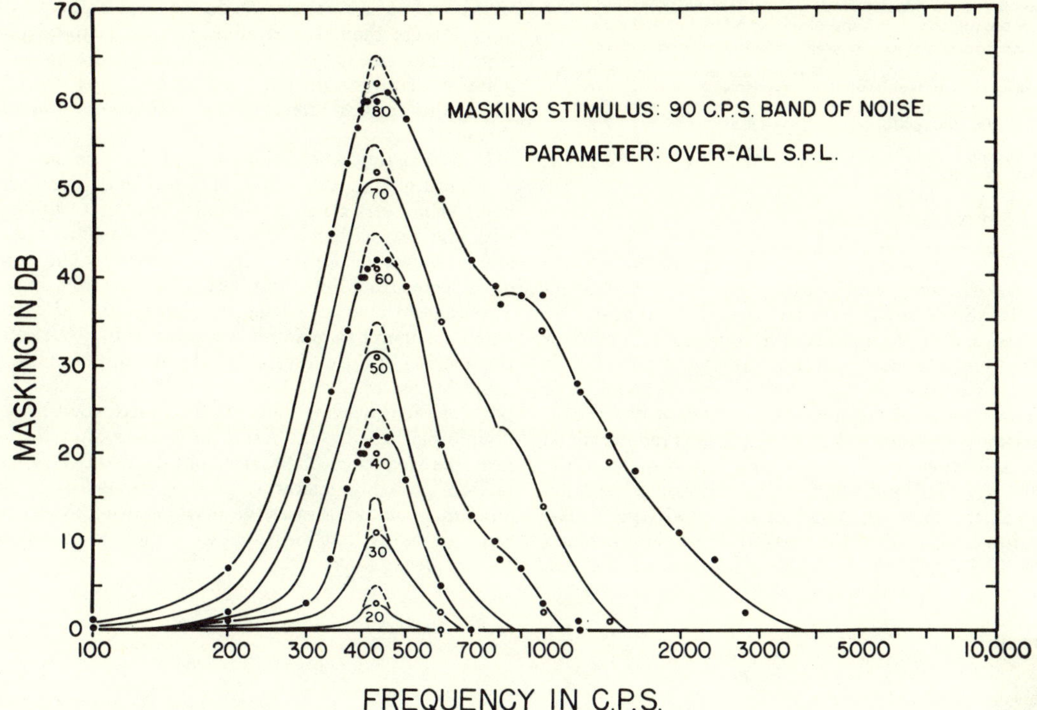

FIG. 8. Masking audiograms of a narrow band of noise (90 c.p.s. wide, centered at 410 c.p.s.) presented at various over-all sound-pressure levels (decibels re 0.0002 dyne/cm²). The pressure spectrum level of the noise may be obtained by subtracting 19.5 db from the corresponding number under the curve. The peak of each masking curve is extended by 4.2 db in order to represent better the amount of excitation near the frequency of the masking stimulus.

The average masking audiogram of a tone of 400 c.p.s. (Fig. 7) was compared with the corresponding data published by Wegel and Lane.[1] With masked stimuli below 400 c.p.s. the agreement is excellent. However, at 450 and 1000 c.p.s. Wegel and Lane found much more masking (by 10–15 db) than that measured in the present experiment. Above 2000 c.p.s. the disagreement is not as marked. Since there are large differences among listeners, it is advisable that the original experiment of Wegel and Lane, which covered such an extensive range of intensities and frequencies of the masking tones, be repeated with several normal ears.

Incidentally, it should be recorded that the value of $\Delta E/E$ obtained with the five *Ss* agrees well with that found by Riesz[6] for the same conditions of measurement. When a pure tone of 400 c.p.s. is the masking stimulus, the values of the masked threshold at 397 and 403 c.p.s. provide one type of measure of the differential threshold for intensity. The value of $\Delta E/E$ found in the present experiment for a 400 c.p.s tone at a sensation level of 65 db is 0.19.

The degree to which a band of noise masks a tone whose frequency is near the center of the band is related to two principal variables: the intensity of the noise and the width of the critical band. If the masking noise is at least as wide as a critical band, then the value of the masked threshold should be given by the following expression: $MT = B + k$, where MT is the masked threshold, B is the intensity/cycle, and k is the width of the critical band. The three values are expressed in decibels with the same reference intensity for MT and B. The maximum value of the average masked threshold for the five *Ss* was 74.5 db (S.P.L.), and the pressure spectrum level of the noise was 60.5 db. In the present experiment the value of k thus turns out to be 14 db. Now, Fletcher[7] as well as Hawkins and Stevens[8] have found that with a wide band of noise k is 17 db at 410 c.p.s., and the difference of 3 db between the values of k found with a narrow and with a wide band of noise is too large to explain away in terms of individual differences or errors of measurement. This difference in the value of k must be attributed to the fact that even with a band of noise,

[6] R. R. Riesz, "Differential intensity sensitivity of the ear for pure tones," Phys. Rev. **31**, 867–875 (1928).

[7] H. Fletcher, "Auditory patterns," Rev. Mod. Phys. **12**, 47–65 (1940).

[8] J. E. Hawkins, Jr. and S. S. Stevens, "The masking of pure tones and of speech by white noise," J. Acous. Soc. Am. **22**, 6–13 (1950).

TABLE I. Standard deviations of masked thresholds of tones heard in the presence of a band of noise centered at 410 c.p.s.

Frequencies of masked tones	*S.D.* of judgments by an average *S*	*S.D.* of means of *Ss*
100, 200, 300, 340	2.9 db	1.2 db
370, 390, 397, 403, 410, 430, 460	1.3	1.8
900, 1000, 1197, 1400, 1597, 2000, 2400	3.6	7.1

the masked tone "beats" with the randomly fluctuating stimulus. Since all subjects reported that the test tone was heard near the masked threshold as a "buzz" or "rattle" it is almost certain that the value of k is underestimated when the masking noise is confined to a narrow band of frequencies. In view of these considerations the value of k at 410 c.p.s. was redetermined using the same five *Ss* and a wider band of noise (0–1000 c.p.s.). This noise had the same pressure spectrum level as the narrower band of noise (90 c.p.s.). The signal-to-noise ratio at the masked threshold was found to be 18.2 db. With the wider band of noise the subjects could not hear the masked tone until it was 4.2 db more intense than that required for the narrow band. It is important to note that with the wider band of noise the subjects do not hear a "buzz" or "rattle" when the masked tone is just above the masked threshold.

It is clear that when masking is used as the measure of excitation the value of k obtained with the wider band of noise is a better estimate than that obtained with the narrow band. Therefore, the masking audiograms shown in Fig. 8 were constructed. The solid circles come from Fig. 2 and the open circles from Fig. 4. The unbroken curves are merely a visual fit to the data with an attempt to maintain a spacing of 10 db between the maxima of the curves. Since the amount of masking near the center of the band of noise is too small, the peak of each masking audiogram was extended by 4.2 db in order to represent better the amount of excitation near the frequency of the masking stimulus. This correction probably makes it possible to interpret the amount of masking near the masking stimulus in the same terms as that measured at distant points along the frequency scale.

22

Reprinted from pages 47-56 of *Rev. Mod. Phys.* **12**:47-65 (1940)

Auditory Patterns*

HARVEY FLETCHER
Bell Telephone Laboratories, New York, New York

DURING the last two decades considerable progress has been made in understanding the hearing processes taking place when we sense a sound. The application of the same instrumentalities that have brought such a wonderful development in the radio and sound pictures to this problem is largely responsible for this progress. Such instrumentalities have made it possible to make accurate measurements which are the basis for understanding any physical process.

To understand this problem then we need to know first how to describe and measure the sound reaching the ears; then we need to know how to describe and measure the sensations of hearing produced by such a sound upon a listener. To do this quantitatively we must also know the degree and kind of hearing ability possessed by the listener. It is with these three phases of the problem that this paper deals.

A pure tone can be defined physically by giving the intensity, the frequency and the phase of vibration at the position where the head of the listener is to be placed. To be precise, this position is taken as the middle of a line connecting the two ears. The measurement of course is made before the head is placed in this listening position. Then the listener faces the source of sound. Any modifications of the sound wave produced by introducing the head to this position are considered as modifications produced by the hearing mechanism. The phase changes are usually unnoticed by the listener, so for most work only the intensity and the frequency are given. A pure tone then is specified by the two coordinates, intensity I and frequency f. In most experimental work on pure tones an endeavor is made to use a free progressive wave or its equivalent, that is, one which is free from reflected waves. Under such circumstances, if I is measured in watts per square centimeter and the corresponding pressure variation in the air wave, expressed in dynes per square centimeter, is p, then I and p are related by the equation[1]

$$I=(p^2/4)\times10^{-8}. \quad (1)$$

The intensity I is usually determined from this equation after making experimental measurements of p. To express the values for all pure tones in the audible range requires a very large range of values of I and p, so a new term called the intensity level and designated by the letter β has been found useful. It is related to I and p by the equation

$$\beta=10 \log (I/I_0)=20 \log (p/p_0), \quad (2)$$

where the values

$$I_0=10^{-16} \text{ watt per square centimeter,}$$
$$p_0=0.0002 \text{ dyne per square centimeter,}$$

have been adopted as international standards. The intensity level is expressed in decibels and varies over a range of only about 130 db when dealing with acoustic problems.

In Fig. 1 is shown a chart on which may be

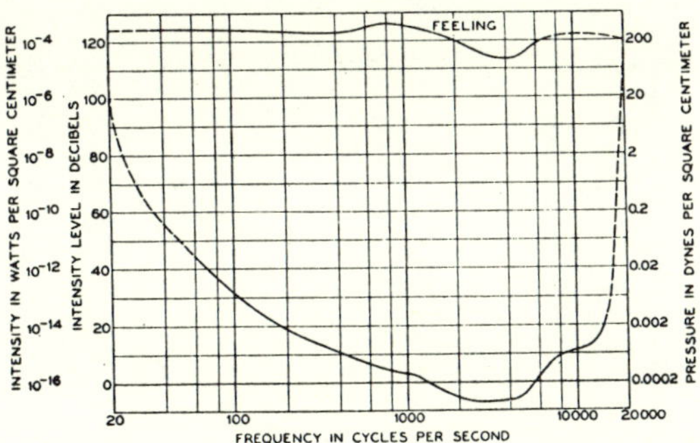

FIG. 1. Auditory area between threshold of feeling and the threshold of hearing.

* From an address given before the joint dinner of the American Physical Society and the American Association of Physics Teachers held in Washington, D. C., on December 28, 1938.

[1] This relation holds exactly for only one temperature and pressure. The variations due to changes in pressure and temperature are small compared to the range in values used in acoustics and for most practical calculations can be neglected.

represented all the pure tones which are audible. It will be noticed that there are three scales for the ordinates and they correspond, respectively, to I, β and p. The values of the frequency f in cycles per second are given by the abscissae. The upper and lower curves enclose the area corresponding to tones which can be sensed as sound. These results are for a young observer having acute hearing. The values of intensity level and pressure are the values obtained in a free air space before the head of the observer is introduced to hear the sound and in a location where the sound waves reflected from walls or other obstacles are negligible. The lower curve gives the faintest sound that such an observer listening with both ears can hear and the upper curve gives the loudest sound that a typical ear can tolerate.

It will be seen from this chart that the pitch range is from 20 cycles per second to 20,000 cycles per second, or a ratio of 1000 to one, and that the intensity range is from 10^{-16} watt per square centimeter to 10^{-4} watt per square centimeter, or a ratio of one thousand billion to one. It will also be seen that the pressure range is from 0.0002 dyne per square centimeter to 200 dynes per square centimeter, or a ratio of one million to one. For a 60-cycle tone, at its maximum tolerable intensity, the amplitude of the air particles is about $\frac{1}{5}$ millimeter. It will be readily seen from these figures that the power necessary to fill a hemisphere 15 meters from a loudspeaker with the maximum sound intensity which can be tolerated by the ear is about 1.5 kilowatts. Of course the electrical power necessary to drive a loudspeaker producing such sounds may be three or four times this value, depending on the efficiency of the loudspeaker. So it is apparent that, although powers involved in sounds are ordinarily very small, still to produce in a large room the loudest sound that the ear can tolerate requires kilowatts of sound power.

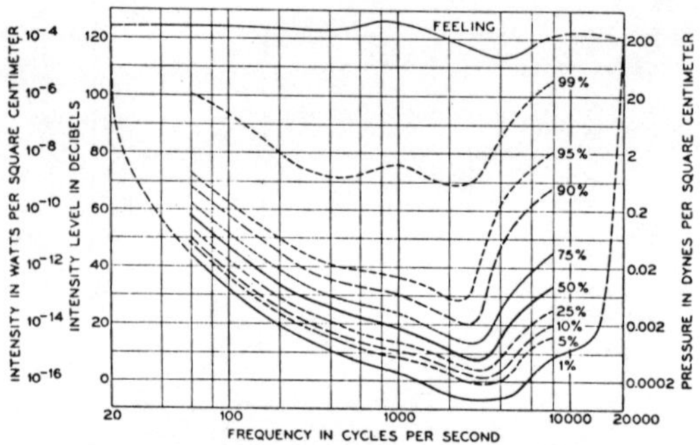

FIG. 2. Auditory areas when hearing is impaired. The curves are indicated by the percent of a typical American group who can hear sounds below the given level.

As stated before, this curve is for an individual having very acute hearing. As a matter of fact about only one in one hundred persons will have as acute hearing as that shown. Recently the Bell Telephone Laboratories cooperated with the U. S. Public Health Service in making a survey of the hearing acuity of a typical American group. The results of this survey have been reported recently by the National Institute of Health in a series of bulletins called the "Hearing Study Series." The results are given in relative intensity levels. Measurements made in our laboratory by Mr. Munson made it possible to reduce these relative levels to absolute intensity levels. From these results the chart shown in Fig. 2 was constructed.

In a general audience, if no noise were present, one percent of the listeners could hear sounds as soft as indicated by the first curve; the next contour line is for 5 percent, and so on for the other curves as indicated. The important curve is the 50 percent curve which is shown by the heavy line. This means that half the people can hear tones at a level as low as indicated by this curve, but the other half must have higher intensities. However, in most auditoriums there is always some background noise. Measurements have shown that in such rooms the threshold values even for acute ears are raised to somewhere near the 50 percent line.

We have thus seen how we can represent a pure tone by a point on the chart such as Fig. 2 by giving the frequency in cycles per second and the intensity level in decibels. Most musical tones have a fundamental and a series of harmonics, so to represent them quantitatively we need to specify the intensity level and frequency for the fundamental and each harmonic. There is a large class of sounds, however, that cannot be specified in such a simple manner. These sounds have components scattered throughout the whole audible range of frequencies. Such sounds are represented physically by giving what is called a spectrogram of the sound. For example, consider a noise like that arising in a busy street. A spectrogram for such a noise is shown in Fig. 3. This spectrogram is determined experi-

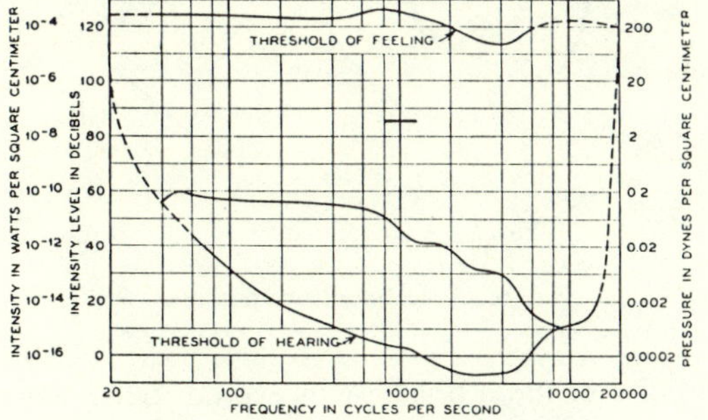

FIG. 3. Spectrogram of street noise.

mentally as follows. The noise is picked up by a microphone, amplified, and then sent through a filter which permits only a small band of frequencies to pass. The sound intensity of this small band is measured and divided by the width of the band in cycles. This result is then reduced to decibels above 10^{-16} watt per square centimeter to obtain the ordinate in our spectrogram. Instruments are available which will read directly the ordinates in such a spectrogram. The total intensity level is given by the solid bar at the 85-db level.

Similarly, it has been found convenient to give a spectrogram for orchestral music. It is true, of course, that such a spectrogram, to be a true representation of the music, would be continually varying. However, when the full orchestra is playing the variations about the spectrogram curve shown in Fig. 4 are only moderate.

Now we will ask ourselves the question, "What is going on in our ears as we sense such sounds?" To understand more clearly what follows it is necessary to give here a brief description of the hearing mechanism.

The main parts of the hearing mechanism are shown in Fig. 5, the inner ear being shown on a very much enlarged scale. As indicated in this diagram, it is usual to divide the mechanism into three parts—the outer ear, the middle ear and the inner ear. The outer ear consists of the external part, or pinna, and the ear canal which leads into the drum. Beyond the drum is the middle ear which contains three small bones called the hammer, the anvil and the stirrup. The stirrup in turn is attached to a little membrane called the oval window which separates the middle ear from the inner ear. The inner ear is filled with a fluid. As illustrated in the diagram the inner ear is composed of two canals separated by a membrane, all of which is wound into the form of a spiral. The nerve endings are scattered along the membrane separating the two canals. Very tiny nerve fibers coming from the main auditory nerve are fanned out so as to reach each of these nerve endings. The arrangement of the nerve fibers is similar to the arrangement of wires in a telephone cable which are fanned out and connected to the jacks in a telephone switchboard. In such a switchboard, used to its full capacity, there are 10,000 jacks and to each one three wires are connected called the tip, ring and sleeve, making a total of 30,000 wire terminals.

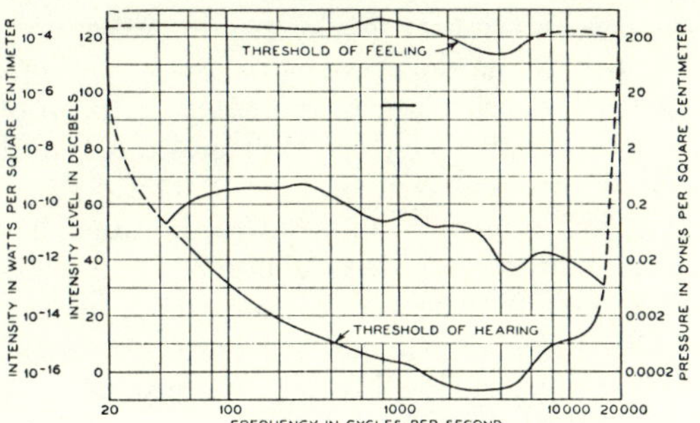

FIG. 4. Spectrogram of orchestral music.

There are approximately this number of nerve terminals along the basilar membrane and nerve fibers leading from them to form a bundle called the auditory nerve. In telephone engineering circles it has been considered a real achievement to have developed a design which permits 30,000 wire terminals to be within the reach of a single operator. The area of such a switchboard panel is about 10,000 square centimeters. Nature has accomplished a similar thing in the hearing mechanizm occupying an area of only $\frac{1}{10}$ of a square centimeter, or only one hundred thousandths of the space in a telephone switchboard. The nerve terminals occupy a space only about $\frac{1}{3}$ millimeter wide and 30 millimeters long. Each one of these tiny nerve endings acts like a telephone transmitter. When they are agitated by the sound waves coming into the inner ear they transmit an electrical current along the nerve fiber. It is these electrical currents which go to the brain and cause the sensation of hearing. The sound wave passes down the ear canal, strikes the drum of the ear at *t*, vibrates the drum, which in turn vibrates the anvil, which in turn vibrates the stirrup. The stirrup then vibrates the oval window which transmits the vibrations to the fluid of the inner ear. This fluid transmits the vibration to the nerve terminals, which in turn converts the vibration into an electrical disturbance which is sent to the brain.

In the following discussion it is not necessary to know the details of this mechanism of hearing. It is important, however, to know that the nerve endings are scattered along a space which is one hundred times as long as it is wide. For this reason we can designate the position of a small group of nerves by a single coordinate. Also, since it is known that this long and narrow membrane containing the nerve endings is wound into a spiral, I have chosen to represent the position of the nerves on such a spiral diagram. A typical form of this is shown in Fig. 6. The distance along this spiral from one end to the other in a typical human cochlea is about 3 centimeters. The numbers along the outside run from zero to 100. In talking about the positions in this cochlear diagram I will refer to these small numbers between zero and 100 as positions of nerve endings, or more briefly as nerve positions. Also for convenience I will speak of a group of nerve endings comprising one percent of the total as a patch of nerves. So the position of each patch is designated by one of the numbers between 0 and 100.

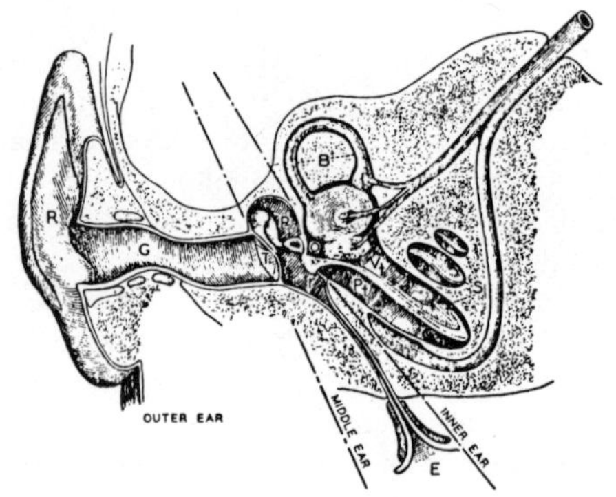

FIG. 5. Semi-diagrammatic section through the right ear (Czermak). *G*—external auditory meatus; *T*—membrana tympani; *P*—tympanic cavity; *o*—fenestra ovalis; *r*—fenestra rotunda; *B*—semi-circular canal; *S*—cochlea; *Vt*—scala vestibuli; *Pt*—scala tympani; *E*—Eustachian tube; *R*—pinna.

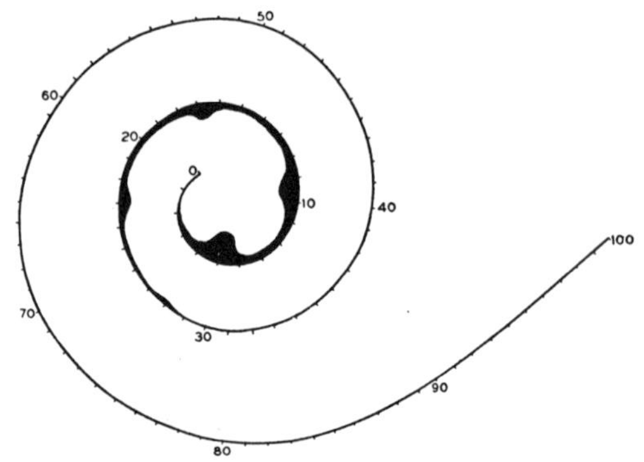

FIG. 6. Typical auditory pattern.

On the chart of Fig. 6 we see a diagram which I will call an auditory pattern. On this spiral diagram representing the cochlea, the height of the dark portion is drawn proportional to the response of the nerves at that position. The pattern shown is that produced in a typical normal ear when a 200-cycle tone is heard at an intensity level of 90 db. The response is measured as the amount of loudness going from each nerve patch at the positions indicated. There is good evidence, although not conclusive, that this loudness is proportional to the number of nerve impulses being sent to the brain per second by each patch of nerves. For example, you see that most of the loudness comes from the region around position 5. However, there is considerable part of the loudness coming from other parts corresponding to the subjective harmonics; for example, at positions $10\frac{1}{2}$, 17, 23 and 28. These subjective harmonics are introduced by the mechanism of hearing. The total loudness corresponds to the total area of the darkened part and this corresponds to the total number of nerve impulses reaching the brain along the auditory nerve.

Later I will discuss methods of deducing such auditory patterns from experimental measurements, but before doing this I wish to present the auditory patterns corresponding to the pure

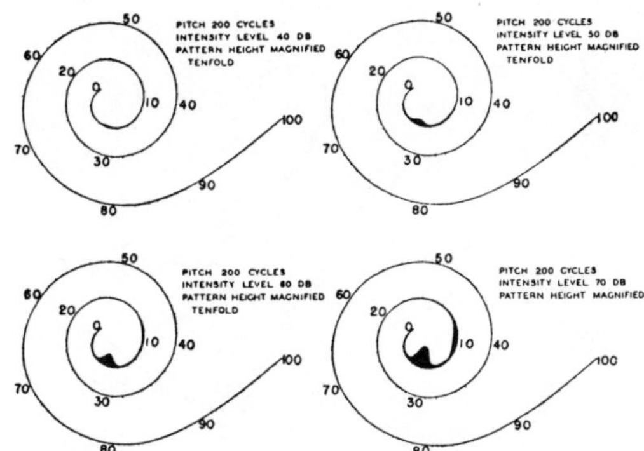

FIG. 7. Auditory patterns for a 200-cycle tone at various intensity levels.

tones. In Figs. 7 and 8 are shown such patterns for a 200-cycle tone at the various intensity levels shown. For intensity levels below 70 decibels the response is confined almost entirely to the positions between 4 and 5. As the intensity level goes above this value it will be seen that more and more subjective harmonics begin to appear until at an intensity level of 110 decibels there is response of the nerves all along the first turn and a half of the cochlea.

In Figs. 9, 10 and 11 are shown the auditory patterns for tones having an intensity level of 90 db but varying in frequency throughout the audible range. It will be seen that the tones of low pitch stimulate the nerves at positions corresponding to low numbers, that is, near the end of the inner spiral called the helicotrema. As the frequency of the tone increases the position of maximum response gradually shifts to positions corresponding to higher and higher numbers. At the same time the position of response due to the harmonics continues to shift as the pitch increases.

How do we know that these auditory patterns correspond to what is taking place in our ears? To determine these patterns we need to know the amount of response as represented by the breadth of the dark portion in the auditory pattern and the position along the spiral where the response is occurring, that is, the nerve position. The fundamental data from which such patterns are drawn are obtained from the masking effect of such sounds. For example, in Fig. 12 are shown such data on the masking produced by pure tones. At the top of this figure is shown the masking produced by a 200-cycle tone. The ordinates give the masking or the number of decibels that the intensity level of a tone having the frequency shown by the abscissa must be raised above its quiet threshold in order to be heard in the presence of this 200-cycle sound. The peaks[2] at 400, 600, 800, 1000 are due to the subjective harmonics. For example, consider the point at 700. The masking here is seen to be 22, which means that a tone of 700 cycles must be raised 22 db above its quiet threshold to be heard in the presence of a 200-cycle tone. Such a curve showing the masking at each frequency is called a noise audiogram.

In the lower part of this figure the masking for several tones of different frequency is given. Only that part near the fundamental is shown. For the sake of clearness the peaks due to the harmonics are omitted. I wish to call attention particularly

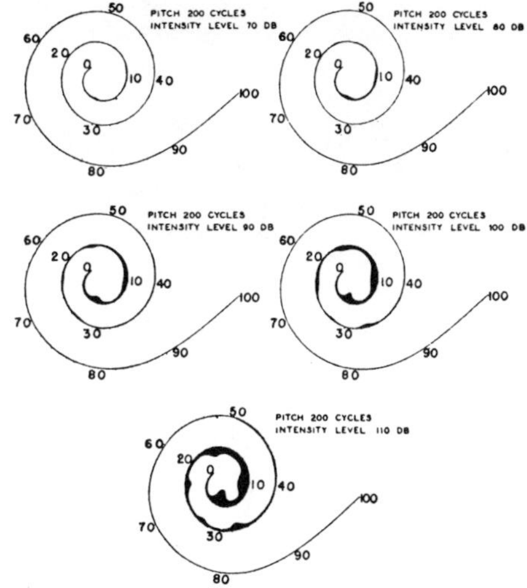

FIG. 8. Auditory patterns for a 200-cycle tone at various intensity levels.

[2] There is an uncertainty of 4 or 5 db in determining these peak values, which is not due to observational error but due to interpretation. When testing the masking at frequencies near the fundamental or any of its subjective harmonics, then beats occur. This new phenomenon makes it much easier to detect the masked tone. The points given are for most distinct beats rather than where the beats just become audible. The points should be somewhere between the best beat and minimum audible beat point. To enter into the discussion here of the best point to take would tend to confuse the main argument of the paper. Changes due to such uncertainty would not change the general shape of the auditory patterns but only alter somewhat the sharpness of the peak.

to the fact that the breadth of these masking curves increases rapidly as the frequency of the tone doing the masking goes above 1000 cycles. Of course this must be related to how the ear mechanism analyzes the sound. The bars at the top of these curves are the minimum frequency band widths of thermal noise for masking these tones and will be discussed later.

In Fig. 13 is shown the masking effect of a noise whose importance will become evident as

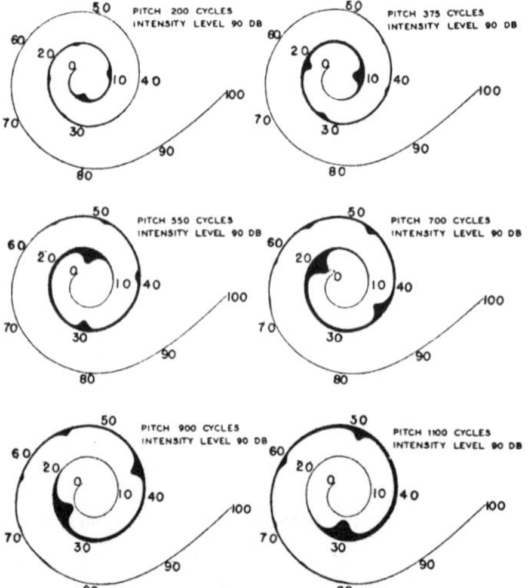

FIG. 9. Auditory patterns at 90 db for various frequencies.

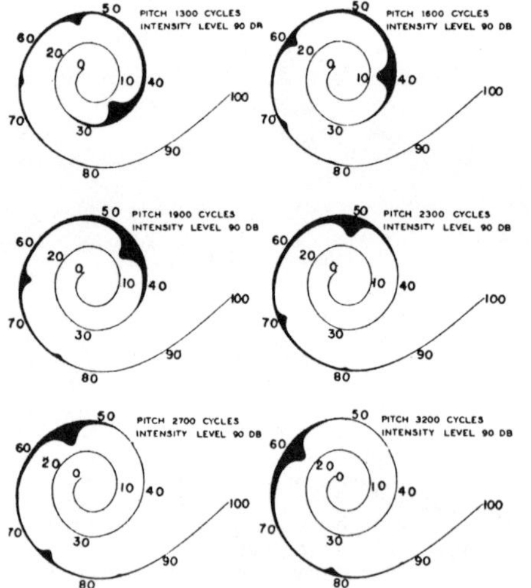

FIG. 10. Auditory patterns at 90 db for various frequencies.

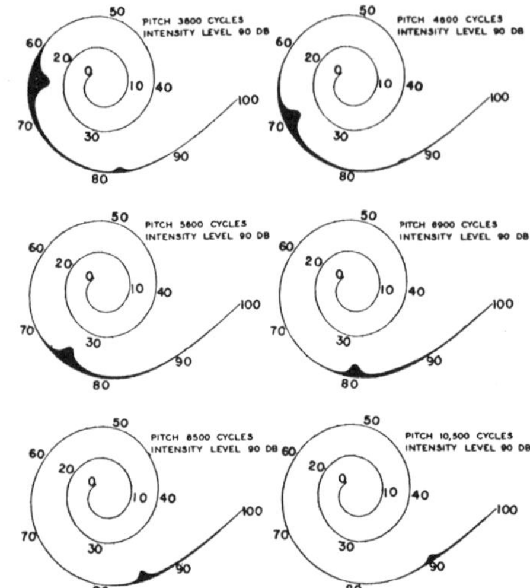

FIG. 11. Auditory patterns at 90 db for various frequencies.

the discussion proceeds. The curve at the bottom of the crosshatched area is the threshold of hearing curve for a quiet place and is taken from Fig. 1. The curve at the top of the hatched area is the spectrogram for this noise. If I_f is the intensity per cycle of the noise for the frequency region f, then the ordinate for this spectrogram curve is given by

$$y = 10 \log (I_f/I_0) \tag{3}$$

and the total sound intensity I of the noise is given by

$$I = \int_0^\infty I_f df = I_0 \int_{20}^{20,000} 10^{(y/10)} df \tag{4}$$

and the intensity level β by

$$\beta = 10 \log \frac{I}{I_0} = \left[10 \log \int_{20}^{20,000} 10^{(y/10)} df \right]. \tag{5}$$

This value calculated from the spectrogram is shown by the solid bar placed across the 1000-cycle ordinate.

The solid dots show the intensity levels of pure tones which are just masked by this noise. The number of decibels these dots are above the threshold curve gives the masking. It will be seen that this is the same for each dot and is equal to 50 db. In other words, the masking for

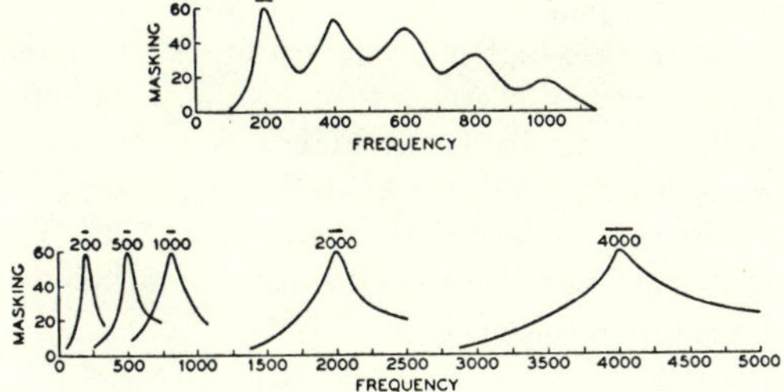

Fig. 12. Noise audiograms of pure tones.

this particular kind of noise is the same for all pure tones. The masking audiogram will then be very simple, that is, a straight line at 50 db for all frequencies.

If we assume that constant masking indicates constant stimulation along the different patches of nerves, then it is evident that the auditory pattern corresponding to this noise giving constant masking for all frequencies is similar to that shown in Fig. 14. It is because such a noise produces a simple pattern that it becomes very important in our discussion.

It is from masking curves like those shown in Fig. 12 and the constancy of the masking by auditory nerves that the auditory patterns can be drawn. To do this we must know how the masking in decibels, that is the ordinate in these audiograms, is related to loudness per patch of nerves, and also how the frequency, that is the abscissae of these audiograms, is related to the nerve position.

First let us consider the data which enable us to determine the relation between the frequency

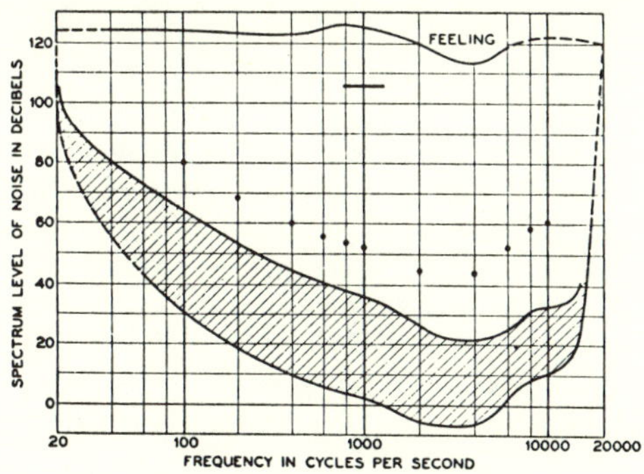

Fig. 13. Masking effect of a noise.

of the sound and the position of maximum stimulation in the cochlea. The nerve position will be designated by the coordinate x (see Fig. 6) going from 0 to 100, and the frequency of the sound will be designated by f. Our problem then is to find the relation between x and f. There are three experiments dealing with quite different phases of audition which give us data from which this relation can be calculated. The first set of data is obtained from experiments on the minimum perceptible differences in pitch. In these experiments the frequency of the tone is varied until the observer perceives a change in pitch. The technique of doing such experiments is

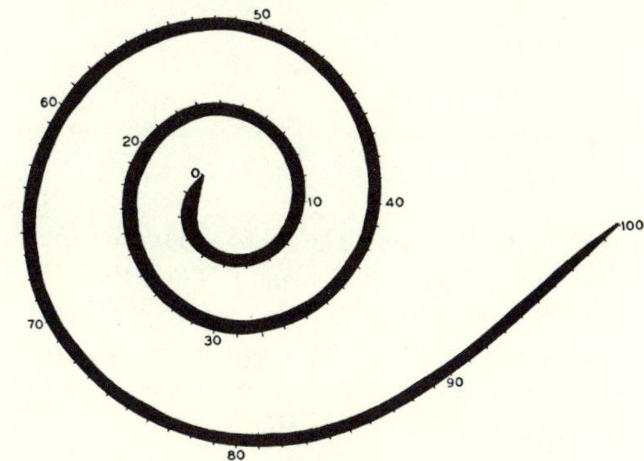

Fig. 14. Auditory pattern stimulation uniform at all frequencies.

described elsewhere.[3] The results obtained by Shower and Biddulph are given in Fig. 15. The ordinate gives the value of the cycles change for a tone to be just audible and the abscissa gives the frequency of the tone. As you will notice, tones whose frequencies are below 1000 cycles require about the same number of cycles for a minimum perceptible change, namely, between 2 and 3 cycles change, while for higher frequencies the fractional rather than the actual increase of frequency is constant and equal to about 0.3 percent. From these data we can derive the desired relation[4] between x and f as follows. It was seen that the position of maximum stimulation shifted as the frequency changed. It seems reasonable to assume that the amount of this shift for a minimum perceptible change in fre-

[3] Shower and Biddulph, J. Acous. Soc. **3**, 275 (1931).

[4] This relation was first derived by Wegel and Lane of the Bell Telephone Laboratories in 1924.

quency is the same for all positions. Therefore if Δx is this shift, then

$$\Delta x=(dx/df)\Delta f=A \tag{6}$$

where A is a constant for all frequencies. With the scale we have chosen it is the percent of the total nerve endings passed over to make the change noticeable. Then

$$x=A\int_0^f \frac{1}{\Delta f}df. \tag{7}$$

The condition $x=100$ when $f=\infty$ determines the constant A, or

$$x=100\frac{\int_0^f \frac{1}{\Delta f}df}{\int_0^\infty \frac{1}{\Delta f}df}. \tag{8}$$

From the curve of Fig. 15 the constant A is determined as 0.08 percent corresponding to about 20 nerve endings.

A second set of data for obtaining this relation is obtained by finding the ratio of the intensity per cycle of the noise to the intensity of the pure tone which is just masked by the noise. If we return again to Fig. 13 it will be noticed that in the region below 1000 cycles the distances between the dots and the spectrogram curve for the noise are about the same and equal to 15 db. In

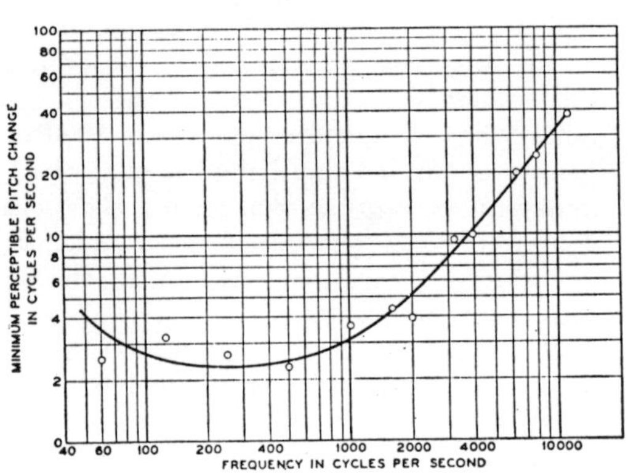

FIG. 15. Minimum perceptible pitch change.

regions above 1000 cycles, however, the distance becomes greater and greater until at 8000 cycles it is 28 db. Now why is this? It is because the frequency positions in the ear are crowded together in this higher pitch region. A wider band of frequencies is going to each patch of nerves corresponding to these higher frequencies and consequently produces a relatively greater stimulation, and consequently greater masking. These ideas can be formulated into a mathematical equation as follows:

Let

ΔI = sound intensity of noise in band between f and $f+\Delta f$;

$I_f=(\Delta I/\Delta f)$ = intensity per cycle of noise at frequency f;

ΔJ = agitating power due to noise on cochlear nerve endings between x and $x+\Delta x$;

$J_x=(\Delta J/\Delta x)$ = agitating power due to noise upon one percent of nerves at position x. It may be called agitation density;

I_m = sound intensity of tone of frequency f which is just perceptible in presence of noise;

J_m = total agitating power on nerve endings at position x by this tone which is masked.

Then if the transmission system is linear $(\Delta I/I_m)=(\Delta J/J_m)$ or, substituting values for ΔI and ΔJ, we have

$$\Delta x=(I_f/I_m)(J_m/J_x)\Delta f. \tag{9}$$

We will now make the following assumption[5]

$$J_m/J_x=C, \tag{10}$$

where C is a constant independent of x and determined by condition $x=0$ when $f=\infty$. Therefore

$$x=C\int_0^f \frac{I_f}{I_m}df \quad \text{and} \quad C=\frac{100}{\int_0^\infty \frac{I_f}{I_m}df}. \tag{11}$$

If we compare the relation given by Eq. (11) to that given by Eq. (8) we must conclude that, since these express the same relation between x and f, the two integrands must be proportional, or

$$\Delta f=k(I_m/I_f), \tag{12}$$

where k is a constant which has been found by experiment to be equal to 20 when dealing with thermal noise.

[5] For a more complete derivation of these relations see Proc. Nat. Acad. Sci. 24, 265–274 (1938).

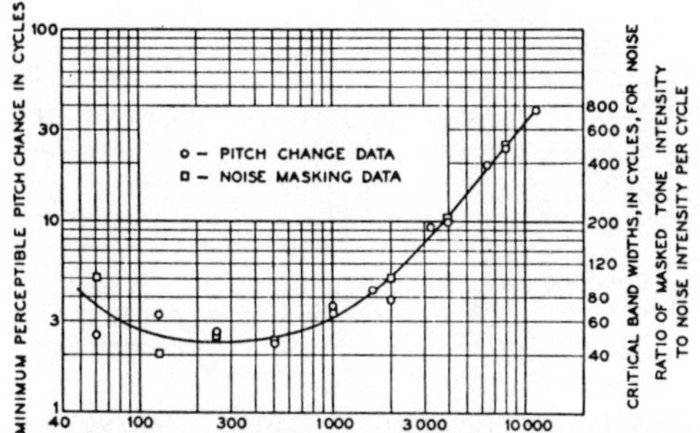

FIG. 16. Plot showing that the minimum perceptible pitch change is proportional to the ratio of the intensity of a tone having the same frequency to the intensity per cycle of the noise which just masks this tone.

In other words, this analysis predicts that the minimum perceptible change in cycles for a tone of any frequency is equal to a constant times the ratio of the intensity of a tone having the same frequency to the intensity per cycle of the noise which just masks this tone. These two sets of experimental data are plotted in Fig. 16 and it will be seen that they do determine the same curve. The masking data were taken from the average of a large number of observations similar to those shown in Fig. 13. If K is the difference in decibels between the dots and the spectrogram curve in this figure, then K is related to I_f/I_m as follows:

$$K = 10 \log (I_m/I_0) - 10 \log (I_f/I_0) \qquad (13)$$

or

$$I_m/I_f = 10^{(K/10)}. \qquad (14)$$

In obtaining these data the question which led to the third type of experiment arose. It is: how does the ratio I_m/I_f vary as the width of the noise band in the neighborhood of the frequency of the masked tone becomes smaller and smaller. It would be expected that when this width became smaller than a certain limiting value, then all of the acoustical intensity could be considered as acting upon the same nerve endings as those stimulated by the tone being masked. Consequently, for band widths smaller than this limiting value, this ratio I_m/I_f becomes smaller and smaller as the band width becomes smaller and smaller. In fact it would be expected that for these smaller band widths the ratio of the intensity of the masked tone to the total intensity of the noise in the small band would be a constant independent of both the band width and the frequency region in which it is placed. Consequently, for these small band widths the ratio I_m/I_f will be proportional to the width of the band. For all values of band widths larger than this critical one this ratio will remain constant.

Experimental tests were made to verify these relations. I will not take the time to describe the apparatus and methods[6] for making this kind of experiment, but will be content however to show the final results, which are given in Fig. 17.

The abscissae give the width of the noise band and the ordinates the ratio of the intensity of the masked tone to the intensity per cycle of the noise. The variable parameter which identifies the different curves is the frequency of the masked tone, which is also the frequency region of the band of noise. It is evident from the results for the 30-cycle band of noise that this ratio is the same for all frequencies and is approximately equal to 30. This result makes the relations very simple. For these smaller bands and for this type of statistical noise, the intensity of the masked tone must be adjusted to be equal to the average intensity of the noise in the band in order for it to be perceived. It will be seen that as the band widths increase, this ratio also increases until the critical band widths are reached, which are indicated by the intersection of the horizontal lines with the 45-degree line.

For example, consider the case for the 2000-cycle tone being masked by variously sized bands

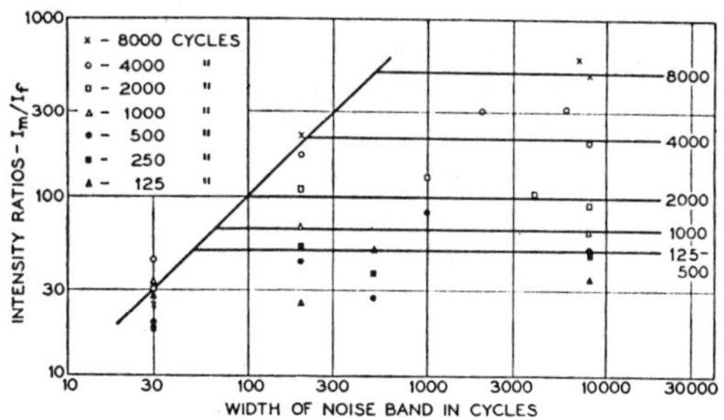

FIG. 17. Ratio of the intensity of the mask tone to the intensity per cycle of the noise plotted against the width of the noise band in cycles. The critical band width in cycles is numerically equal to the ratio of the intensity of the tone masked to the intensity per cycle of the noise producing masking and always corresponds to ½ mm of length on the basilar membrane.

[6] This work will be presented in a future paper.

of noise, indicated by the squares on Fig. 17. It will be seen that the ratio increased until the band width of 100 cycles is reached. Increasing the width beyond this value does not affect the ratio. In other words, increasing the band width[7] beyond 100 cycles does not change the masking at all for hearing the 2000-cycle tone. The horizontal lines were determined from measurements on wide bands of thermal noise and are the same values as were given in Fig. 16. Since their intersection of the 45-degree line determines the critical values of band widths, this very important relation follows:

For this type of noise the critical band width in cycles is numerically equal to the ratio of the intensity of the tone masked to the average intensity per cycle of the noise producing the masking. Regardless of where the band is located, we will see later that these critical widths always correspond to a single element of length on the basilar membrane, namely $\frac{1}{2}$ mm. So we can return again to Fig. 16. The single curve shown can now be given three different interpretations: first, the ordinates can be interpreted as giving the cycles change necessary to produce a perceptible change of pitch; second, when the ordinates are multiplied by 20 they will then give the critical band widths; third, when the ordinates are multiplied by 20 they will give the ratio of the intensity of the masked tone to the intensity per cycle at the frequency of the masked tone of a statistical noise doing the masking. For these reasons we have considerable confidence in the validity of the shape of this curve.

By means of this curve then and either of the formulae developed above, the relationship between x and f can be obtained and is shown in Fig. 18A on a rectangular plot and in Fig. 18B on a spiral diagram. This relation enables us to find the position of maximum stimulation produced by sounds whose power is confined in the region near the frequency f.

Next we will inquire as to what kind of data is used to determine the height of these stimulation patterns. It will be remembered that the height of these auditory patterns is proportional to the loudness being sent to the brain by 1 percent of

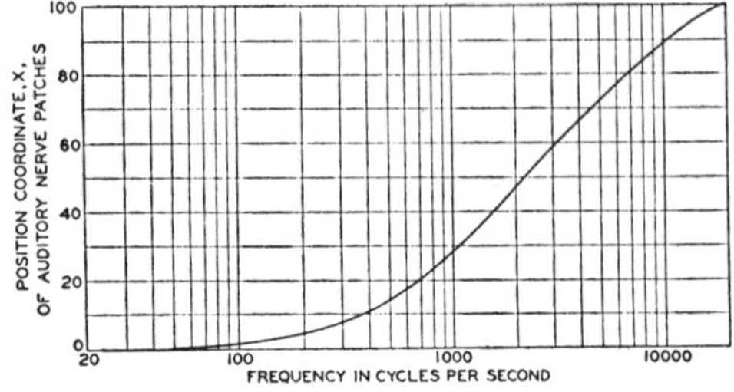

FIG. 18A. Position coordinate X of auditory nerve patches for various frequencies.

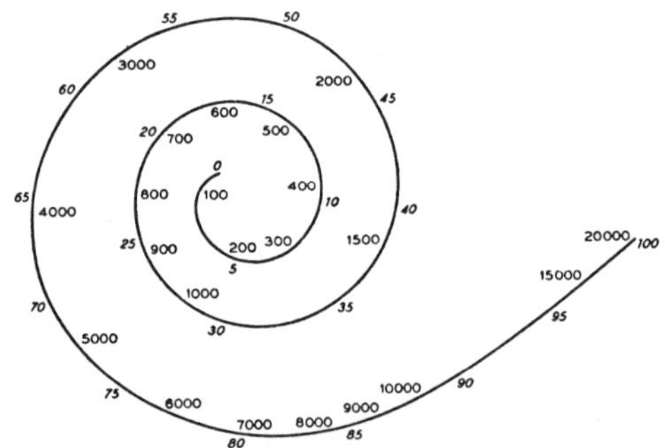

FIG. 18B. Position in the cochlea for maximum response to pure tones.

the nerves at each position. If this is true, then of course the area[8] under the auditory pattern curve will give the total loudness. In order for this to have any meaning we must have a quantitative scale of loudness.

[*Editor's Note:* Material has been omitted at this point.]

[7] It is realized that these critical band widths are not accurately determined from these data. They may be wrong by a factor of 2, but that the bands are the right order there is no question.

[8] For this to be strictly true the patterns should be plotted in rectangular coordinates.

23

Reprinted from *Acoust. Soc. Am. J.* **29**:548-557 (1957)

Critical Band Width in Loudness Summation*

E. Zwicker,† G. Flottorp,‡ and S. S. Stevens
Psycho-Acoustic Laboratory, Harvard University, Cambridge, Massachusetts

(Received February 20, 1957)

THIS paper concerns two problems: how the loudness of a group of tones depends on the spacing of the tones in the complex, and how the loudness of a band of noise of constant sound pressure level depends on the width of the band. Previous experiments by Zwicker and Feldtkeller[1] and by Bauch[2] suggest that an increase in spacing, or in band width, has little or no effect on loudness until a critical band width is reached, after which the loudness increases. In German publications this critical band has been called a *"Frequenzgruppe."* The evidence presented below confirms these findings and suggests, furthermore, that the critical band width observed in loudness summation is consistent with the critical band widths derived from observations on other parameters such as thresholds, masking, and phase relations.[3] These will be discussed in later sections, and the relation of the critical band to other functions will be noted.

Because of the sequence in which our experiments were run, a word needs to be said about the roles of the contributors to these studies. The experiments with pure tones were begun by Stevens early in 1956, with the assistance of Bertram Scharf. During the summer of 1956 Flottorp joined the staff of the laboratory and carried out the major portion of the studies with pure tones, particularly those concerned with the loudness of a four-tone complex. After Flottorp returned to Norway, Zwicker came to the laboratory and carried out the experiments involving the loudness of bands of noise. Since the final draft was prepared by Stevens, and since circumstances made it impossible for all the authors to check on the separate phases of the research, it may or may not be true that all contributors to the enterprise will find themselves agreed on all points.

GENERAL PROCEDURE

In all these experiments the signals were presented binaurally through a pair of PDR-10 earphones (calibrated on a 6-cc coupler) which were mounted in sponge Neoprene cushions MX-41/AR. The subject, seated in an anechoic chamber, adjusted the level of a comparison signal to match the loudness of a standard signal. He did this by turning the knob on a "sone potentiometer," which consisted of two 2000-ohm potentiometers ganged and cascaded. The knob was on the end of a shaft that projected from the control room through the wall into the anechoic chamber. The subjects were instructed to approach their final adjustment by "bracketing," i.e., by setting the comparison signal alternately too high and too low before settling on a final setting.

An electronic switch, keyed by a motor-driven timer, presented the two signals alternately. Each signal lasted about 1 sec and was separated from the next signal by a silent interval of about 0.5 sec.

Figure 1 shows the block diagram for both the experiments with tones and the experiments with noises. The part of the diagram on the right applies to both tones and noises, the upper left-hand section concerns the measurements with noises, the lower left-hand section concerns the measurements with tones. Note that both the standard and the comparison noises were obtained from the same noise generator, and that the only amplification used was common to both channels.

LOUDNESS *VS* TONAL SEPARATION

The major part of the experiment with pure tones involved a complex of four equally intense components supplied by four oscillators (tuned plate circuit).[4] The principal advantage of these oscillators is their stability and the fact that the oscillation of each can be stopped or started by controlling the grid bias. This permits us

* This research was carried out under Contract Nonr-1866(15) between Harvard University and the Office of Naval Research, U. S. Navy (Project Nr142-201, Report PNR-192).

† Dr. Zwicker is at the Institut für Nachrichtentechnik der Technischen Hochschule, Stuttgart.

‡ Dr. Flottorp is at the Audiological Institute, Rikshospitalet, Oslo, Norway.

[1] E. Zwicker and R. Feldtkeller, "Ueber die Lautstärke von gleichformigen Geräuschen," Acustica **5**, 303-316 (1955).

[2] H. Bauch, "Die Bedeutung der Frequenzgruppe für die Lautheit von Klangen," Acustica **6**, 40-45 (1956).

[3] R. Feldtkeller and E. Zwicker, *Das Ohr als Nachrichtenempfänger* (S. Hirzel Verlag, Stuttgart, 1956).

[4] S. S. Stevens and R. Gerbrands, "A twin-oscillator for auditory research," Am. J. Psychol. **49**, 113-115 (1937).

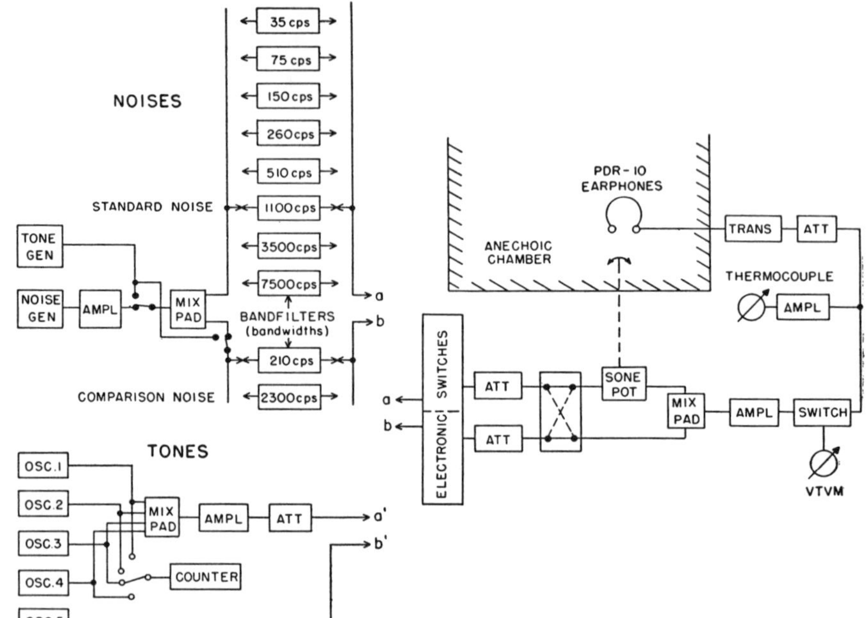

FIG. 1. Block diagram of the apparatus.

to measure the frequency (with a Hewlett-Packard Counter, 522B) as well as the amplitude of each tone without altering the external circuits of the apparatus.

When a subject had adjusted the level of the complex to match the loudness of a single pure tone, the adjusted level was determined by measuring one component in the complex. This gave a steady reading on the voltmeter. Then the median sound-pressure level of the multitone complex was later determined with the aid of a thermocouple. The loudness match made by adjusting the complex was usually complemented by the reverse procedure in which the complex was set at a fixed level and the subjects adjusted the level of a single pure tone to match the loudness of the complex.

The number of subjects who made each match varied from 6 to 22. In general, fewer subjects were used for the easier matches, for which the variability was small, and larger numbers of subjects were used when the variability was large or when an attempt was being made to test effects of spacings that produce only small differences. In all cases the median of the loudness matches was taken as the final measure.

Figure 2 shows the effect on loudness produced by changing the over-all spacing, ΔF, of four tones centered around the frequencies, 500, 1000, and 2000 cps. By over-all spacing is meant the frequency difference between the highest and the lowest tone. The symbols T and C represent the medians obtained under the two procedures: T=single tone adjusted (either 500, 1000, or 2000 cps) and C=complex adjusted. As is usual in loudness balances, the final match depends on which stimulus is adjusted. At the level employed here (57.5 db SPL) the stimulus that is adjusted is set high relative to the match determined when the other stimulus is adjusted. It has been shown elsewhere that at high stimulus levels this constant "error" may reverse its direction.[5] The lines through the data in Fig. 2 are drawn in order to show how well the results agree with the hypothesis that within a critical band the loudness is independent of the spacing of the tones, and that, when the over-all spacing ΔF exceeds a critical value, the loudness increases. The position of the discontinuity, where the two segments of the lines form an angle, was determined independently of these particular data. The values of ΔF predicted for the discontinuities in Fig. 2, and in similar graphs, were derived from measurements of the critical band width in other types of experiments discussed below (see Fig. 12). In this sense the lines in Fig. 2 are predicted values. Although the points do not fit perfectly, it seems clear that their general behavior is in line with the hypothesis.

The points in Fig. 2, represented by the inverted T and C (1000 cps), represent the results of a check experiment run on 12 observers. It was noted that the other points in the vicinity of ΔF values from 50 to 100 cps fall below the horizontal line representing a constant sound pressure level. Since most of the other results (see Fig. 3) suggest that for these values of ΔF the loudness is determined by the sound pressure level, the problem is whether the departure of some of these

[5] S. S. Stevens, "Calculation of the loudness of complex noise," J. Acoust. Soc. Am. 28, 807–832 (1956).

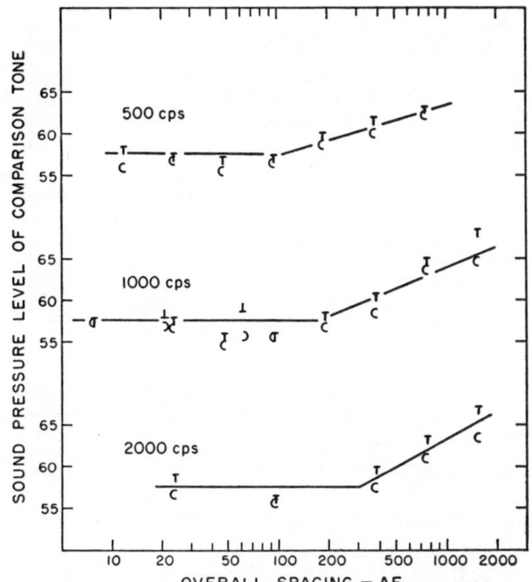

FIG. 2. Dependence of loudness on the spacing of the components in a four-tone complex. The four tones were spaced approximately uniformly in frequency about the center frequency indicated. Loudness balances between the center frequency and the complex were made by groups of from 16 to 22 subjects. *T* means the tone was adjusted and *C* means the complex was adjusted. The lines through the data have a break at the point predicted by the critical-band hypothesis.

points represents a real effect or whether it may be due to experimental variability. Since the inverted points lie more nearly where we would expect them to lie, it seems reasonable to conclude that the other points are probably less representative. In other words, we are not forced to reject the hypothesis that for components lying within a critical band the loudness is determined by the effective sound pressure level.

Figure 3 shows how the loudness of a group of four tones varies with spacing and with sound pressure level. The center frequency was 1000 cps. Here we see that the discontinuity representing the critical band width occurs at the same value of ΔF regardless of the sound pressure level. Another feature that seems evident in Fig. 3 is that the increase in loudness level, as ΔF is made greater than a critical band, is greatest for the medium levels. At the lowest level tested (SPL=17.5 db) there is no apparent increase in loudness level as ΔF increases.

The apparent *decrease* in loudness level at the largest value of ΔF (1536 cps) may have been due to the fact that at this wide spacing some of the individual tones fell below the threshold of some of the subjects. But there is also evidence that some subjects, according to their own statements, feel that they change their criterion for judging loudness when the tones are faint and widely separated. Instead of "integrating" the loudnesses of the components, these subjects feel that they tend to judge the total loudness to be equal to that of a single component in the complex. In other words, it may be that for low levels and wide spacings the "loudness integration," whatever that is, tends to break down. A similar effect was observed in an experiment[5] in which the observer tried to match the loudness of a pair of octave bands of noise widely separated in frequency—a low rumble and a high hiss. It was apparently impossible for at least some subjects to "integrate" the loudnesses of these two disparate sounds.

The data for the lowest level in Fig. 3 suggest an interesting possibility. If the tones in a complex are sufficiently faint, it may be that when their spacing is made greater than a critical band the loudness tends to decrease instead of increase. A corollary of this would be the possibility that at some level (in the vicinity of 20 phons?) the loudness of a complex is independent of the spacing of the components. This problem of the summation of loudness at very low levels needs further exploration.

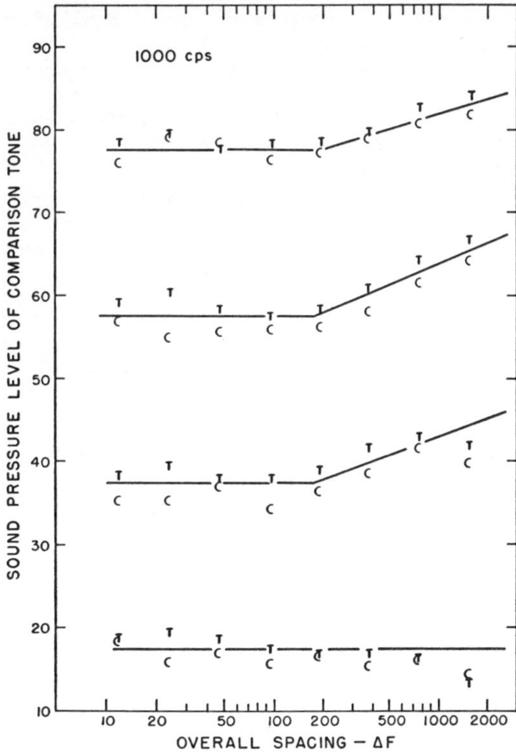

FIG. 3. Dependence of loudness on spacing and level. The critical band width is approximately invariant with level, although little or no loudness summation occurs at levels near threshold. Each point represents the median of two judgments by each of ten listeners. In each experimental session the spacing was kept constant and the levels were tested in irregular order.

Another point should be noted. When the tonal components are so close together that slow beats occur, we would expect the loudness to be judged more in terms of the maximum amplitude of the beat envelope. We did not try to pursue this question, but an effect of this sort is evident in Bauch's results.

EFFECT OF LEVEL

The dependence of loudness summation on level can be seen more clearly in Fig. 4, where some of the data of Fig. 3 are plotted in a different manner. The points represent the average of the T and C values from Fig. 3. The solid points show that when the components lie within a critical band the loudness of the complex is the same as the loudness of a 1000-cy tone having the same sound pressure level as the complex. The unfilled points are for values of ΔF greater than a critical band. The fact that the curves through these points pass through a maximum suggests that loudness summation is greatest for loudness levels in the vicinity of 50 to 60 phons. It will be noted that two of the points do not lie near the curve for the widest spacing (1536 cps). As indicated above, we are not certain of the reason for this discrepancy, although it may well be a real effect rather than an error of measurement.

The crosses in Fig. 4 are from another study[5] and are reproduced for purposes of comparison. These values represent the relative loudness level of a 1000-cy tone interrupted at the rate of 130 per sec. Modulation of this sort turns the single pure tone into a complex consisting of a central frequency (1000 cps) and a group of side bands, and we see that as a function of level the loudness of this complex behaves much like the loudness of a complex of four equally intense tones.

Another set of data, obtained in some of the tests run by Scharf, is shown in Fig. 5, where the loudness level of the complex is plotted as a function of the loudness level of one of the single components of the complex. These results are consistent with those shown in Fig. 4, in that

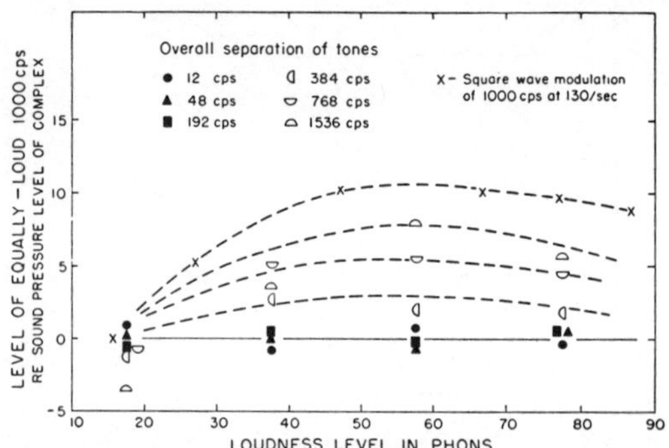

FIG. 4. Relative loudness levels of different complexes as a function of level and spacing. All but the crosses represent data from Fig. 3. The crosses show the relative loudness level of a 1000-cy tone interrupted at a rate of 130 per sec.

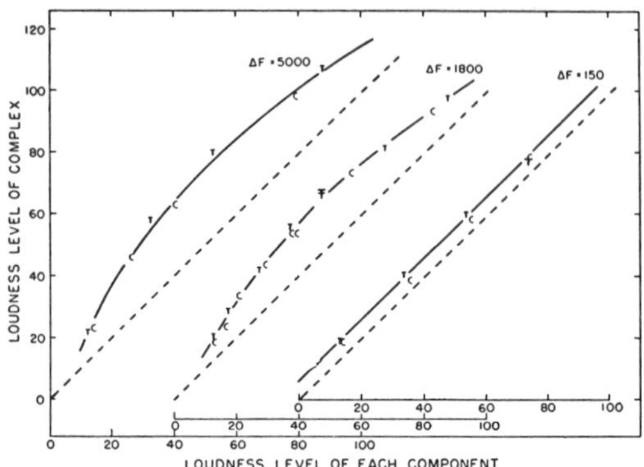

FIG. 5. Loudness levels of various complexes as a function of the level of a single component. The two curves on the left represent complexes of five equally intense tones. The curve on the right is for four tones. The center frequencies of the complexes were 1800, 1250, and 1000 cps for the three curves (from left to right).

loudness summation is greatest at medium levels. The curve at the right is for a group of four tones lying within a critical band ($\Delta F = 150$ cps). Here the loudness level of the complex is proportional to the loudness level of the single component. The other two curves represent complexes of five tones at spacings greater than the critical band width. As we should expect, the loudness level of the complex exceeds that of a single component by a greater amount when the spacing of the components is greater.

EFFECT OF IRREGULAR SPACING

The next question concerns the dependence of loudness on the relative spacing of the tones when the overall spacing ΔF is kept constant. For a given ΔF, does it make any difference how the intermediate tones are spaced in frequency? The answer appears to be that it does, and that uniform spacing produces greater loudness than nonuniform spacing.

Three different experiments were run in which loudness balances were made between a single tone (500, 1000, and 2000 cps) and four-tone complexes in which the relative spacings were as shown in Fig. 6. Groups of 18 to 22 subjects made one balance by adjusting the single tone and one by adjusting the complex. The combined results, giving the sound pressure level of the single tone that matches the loudness of the complex, are listed in Fig. 6.

We see that in each instance the loudness is greatest when the spacing of the tones in the complex is uniform in frequency. Although we did not test the question, there is reason to believe that if the spacing were made proportional to critical band width, which would make the separations approximately equal in mels, the loudness would be slightly greater still. Figure 6 shows also that the more uneven the spacing, the lower the loudness. There is some tendency for the loudness to be

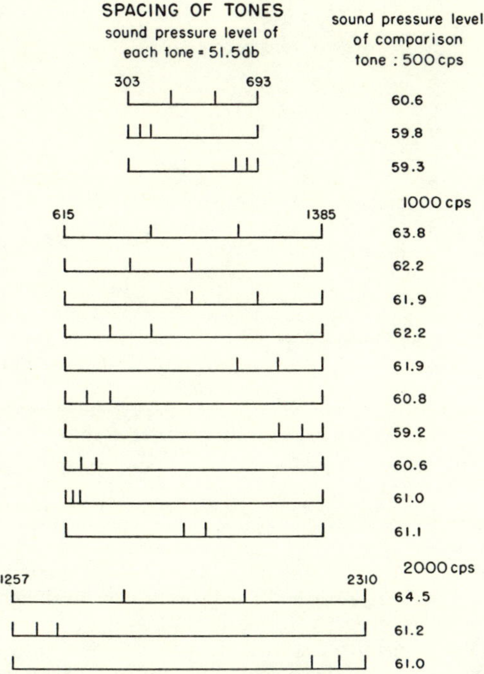

FIG. 6. Loudness as a function of the relative spacing among the four tones in a complex. Three different over-all spacings ΔF were used as indicated. Within a given ΔF the tones were spaced evenly or were bunched in one frequency region or another. The sound pressure level of the tone (center frequency) that was matched in loudness to the complex is listed beside each diagram showing the relative spacings.

slightly greater when the tones are bunched at the low end of the interval than when they are bunched at the high end.

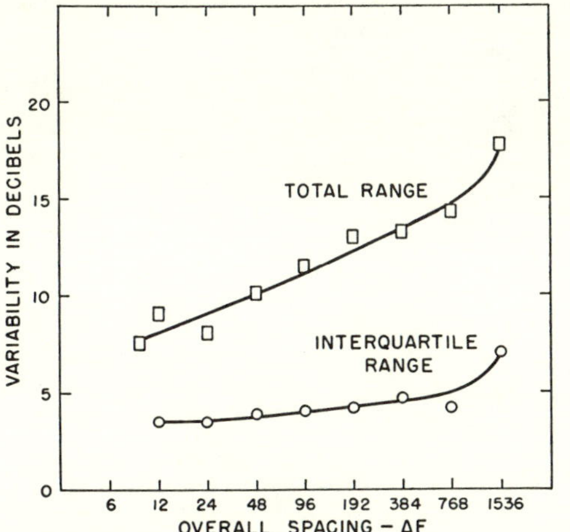

FIG. 7. Showing how the total range and the interquartile range of the loudness balance varies with the over-all spacing of the tones in a complex.

VARIABILITY

When two sounds differ in quality, the matching of their loudnesses is difficult and subject to considerable variability. In general, the variability increases as the difference between the characters of the two sounds increases. Thus when a single tone is matched to a complex, variability increases as the spacing of the tones in the complex is made wider. Evidence for this fact is shown in Fig. 7.

Variability also changes with level. Although there were no significant differences among the three highest levels tested (Fig. 3), the variability was less at the lowest level (17.5 db). On the other hand, for the results shown in Fig. 6 there seemed to be no significant difference in variability for the different spacings of the tones within a constant ΔF.

When the subjects adjusted the complex to match the single tone, the variability was less than when they adjusted the tone to match the complex. The median of the interquartile ranges for all sessions was 4 db when the complex was adjusted, and 4.5 db when the tone was adjusted. This effect has also been noted elsewhere.[5] In addition, there was the systematic tendency already described for the adjusted signal to be set relatively too high.

Although the final results have been reported in terms of medians, the means of the loudness balances were also calculated. The agreement between the two was always within ± 1.9 db, but there was a slight residual skewness in the data, as shown by the fact that the mean values averaged about 0.1 db lower than the median values. The direction of this skewness is what we should expect from the relation between loudness (in sones) and decibels.

One of the persistent difficulties in experiments on loudness is the tendency for different subjects to use different criteria in judging the loudness of a complex. This difference in criterion is especially marked when the tones are faint and widely spaced. Apparently two extreme attitudes may be taken toward the complex: the subject may take an "analytic" attitude and judge in terms of the loudness of a single component, or he may take an "integrative" attitude and judge in terms of a summation of the loudnesses of the components. Different subjects seemed to take these attitudes in different degrees and to hold rather consistently to them. Of course, those who took a more integrative attitude judged the complex to be louder than did those who took a more analytic attitude.

LOUDNESS *VS* BAND WIDTH OF NOISE

The foregoing results concern the loudness of line spectra, and the next question is, how does the loudness of a continuous flat spectrum (white noise) change with band width when the effective sound pressure level is held constant. (In the experiment by Zwicker and Feldtkeller[1] the spectrum studied was uniform masking noise.) In order to test this question it was necessary to design sets of filters having different pass bands centered (geometrically) about a given frequency. Three such sets of filters were used to provide bands of various widths centered about the frequencies 440, 1420, and 5200 cps.

Groups of 12 subjects adjusted a comparison signal (either a band of noise or a tone) to match the loudness of each of the filtered bands. For a given experiment the levels of the filtered bands were held constant in terms of the reading on a thermocouple voltmeter, and after the loudness balance had been made the level of the adjusted signal was read on the same meter. The median results are shown in Figs. 8, 9, and 10.

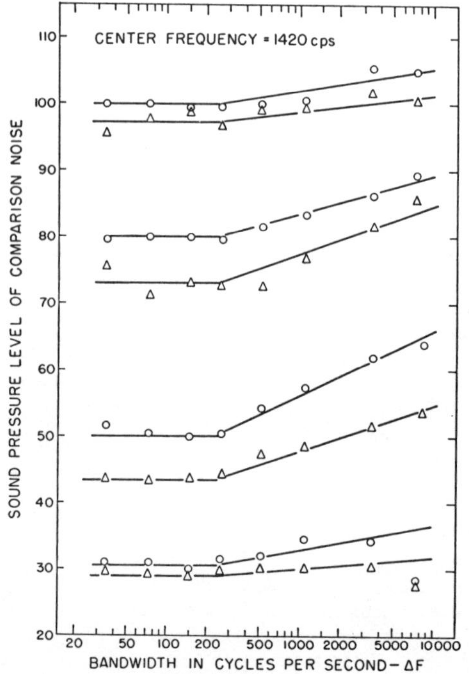

FIG. 8. Dependence of loudness on the band width of a noise of constant SPL having a center frequency of 1420 cps. Comparison noises of two band widths, 210 cps (circles) and 2300 cps (triangles), were matched in loudness to each band width ΔF at a constant SPL.

As in Figs. 2 and 3, the lines through the data were drawn to show the agreement between the data and the critical-band hypothesis. The point at which the two segments of each line form an angle was determined by the critical-band measurements discussed below. It seems clear that the results, taken all together, support the hypothesis that the loudness of a band of noise of constant SPL is invariant with band width provided the band width is smaller than the critical band. When the band width is increased beyond the critical value, the loudness increases. The point at which the increase begins is relatively independent of level.

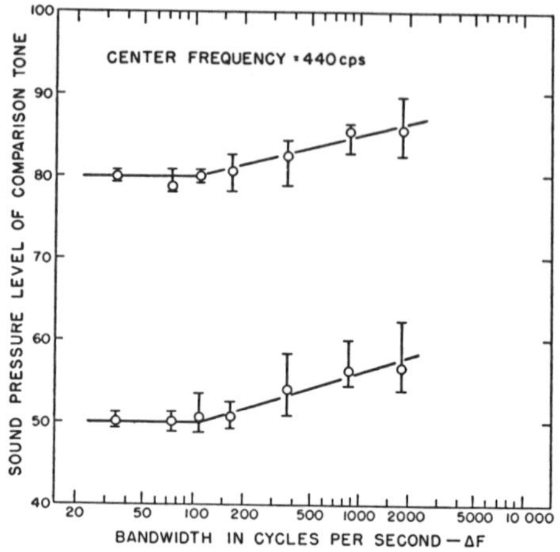

FIG. 9. Dependence of loudness on the band width of a noise of constant SPL having a center frequency of 440 cps. The subjects adjusted a 440-cy tone to match the loudness of each band width ΔF. The vertical bars show the interquartile ranges of the adjustments.

Certain other features of these results also deserve comment. In Fig. 8 four different levels were tested (30, 50, 80, and 100 db) and two different comparison noises were adjusted to match the loudness of the filtered band at each value of ΔF. These comparison noises had band widths of 210 and 2300 cps. Since for the same SPL the wider of these noises is louder, the levels to which the subjects adjusted it (triangles) are lower than the levels to which they adjusted the 210-cy band (circles). The variabilities of the loudness

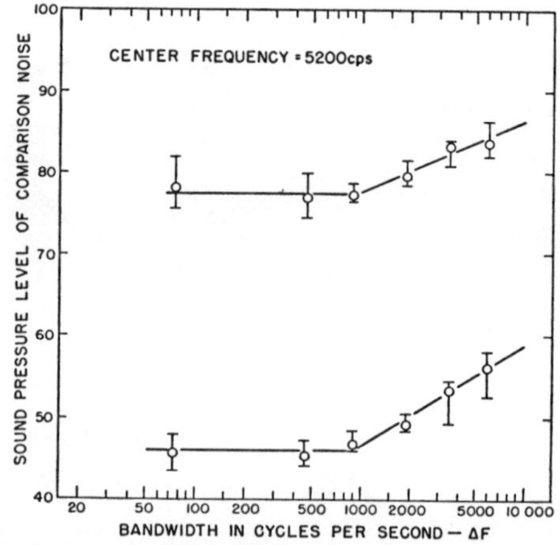

FIG. 10. Dependence of loudness on the band width of a noise of constant SPL having a center frequency of 5200 cps. The subjects adjusted a comparison noise (band width 2500 cps) to match the loudness of each band width ΔF. The vertical bars show the interquartile ranges of the adjustments.

matches showed the expected relations: variability was less when the narrow band was matched to other narrow bands and when the wide band was matched to other wide bands. Consequently, the lower segments of the functions are better determined by the circles (210 cps) and the upper segments by the triangles (2300 cps).

The dependence of loudness summation on level is seen to be rather similar in Fig. 3 (tones) and Fig. 8 (noise). At the highest level (100 db) the growth of loudness, as ΔF is increased beyond the critical band width, is less rapid than at medium levels. And again at very low levels the growth of loudness with ΔF beomes smaller. In fact, at the lowest level tested, the largest value of ΔF (about 7500 cps) seems to be less loud than the narrower bands (see also reference 1). This is reminiscent of the behavior of the lowest curve in Fig. 3, but it is not yet certain that these effects are based on the same causes. The behavior of loudness summation at very low levels still presents many puzzles.

Figure 9 shows the results for bands of noise centered about 440 cps at two levels: 50 and 80 db. In this case the subjects adjusted a pure tone of 440 cps to match the loudness of the bands. The vertical bars through the points indicate the interquartile ranges of the adjustments. In Fig. 10, similar results are shown for bands centered about a frequency of 5200 cps. To match the loudness of these bands the subjects adjusted the level of a comparison noise whose band width was 2500 cps.

CONCEPT OF CRITICAL BANDS

A word is in order regarding the relation between the *Frequenzgruppe*, which we are translating "critical band," and the concept originated by Fletcher. Although a measure called κ was used earlier (1937), it was in his 1940 paper that Fletcher outlined the concept of the critical band as an aid to determining "position coordinates" on the basilar membrane.[6] In order to know how to divide the frequency spectrum into bands of equal effectiveness he wanted to know where on the membrane various frequencies produce excitation. One approach to this problem was via the assumption that successive difference limens for frequency mark off equal steps along the membrane. The other was to assume that masking is proportional to excitation and then to see how effectively different bands of the spectrum produce excitation by determining how pure tones are masked by a broad-band noise. Fletcher assumed that the part of the noise that is effective in masking a tone is the part of the spectrum lying near the tone and containing the same amount of power as the tone. Those parts of the spectrum that are far from the tone contribute no masking. His critical band, then, becomes that width of the spectrum which contains the same acoustic power as the tone that is just masked.

This concept gives us, in effect, a critical band by definition, or by assumption. The masking measurements used to calculate its value have been confirmed in other laboratories,[7] but the direct experimental evidence for the validity of its underlying assumption is not very substantial. Thus far, it seems that a sharp discontinuity has not been found in plots relating the masked threshold of a tone to the band width of a masking noise.[8] Nevertheless, the concept has been a powerful aid in the solution of the problem Fletcher posed, for it turns out that the width of the critical band thus defined varies with frequency in about the same manner as the difference limen. Hence, Fletcher was able to combine information from these two sources and produce a useful "excitation map" of the basilar membrane—one that also agrees with other evidence. A more recent development of this notion is contained in his 1953 book.[9]

Since attempts to determine empirically the width of the critical band by the procedure of masking a tone by bands of noise of different widths have not been definitive, in actual practice the measure of the critical band has usually been taken to be the ratio between the power in the masked tone and the power in a 1-cy band of the masking noise. In other words, the practice rests on a defined quantity or ratio, which might perhaps be called the "critical ratio" or the "critical masking ratio."

Now it happens that the critical band (or ratio) defined by Fletcher leads to a band width that is approximately proportional to the "*Frequenzgruppe*," which is one of the reasons for our suggesting that the *Frequenzgruppe* be called a critical band. This latter critical band has the advantage, however, that it does not rest on assumptions or definitions, but is empirically determined by at least four kinds of independent experiments. The evidence for a critical band in loudness summation has already been presented above, and we will turn now to a brief review of the other types of evidence for it. The four types of experiments that provide direct measures of a critical band width have to do with thresholds, masking, phase, and, as we have seen, loudness summation.

THRESHOLD MEASURES OF THE CRITICAL BAND

In a study by Gässler[10] a critical band width emerges as a discontinuity in the function relating two variables:

[6] H. Fletcher and W. A. Munson, "Relation between loudness and masking," J. Acoust. Soc. Am. **9**, 1–10 (1937); H. Fletcher, "Auditory patterns," Revs. Modern Phys. **12**, 47–65 (1940).

[7] J. E. Hawkins, Jr., and S. S. Stevens, "The masking of pure tones and of speech by white noise," J. Acoust. Soc. Am. **22**, 6–13 (1950).

[8] Schafer, Gales, Shewmaker, and Thompson, "The frequency selectivity of the ear as determined by masking experiments," J. Acoust. Soc. Am. **22**, 490–496 (1950).

[9] H. Fletcher, *Speech and Hearing in Communication* (D. Van Nostrand, Company, Inc., New York, 1953).

[10] G. Gässler, "Ueber die Hörschwelle für Schallereignisse mit verschieden breitem Frequenzspektrum," Acustica **4**, Akust. Beih. **1**, 408–414 (1954).

(1) the level at which a single component in a complex of uniformly spaced tones reaches threshold and (2) the number of tones in the complex. It is assumed that all the components have the same amplitude.

In principle, the procedure is this. We begin with a single pure tone and find its threshold (using the "tracking" procedure of the Békésy audiometer). We then add another tone of the same amplitude but spaced 10 cps lower than the first tone, and again we measure the threshold. We find, of course, that in order to reach threshold the amplitude of each tone can be less for two components than it is for one. We proceed in this fashion to add tones 10 cps apart and to measure the resulting threshold. Up to a certain point, the amplitude of the individual tones decreases as more of them are added, but beyond this point no further decrease occurs. This transition point is a measure of the critical band.

Actually, since the threshold of the typical ear is not flat over a wide range of frequencies, Gässler found it necessary to make the audiogram flat by introducing a uniform masking noise. He was able to show, however, that the behavior at the absolute threshold is similar to the behavior at the masked threshold, regardless of the level of the masked thresholds. Using up to 40 components at various spacings and in various frequency regions, he mapped the width of the critical band in the ears of two observers. The results are shown by two curves in Fig. 11, one for each observer. For purposes of clarity, the curves in Fig. 11 have been separated vertically by one-half of a logarithmic unit.

The crosses represent results with tones under the method just described, and the circles show the results of using an analogous procedure with bands of noise. When the threshold for different band widths of noise is measured, the level per cycle of the noise decreases with bandwidth, up to the critical band. Beyond the critical point, the level per cycle remains constant as the band width is increased. The points in Fig. 11 were determined from the intersections of two line segments on plots that look superficially like those shown in Figs. 2, 3, 8, 9, and 10. In the threshold measurements the slope of the slanting line is such that it represents a constant sound pressure level of the complex.

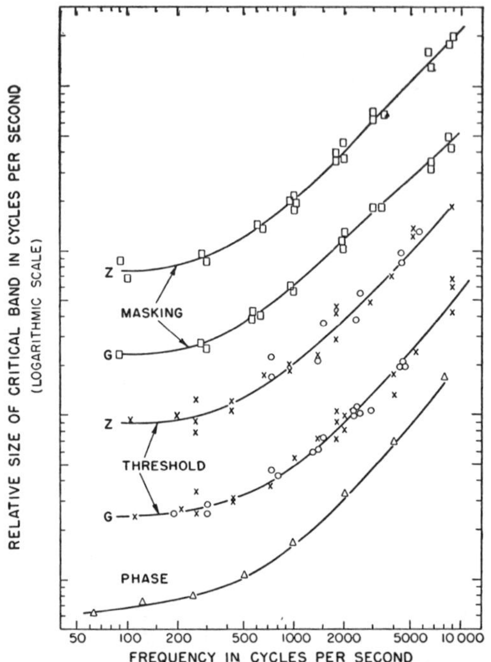

FIG. 11. Functions relating the width of the critical band to frequency, as determined by three experimental methods: masking, threshold, and phase. The letters *Z* and *G* refer to individual observers. On the curves derived from threshold measurements, the crosses represent studies with pure tones and the circles represent studies with bands of noise. The points on the lowest curve represent average values for four observers. For purposes of clarity the curves have been separated by one-half a logarithmic unit.

MASKING

The procedure used to measure the critical band by means of masking is in a sense the inverse of Fletcher's procedure. He used a noise to mask a tone; the inverse experiment[11] uses two tones to mask a noise. A narrow band of noise is placed midway between two pure tones of equal amplitude, and the threshold of the noise is measured. Then the two tones are moved farther apart in frequency, and the threshold of the noise is measured again. It is found that the masked threshold of the noise remains constant until the separation between the two tones reaches a critical value, after which the masked threshold decreases rather abruptly. The point at which this decrease begins is taken as the measure of the critical band.

Critical band widths determined by these transition points for two observers are plotted in Fig. 11 (top two curves). The location of the critical transition points in the masking curves is apparently invariant with level, at least over a range of about 80 db. At high levels a basic asymmetry enters the masking audiogram, which may obscure the effect we are looking for.

PHASE

The manner in which experiments on phase permit us to measure the critical band is through the effect of phase on modulation. To see how this happens we need to note that the difference between a small frequency modulation (FM) and a small amplitude modulation (AM) is essentially a matter of the phase relations among the side bands. When the *frequency* of a tone is modulated sinusoidally through a small range, there results a complex of three principal components: the

[11] E. Zwicker, "Die Verdeckung von Schmalbandgeräuschen durch Sinustöne, Acustica 4, Akust. Beih. 1, 415–420 (1954).

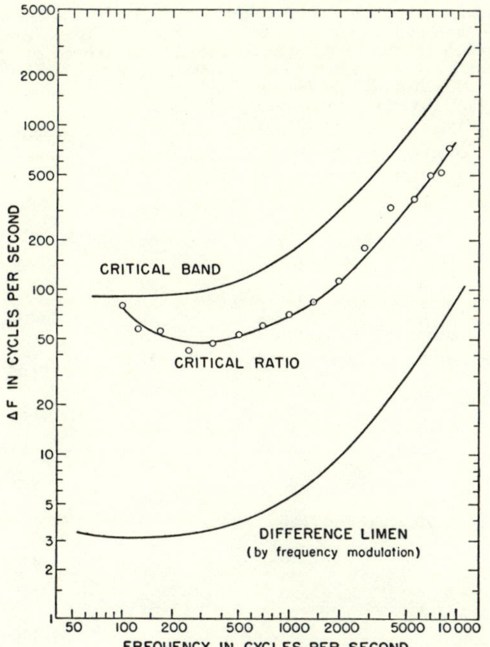

FIG. 12. The top curve, derived from four kinds of experiments, shows the width ΔF of the critical band as a function of the frequency of the center of the band. The middle curve shows the width of the band derived from the "critical ratio," which is defined as the ratio between the intensity per cycle of a noise and the intensity of a pure tone that is just masked by the noise (points are from Hawkins and Stevens). The bottom curve shows the just noticeable range of frequency modulation.

original tone (carrier) and a side band on either side. The spacing between carrier and side band corresponds to the rate (frequency) of the modulation. If the ratio of the range to the rate of modulation is sufficiently small, the side bands beyond the first are negligible. When the *amplitude* of a tone is modulated sinusoidally the same thing happens. There is produced a carrier and two side bands. The difference between AM and FM then is merely one of phase: relative to the phasing of the components produced by AM, under FM one of the side bands is 180° out of phase. In other words, to a first approximation, AM becomes FM if the phase of one of the side bands is reversed.

Now we ask the question, how sensitive is the ear to AM and to FM? When this sensitivity is measured by finding the just detectable amount of modulation—degree of AM and range of FM—an interesting thing is observed.[12] In terms of the amplitudes of the side bands, at low rates of modulation the just detectable AM is less than the just detectable FM. In other words, in order to be heard as a modulation, the amplitude of the side bands must be greater under FM than under AM. However, as the rate of modulation increases, and the side bands are spread wider apart, a point is reached beyond which the just detectable modulation is the same for both FM and AM. At and beyond this point the *phase* of the side bands no longer makes any difference to the ear.

If we take the over-all frequency difference between the two side bands at this critical rate of modulation to be the measure of the critical band, we can use the results of such experiments to measure this band. The bottom curve in Fig. 11 shows the results of such measurements on four observers. The just detectable amounts of AM and FM were measured at various carrier frequencies, at various rates of modulation (from 1 to 6000 per sec), and at loudness levels ranging from 30 to 80 phons. As was true with the other measures of the critical band width (threshold, masking, and loudness summation) the critical band determined by phase sensitivity turns out to be independent of level over the ranges tested.

As is evident in Fig. 11, the width of the critical band determined by these various methods is approximately the same, and its dependence on frequency follows a similar course. Over the low-frequency range the critical band tends to remain constant at a width of about 90 cps, but with increasing frequency it grows rapidly until in the vicinity of 10 000 cps its width is about 2000 cps.

[12] E. Zwicker, "Die Grenzen der Hörbarkeit der Amplitudenmodulation und der Frequenzmodulation eines Tones," Acustica **2**, Akust. Beih. **3**, 125–133 (1952).

RELATIONS TO OTHER FUNCTIONS

On the basis of the evidence available from the direct methods for measuring the critical band, an attempt has been made to construct a function relating its width ΔF to frequency. This function, shown as the top curve in Fig. 12, represents our present best estimate of the size of the critical band (ordinate), as a function of the frequency of the center of the band (abscissa). As we have seen, this curve is derived from four types of experiments. At very low frequencies the width of the critical band becomes indeterminate, for its lower limit falls, so to speak, beyond the bottom end of the scale.

Approximate values for two sets of critical band widths are listed in Table I. Since we are free to choose either the lower or the upper cut-off frequency of a critical band, other sets of values could be tabled with the aid of Fig. 12.

We have already mentioned the fact that the critical band measured by direct methods is approximately proportional to the size of the band derived by Fletcher from the "critical ratio." As can be seen from the middle curve in Fig. 12, the directly measured band is about two-and-a-half times as wide as Fletcher's band. Since over most of the frequency range the forms of these two functions are similar, it seems reasonable to suppose that they may reflect aspects of the same underlying process. The two functions differ mainly at the lower end, where the "critical ratio" curve turns up. A possible explanation of this upturn is that at low frequencies, where the critical band is narrow, the masked threshold tends to rise because the "envelope" of a narrow (critical) band of noise is not as steady, relative to the time constant of the ear, as the envelope of a wide band of noise.[13] With narrow bands the ear begins to hear the amplitude irregularity of the envelope and this irregularity may contribute to the masking of a tone.

The critical band seems also to bear a relation to certain other auditory phenomena such as the difference limen for frequency, the function relating frequency to subjective pitch in mels, and the function relating frequency to the position of stimulation on the basilar membrane.

That the difference limen for frequency approximates a constant fraction of a critical band is shown by the bottom curve in Fig. 12. This bottom curve has about the same form as the top curve. The bottom curve represents the just detectable change in frequency as measured by the detectable range of frequency modulation when the rate of modulation is about 4 per sec.[13] This curve, for an SPL of 80 db, is based on measurements on four observers who used the method of "tracking" to determine the difference limen, defined as the total range of the just detectable frequency modulation. These values agree reasonably well with those of Shower and Biddulph.[14]

An interesting relation between the critical band and the mel scale[15] of pitch is suggested by the fact that over most of the frequency range the width of the critical band approximates a constant number of mels. The average width of the critical band is about 137 mels. It varies from about 100 mels at low frequencies to about 180 mels at high frequencies. In view of the difficulty of determining the pitch scale with great precision, this degree of agreement between critical bands and intervals of subjective pitch makes it reasonable to entertain the hypothesis that the two may be closely related. If we were to plot in Fig. 12 a curve showing the ΔF corresponding to a constant interval of pitch, we would obtain a curve not greatly unlike the others shown there (see, for example, Licklider's Fig. 18[16]).

Finally, as has been pointed out elsewhere,[17] Békésy's determinations of the positions at which various frequencies produce a maximum vibration of the basilar membrane result in a cochlear map that suggests an additional interesting hypothesis. Critical bands, equal mel intervals, and difference limens may correspond to equal distances along the basilar membrane. The precision with which some of these things can be measured does not yet permit a precise test of this possibility, but the general similarity of the several functions justifies our using it as a working hypothesis.

TABLE I. Examples of critical band widths ΔF. The left-hand center column gives the cut-off frequencies of bands whose center frequencies are listed in the right-hand center column, and vice versa. Example: The band 900 to 1060 has a width ΔF of 160 and a center frequency of 980 cps. The band 830 to 980 has a width ΔF of 150 and a center frequency of 900 cps.

ΔF	Center and cut-off frequencies		ΔF
	20		
90		65	
	110		90
90		155	
	200		95
95		250	
	295		95
100		345	
	395		105
108		450	
	503		110
120		560	
	625		130
130		690	
	755		140
145		830	
	900		150
160		980	
	1060		175
190		1155	
	1250		200
210		1355	
	1460		225
240		1580	
	1700		255
270		1835	
	1970		295
320		2130	
	2290		350
380		2480	
	2670		420
450		2900	
	3120		500
560		3400	
	3680		620
680		4020	
	4360		760
840		4780	
	5200		920
1000		5700	
	6200		1150
1300		6850	
	7500		1550
1800		8400	
	9300		2100
2400		10500	
	11700		2800
3300		13300	
	15000		4000
		17300	

[13] E. Zwicker, "Die elementaren Grundlagen zur Bestimmung der Informationskapazität des Gehörs," Acustica **6**, 365–381 (1956).

[14] E. G. Shower and R. Biddulph, "Differential pitch sensitivity of the ear," J. Acoust. Soc. Am. **3**, 275–287 (1931).

[15] S. S. Stevens and J. Volkmann, "The relation of pitch to frequency: a revised scale," Am. J. Psychol. **53**, 329–353 (1940).

[16] J. C. R. Licklider, "Basic correlates of the auditory stimulus," S. S. Stevens, editor, *Handbook of Experimental Psychology* (John Wiley and Sons, Inc., New York, 1951).

[17] G. von Békésy and W. A. Rosenblith, "The mechanical properties of the ear," S. S. Stevens, editor, *Handbook of Experimental Psychology* (John Wiley and Sons, Inc., New York, 1951).

24

Reprinted from *IEEE Proc.* 58:713–723 (1970)

Application of Detection Theory in Psychophysics

DAVID M. GREEN

Invited Paper

Abstract—The paper reviews how current developments in detection theory have contributed to our understanding of human sensory processes. The first section of the paper emphasizes the methodological contributions of detection theory and how the theory is useful in the analysis of discrimination data. Next, a brief discussion of the substantive contribution of the theory in auditory research is considered. Energy detection, internal and external fluctuation, and some recent work using a Poisson model, illustrate these substantive applications of detection theory.

Introduction

THE HUMAN senses are remarkable information-processing systems. It is, I am sure, unnecessary to recount their several virtues or to extol their remarkable accomplishments to the readership of the PROCEEDINGS. The fascination of the human senses for people interested in communication and information processing is evident in the many applications of communication and information concepts in the analysis of these systems. One reason for this fascination is that the functioning of the entire sensory system often seems to transcend the apparent limitations of its particular parts. The astronaut's visual acuity, for example, seemed incredible, given the rather simple lens of the eye. Similarly, the auditory system provides a remarkably detailed frequency analysis of the acoustic waveform despite the lack of any very sharp resonance structures and, paradoxically, this fine spectral resolution is coupled with remarkably acute temporal resolution.

Further examples could be listed but they hardly seem necessary since we probably all agree that it would be interesting and, perhaps, useful to understand how human and animal sensory systems operate. There probably is less widespread agreement about how we should try to gain such an understanding. Some will immediately opt for a molecular approach, feeling that the only way to proceed is to take the system apart, piece by piece, and study the various parts and their interactions. There is much to recommend such a mode of attack, but there are also some serious drawbacks, especially if the system is large, complicated, and strongly interconnected, as all sensory systems are. For this reason we will follow a more system-oriented approach in this paper. We will deal with the intact human being, and by asking him questions about what he senses, in a carefully contrived and controlled experimental situation, we attempt to arrive at a picture of how at least some aspects of the system operate. The basic shortcoming of this approach is that a limited set of data can always be explained by a number of quite different theories or hypotheses. More discouraging is the fact that a detailed theory built from careful observations in one experimental setting may show little value in understanding the results obtained in other experimental situations. For this reason, most psychologists show a keen interest in the results of research on more molecular levels. Sometimes a psychologist's theory is specifically designed to accord with some aspect of physiological theory or data. The reverse is also true. Further work on both system and molecular levels will be needed before we achieve anything near a complete understanding of the entire process.

Manuscript received January 19, 1970. This work was supported in part by the National Institutes of Health, Public Health Service, U. S. Department of Health, Education, and Welfare; and in part by the National Science Foundation.

The author is with the Department of Psychology, University of California at San Diego, La Jolla, Calif. 92037.

Outline of the Paper

This paper is a brief review of how some of the current developments in communication theory, especially detection and decision theory, have contributed to our understanding of the sensory systems. The paper is tutorial in nature; we will not review any of the ideas in great detail. Rather, the paper will try to explain the major motivation of the research and cite some of the principal results. While the emphasis will be on the contribution of detection theory, it will also become apparent that many disciplines—anatomy, physiology, and psychology, as well as the communication sciences—have made, and are continuing to make, a contribution to our understanding of the human senses.

Historically, the system approach to the study of the human senses has been called psychophysics since the original aim was to relate some physical dimension of the stimulus, such as the power or frequency of a sinusoid, to a so-called psychological attribute, such as the apparent loudness or pitch. At present, a majority of the research in psychophysics is based on the results of discrimination experiments. In such experiments, one attempts to learn something about the sensory system by determining just how small a change in some aspect of the stimulus can be reliably detected. Formally, it is simple to treat a discrimination experiment from the viewpoint of detection theory. The small change in the stimulus is the signal. The noise is either the physical variability of the stimulus itself or variability within the processing mechanism, or both. Once the statistics of the noise and character of the signal are described, it is straightforward to apply the formal apparatus of detection theory.

The first part of the paper will review the description of the process of discrimination generated by detection theory. A central feature of that description is to treat the criterion that the subject uses in deciding whether or not a signal is present as explicitly distinct from his sensory capabilities. A method is presented for analyzing discrimination data which attempts to separate the sensory and nonsensory variables. The second part of the paper is more substantively oriented. It will review the use of discrimination data in an attempt to understand a particular sensory system, namely, the human auditory system, and will briefly describe two specific models of this system.

Analysis of Human Detection Data

Experimental Task

The essentials of a detection or discrimination experiment are quite simple. We present the subject with two stimuli that differ in some small way. By associating arbitrary labels with these stimuli we can ask him to demonstrate his ability to distinguish between the two stimuli. By correlating the reliability of his discrimination performance with the size of the stimulus differences we can make some inferences about his sensory processing. Often, the smallest change in the stimulus that the subject can reliably detect is used as the fundamental datum.

Sad experience has taught us that the subject's judgments in such experiments are often influenced by a variety of nonsensory variables, including 1) how anxious he is to please the experimenter, 2) whether he wants to establish that he is a sensitive and discerning individual, and 3) how reluctant he is to say something is present when it is not.

Thus, an essential part of the analysis of such data is a means of separating the sensory factors from all the other factors operating in the discrimination experiment so that inferences based on the data can be directly related to the sensory system itself and not contaminated by the presence of various other variables, such as the personality characteristics of the subject, whether he is conservative or inclined to take risk, how he has interpreted the instruction of the experimenter, and the like.

To pursue this problem in more detail, let us consider the analysis of some typical discrimination data, in particular the data collected in a simple detection experiment. This example will illustrate the essential features of the discrimination task and permit us to present the various theories of the discrimination process in terms of a concrete example.

Some Typical Detection Data

In the simple detection experiment, also called a Yes-No procedure, there are two possible stimulus alternatives on each trial, either noise alone, n, or a signal added to the noise, $s+n$. The noise might be broad-band audio noise, and the signal a sinusoid of definite duration, frequency, phase, and starting time. The subject responds *yes* if he believes he hears the signal and *no* otherwise. We denote these responses by the capital letters Y and N. In such a task, one of four distinct events occurs on each trial and the probabilities P associated with each event are indicated in the matrix of Table I. We note the constraint on these probabilities as indicated below the matrix in Table I, namely, given that either noise or signal-plus-noise was presented, the probability of a *yes* or *no* response is unity. Thus, the basic matrix from a simple-detection task contains only two independent probabilities—the probability of a *yes* response, given noise alone, and the probability of a *yes* response, given signal-plus-noise. These are called the *false-alarm* and *hit* probabilities, respectively.

TABLE I

		Response: Y	Response: N
Stimulus condition	$s+n$	$P(\mathrm{Y}\mid s+n)$ a hit	$P(\mathrm{N}\mid s+n)$
	n	$P(\mathrm{Y}\mid n)$ false alarm	$P(\mathrm{N}\mid n)$

$$P(\mathrm{Y}\mid s+n)+P(\mathrm{N}\mid s+n)=1.00$$
$$P(\mathrm{Y}\mid n)+P(\mathrm{N}\mid n)=1.00$$

In addition to this formal definition of the simple-detection task, we might also indicate something about the typical experimental situation. Our subjects are, as you might expect, largely undergraduate students with normal hearing. The subject wears earphones and may hear a constant background noise generated by a white-noise generator. He views a display board where small lights indicate when the auditory signal, if it is presented, will occur. Other lights tell him when to respond, indicate if his answer was correct, and warn him that the next trial is about to begin. A single trial might last 5 seconds and consist of the following sequence: warning light (0.1 second), pause (0.9 second), observation interval (0.1 second), pause (1.9 seconds), answer interval (1.0 second), pause (0.5 second), feedback (0.1 second), pause (0.4 second), begin the next trial. Perhaps 100 such trials constitute a single experimental condition and perhaps 10 such conditions are run each day. So, typically, a daily session consists of about 1000 observations and lasts about 2 hours. Each subject observes for many daily sessions, often for a semester or longer.

For each condition we hold constant all physical parameters, signal-to-noise ratio, etc. During the signal interval, either we present the signal (say, a gated sinusoid added to the noise) or we do not, and the subject's response, *yes* or *no*, is recorded. From these data we estimate the probabilities indicated in the table, simply from the corresponding frequencies, assuming the trials are independent.

Following Peterson, Birdsall, and Fox [20] these estimated probabilities of a false alarm and hit are plotted on the x and y axes of the unit square. If the subject can discriminate

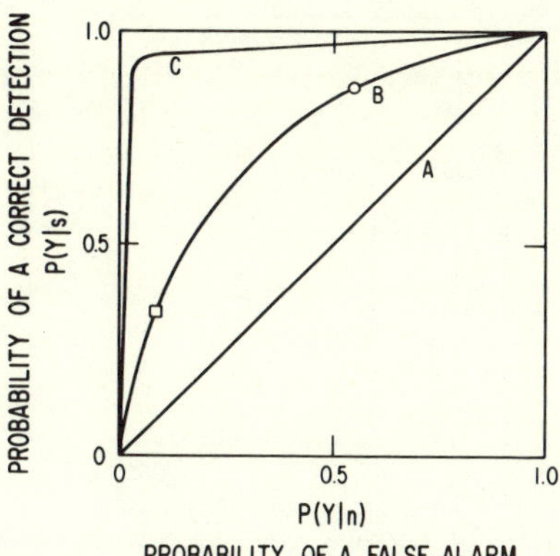

Fig. 1. A receiver-operating-characteristic (ROC) graph and some ROC curves. The notation for the coordinates is the same as that used in Table I.

not at all, then the probability of a hit and a false alarm will be equal, independent of the particular value—that is, the performance will yield a point somewhere along the major diagonal in the unit square (line A, Fig. 1). To the extent that the signal is discriminable in the noise, the point will move toward the upper-left corner of the unit square. The upper-left corner itself represents a special case in which the signal is detected whenever it is presented and no false alarms are ever made.

Suppose we hold everything constant but systematically vary the subject's disposition to respond, either by manipulating the payoffs associated with each of the stimulus-response outcomes, or by simply instructing him to change his criterion for deciding whether or not he says a signal is present. We then obtain a systematic set of points that appear to lie along a single curve. A typical example of such a curve, called a receiver-operating characteristic curve (ROC curve), is labeled B in Fig. 1.

The two points marked on curve B might represent the performance of two different subjects who have identical sensory capabilities but quite different criteria for what they call "detecting the signal." The circle represents a subject with a liberal criterion; the square represents a subject using a more stringent or conservative criterion. On the other hand, if one subject is genuinely different from another subject in his sensory capabilities, and if an entire curve is generated for each subject by varying his criteria and measuring the several hit and false-alarm probabilities necessary to estimate an entire ROC curve, then one might find the more acute subject produces data following curve C in Fig. 1, and the less sensitive subject produces data following curve B. Since we are mostly interested in the differences in sensory capabilities and not differences in various subjects' criteria, the area under the ROC curve provides a useful index of sensory differences.

Before signal-detection theory and the ROC curve analysis were suggested, several psychologists advocated using *forced-choice* procedures, rather than the simple Yes-No procedure outlined above, because they found the latter gave unstable estimates of the probability P of detecting a signal, $P(Y|s)$, as we might expect. The simplest example of this alternate procedure is a two-interval forced-choice task. The subject listens to two successive time intervals, only one of which contains the signal. We ask the subject to identify which interval he believes contained the signal. As the signal becomes easier to hear, the percentage of correct responses approaches 100; as the signal becomes harder to hear, the subject approaches a chance score, or 50 percent. The range of possible scores in a two-alternative task has the same range as the area under the ROC curve in the more conventional Yes-No procedure. In fact, under quite general assumptions one can show that the area under the Yes-No ROC curve is exactly equal to the expected percentage of correct responses in the two-alternative forced-choice task [7]. The variability of the area measure has also been studied [22].

Several people have argued that because subjects seldom have any strong bias toward choosing the first or second time interval of the forced-choice task, and precisely because the procedure merely requires a judgment as to which of the two intervals is more likely to contain the signal, the forced-choice procedure avoids many of the problems inherent in the more traditional Yes-No psychophysical procedures [16].

Probably for these reasons the forced-choice procedure is widely used in studying sensory aspects of the discrimination process. It is also more efficient, since all the data of a session can be used to estimate a single percentage rather than using the data of several sessions to generate the separate points needed to estimate the entire ROC curve and its area. However, the Yes-No ROC curve, especially its shape, is often studied because it may provide considerable information about the essential features of the discrimination mechanism. There is still considerable argument about the exact shape of the curve in different experimental settings and equally strong opinion about what inferences concerning the basic mechanism of discrimination can be drawn from such curves. To understand this controversy we need to consider briefly the threshold problem and review how detection theory has contributed to the analysis of the various theories in this area.

The Threshold Problem

Classical Threshold Theory: In the earliest studies of detection, no explicit, external, interfering noise was present. The subject listened in a room that sounded absolutely quiet, and as the amplitude of a signal was raised, eventually it could be reliably detected. Since there was no obvious background noise or interference, it is not surprising that the earliest theory treated the process of detection or discrimination of the signal in such an environment as essentially a matter of exceeding some internal energy or amplitude threshold. Thus, signals with sufficiently large amplitude were detected and those with sufficiently low amplitude remained undetected. The very fact that the subject did not detect signals when signals were not being presented indicated that the probability of a false detection (that is, a false alarm triggered by any residual background noise) was very nearly zero. In fact, this belief was incorporated into the theory as a premise of the experimental procedure and observers were severely reprimanded for reporting signals when none were presented. If the subject reported more than a few false alarms in the course of an entire experimental session, he was thought to be confused or not paying proper attention to the experimental task. A description of these experiments might involve statements such as: "The probability of a false alarm was lower than 1 percent." Or: "In the entire sequence of 10 000 observations, only three false alarms occurred." Another reason for an incredibly low false-alarm rate was that the experimental procedure did not allow much opportunity for such occurrences. The experimenter seldom presented trials in which signals were not presented since, from his point of view, they wasted experimental time. The estimates of these low false-alarm rates are therefore extremely unstable.

Continuous Theory: It is probably safe to say that no one actually believed the classical threshold position, yet a viable alternative to this formulation of the discrimination process was not available until fairly recently. Some of the pioneering papers on this topic occurred shortly after World War II when, for example, Smith and Wilson [29] at Lincoln Laboratory showed that some obvious implications of the classical threshold theory were incorrect. Munson and Karlin [18] at Bell Telephone Laboratories also challenged some of the basic assumptions of the classical threshold theory. The first complete statement of an alternative to the classical threshold model was made by Tanner and Swets [31] at the University of Michigan. Their theory was essentially an adaptation of the early work on physical detection theory by Peterson and Birdsall [19]. The central idea of the Tanner-Swets theory was the assumption that noise is present in all discrimination tasks. If there was no obvious external noise, then internal noise must be assumed. The process of discrimination or detection of the signal is pictured as consisting of two parts: 1) the calculation of likelihood ratio (the likelihood that the signal was present divided by the likelihood of noise alone), and 2) a straightforward decision procedure based on this calculated likelihold ratio (that is, the subject says *yes* if the likelihood ratio exceeds a predetermined criterion value). The general assumption made in the initial statements of this theory was that some transformation of the likelihood ratio is Gaussian under both noise and signal-plus-noise hypotheses. To psychologists, these assumptions were very similar to those made in Thurstonian scaling [32].

The only threshold in the Tanner-Swets theory was a threshold on likelihood ratio, that is, the cut on the likelihood-ratio continuum that led to either a *yes* or *no* response. Continuous theory has no sensory threshold as such, but only a response threshold. It is continuous in the sense that, in theory, any likelihood ratio can arise and could potentially be used as a response threshold. One should be able to judge how near the observed likelihood had been to the response threshold even when the ratio led to a "no, I did not hear it" response. Thus, the crucial difference between

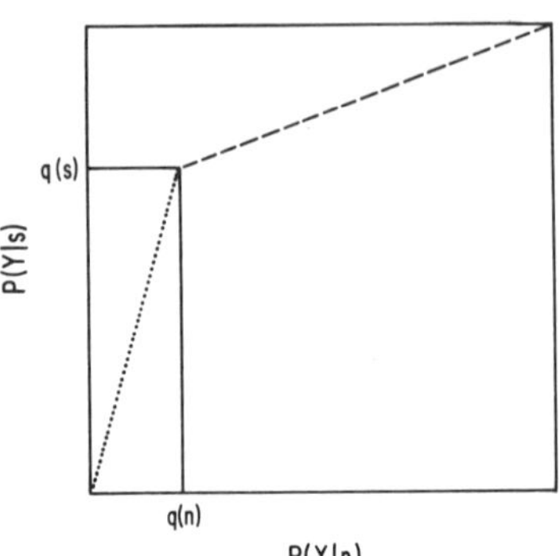

Fig. 2. The ROC curve according to two-state theory.

the classical threshold theory and the continuous or likelihood-ratio theory is that the observer is assumed to make an almost infinite gradation of the sensory input, even distinguishing among those inputs that he reports he does not hear! According to classical threshold theory, anything the observer failed to detect should convey no information.

Given only these two contenders, there really was not much of a contest. It was easy to derive certain predictions from classical threshold theory which practically all data reject, and though several nontrivial modifications of the continuous theory needed to be made, especially some rather awkward assumptions concerning the relative size of the variance of the signal and noise distributions, practically all the data supported the continuous theory. The contest was rejoined, however, in 1963 when Luce presented, in complete form, a viable alternative which still preserved a sensory threshold and yet avoided almost all of the obvious failings of classical threshold theory.

Two-State Theory: The essential modification of classical threshold theory which Luce incorporated in his two-state theory was the assumption of a nonzero false-alarm rate. Thus, even when the signal is not presented, there is some nonzero probability that the subject would "detect" the signal. Let us denote this probability that a detect state occurs, given that there is no signal, as $q(n)$. Similarly, we define the probability of a detect state, given that the signal is present, as $q(s)$. Suppose the subject says *yes* if, and only if, the detect state occurs, and says *no* if, and only if, the nondetect state occurs; then obviously the hit and false-alarm rates would be $q(s)$ and $q(n)$, respectively. Fig. 2 shows the point on the ROC curve corresponding to this decision procedure.

To explain how motivation, instructions, and other nonsensory factors might influence the observer's performance in a detection task, Luce assumed a simple decision procedure in which the subject biases his *yes* and *no* responses, given the binary sensory information (detect or nondetect). These biases can be regarded as a mixture of two strategies. One strategy is to rely on the sensory information and to report *yes* if a detect state occurs and *no* if it does not. The other strategy is a pure strategy, that is, to always say *yes* or always say *no*. This pure strategy is used to either increase or decrease the toal number of *yes* responses. If any two strategies are randomly mixed, it is easy to derive that the resulting behavior will fall on a line connecting the points represented by each strategy separately. Thus, the dashed line in Fig. 2 represents the locus of all points that can be obtained by mixing a pure *yes* response strategy with the sensory information leading to the hit rate of $q(s)$ and the false-alarm rate of $q(n)$. Similarly, the dotted line running from [0, 0] to $[q(s), q(n)]$ is the locus of all points generated by the mix of a pure *no* response strategy and one influenced only by the sensory information. In fact, if the mix is an equal proportion of each strategy, then the resultant point will fall halfway between the points corresponding to the two separate strategies.

Evaluation of the Theories

Given these three theories, which accords best with the experimental data? Classical threshold theory is a special case of two-state theory, with $q(n)=0$, and so the ROC curve predicted by that theory is a single straight line running from the point $[q(s), 0]$ to the upper-right corner of the graph, the point [1, 1]. Since practically no data ever follow such a line, especially near the lower-left corner, we can reject classical theory without further consideration.

Of the two remaining theories it is indeed remarkable that little evidence can be marshaled to indicate clearly which is in best accord with detection data. Although the differences in assumptions of the two theories are quite striking—the sensory continuum is assumed to contain two states in one theory or an infinity of states in the other—their predictions are remarkably similar. It is difficult to find data that clearly support one theory and reject the other. Certainly, two-state theory is, at the very least, a good approximation to a great deal of psychophysical data, and the simplicity inherent in such a theory is attractive if one is primarily interested in other factors, such as learning or motivation, rather than in details of the sensory mechanism. As one might expect, it is even more difficult to reject a three-state model, such as that recently suggested by Krantz [12] which seems to avoid what some might regard as minor failings of Luce's two-state theory. Krantz's paper also provides a clear statement of the attempts to decide between the theories and what evidence is crucial.

The ROC curve is therefore useful in summarizing the data of a discrimination experiment, but it is not possible to use the shape of the curve to determine which theory of the detection process is correct. The difficulty is most easily seen if we consider the expected ROC curve for the major theories. One need only compare the ROC curve of Fig. 1 (curve B), based on the Gaussian assumption, with the two-line segment curve shown in Fig. 2 to realize the difficulty one would have in trying to pick among the theories based on experimental data. These two ROC curves (curve B in Fig. 1, and Fig. 2) represent about the largest differences in prediction that one can achieve. To determine the shape of an ROC curve, one must estimate 5 to 10 separate points and overcome the binomial variability inherent in the estimate of both coordinates of each point. One can calculate that about 2000 observations would be needed to estimate each point on the ROC curve to an accuracy of 1 percent, and thus about 2 to 4 weeks of observation would be needed to determine the entire curve. Over a time period of a month, I am absolutely certain that we cannot bank on the binomial assumptions. For these reasons the fundamental nature of the detection or discrimination process remains in doubt. According to the two prominent theories, it is either continuous or extremely discrete and there is remarkably little evidence that is decisive on this point.

Nonetheless, the predictions based on either theory are similar enough to encourage us to believe that many inferences about the sensory mechanisms can proceed relatively independent of a variety of nonsensory factors. In particular, the Yes-No and forced-choice methods allow us to compare results from different laboratories, confident that differences in instruction and differences among the subjects' criteria are not exerting a strong influence on the sensory measurements. Despite large differences in criteria among different subjects, the ROC curve has helped to indicate that by and large the subject's sensory abilities are not very different. In detecting a sinusoidal signal in noise, for example, the differences among subjects with no obvious hearing deficit is probably less than 1 dB.

A Substantive Application of Detection Theory

Let us now consider the more substantive problem of how the auditory system operates to detect weak signals. Although we might consider this problem for a variety of signals and a number of psychophysical tasks, we will restrict our attention to the auditory detection of a sinusoidal signal added to a steady background of noise. This problem is, of course, ideally suited to an analysis from the viewpoint of detection theory since the detection of a definite waveform in Gaussian noise is a standard problem in that area.

Unencumbered by any facts, we might imagine the auditory-detection process to be like any number of detection systems. It might be analogous to a cross correlator, an autocorrelator, a simple energy detector, or other detection systems. To understand why several investigators have ignored some of these alternatives and instead are exploring a class of detectors largely insensitive to details of the waveform and having a strong Poisson flavor, let us review something of what we know about the anatomy and physiology of the auditory system. This will somewhat restrict our more fanciful theories and will provide a more concrete framework from which to understand the later discussions of auditory-detection models. This review will be brief; for more specific information see [2], [24], and [33].

Anatomy and Physiology of the Auditory System

For present purposes, we treat the acoustic stimulus as simply a pressure waveform $p(t)$. This waveform enters the external ear channel, displaces the tympanic membrane (see Fig. 3), which in turn displaces the three small bones of the

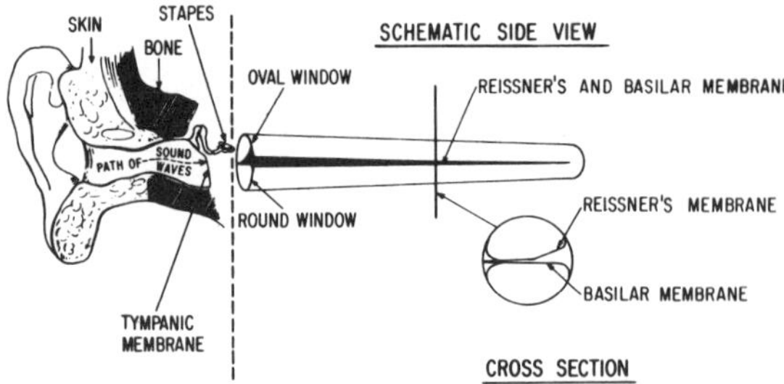

Fig. 3. Basic anatomy of hearing. To the right of the dotted line the cochlea has been uncoiled and the scale considerably expanded.

middle ear. The last of these, the stapes, displaces a thin membrane covering the oval window. The oval window is one of two small holes (the other being the round window) that provide access to the fluid-filled space in which the semicircular canals and the inner ear are located. For moderate stimulus intensities the movement of the stapes is apparently a linear function of the input pressure waveform. Thus, one may express the displacement of the stapes as a convolution of the input pressure waveform $p(t)$ with $h(t)$, the impulse response of the entire system up to the oval window. These mechanical transformations summarized by the impulse response $h(t)$ achieve an impedance match between the air and the liquid of the inner ear, and also limit the very high and very low frequency response of the system. Essentially, this part of the transmission path acts as a broadly tuned bandpass filter.

The movement of the stapes produces sound waves in the fluids of the inner ear, or cochlea. The cochlea is a coiled tapered structure that encloses a fluid-filled tube. Through the middle of this tube run two thin membranes called the *Reissner's* and *basilar* membrane. Fig. 3 schematizes the side view and cross section of the uncoiled cochlea. As the membrane covering the oval window is displaced by the motion of the stapes, the fluids in the cochlear tube cause the membrane covering the round window to bulge outward. Because of the wave disturbance in the fluids of the cochlea, produced by the motion at the oval window, the two delicate membranes located between the two fluid columns vibrate. Our information about how they vibrate, and the way the patterns of vibration change as a function of frequency of the acoustic stimulus, is due almost entirely to the classic work of von Békésy [2]. He solved the multitude of technical problems connected with observing the interior structures while preserving their integrity, and measured characteristics of the vibration pattern of the basilar membranes when excited by sound stimuli. We may briefly summarize von Békésy's observation as follows.

If the sound is a continuous sinusoid, a wave travels along the basilar membrane moving from the oval window down the cochlear partition. At each point the up and down motion of the basilar membrane is sinusoidal and the frequency of this motion equals that of the input sinusoid. The amplitude of the motion, however, is quite different at different points along the partition. At some position the amplitude is maximal and its location correlated with the frequency of the signal. The maximum for the high frequencies is near the oval window, whereas for the lower frequencies it is near the end of the cochlear duct. Roughly, the vibration of the basilar membrane is similar to the waves produced in a rope that is tied at one end and is rapidly vibrated up and down at the other. This analogy is, however, faulty in several respects. First, the cochlear partition is not uniform in any of the important physical dimensions as a function of length. The important implication of this fact is that as the wave travels toward the end of the cochlear duct its energy is absorbed before reaching the end, and hence no standing waves occur. Second, the variation in the critical physical parameters causes the place of maximum vibration to vary with frequency. Thus, the rope analogy is particularly poor because the traveling wave in the rope diminishes slightly in amplitude as it travels from the source to the opposite end, whereas in the ear a low-frequency sound induces a traveling wave whose maximum amplitude is largest at the far end of the basilar membrane while less apparent motion occurs at what would appear to be the source.

The vibrations of the basilar membrane are transformed into nerve impulses by the approximately 25 000 nerve cells, called "hair cells," located within a structure that rests on top of the basilar membrane. The exact mode of excitation of these primary receptors is still a matter of some argument but a mechanical force, presumably a shear force, excites the hair cells. The neural impulses initiated in the hair cells travel up the eighth nerve and, after synapsing at two or three way stations, arrive at the cortex. Since nerve impulses are discrete, all-or-none signals, the information relayed by the individual hair cells is essentially digital and may be considered a series of discrete pulses. The character of the encoding of the receptor elements has been a topic of intense interest for the last 30 years. In 1943 Galambos and Davis [3] recorded with microelectrodes from individual fibers and revealed that the neural impulses are phase-locked to the acoustic input, at least at low frequencies. That is, the nervous impulse originates at a time corresponding to a particular phase of the sinusoidal input and at no other time. The unit might not fire on every cycle—it might skip one, two, or more—but when it fires, it fires at a particular phase of the stimulating sinusoid.

A recent monograph by Kiang [11] provides the most complete and thorough summary of the action of these primary fibers, giving detailed information about the statistical characteristics of the activity of single neural elements when excited by either sinusoidal or impulsive stimuli. Of many important conclusions in this impressive work, we stress only two. First, as others have observed, the nerve fibers are spontaneously active, even in the absence of any apparent acoustic stimulus. Kiang found that the time intervals between successive impulses appear to be random, that is, the distribution of these "latencies" appears to have an exponential tail. Only the tail is exponential because nerves exhibit a lockout phenomenon, that is, one does not find two impulses within some brief period of time (approximately 1 ms) called the absolute refractory period of the fiber. Second, when a continuous acoustic signal, such as a sinusoid, is introduced, the average rate of firing increases. If the signal frequency is very high, above 4000 Hz, the interval between successive neural impulses appears to be random, but the exponential parameter is much larger than for spontaneous activity. Thus, when the signal is present, the mean time interval between successive impulses becomes smaller. There is a definite transient response, a high rate of firing at onset, but this usually diminishes and a constant, steady-state rate is reached in about 10 ms. At lower frequencies, say 500 Hz, the phase-locked principle is also clearly evident; the intervals between impulses are almost all integer multiples of the period of the sinusoidal stimulus. The distribution of times between successive impulses is then essentially discrete and appears to approximate a geometric distribution.

Models of the Auditory Detection System

The preceding facts have led some investigators to conclude that a reasonable detection model is a bandpass filter followed by some sort of energy detector. The output of this detector drives the mean rate of a Poisson process. The detection of a signal in a background noise is determined jointly by the statistics of the acoustic waveforms and the fluctuation introduced by the Poisson process.

Both McGill [14] and Siebert [27] have elaborated this general model in recent papers. There are many ramifications of this type of model and we will explore only some of their essential features. Specific assumptions and particular functional relations assumed by the individual models are presented in the original papers.

Let us begin by analyzing the problem faced by an observer trying to detect a small signal added to Gaussian noise. Assume the signal is presented for a duration T and that the noise either has bandwidth W or that the first-stage filtering of the observer restricts the noise to a band W. Using a simple model of the noise process, one can show that the distribution of energy at the input to the Poisson process is essentially Gaussian and has the form shown in Fig. 4 [8]. The total number of counts, N, generated by an input energy E, is assumed to be a monotonic increasing function of signal energy, $N=f(E)$. The brain, which is presumably monitoring the number of counts, N, is then faced with the detection problem sketched on the y axis of Fig. 4. If, as the figure illustrates, the derivative of f changes little over the range of input fluctuations, then f can be treated as locally linear and its exact form is unimportant. One crucial detection quantity is the variability of the input compared to its mean. This mean-to-sigma ratio is approximately equal to the square root of the degrees of freedom in the noise process. As Fig. 4 shows, the mean-to-sigma ratio, given noise alone, is equal to the square root of the product of bandwidth and duration, WT.

Even if WT is large, so that the exact form of f is unimportant, the distribution of counts will show a greater variability distribution of input energy because of the variability inherent in the Poisson process. The relative influence of fluctuation in the Poisson process, compared with the fluctuation in energy, depends on N. The stability of a Poisson process (m/σ) is proportional to the square root of the total number of counts. If N is very large, then N is a very precise estimate of the energy at the input; for example, the precision is 1 percent if $N=10\,000$. If N is very small, however, the precision of the estimate is much less. In that case, the distributions drawn on the y axis in Fig. 5 would not be correct; one should draw a histogram to illustrate the discrete nature of the Poisson process. Even for moderate N the signal is bound to be more difficult to detect at the output of the Poisson process than at the input.

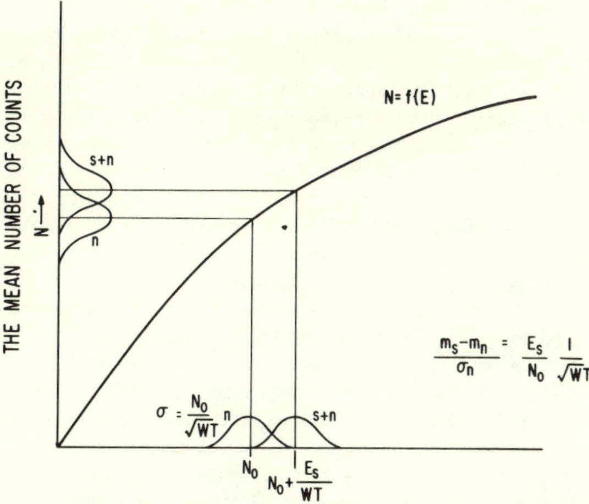

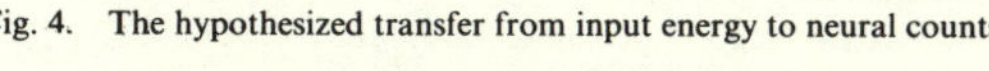

Fig. 4. The hypothesized transfer from input energy to neural counts.

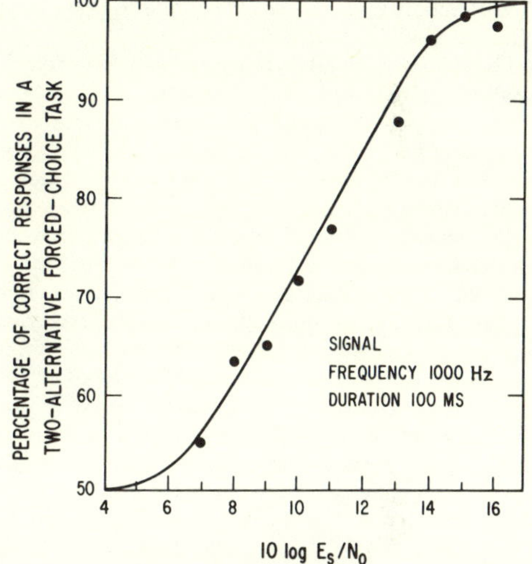

Fig. 5. Some typical detection data.

Data on the Detection of a Sinusoid in Noise

Before continuing our discussion of the Poisson model,

we might pause to show that at least some aspects of this model are in accord with actual detection data. Suppose we assume that the mean number of counts is moderately large and that the function f is locally linear. With these assumptions it is easy to calculate the expected probability of a correct response in a two-alternative forced-choice task. This probability depends on the signal energy E_s, the spectral level of the noise N_0 (watt/hertz), the signal duration T, and the noise bandwidth W. Fig. 5 shows how this predicted probability varies with the ratio E_s/N_0 along with some typical data from a single subject. The duration of the signal in this experiment was 0.1 second. The solid line fitted to the data is based on the assumption that the observer is listening to the noise with a bandwidth of about 1000 Hz ($WT=100$). This bandwidth is much larger than we would wish it to be. Other experiments suggest that the bandwidth should be nearly an order of magnitude smaller. To describe the discrepancy in terms of signal-to-noise ratio, the observer is about 5 dB poorer than we would expect [8, ch. 10]. Nor is this discrepancy unique to the experimental conditions used to obtain the data of Fig. 5. The value of $E_s/N_0=10$ for approximately 75 percent-correct detection for a 0.1 second signal at 1000 Hz has become nearly a standard in the field.

A discrepancy of 5 dB is too large to blame solely on internal fluctuations and a variety of other alternatives are presently being investigated in an attempt to explain the discrepancy. One reasonable explanation for the poor performance is that the observer does not know the exact time interval in which the signal may occur. In a typical experiment the noise is continuous and the possible signal intervals are marked by flashing lights; thus, the observer may be listening over an interval longer than T seconds, and hence integrating more noise energy than necessary. One might attempt to remove this uncertainty by presenting the noise background only for the duration of the observation interval, a so-called "gated" presentation procedure. In the gated version of the two-alternative forced-choice procedure the subject hears two noise bursts, each T seconds in duration. The signal is added to one of the noise bursts.

This gated procedure has created almost as many problems as it was expected to solve. For the case of sinusoidal signals in noise, there is little difference between the performance of observers in the gated and continuous procedures so long as the signal duration is moderate, about 0.1 second. However, if the signal is brief, say 0.01 second, then, contrary to hypothesis, the gated procedure produces much poorer performance than the continuous procedure, especially if the signal frequency is above 2000 Hz. The single instance in which the gated procedure has produced an effect consistent with the uncertainty hypothesis is the detection of an increment in the power of the noise. If one plots a curve analogous to that displayed in Fig. 5 for this situation one finds consistent, but small, differences in the shape of that curve when comparing the gated and the continuous conditions [5]. The direction of these changes is consistent with the hypothesis that the observer is uncertain about the duration and starting time of the signal interval.

Trial-by-Trial Analysis

The Poisson model illustrates the importance of two kinds of fluctuations and the role each plays in limiting the detectability of faint signals. One source of fluctuation is external noise, the random fluctuation of the pressure wave to which the signal is added. The other source of fluctuation is internal or biological noise, which is modeled as a Poisson process. It arises in the course of signal processing and is independent of the acoustic waveform. If the processing were completely noiseless, then in principle one could predict the trial-by-trial performance of the subject. Even if a large proportion of the noise is internal, we could repeat the same acoustic waveform on several trials and attempt to predict the subjects' average response to that waveform. Alternatively, we might have a group of subjects listen to the same waveform. Since any internal noise should be independent from one observer to the next, the average response of the group should be predictable from a knowledge of the particular waveform presented on a given trial.

The main motivation for a trial-by-trial analysis is simply that this level of analysis allows one to investigate details of the detection mechanism which will always be obscure as long as one deals with average responses to average stimuli. Imagine the difficulty one would have in trying to determine if a detector were using a full- or half-wave rectifier if one could only measure the average detectability of a signal over many independent noise samples. Measuring the detection of signals in particular noise samples affords the opportunity to answer questions that are far beyond the limits of experimental precision using conventional procedures.

The first to explore this area experimentally were Sherwin, Kodman, Kovaly, Prothe, and Melrose [26]. They reported only a very modest correlation between the responses of human observers trying to detect a sinusoid added to noise and various energy-like quantities calculated from the individual waveforms. Green [6] used an analog tape recorder and after simply recording a sequence of many trials compared subjects' responses as they listened to the same tape on different occasions. At low signal levels, any correlation among the responses would indicate that the physical fluctuations in the noise waveforms were larger than the fluctuations in the sensory processing. A simple model was presented which allowed one to estimate relative amounts of internal and external variability from the consistency of the repeated responses. According to this model, the internal and external variability were roughly equal in size. The result was remarkably uniform despite changes in various stimulus parameters, such as the overall intensity level of the noise, the signal frequency, and the signal duration.

A more elegant way to conduct such investigation is to store the noise waveforms in digital form and to use the computer to generate the waveforms. Pfafflin and Mathews [21] were the first to investigate the problem in this way. Because of the small size of their computer's memory, they employed rather few (12) noise waveforms. Like Sherwin *et al.*, they found only a slight correlation between obvious physical characteristics of the noise waveform (for example, the total energy in a band centered at the signal frequency) and the observer's detection behavior. Other investigators have also confirmed this finding [1], [17], and [23].

Recent work by J. Patterson in our laboratory has illuminated some other aspects of this situation. Given that the energy in the noise waveform can explain only part of the subject's responses, we wanted a set of waveforms that were identical with respect to the energy spectrum and differed only in other ways. Huffman [9] has suggested a technique for generating a set of such waveforms. Each waveform is nonzero over a finite interval T. The power spectrum of each waveform in the set is the same; only the phase spectrum differs. The set of waveforms is generated by passing transients through all-pass filters that differ only in the locus and number of their phase singularities. We call each waveform in the set a "Huffman sequence."

In the first experiment the same Huffman sequence was used as the "noise" waveform in the two intervals of the forced-choice task. In the result we shall describe, the duration of the waveform was 10 ms. The signal, a sinusoid (also 10 ms in duration), was added in one or the other interval. The detectability of a sinusoid in these brief noise-like waveforms depends heavily on the particular waveform used, despite the fact that all the waveforms have identical power spectra. These Huffman sequences vary as maskers of sinusoidal signals by 30 dB!

Although the results are just beginning to accumulate, and several aspects of the problem have not yet been explored, it is clear that both the number of phase singularities and their location in the spectrum are important variables. Increasing the number of singularities produces a more uniform distribution of energy within the 10-ms interval and therefore decreases the chances of an extremely favorable signal-to-noise ratio appearing at some point within the 10-ms interval. Perhaps, for the same reason, the distribution of singularities within the spectrum is an influential variable, even if the total number of singularities is the same. The general rule seems to be that if the Huffman sequence has a phase singularity near the signal frequency, then the signal is less detectable (by perhaps 10 to 15 dB) than if the masker has no rapid phase change in this region.

There is clearly a great deal of work to be done before the entire picture becomes clear but the results thus far have already upset some of our previous notions of the auditory-detection mechanisms. In particular, thinking in terms of an integration time of 100 ms simply does not appear to be reasonable. Such an integration time may be useful on some system level in summarizing average responses to many different waveforms, but it does not appear to be useful when trying to understand the detection of sinusoids in particular noise samples.

Weber's Law—Detection of an Increment in a Sinusoid

To the extent that a theory emphasizes the variation in the *external* noise as setting the limits on detection, we might describe the theory as "stimulus-oriented" following a designation suggested by Jeffress [10]. The papers of Green [4], Jeffress [10], Pfafflin and Mathews [21], and Ronken [25] illustrate this type of approach. Basically, a stimulus-oriented theory attempts to account for an observer's detection performance by considering the detailed characteristics, especially the fluctuations, of the stimulus. The sensory processing is assumed to be essentially noiseless or, if noisy, equivalent to introducing an additive independent noise component at the input. The Poisson models, on the other hand, tend to emphasize fluctuations in the processing of the sensory information. As our final topic in this review of the applications of detection theory to the analysis of sensory systems, we consider a fundamental difficulty that has bedeviled practically the entire class of models, both the stimulus-oriented models and the Poisson models.

Suppose, instead of noise, one uses a sinusoid of fixed intensity I, and determines the smallest increment that the subject can reliably detect—call that increment ΔI. Thus, a steady sinusoid replaces the external noise and the signal is an increment in this sinusoid. As a rough rule, we find that $\Delta I/I$ is constant, about 0.1. This relation is called Weber's law and has been known for over a century. One can find small but consistent departures from this rule [15], but as a first approximation, Weber's law holds over a range of about eight orders of magnitude in I. For high levels of I any fluctuation in the stimulus is at least 60 dB below I, so ΔI, which is a constant fraction of I, is enormous compared with any background fluctuation. Therefore, from the viewpoint of stimulus-oriented theories (for example, energy detector, envelope detector, or others) the detector becomes less and less efficient as the level of the steady sinusoid is increased, and predictions of detection performance based on stimulus characteristics alone become more and more inaccurate. There are only two means of escape: 1) assume some internal noise that grows with I, or 2) assume that the detection process can only distinguish between energy or envelope levels that differ by more than certain fixed amounts, that is, quantum assumptions. The ad hoc character of each of these routes is obvious. The Poisson model offers a third avenue of escape, and this alternative has some interesting implications.

The crux of this argument can be understood by again referring to Fig. 4. The input now is a sinusoid of intensity I. Since, by hypothesis, I is large compared with the background fluctuation, the distribution of energy along the x axis is essentially a line. When the signal is added to the constant sinusoid, the distribution of energy, still a line, moves to location $I+\Delta I$. Two distributions of neural counts are thereby produced. These two distributions will have means of $f(I)$ and $f(I+\Delta I)$. (See y axis of Fig. 4.) The detectability of the increment then depends solely on the variability of the number of counts. If f were nearly linear over its entire range, then the variability in the number of counts would decrease with I. Specifically, because the m/σ of a Poisson process is proportional to the square root of the number of counts, we would expect the m/σ to be proportional to I. Hence, if f were linear and detectability determined solely by internal fluctuation, then we would not expect $\Delta I/I$ to be constant, but rather to decrease as $I^{-\frac{1}{2}}$. If, however, f is some nonlinear function of I and, in particular, if f increases more slowly than the square-root relation, then $\Delta I/I$ will not decrease as I increases and one might hope to predict a relation such as Weber's law. The specific assumption about the form of f is of course also ad hoc, but the assumption of a particular nonlinear relation has a multitude of interesting implications.

Siebert fits his model to some of Kiang's data on frequency of firing versus intensity and suggests that the mean rate asymptotes rather sharply after only a two-order-of-magnitude change in I. Whitfield [34] reaches the same conclusion, using older data from Galambos and Davis [3]. Whitfield presented some qualitative speculations based on this "saturation" hypothesis and these speculations are similar to those suggested by Siebert in a more quantitative manner. The effect of this assumption of rather severe saturation has several interesting properties which Siebert is presently exploring in his more recent papers. McGill estimates the nonlinear transfer from energy to mean rate by fitting data relating ΔI to I. He concludes that the mean rate varies as $I^{\frac{1}{3}}$. This last relation is rather remarkable since it is almost exactly the transfer relation that Stevens [30] finds by asking subjects to judge the apparent growth of "loudness" as a function of intensity.

The study of the Poisson model has clearly just begun. In the near future we can expect to see a number of theoretical papers that will pursue the various implications of specific assumptions. We can also expect to see a number of experimental studies, especially those involving measurements of the Weber fraction in a variety of different detection situations.

Summary

We have reviewed some of the ways in which detection-theory analysis has been useful in trying to understand how a human sensory processing works. The first section of the paper emphasized its methodological contribution and how detection theory has been used to provide an analytic separation of the sensory and nonsensory variables. However, the fundamental nature of the detection or discrimination process, whether continuous or discrete, still remains in doubt. Next, after a brief review of the anatomy and physiology of the auditory system, we considered how detection theory has been used in the analysis of the auditory-detection process. The Poisson models were emphasized since they provide an explicit recognition of both internal and external fluctuation. Attempts to analyze trial-by-trial performance and the problem of Weber's law provided topics that illustrate the current application of detection theory.

The review has covered the several areas in varying degrees of detail. I hope I have indicated some of the major areas of research and the motivation behind these efforts as well as emphasized the variety of disciplines currently engaged in trying to understand the human senses.

Acknowledgment

The author wishes to thank G. Mandler, R. D. Luce, F. Wightman, and J. A. Swets for reading and criticizing an earlier draft of this paper, and D. E. Rumelhart for several lengthy discussions. Many of Dr. Rumelhart's ideas are present in the discussion of Weber's law.

References

[1] A. Ahumada, Jr., "Detection of tones masked by noise," Ph.D. dissertation, Dept. of Psychol., University of California, Los Angeles, 1967 (presented at 76th Meeting of the Acoustical Society of America).

[2] G. von Békésy, *Experiments in Hearing*, E. G. Wever, Ed. New York: McGraw-Hill, 1960.

[3] R. Galambos and H. Davis, "The response of single auditory-nerve fibers to acoustic stimulation," *J. Neurophysiol.*, vol. 6, pp. 39–57, 1943.

[4] D. M. Green, "Auditory detection of a noise signal," *J. Acoust. Soc. Am.*, vol. 32, pp. 121–131, 1960.

[5] D. M. Green and S. T. Sewall, "Effects of background noise on auditory detection of noise bursts," *J. Acoust. Soc. Am.*, vol. 34, pp. 1207–1216, 1962.

[6] D. M. Green, "Consistency of auditory detection judgments," *Psychol. Rev.*, vol. 71, pp. 392–407, 1964.

[7] D. M. Green and F. L. Moses, "On the equivalence of two recognition measures of short-term memory," *Psychol. Bull.*, vol. 66, pp. pp. 228–234, 1966.

[8] D. M. Green and J. A. Swets, *Signal Detection Theory and Psychophysics*. New York: Wiley, 1966.

[9] D. A. Huffman, "The generation of impulse-equivalent pulse trains," *IRE Trans. Information Theory*, vol. IT-8, pp. S10–S16, September 1962.

[10] L. A. Jeffress, "Stimulus-oriented approach to detection," *J. Acoust. Soc. Am.*, vol. 36, pp. 766–774, 1964.

[11] N. Y. S. Kiang, with assistance of T. Watanabe, E. C. Thomas, and L. F. Clarke, Cambridge, Mass.: M.I.T. Press, Research Monograph no. 35, 1966.

[12] D. H. Krantz, "Threshold theories of signal detection," *Psychol. Rev.*, vol. 76, no. 3, pp. 308–324, 1969.

[13] R. D. Luce, "A threshold theory for simple detection experiments," *Psychol. Rev.*, vol. 70, pp. 61–79, 1963.

[14] W. J. McGill, "Neural counting mechanisms and energy detection in audition," *J. Math. Psychol.*, vol. 4, pp. 351–376, 1967.

[15] W. J. McGill and J. P. Goldberg, "Pure-tone intensity discrimination and energy detection," *J. Acoust. Soc. Am.*, vol. 44, pp. 576–581, 1968.

[16] T. M. Marill, "Detection theory and psychophysics," M.I.T. Res. Lab. of Electronics, Cambridge, Mass., Tech. Rept. 319, 1956.

[17] J. Markowitz and J. A. Swets, "Signal detection with a fixed sample of masking noise," *J. Acoust. Soc. Am.*, vol. 42, p. 1194(A), 1967.

[18] W. A. Munson and J. E. Karlin, "The measurement of human channel transmission characteristics," *J. Acoust. Soc. Am.*, vol. 26, pp. 542–553, 1954.

[19] W. W. Peterson and T. G. Birdsall, "The theory of signal detectability," Electronic Defense Group, University of Michigan, Ann Arbor, Tech. Rept. 13, 1953.

[20] W. W. Peterson, T. G. Birdsall, and W. C. Fox, "The theory of signal detectability," *IRE Trans. Information Theory*, vol. PGIT-4, pp. 171–212, September 1954.

[21] S. M. Pfafflin and M. V. Mathews, "Detection of auditory signals in reproducible noise," *J. Acoust. Soc. Am.*, vol. 39, pp. 340–345, 1966.

[22] I. Pollack and R. Hsieh, "Sampling variability of the area under the ROC curve and d_e'," *Psychol. Bull.*, vol. 71, pp. 161–173, 1969.

[23] D. H. Raab and B. Leshowitz, "Use of an average response computer to provide reproducible bursts of noise," *J. Acoust. Soc. Am.*, vol. 44, pp. 282–283, 1968.

[24] G. L. Rasmussen and W. F. Windle, *Neural Mechanisms of the Auditory and Vestibular Systems*. Springfield, Ill.: Thomas, 1960.

[25] D. A. Ronken, "Intensity discrimination of Rayleigh noise," *J. Acoust. Soc. Am.*, vol. 45, pp. 54–57, 1969.

[26] C. W. Sherwin, F. Kodman, Jr., J. J. Kovaly, W. C. Prothe, and J. Melrose, "Detection of signals in noise: a comparison between the

human detector and an electronic detector," *J. Acoust. Soc. Am.*, vol. 28, pp. 617–622, 1956.

[27] W. M. Siebert, "Some implications of the stochastic behavior of primary auditory neurons," *Kybernetik*, vol. 2, pp. 206–215, 1965.

[28] ——, "Stimulus transformations in the peripheral auditory system," in *Recognizing Patterns*, P. A. Kolers and M. Eden, Eds. Cambridge, Mass.: M.I.T. Press, 1968.

[29] M. Smith and E. A. Wilson, "A model of the auditory threshold and its application to the problem of the multiple observer," *Psychol. Monogr.*, vol. 67, no. 9 (whole no. 359), 1953.

[30] S. S. Stevens, "On the psychophysical law," *Psychol. Rev.*, vol. 64, no. 3, pp. 153–181, 1957.

[31] W. P. Tanner, Jr., and J. A. Swets, "A new theory of visual detection," Electronic Defense Group, University of Michigan, Ann Arbor, Tech. Rept. 18, 1953.

[32] L. L. Thurstone, "A law of comparative judgment," *Psychol. Rev.*, vol. 34, pp. 273–286, 1927

[33] E. G. Wever and M. Lawrence, *Physiological Acoustics*. Princeton, N. J.: Princeton University Press, 1954.

[34] I. C. Whitfield, *The Auditory Pathway*. London: E. Arnold, 1967.

Part V

TIME RESOLUTION

Editor's Comments on Papers 25 Through 31

25 HAAS
The Influence of a Single Echo on the Audibility of Speech

26 RONKEN
Monaural Detection of a Phase Difference between Clicks

27 MILLER
Masking Effect of Periodically Pulsed Tones as a Function of Time and Frequency

28 ELLIOTT
Backward and Forward Masking of Probe Tones of Different Frequencies

29 PLOMP
Rate of Decay of Auditory Sensation

30 CRAIG and JEFFRESS
Effect of Phase on the Quality of a Two-Component Tone

31 HIRSH
Auditory Perception of Temporal Order

Obviously the auditory sense is time oriented. In contrast to the visual system, where ambient light is reflected continually from many contrasting patterns, most of the sources that furnish information to the auditory sense vibrate only when driven, and frequently the driving energy is an impulse or an impulse pattern. Such events can occur in very rapid succession, so that a basic question for the auditory system concerns the shortest time interval that can be perceived between two auditory events.

In the early 1930s, the question was raised in two very practical settings. The first concerned how sensitive the ear might be to the smearing of temporal patterns occasioned by reverberation in ordinary listening environments. According to Haas (Paper 25), Pezold, as early as 1927, had set 50msec as the auditory time threshold for "deterioration" of sound because of the mixing of reflections. Subsequent studies reveal that a single time constant will not suffice, though Atal, Schroeder, and Kuttruff (1962) devised an impressive method for deriving an auditory time constant from a prototypical signal. They used computer simulation to create the kind of rippled spectrum that single prominent echos produce from broad-band noise. From perceptual discrimination of the spectral ripples, they derived a time constant (1/e) of 9msec for the exponential weighting function of the auditory system's short-term power spectrum analysis.

The second practical application involved the fact that similar perceptual deterioration of rapidly changing complex sounds could occur if different frequencies were delayed by different amounts in telephone transmission (Steinberg, 1930). Bürck, Kotowski, and Lichte (1935) recognized that what mattered in such a case is the point at which the ear reacts to this as time distortion. In our discussion of pitch, we noted that these same authors tested the minimum onset separation at which two tones of similar frequency (f_1/f_2 = 1.1) would no longer sound coincident. In the mid-frequency range (.5–5kHz), the tone onsets could be separated by10msec before they no longer sounded simultaneous. At frequencies above or below this range, the time separation could be greater. Now we know that the frequency separations Bürck, Kotowski, and Lichte used are less than the width of the auditory critical band, and the results might differ for more widely separated signals. Patterson and Green (1970, appendix C) performed a highly similar experiment. With a much more sensitive technique, they got their subjects to recognize onset differences of less than 2msec when the frequency separations were large. But for tones within one critical band, subjects needed at least 8msec to discern temporal order of the two tones. The fact that this same kind of temporal distortion between widely separated frequencies can be detected by the auditory system in everyday listening was discovered almost accidentally.

In the process of developing wide-range loudspeaker systems with crossover network for different frequency ranges, careful listening revealed that the ear hears smaller timing discrepancies between frequency ranges than previously suspected. In such systems, without proper precaution, the low-frequency range may be delayed by as much as a millisecond more than the rest of the spectrum and, for familiar complex sounds, this does lead to the perception of time distortion in the sound (Hilliard, 1964).

On the other hand, Steinberg (1936) demonstrated that much

longer differences in delay between frequency bands on telephone transmission lines could be tolerated by the ear without appreciable loss of speech intelligibility. The system's versatility and adaptability continue to defy our attempts at a simple specification of its properties.

It should be noted that reflections from a wall had long before raised the question of a time-pattern response from the auditory system. Huygens in 1963 heard a pitch attributable to the time separation between the direct sound and the reflected sound from a nearby fountain. (See Bilsen, 1970, for the sequel to this kind of observation.) The processing of direct and reflected waves is a commonplace occurrence for the auditory system. Whether the auditory response to different spacings of reflected repetitions is mediated by spectral clues, temporal clues, or both is an open question in most instances.

The response made by the auditory system when it receives two temporally spaced copies of a waveform seems to be strongly a function of context. Room-acoustics coloration is probably the most frequent response, but when the spacing is around one to ten milliseconds, it is also easy to elicit the pitch response. This may arise from the damped-sinusoid response of a room's resonant frequency. But it may also have some relevance to our current discussion of time processing in the ear since it resembles the pitch associated with the period of a single pulse-pair spacing (McClellan and Small, 1967), the pitch change occasioned by shifting the polarity of the second pulse of a single-pulse pair (Nordmark, 1963), and the pitch response to small changes in the time interval between a single pair of tone bursts (Hiesey and Schubert, 1972). These all point toward the pulse pattern as the pitch clue when pulse spacings are of the order of a few milliseconds.

The spacing of waveform repetitions of the order of 10msec and longer represents those most frequently encountered in room listening, but the object of very little formal study until the development of tape recording made it practical to do the Haas experiments reported in Paper 25. At these intervals, where the system ought to separate individual pulses quite readily, a single fused image is the rule until the spacing is quite large—as the Haas study shows. Lochner and Burger (1958) verified Haas' results for speech and showed that tone bursts of 100msec duration behaved in a somewhat similar fashion.

As Gardner (1968) notes in his scholarly account of the background of the Haas effect, auditory reaction to physical echo spacings of a few milliseconds was recognized in the late nineteenth century. There is an abundance of subsequent experimental evidence that this order of time resolution is well within the capability of the system. We must consider, then, that the failure to hear an echo until the spacing reaches 30msec to 50msec is the result of an active fusing of the two copies, not an inability to separate them.

This fusing of similar waveforms is truly one of the remarkable talents of the auditory system, particularly in view of its facility in separating two different signals. It is probably, however, also at the root of our inability to discern easily its limits of temporal resolution. Possibly the most straightforward experimental pattern one could envision for ascertaining the minimum time separation discernible by the system is to take the signal most nearly punctate in time—a sharp click—and discover at what spacing the ear reports two signals rather than one. But in many settings, the most useful behavior for the system is to fuse these two identical signals into one image rather than report a double one. How much this influences the laboratory judgment of a single versus double click perception is difficult to determine.

In a study of the way in which a short auditory stimulus affects an immediately following one, Buytendijk and Meesters (1942) used pairs of clicks with varied spacing. When the clicks were separated by about 2msec, the listeners reported a slight roughness, at 3msec a decided "fluttering," and at 4msec to 7msec an "ever more distinct" double click. But they also reported that at a spacing of 10msec and beyond, the second click appeared louder than the first, and at 10msec it took about 12dB of attenuation of the second to make the two clicks subjectively equal. These results held whether both clicks were presented to the same ear or each to a different ear. It can be seen from the Haas study that this corresponds but poorly with the behavior of speech signals from loudspeakers with the same order of spacing between repetitions.

In connection with their study of binaural responses to click configurations, Wallach, Newman, and Rosenzweig (Paper 33) determined at what spacing a listener would hear a pair of monaural clicks as double. They discovered that if the temporal interval was gradually increasing (from that which gave a single impression), the spacing required to yield a clearly double sound was 6msec. If the interval was gradually decreased from a spacing that was clearly double, then the image remained double until the spacing was 3msec. Gescheider (1966) found that monaurally presented click pairs led to a report of a different image when the spacing was 1.6msec. His subjects were not instructed to wait for the perception of two separate parts but to report "double" when they "perceived a rough rather than a smooth sensation." This image emerged for a closer spacing—their time resolution was best—when the first click was 5dB to 10dB less than the second, possibly indicating that the tendency to fuse the images operates less strongly when the copy does not appear to be an attenuated reflection. Whether there exists a contradiction to the Haas effect in the click separation results is not easy to say, since the click experiments have used quite different response criteria, no one has repeated the Haas study with signals covering the range of durations from a few milliseconds to seconds, and—perhaps most important of all—we do not know whether the Haas effect is solely binaural or more general.

Judgments of click separation are not at all simple, nor is there general agreement among subjects. With small separations, (a millisecond or two), the quality of the click changes in ways that subjects describe differently, although they agree that it is a quality (sometimes pitch) difference. With separations ranging even up to 50msec or so, the stimulus has a rougher, perhaps two-peaked sort of sound, but still not always two cleanly separated clicks. This latter does not come about for most listeners until the separation is beyond 50msec to 60msec. Thus, from anecdotal reports, clicks do behave very much like the longer signals of Haas. The situation is made even more complex by Hirsh's report (Paper 31) that for dissimilar (differently filtered) clicks, the time separation required for the judgment of "double" was approximately the same as for similar ones. Possibly some minimal duration or some requisite waveform similarity is necessary before the fusion mechanism takes effect.

A modern approach to the two-click threshold is reported by Leshowitz (1971), who had his subjects compare the sound of a 20μsec click* with two 10μsec clicks moved from temporal contiguity (same as a 20μsec click) to a spacing wide enough to hear a difference between the 10-μsec pair and the single 20μsec click. Surprisingly he found that a 10μsec (silent) spacing between the clicks was enough for his observers to hear the difference 75 percent of the time.

Unfortunately if one is looking, by this method, for the ultimate time resolution, an alternate interpretation (preferred by Leshowitz) is that the two signals being compared differ in amplitude spectrum, and this is the cue being used by the auditory system. Of course, though it is of great theoretical interest which clue is being used, the practical implication is that two signals differing in only a microinterval of time differ also in perceptual response.

For a limited class of signals, Ronken (Paper 26) showed that it is possible to restrict the decision to a time clue alone. The paper is included here because it is an ingenious solution to the two problems: one of not depending on the subject's perception of two images, the second of matching all relevant aspects of the signal except its time course (phase spectrum). Resnick and Feth (1975) adopted the same idea but employed improved psychoacoustic technique and a wider variety of click patterns. With optimum choice of both overall level and difference between levels of the two clicks composing the pair,

*These are specifications of the driving waveform at the input to the phone.

their listeners could discern click-pair reversals when the spacing was 0.5msec, the smallest spacing they reported. Hall and Lummis (1973) were able to show differences in detectability of a click pair and its time reversal when the total waveform duration of the click pair plus gap (electrically) was only 350μsec. Since they used a very wide-range transducer (one-inch condenser microphone), the acoustic waveforms were presumably also very short. Hall and Lummis advanced as the most likely explanation of this difference in detectability the fact that the normal and the reversed waveform of such a click pair would have a different peak pressure (even though total energy is the same), but at least this would indicate a time-sensitive processing in the sense that energy is not simply integrated by the auditory system over the entire 350μsec duration. Ideally the set of equal-energy, matched-duration signals generated by Patterson and Green (1970) as Huffman sequences should be the generalization of the two-click experimental pattern. Using a class of signals that have the same spectrum, same total energy, and same duration, they made at least a beginning in exploring what kinds of differences can be discriminated by the auditory analyzer for very short signals. (See Green, 1971, for a concise review.)

Apparently these various bits of evidence indicate that the system *can* follow some rapid changes. What exacerbates the theoretical problem is that its most adaptive behavior as a sensory system consists in ignoring changes not likely to be preserved in most of its listening environments.

Life would be simpler for the auditory theorist if the auditory system could be viewed as a passive, stationary analyzer. But evidence abounds that its responses are frequently influenced by its immediate past history or even its long-term experience. Thus our analysis of the temporal resolution of the system is complicated by the fact that masking phenomena extend both directions in time.

Two studies reported in 1947 moved our understanding of the nature of auditory interference of closely spaced sounds much further ahead. In an extensive study of the "decay of sensation" for the auditory system, Lüscher and Zwislocki (1947) plotted the amount of threshold shift for a short tone burst (20msec) following a tone of 400msec at various sound pressure levels. Typical of these results is a curve showing that for a 60dB SPL tone at 1kHz lasting 400msec, the threshold for the 20msec burst twenty milliseconds after cessation of the first tone is 22dB above normal; and even though initial recovery appears to be taking place at a rapid rate (400dB/sec), it will still be about 0.2sec before sensitivity is back to normal.

Shortly after, Munson and Gardner (1950), apparently without knowledge of the Lüscher and Zwislocki work, measured the amount of threshold shift for a short probe tone that ended 98msec after the end of the masking tone. They called the shift of the second tone *residual* masking.

At about the same time, R. L. Miller (Paper 27) explored the amount that a short tone burst was shifted in threshold by another tone burst of different but adjacent frequency as its time relation to the original burst varied over several milliseconds. He showed that an interfering tone can have an effect on a test tone that acually occurred a few milliseconds earlier—an unexpected outcome. Although Miller did not use the term, these are the data that gave rise to the concept of backward masking.

These two types of interference between temporally contiguous signals have been exhaustively studied since those early attempts and are now known as forward and backward masking, respectively. A capsule view of the effects of these two forms of interference is afforded in Paper 28 by Elliott. This brief synopsis is all that space permits here, but it does not do justice to the imagination and vigor that characterize the work on nonsimultaneous masking. The interested reader should consult other work by Elliott (1962, 1971) and others (Duifhuis, 1973; Penner, 1974).

Recently Zwicker (1976a, b) has also developed a technique for exploring the more dynamic aspects of the masking of high frequencies by low-frequency signals of various shapes. Invoking the analog of time-locked average techniques, he records the amount of masking as a high-frequency probe is made to occupy various positions in the cycle of the low-frequency masker. He reports slopes of the masking period as high as 10dB/msec. It is apparent that a rather complex form of interference between temporally contiguous signals operates to determine the eventual temporal resolution of the ear.

Since we know so few of the details of auditory processing, perhaps the most practical question to pose in assessing temporal resolution is a very simple one: How long does it take for the excitation pattern for a given signal to die away (that is, for what period is the system preoccupied with the processing of the previous signal)? Békésy (1929) addressed this problem by finding the decay rate for which subjects could not tell the difference between an abrupt and a gradual decay and concluded that regardless of level, the excitation pattern died to threshold level in 140msec. Miller (1948), using essentially the same approach, arrived at a figure roughly half as long but still endorsed the same principle: that the time taken for remaining excitation to disappear is independent of level. But Plomp, noting that if one plots Miller's data with log time as the abscissa and looking also at the numerous studies attempting to portray the immediately postsignal behavior of the auditory system, took quite a different view of what constitutes minimum separation time between two signals (Paper 29).

Plomp's figure 8 is especially interesting; it indicates that even for signals of long duration compared with clicks (200msec), the effect of the second signal can be discerned for medium-level signals when the separation is only two or three milliseconds. Thus though the work of Lüscher and Zwislocki has shown that after a medium-duration signal, it does take time for the system to recover to completely normal (pre-signal) sensitivity, the Plomp data suggest that the system can still make a useful response within a much shorter interval. Penner's work (1977) pursues this type of resolution closer to the ultimate and indicates that subjects can detect a gap of approximately 0.5msec between two 2msec bursts of random noise.

In searching for evidence of the capability of the auditory system to recognize timing patterns, one must include the evidence that the system discriminates between simple intraperiod monaural phase patterns. The report by Craig and Jeffress (Paper 30) is the classic paper on this aspect of monaural processing. Later Nixon, Raiford, and Schubert (1970) proposed a technique whereby phase changes can be readily heard, and Raiford and Schubert (1971) demonstrated that some subjects can hear changes of thirty degrees, corresponding to a time-pattern change—at the frequencies used—of 167μsec. Detection of monaural phase changes—historically a controversial area—may yet prove to be a good mechanism for exploring one form of time resolution capability.

It must be eminently apparent that what we arrive at as the limit of time-pattern resolution is dependent on the signals used and the questions asked of the listener. Hirsh asked his listeners to tell which of two signals began earliest and got the oft-cited result (see Paper 31) that seventeen to twenty milliseconds difference in onset time is required. Broadbent and Ladefoged cited evidence in a brief note (1959) and offered persuasive logic for the view that continued experience with rapid sequences has a dramatic effect. Warren (1969) later sampled the other end of this order-perceiving dimension when he exposed subjects to four unrelated sounds (high tone, low tone, hiss, buzz) and found that to get subjects to recognize their order of occurrence on first exposure, the onsets had to be separated by as much as 700msec. Neisser and Hirst (1974) have since demonstrated that, with practice, recognition of sequence with signals of the sort used by Warren can be achieved when the signals are of the order of 25msec in length—close to the length of individual phonemes of speech, which, of course, are even more highly practiced (if, indeed, they continue to be processed as individual phonemes).

Patterson and Green (1970, appendix C) repeated part of the Hirsh experiment with long tones (500msec) and got essentially the Hirsh result. By contrast, with their short-tone bursts (10msec), they found that starting time discrepancies of about 2msec led to a difference in perception when one tone rather than the other preceded. Efron (1973) has confirmed the value of about 2msec as sufficient for recognizing which of two short tone bursts of different frequency began earlier.

We now know also from the work of Divenyi and Hirsh (1975) on short melodic sequences, from Watson et al. (1975) on rapid tonal patterns, and from the effect of changes in voice onset time (Lisker and Abramson, 1967) that the system frequently makes use of time separations of the order of twenty to forty milliseconds. Again, however, on closer scrutiny of a particular behavior, the reaction of the system turns out to be dependent on the nature of the specific signal and frequently on the previous history of the auditory system.

REFERENCES

Atal, B. S., M. R. Schroeder, and K. H. Kuttruff. 1962. Perception of coloration in filtered Gaussian noise—Short-time spectral analysis by the ear. *Fourth Int. Cong. Acoust., Copenhagen, Paper H31.*

Békésy, G. V. 1929. Zur theorie des Hörens; über die eben merkbare amplituden- und frequenz-änderung eines tones; die theorie des schwebungen. *Physik. Zeitschrift* **30**:721-745.

Bilsen, F. A. 1970. Repetition pitch; Its implication for hearing theory and room acoustics. In *Frequency analysis and periodicity detection in hearing,* ed. R. Plomp and G. F. Smoorenburg, pp. 291-299. Leiden: Sijthoff.

Broadbent, D. E., and P. Ladefoged, 1959. Auditory perception of temporal order. *Acoust. Soc. Am. J.* **31**:1539(L).

Bürck, W., P. Kotowski, and H. Lichte. 1935. Die hörbarkeit von laufzeitdifferenzen. *Elektr. Nachr. Tec.* **12**:355-367.

Buytendijk, F. J. J., and A. Meesters, 1942. Duration and course of the auditory sensation. *Commentat. Pontif. Acad. Sci.* **6**:557-576.

Divenyi, P. L., and I. J. Hirsh. 1975. The effect of blanking on the identification of temporal order in three-tone sequences. *Percept. Psychophys.* **17**:246-252.

Duifhuis, H. 1973. Consequences of peripheral frequency selectivity for nonsimultaneous masking. *Acoust. Soc. Am. J.* **54**:1471-1488.

Efron, R. 1973. Conservation of temporal information by perceptual systems. *Percept. Psychophys.* **14**:518-530.

Elliot, L. L. 1962. Backward masking: monotic and dichotic conditions. *Acoust. Soc. Am. J.* **34**:1108-1115.

Elliott, L. L. 1971. Forward and backward masking. *Audiol.* **10**:65-76.

Gardner, M. B. 1968. Historical background of the Haas and/or precedence effect. *Acoust. Soc. Amer. J.* **43**:1243-1248.

Gescheider, G. 1966. Resolving of successive clicks by the ears and skin. *J. Exp. Psychol.* **71**:378-381.

Green, D. M. 1971. Temporal auditory acuity. *Psychol. Rev.* **78**:540-551.

Hall, J. L., and R. C. Lummis. 1973. Thresholds for click pairs masked by bandstop noise. *Acoust. Soc. Am. J.* **54**:593-599.

Hiesey, R. W., and E. D. Schubert, 1972. Cochlear resonance and phase-reversed signals, *Acoust. Soc. Am. J.* **51**:518-519.

Hilliard, J. K. 1964. Notes on how phase and delay distortion affect the sound quality of speech, music and sound effects. *IEEE Trans. Acoust.* **AU-12**: 23–25.

Leshowitz, B. 1971. Measurement of the two-click threshold. *Acoust. Soc. Am. J.* **49**:462–466.

Lisker, L., and A. S. Abramson, 1967. The voicing dimension: Some experiments in comparative phonetics. *Sixth Int. Cong. Phon. Sci., Prague, Proc.*, 563–567.

Lochner, J. P. A., and J. F. Burger, 1958. The subjective masking of short-time delayed echoes by their primary sounds and their contribution to the intelligibility of speech. *Acustica* **8**:1–10.

Lüscher, E., and J. Zwislocki. 1947. The decay of sensation and the remainder of adaptation after short pure-tone impulses on the ear. *Acta Otolaryngol.* **35**: 428–445.

McClellan, M. E., and A. M. Small, Jr. 1967. Pitch perception of pulse pairs with random repetition rate. *Acoust. Soc. Am. J.* **41**:690–699.

Miller, G. A. 1948. The perception of short bursts of noise. *Acoust. Soc. Am. J.* **20**: 160–170.

Munson, W. A., and Gardner, M. B. 1950. Loudness patterns—a new approach. *Acoust. Soc. Am. J.* **22**:177–188.

Neisser, U., and Hirst, W. 1974. Effect of practice on the identification of auditory sequences. *Percept. Psychophys.* **15**:391–398.

Nixon, J. C., C. A. Raiford, and E. D. Schubert. 1970. Technique for investigating monaural phase effects. *Acoust. Soc. Am. J.* **48**:554–556.

Nordmark, J. O. 1963. Some analogies between pitch and laterilzation phenomena. *Acoust. Soc. Am. J.* **35**:1544–1547.

Patterson, J. H., and D. M. Green. 1970. Discrimination of transient signals having identical energy spectra. *Acoust. Soc. Am. J.* **48**:894–905.

Penner, M. J. 1974. Effect of masker duration and masker level on forward and backward masking. *Acoust. Soc. Am. J.* **56**:179–182.

Penner, M. J. 1977. Detection of temporal gaps in noise as a measure of the decay of auditory sensation. *Acoust. Soc. Am. J.* **61**:552–557.

Raiford, C. A., and E. D. Schubert, 1971. Recognition of phase changes in octave complexes. *Acoust. Soc. Am. J.* **50**:559–567.

Resnick, S. B., and Feth, L. L. 1975. Discriminability of time-reversed click pairs: Intensity effects. *Acoust. Soc. Am. J.* **57**:1493–1499.

Steinberg, J. C. 1930. Effects of phase distortion on telephone quality. *Bell Syst. Tech. J.* **9**:550–566.

Steinberg, J. C. 1936. The sense of hearing, speech and music, and effects of distortion. In *Electrical engineers' handbook,* 3d ed., H. Pender and K. McIlwain, pp. 9–32. New York: Wiley.

Warren, R. M., C. J. Obusek, R. M. Farmer, and R. P. Warren. 1969. Auditory sequence: Confusion of patterns other than speech and music. *Science* **164**: 586–587.

Watson, C. S., H. W. Wroton, W. J. Kelly, and C. A. Benbassat. 1975. Factors in the discrimination of tonal patterns. I: Component frequency, temporal position, and silent intervals. *Acoust. Soc. Am. J.* **57**:1175–1185.

Zwicker, E. 1976a. Psychoacoustic equivalent of period histograms. *Acoust. Soc. Am. J.* **59**:166–175.

Zwicker, E. 1976b. Masking period patterns of harmonic complex tones. *Acoust. Soc. Am. J.* **60**:429–439.

25

Reprinted from *Audio Eng. Soc. J.* **20**:146–159 (1972)

The Influence of a Single Echo on the Audibility of Speech*

HELMUT HAAS

A thorough investigation was made of the influence of a single echo as a function of different parameters on the audibility of speech. An apparatus was built for the artificial generation of echoes and measurements were made with a large number of observers under specified conditions.

Editor's Note: Through the efforts of Edward M. Long, whose paper appears earlier in this issue, we are pleased indeed to publish the English translation of Dr. Haas' now-famous paper. To the best of our knowledge, this dissertation has never been published in the United States, and we are certain that many working in the field would benefit from reading the "Haas Effect."

INTRODUCTION: Sounds produced in rooms suffer numerous reflections from boundary surfaces and furniture. A reflected sound reaches the observer later than the direct sound, and major path differences or delay time (transit time) differences may impair or even spoil the acoustical effect. A sufficiently long time difference causes the direct sound and the reflected sound to be heard separately, that is to say, one hears an echo in the usual sense of the word. In the present paper the term "echo" will cover all reflections of sounds, independent of the magnitude of the delay time.

The threshold value of the delay time, above which a noticeable deterioration of the acoustical impression occurs, has been called "threshold of masking" by Petzold [1]. He gave as the value for speech.

$$t = 0.05 \pm 0.01 \text{ second}$$

corresponding to a path difference in air $s = 17 \pm 3$ m.

In rather small rooms such a difference would occur only after many reflections. No disturbance due to echo is to be expected because the intensity of the often reflected sound is very much reduced after 50 ms. Besides, the ear receives in quick succession a great number of reflections, decreasing in intensity, and the hearer is not capable of perceiving them separately. This gradual decay of sounds in rooms is called reverberation. A certain reverberation time is even advantageous for audibility, since it entails an intensification of the sound as well as a pleasant modification of the character of the tone.

The critical delay time can easily be exceeded in large rooms, after only one reflection, or after a few reflections. A bad effect upon the representation is likely to result if the energy of the reflected sound is sufficiently high to accentuate certain points in the reverberation curve of a gradually decaying sound. In the extreme case a real echo will be heard.

The possibility of estimating in advance the extent of likely disturbances due to echoes is of paramount importance in the design and construction of buildings. Irritating echo phenomena caused by sufficiently great time differences can also occur in connection with the arti-

* This paper was submitted as a dissertation toward the doctor's degree to the University of Gottingen, Gottingen, Germany, under the title, "Über den Einfluss des Einfachechos auf die Horsamkeit von Sprache." The present translation from the German by Dr. Ing. K.P.R. Ehrenberg is reprinted with permission from the Building Research Station, Watford, Herts., England, Library Communication no. 363, December 1949.

ficial amplification of sounds indoors, or with the transmission of sounds by means of several loudspeakers placed at distances from each other. Lastly, echo phenomena occur with disturbing effects under certain conditions in telecommunications.

The object of the following investigation is to determine the influence of echoes on the audibility of speech in binaural hearing, as a function of various parameters, viz., delay time, intensity, timbre, and direction. The investigation has been confined to single echoes, i.e., only one repetition following the direct sound, in order to obtain simpler conditions, and to limit the experimental requirements. Measurements have been made as far as the results are of practical significance. No previous investigations on such a scale with a large number of observers taking part have been made in this field. Decker [2] studied echo phenomena occurring in telephone connections over long cables. When the intensity of the echo was equal to that of the primary sound, 50% of 50 pairs of observers felt disturbed in the flow of their conversation when the delay time difference was 100 ms. The critical difference rose to 150 ms when the echo amplitude was only 60% of the amplitude of the primary sound.

Stumpp [3] studied in the open air the influence of different directions of the incidence of a single echo equal in intensity to the primary sound. The critical delay time difference was 80 ms for speech and echo coming from the same lateral direction, but 50 ms for opposite lateral directions.

DESCRIPTION OF EQUIPMENT FOR ARTIFICIAL GENERATION OF ECHOES

An accurate control of the properties of reflected sound necessitates a device for the artificial generation of echoes, capable of repeating a sound phenomenon after a fixed time. This problem can be tackled in different ways.

1) Delay by electrical network. This solution is excluded because of the order of magnitude of the time differences required, and because of the wide frequency range involved.

2) Delay by using the finite velocity of sound in a medium, e.g., air in a long tube. Such an apparatus would be very cumbersome, varying the delay time by small steps would be difficult, but, most important, already an upper limiting frequency of 5,000 Hz and a delay time of 200 ms (length of the tube conduit 68 m) would cause very high damping [4], which hardly could be compensated without special expenditure.

3) Delay by using two pickups from a single record, or by staggered pickup from two identical records. At first sight this simple solution appeared appropriate, but further examination proved the apparatus to be rather complex, if convenient and exact working was to be achieved, even apart from the poor frequency range of the phonograph method.

4) Delay by the magnetophone method. Although this is expensive, it has been chosen because it best fulfills the requirements. The idea is that the sound process to be delayed is magnetically recorded on a tape, from which the direct sound and the echo can be picked up with any delay needed in practice.

Fig. 1 shows the block diagram of this installation. The microphone M transforms the sound, in the following investigation chiefly speech, into voltage modulations, to be amplified and conducted to the recording channels of the magnetophone apparatus. If the same text is to be used repeatedly for certain measurements, it can be recorded and played back by means of a magnetic tape apparatus. The changeover switch after the microphone amplifier is used to select direct or indirect reproduction. The level is controlled, and kept constant by means of a level monitor.

The actual delay of sound is produced by an endless-tape magnetophone apparatus, sketched on top of Fig. 1, and registered by the high-frequency method.

Two pivoted guide rollers R, 150 mm in diameter, carrying a loop of normal magnetic tape, are fixed at a distance of 1 m. A rubber roller presses the tape against the shaft of a synchronous motor (n = 1500 r/min),

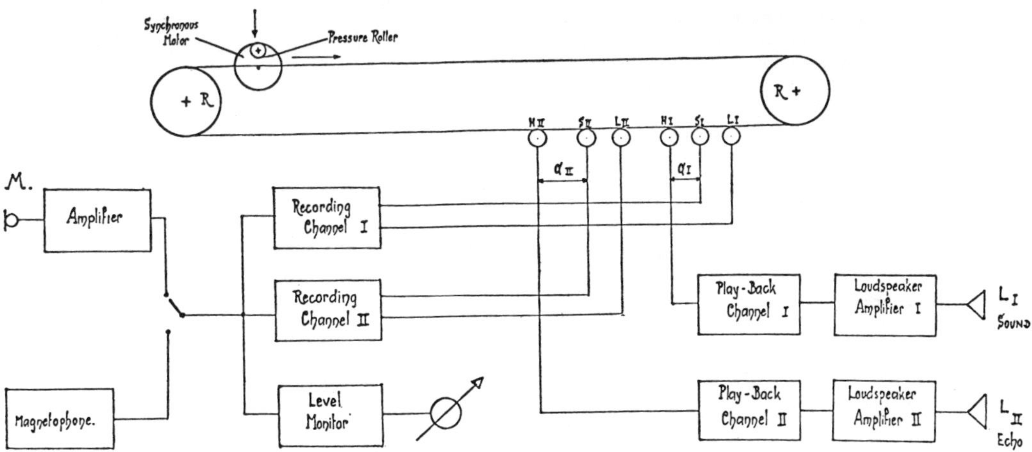

Fig. 1. Block diagram of echo apparatus.

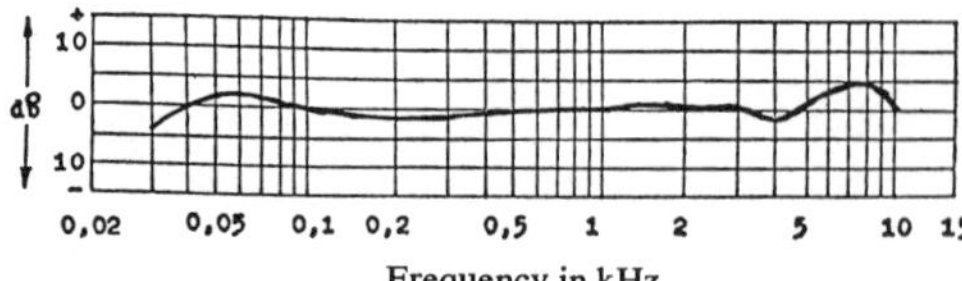

Fig. 2. Frequency response curve of microphone (according to manufacturer).

which drives it at a speed of 77 cm/s in the direction of the arrow. Circles indicate the wiping heads L_I and L_{II}, playback heads H_I and H_{II}, and the recording heads S_I and S_{II}, all fixed on an optical bench, H_{II} being movable along the line of the tape.

The equipment operates in the following manner. L_I and L_{II}, fed with high frequency (about 80000 Hz) from the recording heads, wipe out the magnetic records on the tape. S_I and S_{II} are excited from the recording channels I and II, which on the input side are connected in parallel. This signal is then picked up by the playback heads H_I and H_{II}. The delay difference Δt is determined by

$$\Delta t \approx (a_{II} - a_I)/v$$

where a_I denotes the distance between the gaps of S_I–H_I, a_{II} the corresponding distance S_{II}–H_{II}, and v the speed of the tape. The transit difference is $\Delta t = 0$ for $a_I = a_{II}$, i.e., the sound phenomena are picked up simultaneously as they were recorded. The echo delays are adjusted by moving H_{II} along a scale calibrated in milliseconds.

It was originally thought that an echo could be obtained from the time difference between the direct sound and a simple recording via the playback head, but it would not then have been possible to reduce a_I, and with it the delay difference, to a very small value. Double recording was therefore necessary.

The levels induced by the moving magnetic tape at H_I and H_{II} are fed to two separate playback channels I and II and amplified. The loudspeaker L_I emits the original sound, and L_{II} the same sound delayed in time, i.e., the echo.

The first sound phenomenon, hereafter called "direct sound" or "primary sound," is also produced from a loudspeaker. This appeared expedient in order to prevent acoustical feedback and to avoid any disturbing effect of the echo on the speaker.

Special consideration was given to appropriate dimensions with a view to excluding as far as possible inaccurate results due to the reproducing apparatus.

The recording microphone was a dynamic one, with a frequency response curve, according to information obtained from the manufacturer, as shown in Fig. 2 (output level across 200 ohms for constant sound pressure at the microphone as a function of frequency).

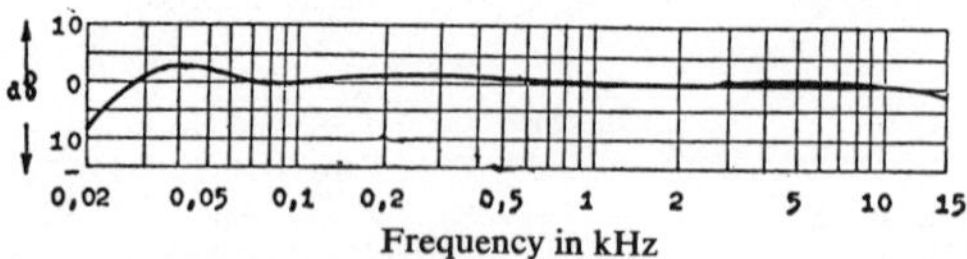

Fig. 3. Frequency response curve of magnetophone apparatus.

The reproduction is most favorable for high frequencies above 5000 Hz, provided that the direction of the speech is suitable.

The frequency response characteristic of the microphone amplifier is perfectly flat over the relevant range. The magnetic recording and reproducing equipment is also flat. The overall frequency response characteristics of both magnetophone channels are practically identical; they are given in Fig. 3 for the use of a *c* tape. The output level of the playback head for constant level of the recording channel is measured as a function of frequency. Curve I on Fig. 4 is the frequency response curve of the loudspeaker amplifier, the output level being plotted for loading and a constant input level. The resistance frequency characteristic I of this amplifier can be altered in steps according to curves II and III. Again care was taken to obtain identical frequency response curves for both amplifiers.

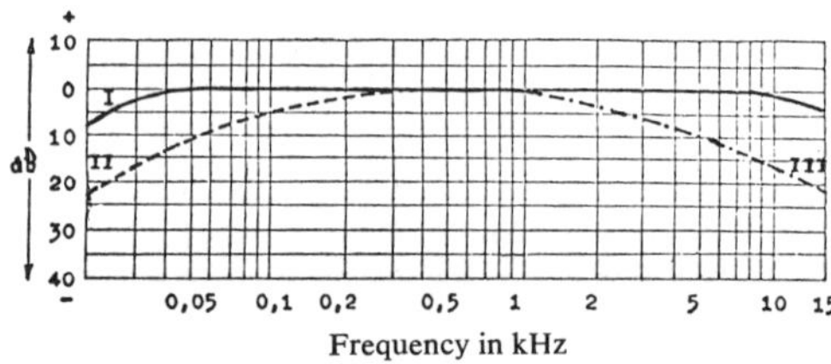

Fig. 4. Frequency response curve of loudspeaker amplifier.

The weakest link in the system is the loudspeaker. Numerous types, made by different manufacturers, were tested. Finally a dynamic 12.5-W loudspeaker (30-cm diameter of diaphragm) with a permanent magnet was chosen, and the two specimens selected were as near to uniformity as possible. These loudspeakers were placed in small, square baffle boards (40 by 40 cm), supported by easily transportable racks so that they were at the height of the observer's head. The baffle boards were used to prevent reflections from large walls when the loudspeakers stood opposite each other. The large diameter of the diaphragm was chosen in order to obtain sufficient emission of low frequencies, even with small baffle boards. A special system for the emission of high frequencies was not used, since the expenditure was not thought to be justified. Such piezoelectric loudspeakers as were tested showed a great number of very pronounced resonance points within the important range. The emission of high frequencies from small dynamic loudspeakers was very little superior to that of the large type actually used.

Fig. 5 shows the sound pressure as a function of frequency for one of the loudspeakers employed for the measurements described hereafter, at a distance of 2 m on the axis and in the 40- by 40-cm baffle board. The loudspeaker was driven from the loudspeaker amplifier, the input terminals of which were fed with an ac voltage of constant amplitude.

As no damped sound room was available, the measurements were made in the open air, on the roof of the Institute. Interference due to reflections from the floor was eliminated by placing the baffle board immediately upon the roof, viz., so that the axis of the loudspeaker

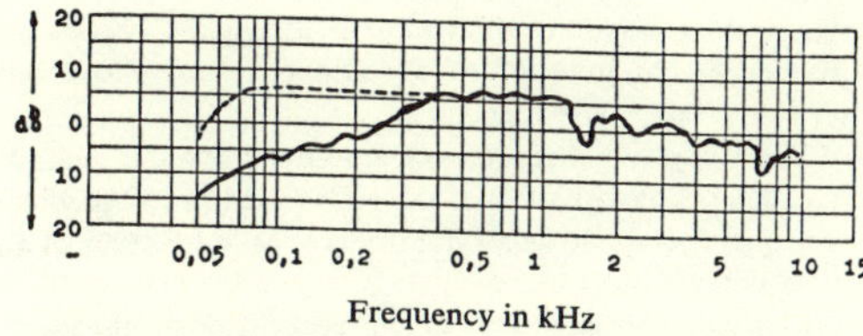

Fig. 5. Frequency response curve of loudspeaker (sound pressure on median line).

was focused upon the measuring microphone which was close to the floor. The sound pressure was measured by a calibrated spherical condenser microphone, 3.5 m in diameter, with its sound pressure response compensated by electrical filters. The sound pressure as a function of frequency was taken with a Neumann level recorder.

The dashed curve in Fig. 5 indicates the sound pressure curve for the same loudspeaker when used in a baffle board of infinite size (the wall of a house). The distance to the microphone was again 2 m in the axis.

The overall frequency response characteristic of the echo system, combined from Figs. 2–5, is shown in Fig. 6. The sound pressure at a distance of 2 m from the playback loudspeaker in the direction of its axis is plotted against frequency for constant sound pressure at the receiving microphone. It is seen that the greatest deviations within the frequency range from 100 to 10 000 Hz amount to ± 7 dB.

No nonlinear distortions could be detected in the oscillogram of a pure tone of 1000 Hz. Since the loudspeaker amplifier and the loudspeaker have been dimensioned with a sufficient margin, it follows that the magnitude of the distortion factor is determined essentially by the magnetophone equipment. The value is given in the literature as < 3% at 800 Hz.

The results obtained from objective measurements made it appear that the installation was quite suitable for the transmission of natural speech. This has been confirmed by subjective measurements. A trained team reached 96% intelligibility for syllables across the whole installation. This value is also the maximum for direct transmission between mouth and ear. The remaining 4% are explained by occasional inattention of observers or poor articulation by the speaker.

The slight linear distortions of the system can affect the timbre of the speaker, but they do not reduce the intelligibility and are therefore not detrimental.

EXPERIMENTS WITH SMALL DIFFERENCES

Auditory performances in smaller rooms are always connected with echoes following the direct sound after a brief interval. Let us imagine a conversation in a normal living room where the smooth surface of the ceiling will reflect sound. For simplification, the walls and the floor can be assumed to be more or less sound absorbing. The regular decay of the reverberation will then be replaced by individual echoes. Such echoes arriving after a short time are not disturbing, in spite of the fact that the energy of the reflected sound is not appreciably lower than that of the direct sound. On the contrary, conversations without such small reflections are felt to be more tiring and less natural; this can be observed, for instance, in a damped room, or outdoors in the presence of a deep cover of fresh snow.

This experience shows that our organ of hearing accepts as an entirely natural process the integration of the direct sound impressions together with their immediately following reflections. The question arises then, how the hearing of a sound without reflections differs from one with slightly delayed echoes. The following experimental arrangement has been devised for the solution of this problem.

In the absence of a dead room the investigation had to be made outdoors, and the flat roof of the Institute, a detached building, proved suitable. Some projecting parts were covered with inclined timber walls to deflect the incident sound upwards.

The positions for loudspeaker and observer were chosen with a view to reducing to a minimum echoes from an annex about 20 m distant. Points were determined by giving short sound impulses from a loudspeaker, and receiving the reflections in a microphone at the observer's eventual stand, with oscillographical registration.

The influence of reflections from the surface of the roof was eliminated by placing the loudspeaker, focused on the observer's head, immediately upon the roof in a 40- by 40-cm baffle board. However, this reflection from the ground was found to have no effect on the results of the measurements, so that afterwards the loudspeakers were always placed at the height of the observer's head, a procedure closer to practical conditions.

Two loudspeakers of the same type were placed 3 m distant from the observer at an angle of 45°, half to the right and half to the left of him. The only reason for this particular arrangement was that it proved to be the best for balancing. The loudspeaker axes were focused on the observer in order to prevent a fall in the high frequencies owing to the directional characteristics of the loudspeakers. Both loudspeakers were then at the same intensity; the loudness at the observer's position was about 50 phon, checked by comparing the loudness with the reference tone and a calibrated microphone.

Prior to the start of the measurements, the delay difference is set at zero, and the position of the head of the observer is chosen so that the sound appears to arrive directly from the front. (See also the remark on directional hearing below.) The observer maintains his position during the subsequent measurements. The imaginary sound source which for the zero difference had been located directly in front was found to move gradually in the direction of the primary loudspeaker when differences between zero and 1 ms were tried, i.e., very small differences influence the directional impression. Now let the speech from the echo loudspeaker be delayed by 10 ms, corresponding to a path difference in air of approximately 3.4 m. This has the remarkable effect that

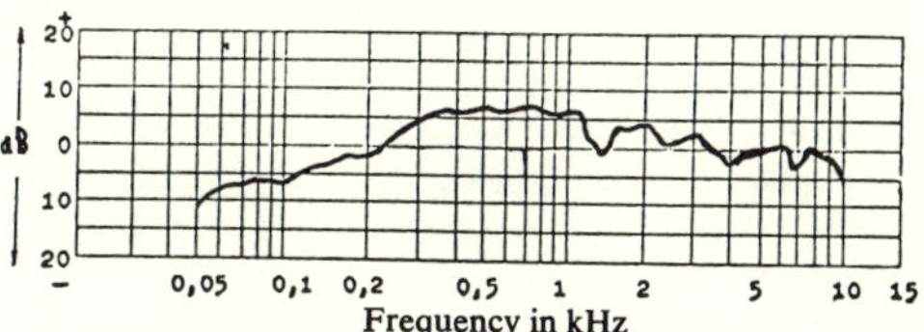

Fig. 6. Total frequency response curve of echo apparatus.

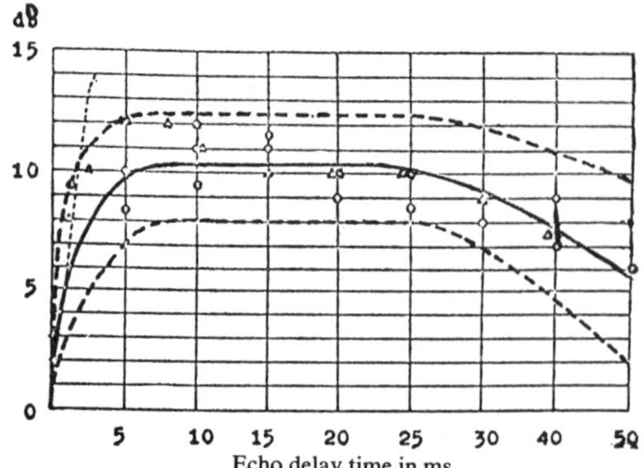

Fig. 7. Echo suppression effect as a function of delay time for speech.

the echo loudspeaker is not heard at all, although its energy is equal to that of the primary loudspeaker. Apparently the speech issues only from the latter. An explanation for this phenomenon cannot be given. It is probably due to a function of our central nervous system, and a possible explanation may be some kind of blocking reaction, caused by the first sound impression, preventing the separate perception of repetitions of the same impression following after brief intervals. Possibly the rise with time of the nerve reaction currents contributes to directional hearing.

The factors which acoustically enable us to state the direction of a sound reaching the ears have been studied thoroughly by v. Bekesy [5], Reich and Behrens [6], de Boer [7] and Warnecke [8]. These authors discovered that the directional discrimination is produced by differences of transit time and intensity as the sound reaches the two ears. However, the differences observed by these workers were mostly in the range between zero and 0.62 ms, corresponding to a path difference in air up to 21 cm. This is nearly the largest path difference with which sound impressions from a single source can reach our ears. Further increases of the path difference do not affect the directional impression.

What then can be observed when the difference is further increased? Hearing both loudspeakers with differences from 1 to 30 ms differs from hearing only one of them by a modification of the quality of the sound and a greater loudness, which will be discussed at a later stage. The impression is that of more "liveliness," the sound is growing in "body," and the sound source gains volume. This "pseudostereophonic" effect has been known for some time and was utilized as early as 1926 for the construction of the ultraphone [9], that is a normal disc recorder with two mechanical pickup heads arranged to pick up from the same disc with a time difference of 1/15–1/30 s. The same effect can be achieved with two loudspeakers operating simultaneously while the transit time difference is obtained by different distances between the two loudspeakers and the observer.

This condition is obtained without marked modification between 1- and 30-ms differences. Only when the difference reaches a value around 40 ms is the loudspeaker recognized as an additional sound source, but the sound source is still located at the position of the primary loudspeaker. A further increase beyond 50 ms makes it possible to discriminate a separate echo, but the "center of gravity" of the sound emission still rests on the primary loudspeaker.

The following method was employed for the quantitative determination of the subjective "suppression effect" observed for small delay differences, as a function of the echo delay time.

Both loudspeakers, arranged according to the above description, gave a continuous spoken text. The delay difference was statistically altered, in steps, from 1 to 40 ms.

An attenuator, calibrated in dB, enabled the observer to reduce the intensity of the primary loudspeaker until both appeared to be heard at the same loudness. This does not produce any "direct-in-front" impression as in the case of very small differences. Rather the sensation of two sound sources emitting from different directions, coinciding with the position of the loudspeakers, is produced. No difficulty was encountered by the observers in adjusting both sound sources to equal loudness of a spoken text, and scattering was relatively small. The location of both sound sources at an angle of 45° to the left and right side of the observer proved particularly favorable for loudness balancing.

The results obtained with 15 observers are shown in Fig. 7, where the difference of intensities in dB is plotted as a function of the delay time, that is, the reduction of the intensity of the primary loudspeaker required to produce the sensation of equal loudness for both sources. The full-line curve gives the mean value of all measuring points, the dashed lines show the limits of the deviations.

A distinction has been made between the points obtained from two different observers, with the purpose of showing the quantity of the deviations for individual observers.

De Boer gave the data on which the thin dotted line was based, but he obtained them by a different, indirect, method. His starting point was the perception that differences of time as well as of intensity reaching the ears of the observer bring about a directional impression. He placed two loudspeakers 3.5 m from each other, behind a canvas screen, focused on an observer standing in the direction of the median line to the connecting line of the two loudspeakers, at a distance of 3 m from the screen, which was used only in order to conceal the

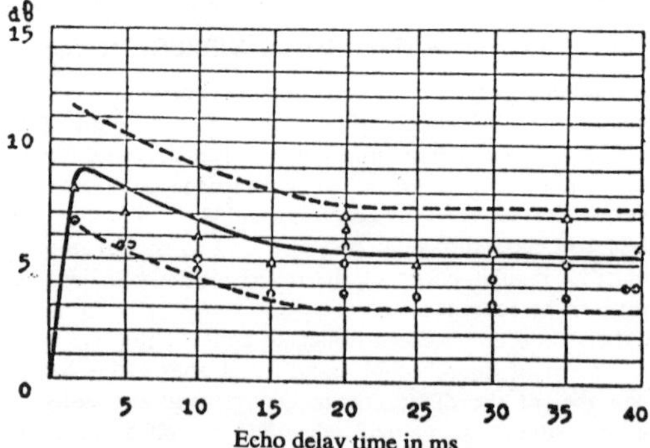

Fig. 8. Echo suppression effect as a function of delay time for noise with frequencies between 200 and 400 Hz.

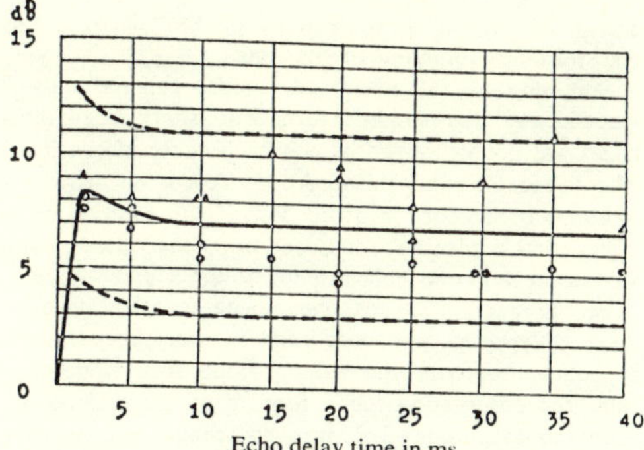

Fig. 9. Echo suppression effect as a function of delay time for noise with frequencies from 3200 to 6400 Hz.

loudspeakers from the observer. Both loudspeakers were excited simultaneously from a record and were adjusted to equal loudness, and in a first test the intensity of one loudspeaker was varied by means of a calibrated potentiometer. It was found that the hearer received different directional impressions according to the ratio of the intensities. The particular directional sensation belonging to each intensity ratio was drawn in a diagram.

A second test was based on equal intensities, where various small time differences were obtained by one loudspeaker being moved away from the observer. Again the different directions corresponding to delay differences were drawn in a diagram.

From both sets of measurements de Boer derived his curve shown in Fig. 7. He eliminated the directional impression and plotted intensity difference against time difference belonging to the same directional impression.

The agreement with our curve, obtained by a different method, is quite satisfactory, taking into account the wide scattering to be expected for subjective measurements. It appears from Fig. 7 that for differences from 5 to 30 ms the intensity of the echo loudspeaker must be ten times greater than that of the primary loudspeaker, i.e., against 10 dB, in order to create the impression of equal loudness. Above 30 ms the intensity difference drops slightly and the points are more scattered.

The experiment was repeated with the speech replaced by two noise spectra of different frequencies. For this purpose a white-noise generator was constructed with a gas-filled triode. Frequency ranges, as required, were obtained from the spectrum with an octave bandpass filter; they were then transmitted to the loudspeakers over the echo apparatus. The results are shown in Fig. 8 for a frequency range from 200 to 400 Hz and in Fig. 9 for a frequency range from 3200 to 6400 Hz. The mode of presentation and the measuring points correspond to Fig. 7. It is seen that the shape of the curves differs considerably from that in Fig. 7. The explanation may be that the effect in question is conditioned by a pronounced character and transit time difference of the sound impressions. These demands are fulfilled far less by noise spectra than by speech, and that may account for the rapid decline of the curves in Figs. 8 and 9, especially for high frequencies. Hence the balancing of the loudness was much more difficult than for speech, especially for the high frequencies, as is obvious from the wider scattering of the measurements. It is likely that this effect of the auditory suppression of echoes with a brief time difference enables us to discriminate directions in enclosed spaces where the hearing mechanism integrates only the first impression, that from the direct sound.

This effect is particularly conspicuous when loudspeaker arrangements operate in the open air, as for instance in large public meetings. As a rule, several loudspeakers of the same type, emitting equally in all directions (for instance mushroom loudspeakers), are fed simultaneously with the same signal. An observer moving from the vicinity of one loudspeaker in the direction of another one hears at first only the nearer loudspeaker. This may be explained by the ratio of energies. The impression persists unambiguously when the hearer moves on toward the second loudspeaker, although at this stage the energies emitted from both sources are almost equal, so that both should be heard.

However, as soon as the middle of the distance has been passed, if only by a few centimeters, the sensation passes suddenly to the other loudspeaker, with the impression that the sound comes from this direction only. This abrupt change of the impression is due entirely to delay phenomena.

A further test, based on speech, concerned the possible influence of the direction of the echo on the suppression reaction. No influence was found to exceed the limits of deviations in Fig. 7. This agrees with experience. Briefly delayed echoes in enclosed spaces may come from all directions without a disturbing effect. We mention in this connection a technical application of the suppression effect of briefly delayed echoes pointed out already by Cremer [10]. It is quite feasible to amplify sounds by 10 dB, possibly more, without the amplifying source being perceived, if the hearers are at the same time distracted by a further, e.g., optical, impression.

We will now discuss the increase in loudness caused by echoes with brief delay differences. In our case the echo has the same intensity as the direct sound, and the hearing organ receives therefore twice a certain, equal, energy, separated by the transit time difference. Our susceptibility to sounds is conditioned by a certain inherent inertia. For instance, according to v. Bekesy [11] the end value of the loudness perceived is reached only 200 ms after the tone has been switched on. On the other hand, investigations made by Steudel [12] showed that after the sudden switch-off of a tone the subjectively felt loudness decays only gradually. Bürck *et al.* [13], in conjunction with their development of an objective registering loudness meter, determined the time constants of the subjective building-up and decay sensation from the measurements made by v. Bekesy and Steudel. The mean values were 130 ms for v. Bekesy and 50 ms for Steudel. The conclusion suggests itself that our hearing mechanism integrates the sound intensities over short time intervals similar, as it were, to a ballistic measuring instrument. If we apply the law of the addition of energies to the echo with a short time difference, we obtain for double sound intensity a loudness increase of 3 phon, taking into account the nearly logarithmic sensitivity of the ear. Measurements with speech and music undertaken by Aigner and Strutt [14] confirmed this, provided that primary sound and echo had the same timbre. However, when their timbres were markedly distinct, the authors reported an increase in subjectively felt loudness exceeding by 6–9 phon the value according to the law of the addition of energies.

Lübcke [15] repeated with noises the tests made by Aigner and Strutt and found, even in the case of equal timbre, for small path differences and equal intensities of primary sound and echo a subjective increase in loudness of 5–6 phon, i.e., 2–3 phon above the value to be expected according to the said law.

The first two authors used radio receiving sets as sound sources. The difference in transit time was produced either by different distances from the observer or, with equal distances, by double staggered pickup from discs. Lübcke placed the loudspeakers at the same distance and obtained the difference in time by the insertion of an air interval in a transmission channel.

The measurements of the subjective loudness were made in both investigations with a Barkhausen noise meter [16], i.e., by comparing the loudness with a 800-Hz sound.

Aigner and Lübcke stated that the magnitude of the said effect was very little influenced by the delay difference, provided that this was below the threshold of masking. Nevertheless, it is proposed to discuss here also the influence of different transit time differences. We used the same apparatus as for the study of the suppression effect. The increase in loudness was not measured with a loudness meter, but by direct comparison of the sound impressions with and without echo.

To this end the observer was provided with a switch to disconnect the echo loudspeaker and to vary the energy of the primary loudspeaker in this position of the switch. By switching back he restored the initial state, i.e., both loudspeakers emitting the same intensity. It proved quite feasible to balance the subjectively felt loudness for both cases by repeated operation of the switch.

The effect of an echo-loudspeaker sounding with small delay differences has been defined before as an alteration of the timbre without alteration of the directional impression, i.e., without acoustical perception of the second loudspeaker.

Our tests produced the surprising result that there was no increase in loudness beyond the value to be expected from the law of the addition of energies, i.e., 3 phon.

We tried all kinds of changes: alteration of the delay difference below the threshold of masking, variation of the directions of the incidence of direct sound and echo; the timbre of the echo was modified while the impression of equal loudness of both loudspeakers was maintained. The experiments were made in enclosed and open spaces and with different observers. Invariably the increase due to echo of the same intensity was 3 phon. The greatest deviations under different conditions and with different observers were $\pm$ 1 phon, i.e., such as are to be expected in subjective measurements.

A possible explanation of this discrepancy between the results of our and earlier investigations may be found in the method of measuring the increase in loudness. A direct comparison of the sound impressions in our case should be more reliable than the comparison of the single impression with a noise the intensity of which, according to Aigner–Strutt, could be changed only in steps of 5 phon. It is also surprising that none of the authors mentioned that the echo loudspeaker could not be located acoustically. The earlier findings may also to some extent be due to imperfections of the electroacoustic transmitting equipment of the time.

Summing up the results of the foregoing discussions we can say that single echoes with short delay differences are not perceived as echoes because of the inertia of our hearing mechanism. All we feel is an increase in loudness in concord with the law of the addition of energies, and a pleasant modification of the quality of the sound, an apparent enlargement of the sound source.

Before passing on to phenomena created by longer delay differences, we must point out an effect observed in connection with the study of the small differences, since the observation has a bearing on the technique of telecommunications. Let primary sound and echo be emitted from the same loudspeaker, e.g., by series connection of the output terminals of the playback channels I and II (Fig. 1), consequently operating only one loudspeaker amplifier and loudspeaker. This causes intense distortions of speech for delay differences up to approximately 20 ms, but they disappear almost entirely with greater differences.

This phenomenon is due to interference between primary sound and echo in electrical superposition, resulting in large linear distortions of the tone. According to the particular delay difference of the echo, certain frequency ranges are very much reinforced whereas others are completely wiped out, assuming equal intensities of sound and echo.

Strongly pronounced interference effects are less liable to occur when the delay difference exceeds the average duration of the single sounds in speech; practically no disturbance is experienced then. The said phenomenon has to be borne in mind, for instance, when a performance is recorded by several microphones and then played back on a single loudspeaker. As a rule, the sound will reach the microphones with a certain path difference. Distortions of the reproduced sound can be avoided by placing the microphones so that the value of the differences is either zero or lies between 20 and 40 ms, corresponding to a microphone distance of about 6–12 m. Another method of avoiding interference effects makes use of directional microphones, arranged so that in each case the impression is recorded mainly by a single microphone.

Interferences are not perceived in binaural hearing of sound and echo from two loudspeakers, i.e., with acoustical superposition, because the distance between the ears makes us always hear simultaneously at two different points of the sound field. Also there is shielding from head and body, and if reflections occur, as in practice they always do, such pronounced interference phenomena as in electric transmissions cannot arise.

Only consequence of small delay differences in acoustic superposition is the described directional impression.

EXPERIMENTS WITH LARGE DELAY DIFFERENCES

We now pass on to the investigation of the influence of single echoes with greater delay differences on the audibility of speech. Beyond a certain difference value we perceive primary sound and echo separate. Further extension of the interval impairs the clearness of the acoustical impression or, in the case of speech, the intelligibility. Although our capability of concentration enables us to overcome to a degree this disturbance, it will certainly render prolonged listening very tiring. Still further increase of the delay difference leads to rapid deterioration of the intelligibility.

The appropriate method for the study of the influence of an echo on the intelligibility of speech appeared to be the use of syllables, a method which has stood the test in judging telephone communications, and in some investigations on the acoustics of rooms [17].

Such measurements are based on the transmission of a number of logatoms (syllables devoid of meaning in ordinary language). They are read by a speaker and heard and written down by a number of observers. The percentage of correctly understood logatoms determines the intelligibility of syllables or logatoms. Since the lists of logatoms edited by CCIF [18] were not available, new lists have been prepared according to the frequency of the various sounds in the German language [19].

They are composed of one or two consonants as initial sounds, followed by a vowel, with one or two consonants at the end (e.g., gan, pris, murt, schlerm). A test text always has 50 logatoms. Numerous lists have been compiled, in order to prevent the observers from getting accustomed to the syllables and causing errors.

Our measurements took place on the roof of the Institute, so that room influences were avoided. The logatoms were always carefully spoken by the same speaker, and were written down by five observers. Every syllable undisturbed by echo was followed by one with echo, in order to make provision for fatigue or for alterations in the conditions of the team.

The observers themselves evaluated the measurements immediately. The procedure yielded two results for each measurement, viz., the intelligibility of the syllables for undisturbed and disturbed reproduction.

However, the very first preliminary experiments revealed that the conventional monosyllable logatoms are not suitable for the study of echo effects. The single echo is briefly delayed, so that the first echo sound will coincide in the most favorable case, i.e., at a certain speed of the speech, with the second direct sound when a logatom consists of three sounds. Thus the first direct sound will be heard clearly at any rate. The second sound, a vowel, will always be understood easily because its sound energy is much greater than that of the superimposed consonant. On the third sound of the direct speech the vowel of the echo is superimposed; it is therefore quite often not understood, but it is heard again, this time undisturbed, after the decay of the primary syllable. This conclusion has been confirmed by elaborate tests, that is to say, it is not possible to impair the intelligibility of monosyllable logatoms by single echos of any delay difference.

A superimposed noise merely causes equal deterioration of the intelligibility of undisturbed and disturbed texts.

Intelligibility tests in large (reverberant) rooms are sometimes made by speaking several words before and after the logatom, e.g., "Schreiben Sie bitte—klas—sorgfältig auf" (please write—klas—down carefully). This cannot be done in our case because the time interval between preceding and closing text cannot be kept sufficiently short owing to the rather difficult pronunciation of the logatoms. Besides, the capability of concentration enables the observers to suppress in their perception the framing text and to focus their attention on the logatom, a reaction that is bound to counteract the effect to be measured. Another procedure could be to engage the observer in some other distracting occupation, e.g., summing up columns of numbers, but it would hardly be possible to determine the degree of that distraction.

The next attempt was made with multisyllable logatoms. Some effects of the echoes were observed, but the reduction of the intelligibility appeared only in the case of delay differences far beyond the threshold of masking. This is due to the different speeds of speech which essentially determine the maximum of the admissible echo difference, as will be demonstrated later on. About 5 syllables per second are spoken in normal conversation, but the speed has to be reduced to a mere 1.5 syllables per second when logatom texts are to be spoken in such a manner that single sounds can be understood. Such measurements with a speed differing so considerably from normal speech would yield results whose conversion into data valid for normal speaking would necessitate special comprehensive investigations. We therefore definitely abandoned the method of the intelligibility of syllables for the present investigation.

Measurements yielding results suitable for direct practical application must be based on the transmission of a text spoken at the normal speed. A first attempt was made with numbers, still with a view to copying the logatom method in so far that the numbers were to be written by the observers, an easy task if the speed of the transmission is 4 syllables per second. This experiment became another failure due to the restricted quantity of numbers (zero to ten) and because generally they are easily recognized from their vowel. This leads to practically 100-percent intelligibility, even for extremely long echo delay differences.

The only possible expedient was therefore to give a continuous text true to practical conditions and with various echo disturbances, and then to leave to the observers the decision whether they felt disturbed or not. An echo was characterized as disturbing when listening became unpleasantly strained, although the text might still be fully understood.

The experiments were made by altering the delay difference in steps. A very long or very short interval allowed a practically instantaneous judgment, while near to the threshold of masking it took the observers about a minute to make up their mind.

The objection could be made that such a time is too short, and that listening for a longer period even to a slightly disturbed text would be far more straining and very tiring, so that measurements of this kind would show admissible echo delay differences which were too high. In practice, however, other circumstances exert an opposite and nuisance-reducing influence, for instance, we receive and integrate as a rule a visual beside an acoustical impression and we divide our attention between both impressions. A disturbance is felt less in such a case than when only one type of sensation is to be integrated.

This effect may be illustrated by the following example. The loudspeaker for the reproduction of sounds in cinemas is usually placed behind the middle of the screen. When an actor speaks from one side of the screen the

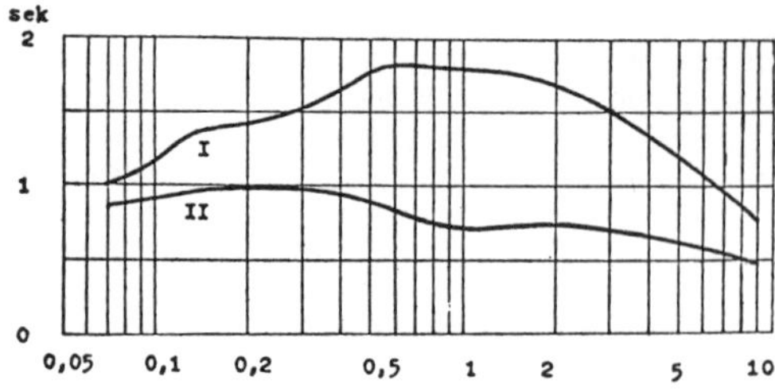

Fig. 10. Reverberation time of room used for measurements plotted against frequency. Curve I—empty; curve II—fully occupied.

sound is easily localized on the speaker. We do not realize at all that it arrives in fact from a quite different direction.

The assumption appeared therefore justified that useful results could be obtained in the manner described above, the more so as for statistical reasons the number of observers was raised to 50–100. Possible consequences of fatigue were reduced by restricting the time of intense attention to 30 minutes at the longest. The observers were mainly university students or scholars of higher schools.

The success of these measurements depends essentially on the order of the delay time alterations, particularly in the critical range. For instance, let a certain delay difference cause 50% of the observers to feel disturbed. If this particular difference had been preceded by one less effective, the number of the disturbed observers would have been greater than if the previous difference had produced a more effective disturbance. We therefore always made two straddling measurements in the critical range for each degree of the disturbance, defined by the number of observers who felt disturbed. The mean of those two measurements gave a fairly good criterion for the real condition. It was not always possible to determine in a single series of measurements the influence of a particular parameter. In the case of a further series it was important that the other parameters remain unchanged. To that end texts with a neutral meaning were recorded on magnetophone tape in order to eliminate influences of differences in the manner of speaking. During recording in the open air we took special care to maintain the same loudness and a constant speed of speech. Before every measurement the loudness of the primary loudspeaker and the echo loudspeaker were adjusted.

The results obtained with such precautions for the same acoustical conditions from different observers did not diverge by more than 10%. This applies even to small groups of six persons, not only to physicists who had taken part several times already in echo tests but also, after a short time of training, to members of the industrial staff of the Institute who for the first time took part in such tests.

Such limits are relatively narrow for subjective measurements, and it is surprising that they could be maintained by introducing the definition of "feeling disturbed," considering that the degree of a disturbance might have been judged very differently by individual observers, and that also the character of the disturbance varied considerably, corresponding to the particular circumstances. However, the method proved successful in all its applications, and it can therefore be definitely accepted as suitable for the estimation of echo effects.

Technical reasons (extension and loadbearing capacity of the roof of the Institute building) made it necessary to transfer the tests to a closed space. We are nevertheless confident that the results obtained there can be applied in practice, because in most cases where echos with long time differences occur in rooms, they will be accompanied by reverberation. The influence of the reverberation time will be discussed in detail at a later stage.

The room used for these measurements was an auditorium, 12.5 m long, 6.0 m wide, and 4.5 m high, with 80 built-in folding seats of plywood, rising in ten stepped rows. The volume is about 290 m^3. Fig. 10 gives the reverberation time as a function of frequency for the empty and fully occupied room. The average reverberation time for speech is 0.8 second for the full room.

The two loudspeakers had to be placed at a small distance in order to obtain, as far as possible, equal energy conditions and the same transit time differences all over the room. They were placed in the middle of one of the small sides in front of the blackboard, 4 m distant from the first row of seats, 160 cm above the floor, and were focused on the hearers.

It seemed advisable to get an idea of the effect the particular position of an observer might have on the results of the measurements. This was achieved by separating for one set of measurements the results obtained from observers in the front rows from those from observers in the rear. The deviations were found much smaller than the scattering between the measured points in general, i.e., they were negligible.

A recorded text spoken at a speed of 5.3 syllables per second, that is, similar to normal speech, was used for all investigations, except those on the influence of the speed.

For practical purposes the loudness of the primary loudspeaker could be considered constant over the whole lecture room because of the considerable distance from the first row of hearers. The loudness was maintained for the occupied room at 55 phon, except when the influence of the loudness itself was tested. It was controlled, as before, by comparison with the reference tone.

The foregoing conditions provided the basis for studying the disturbances caused by echoes as a function of various parameters.

Influence of the Speed of Speaking

The influence of the speed of speech was investigated for equal intensity and timbre of direct sound and echo.

Three sets of measurements were taken with speeds of 3.5, 5.3 and 7.4 syllables per second, i.e., within the limits found for normal speech. The continuous text was disturbed by altering in steps either transit time difference between direct sound and echo, or any other parameter.

The hearer had to decide whether he felt disturbed by the echo by answering "yes" or "no." The percentage of disturbed observers plotted against the echo delay differences is seen in Fig. 11. An inspection of the figure indicates a rapid rise of the percentage above 40 ms, to reach 100% at 100 ms. The measured points for curve II, i.e., 5.3 syllables per second, are given separated for two

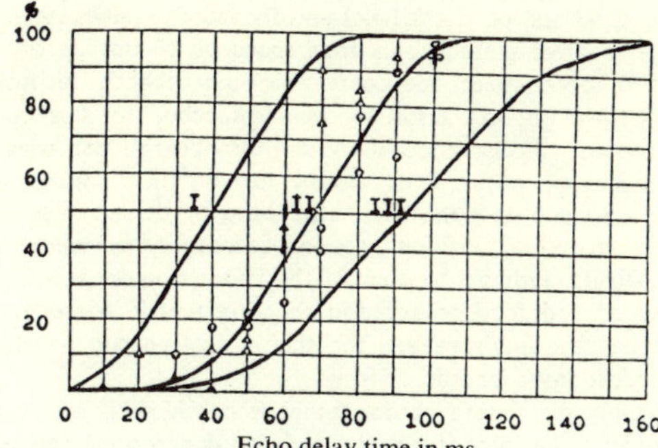

Fig. 11. Echo disturbance as a function of speed of speech. Curve I—7.4 syllables per second; curve II—5.3 syllables per second; curve III—3.5 syllables per second.

measurements under equal conditions, but with different observers, as is indicated by the round and triangular dots.

The evaluation of these results might be on the following lines. A critical difference would be assumed where 10–20% of the hearers felt disturbed, that is, 40 or 50 ms. Then follows a zone of relatively quick rise of the number of disturbed persons, due to differences in the individual judgment or to doubts about the decision. Differences above 80 ms to 90 ms cause 80 to 90% of the hearers to indicate disturbance, and it is a fair assumption that such echo delay times are certainly too long for satisfactory intelligibility.

The statement derived from those results would then be an admissible delay difference of 45 ms and a disturbing difference of 85 ms. However, the value of 45 ms would certainly be too low in practice, when the circumstances mentioned in the preceding are taken into account. We dealt here with wholly acoustical observations where the attention is concentrated on the hearing organ, whereas in the normal case optical impressions compensate to a certain degree for acoustical disturbances.

We considered this factor by drawing a curve with the closest possible approach to the points of the measurements, being a straight line in its middle section. The critical ratio of the delay differences is where 50% of the observers feel disturbed, that is, for curve II, 68 ms. This quantity is fairly close to the arithmetical mean between 45 and 85 ms and should serve as a good characteristic for the prevailing conditions.

The scattering of the measurements is rather small, considering their origins from two sets with different observers, and also the abrupt alterations of the degree of the disturbance. Greater deviations, e.g., in Fig. 11 those for 70 ms, are probably due to disturbing noises in the recorded text, erroneously taken as echo effects by some observers. Such incidental noises could not entirely be excluded, although the recording took place during the night hours (in the open air, in order to avoid room influences), e.g., sounds from aeroplanes, motor vehicles, and railways. On the whole they did not affect the results unduly.

The critical difference of 68 ms would not be affected appreciably when two separate curves would be drawn for the circular and triangular dots. The statistical demands are complied largely by the number of 2000 judgments derived from 80 observers in 25 measurements.

One item is worth mentioning. During all measurements made in the auditorium the first question was "when does the echo disturb you?" and a second question ran, "when do you hear an echo?" Again the answer was to be "yes" or "no," indicating whether the hearer was able to discriminate a difference at all from the anechoic transmission which started each set of measurements.

The answers to the second question showed no clear tendency, especially for small differences, and the results could not be evaluated. This failure is due probably partly to reverberation and partly to a psychological factor, i.e., the observer thought that almost always an echo was transmitted, as it was indeed, and he endeavored therefore to avoid the blame of being inattentive.

Fig. 11 makes clear how the critical delay difference depends on the speed of speaking. The value is 40 ms for high speed (7.4 syllables per second), 68 ms for normal speed (5.3 syllables per second), and 92 ms for slow (solemn) speech (3.5 syllables per second). That is to say, the critical difference is nearly inversely proportional to the speed of speaking. Of course, these statements should not be taken too rigidly, because the structure of speech is very involved and the above values are valid only for a certain range of speeds.

It is evident from these measurements that hearers may well follow without difficulty a slow speech in a room, whereas disturbances will arise with increasing speed of speaking.

Influence of the Intensity of the Echo

The next parameter to be varied was the intensity of the echo. The speed of speech for these tests was 5.3 syllables per second, the timbre of direct sound and echo was the same.

The intensity was altered in steps, the difference between the intensities of direct sound and echo being in turn + 10 dB, 0 dB, − 3 dB, − 6 dB, and − 10 dB. This investigation was divided into two series, the first with fluctuations between + 10 dB, 0 dB, and − 10 dB, and the second with fluctuations between 0 dB, − 3 dB, and − 6 dB.

Again the echo disturbance was altered abruptly, but its measure was now conditioned by differences of time as well as of intensity. The three sets of measurements were, as it was, interlocked. For instance, an echo disturbance defined as a delay difference of 60 ms and an intensity difference of − 6 dB were followed by one with 80 ms and 0 dB, these by 30 ms and − 3 dB, and so on. Deviations were not greater than in previous measurements, a further proof of the usefulness of the method.

The results are plotted in Fig. 12, indicating quantitatively how the nuisance effect of an echo can be reduced by lower intensity, as it is indeed normally in practice, viz., by covering reflecting surfaces with sound-absorbing materials.

The critical delay time, being again 68 ms for equal intensities of both loudspeakers, rises rapidly to 108 ms when the intensity of the echo is reduced by 3 dB and to 175 ms for 6 dB, while almost no disturbance at all

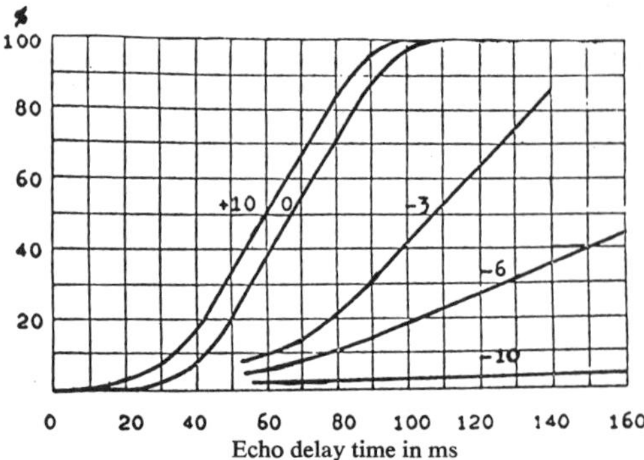

Fig. 12. Echo disturbance as a function of intensity of reflected sound. The numbers show the difference between the intensities of sound and echo in dB.

is felt when the reduction amounts to 10 dB. This value of 10 dB obtained for the complete stopping of the disturbance by reduction of the echo intensity is exactly the same as the magnitude of the echo-suppression effect for small differences (see Fig. 7).

An increase of the echo intensity by 10 dB occurs, for instance, through concentration of sound from curved surfaces, as in domes and planetariums of an out-of-date design. In such a case the critical delay time is reduced only from 68 to 60 ms.

Influence of the Timbre of the Echo

We now propose to show the effect of the timbre of an echo and that its influence on the subjectively felt disturbance cannot be neglected. We begin with the description of an experiment that is very suitable for demonstration and can easily be arranged by using a commercial magnetophone apparatus.

Two loudspeakers L_I and L_{II} are placed at a distance of several meters opposite each other and set at equal loudness (Fig. 13). Let L_I be the primary source and L_{II} the echo, with a delay difference of 60–80 ms. This can be produced with normal magnetophone equipment by feeding L_I with the level furnished to the recording channel, whereas L_{II} receives the level induced during the recording operation in the playback head. The delay difference is determined by the distance between recording head and playback head and its value usually reaches the required amount at a tape speed of 77 cm/s.

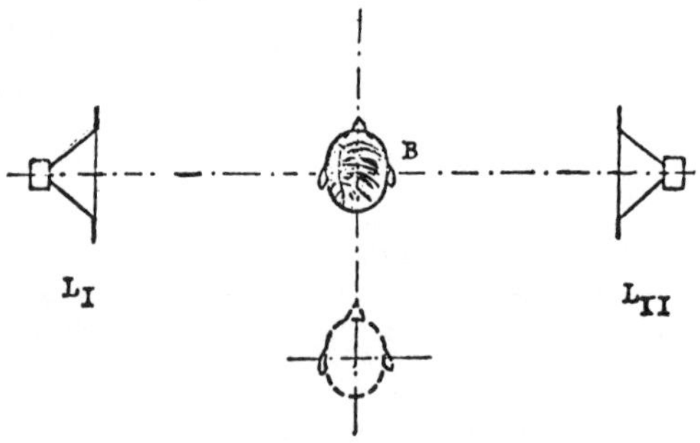

Fig. 13. Scheme of experiment proving dependence of echo disturbance on timbre.

An observer on the connecting line between the two loudspeakers will distinctly hear an echo, but this impression will decay gradually and disappear at last, when the hearer moves away on the median line. The delay difference is still the same, the ratio of the energies at the observer's position remains constant. The loudness is slightly reduced because of the larger distance between hearer and loudspeaker and the directional characteristics of the loudspeakers, but this is not relevant for the present investigation.

Only the timbre of the sound is considerably affected because the intensity of the higher frequencies decreases more and more when the distance from the connecting line grows, owing to their directional emission. The reduction of the echo nuisance must therefore be due to the absence of the high frequencies in the sound. The disturbance returns at once when the echo source, or both loudspeakers, are focused on the observer. The echo nuisance can be reduced also for an observer between both loudspeakers when the high frequencies are attenuated in the transmission channel to the echo loudspeaker.

This experiment reveals the importance of a high-class transmitting equipment for all previous investigations. The results would have been very much impaired by using disc reproduction with an upper limiting frequency of 5000 Hz.

The above experimental arrangement is not suitable for quantitative evaluation, because the directional characteristics of a cone loudspeaker as functions of frequency show a very complex and irregular pattern.

The difficulties of a quantitative evaluation, due to the appearance of numerous secondary maxima in case of the emitter being large in relation to the wavelength, had to be expected already from the directional characteristics computed for a piston diaphragm [20]. Nevertheless, we investigated how far those computed curves would agree with measured curves for a cone loudspeaker. The directional characteristics of one of the loudspeakers used in the above tests (diameter of diaphragm 30 cm) were recorded as a function of frequency. There is very poor agreement, especially for higher frequencies.

While the expected figure of an 8 was indeed measured for the directional characteristics at frequencies up to about 1000 Hz (diameter of emitter $\approx$ 1 wavelength), the curves measured for higher frequencies differed very much from the theoretical curves. This is due to unequal vibrations of different sections of the diaphragm, and to deflections of the baffle board and parts of the loudspeaker. The conditions become so involved that only the maximum fluctuations of the intensity in the region of a certain angle can be given.

In our particular case the fluctuation in intensity due to the directional effect, for instance for frequencies between 80 and 1000 Hz, kept below 10 dB only in the region of an angle of $\pm$ 20°. In the region between 0° and 180° we found fluctuations up to 40 dB.

Echoes for the quantitative investigation of timbre modifications were produced electrically by distortion of the transmission characteristic (Fig. 4) of the loudspeaker amplifier in the echo channel. This measurement was likewise made in the auditorium and with numerous ob-

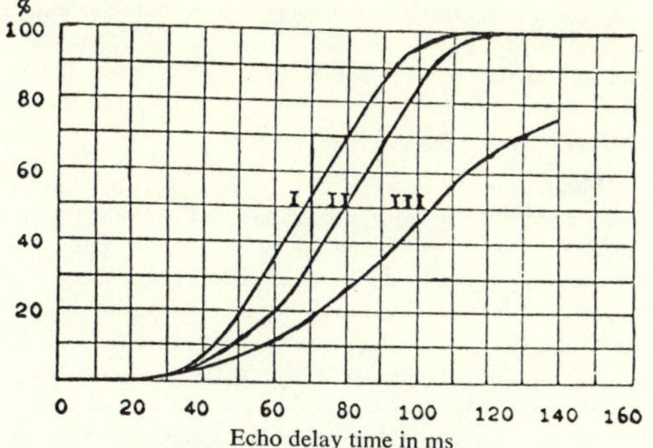

Fig. 14. Echo disturbance as a function of timbre of echo. Curve I—equal timbre of sound and echo; curve II—low frequencies of echo attenuated; curve III—high frequencies of echo attenuated.

servers. The speed of speech was 5.3 syllables per second; both loudspeakers had the same intensity.

The timbre of the echo from curve I in Fig. 4 was modified according to curves II and III, and again timbre differences and delay time differences were interlocked. The attenuation characteristic was intentionally chosen with a gradual rise at either the high or the low frequencies, as it agrees with practical conditions. In practice, attenuation of low frequencies similar to curve II in Fig. 4 would ensue from the use of resonance absorbers, an attenuation of the high frequencies according to curve III in Fig. 4 from porous absorbing materials.

Fig. 14 gives the results of the measurements. Curve I applies to equal timbre of sound and echo, the critical difference being again 68 ms. Curve II, obtained by attenuation of the low frequencies, gave a critical difference of 105 ms.

The objection could be put forward to the shape of the curves drawn in Fig. 14 that they indicate not so much alterations of timbre but rather the decrease in loudness connected with it, since this determines the critical difference (see Fig. 12). We checked this by comparing the subjectively felt loudness of a text transmitted according to curve I of Fig. 4 with a transmission according to curves II and III. The finding was that in both cases the decrease in loudness, caused by attenuating part of the transmitted frequency range, was less than 1 phon. An exacter result cannot be obtained by subjective measurements because of the physiological properties of our ear, but a quantitative estimate of the reduction in loudness can be derived from the following deliberation.

The spectral distribution of the energy in speech is highly frequency conditioned [7, Fig. 4]. The energy content per cycle in the frequency range from 100 to 1000 Hz is almost constant, but it decreases rapidly at higher frequencies, to become about 80 dB lower at 10 000 Hz than for 1000 Hz. An inspection of the transmission characteristics we used for effecting the timbre modulations (Fig. 4) indicates that curve II attenuates mainly regions of a high energy content and is apt to have a greater influence on the overall intensity than curve III which produces attenuation only in the frequency ranges of lower speech intensity.

Based on this argument we assume, in agreement with our loudness comparison, a reduction in loudness by 1 phon through damping of the low frequencies and we correct curve II in Fig. 14 according to the results plotted in Fig. 12. The result is that the curve now becomes almost identical with curve I of Fig. 14.

Let the decrease in loudness for curve III (Fig. 14) be assumed to be 0.5 phon. The correction according to Fig. 12 gives likewise a reduction of the critical delay difference, viz., from 105 to 95 ms approximately, but this is still much higher than the value of 68 ms for curves I and II. A conclusion from the foregoing consideration is therefore that the high frequencies of the echo certainly cause greater subjective disturbance than the low frequencies. However, the results shown in Fig. 14 have a direct practical bearing because a timbre modulation is almost always accompanied by a reduction in energy (frequency-dependent sound absorption).

Fig. 14 provides the quantitative foundation for the familiar experience that disturbances from echoes are reduced by covering the disturbing reflecting surface with porous absorbers in order to absorb mainly the high frequencies.

The reason for the dependence on frequency of the susceptibility of the human ear to echo disturbances is not yet known. The phenomenon might be due to a frequency-dependent time factor of the build-up and decay process.

A noticeable observation in echo experiments, particularly in the open air, was the impression of hearing from the echo loudspeaker, after it had not been perceived at all at small delay differences, at first only high frequencies, that is, in speech chiefly sibilants.

Influence of Loudness

So far the loudness of the primary loudspeaker had been maintained at approximately 55 phon, and only parameters of the echo had been altered. We now investigated the disturbing effect of the echo as a function of the general loudness. In this measurement the speed of speech was again 5.3 syllables per second; both loudspeakers had the same intensity and timbre.

The intensities of the two loudspeakers were varied in steps simultaneously, viz., toward lower degrees of loudness, between 55 phon, 45 phon, and 35 phon, to keep close to practical conditions. This was done by diminishing the amplifier output that produced 55 phon by 10 and 20 dB. It was found that the modification of the loudness in the said range exerted no influence on the subjectively felt disturbance.

Influence of the Angle of Incidence of the Echo

Stumpp [3] found an influence of the direction of the origin of the echo on the subjective disturbance value. His investigation dealt only with lateral incidence of the primary sound, while the echo arrived either from the same or from the opposite direction. The common experience, however, is that the sound comes from the front, while the echo may come from any direction. In our tests this was taken into account.

The measurements described so far had been made

with numerous observers in a closed space, with primary sound and echo coming from the same direction, direct in front. This was necessary in order to create, as far as possible, uniform experimental conditions, independent of the position of the individual observer. Such a state would not obtain if for instance the loudspeaker was placed at a side wall or rear wall, because the intensities and delay differences would vary very much for different parts of the room, so that in such a case the observers ought to be concentrated as near as possible to a single point. Instead of 100 persons taking part we had to cut down the number of observers to a few. On the other hand, a small number makes it possible to operate on the roof of the Institute, where conditions are very favorable, an important factor, especially when the influence of direction comes into play.

We first tried direct comparisons between two different sound impressions, the method which had been applied so successfully in our previous tests. A single observer was asked to compare directly a constant reference disturbance from an echo in front of him with the sensations caused by echoes incident from various directions. The two degrees of disturbance had to be balanced by adjusting the delay difference of the random echo.

The experiment proved that such a direct comparison is not feasible because these sound impressions differ too much. To give a somewhat exaggerated illustration, let a frontal echo with a certain delay difference convey the impression of a stammering speaker. The lateral echo would, for example, produce the effect of two speakers talking at the same time. Monaural hearing would have made the two sound impressions comparable, but would not agree with practical conditions.

We tackled the problem in the following way. A group of six observers was concentrated on the smallest possible area, their eyes focused on the primary loudspeaker standing at a distance of two meters, level with their heads. Intensity and timbre were equal to those of the echo loudspeaker, placed anywhere on a circle of a 2-m radius, focused always on the hearers.

The delay difference of the echo was changed abruptly, within the interesting range, for different positions of the echo loudspeaker, as was done before in the auditorium tests, in order to obtain curves of the disturbance values. All measurements were made with two groups formed as before; the second group was again composed of members of the industrial staff to whom these measurements were entirely new.

The results obtained by group I showed no more scatter than with numerous observers used earlier in the lecture room, in spite of the small number of observers and the great difference in the impressions of the sounds. The deviations observed in the results obtained from group II decreased rapidly after a short exercise, for practical purposes reaching the level of group I. At that stage the values derived from both groups agreed to an astonishing measure, a proof of the correctness of results obtained even with so small a number of observers. Table I gives the results, viz., the critical delay difference as it corresponds to different angles of incidence, first separated for both groups, then combined. These values indicate a relatively small influence of the direction of the echo. The rise of the critical delay difference for lateral incidence is probably due to the decrease of the intensity at the remote ear compared with that of the direct sound.

Influence of Room Reverberation

The difference between the values of the critical delay difference obtained in the open air and in the fully occupied auditorium is considerable, i.e., 44 ms and 68 ms, respectively, for frontal incidence of both sounds and equal conditions. This leads to the conclusion that the reverberation time influences the critical difference.

The question arose whether further increase of the room reverberation time would be accompanied by higher critical delay differences. Measurements were taken with different groups, each of six observers, in the empty auditorium, having an average reverberation time of about 1.6 s (see Fig. 10).

Primary loudspeaker and echo loudspeaker emitted the same intensity and timbre, so that the loudness at the place of the observer was about 55 phon, the speaking speed was 5.3 syllables per second, the listeners were seated in two middle rows.

In these measurements the decision on the degree of disturbance was complicated because the reverberation time itself exerted an unfavorable effect on the reproduction of the speech. This was indicated by widely scattered results from less experienced observers. We selected therefore a number of discriminating listeners who were capable of judging with certainty the deterioration in audibility purely due to the echo, in spite of the disturbance caused by reverberation. In this way a critical transit time difference of 78 ms was obtained.

Table I

Direction and Angle of Incidence		Critical Transit Time Difference (ms) Group I	Group II	Groups I and II
Horizontal (frontal)	0°	46	42	44
	45°	53	50	52
Horizontal (lateral)	90°	52	51	52
	135°	50	52	52
Horizontal (from the rear)	180°	53	57	55
At 45° inclined from above	0°	49	45	47
	45°	59	53	55
	90°	60	56	56
	135°	58	59	58
	180°	62	57	59
Vertical from overhead		55	50	50

The effect of the reverberation time on the magnitude of the subjectively felt echo disturbance is plotted in Fig. 15. The critical delay difference increases with the reverberation time. Small delay differences seem to be veiled by the reverberation, so that their recognition becomes difficult.

CONCLUSION

A thorough investigation has been made of the influence of a single echo as a function of different parameters on the audibility of speech. An apparatus was built for the artificial generation of echoes with a time difference to the direct sound which could be varied. The

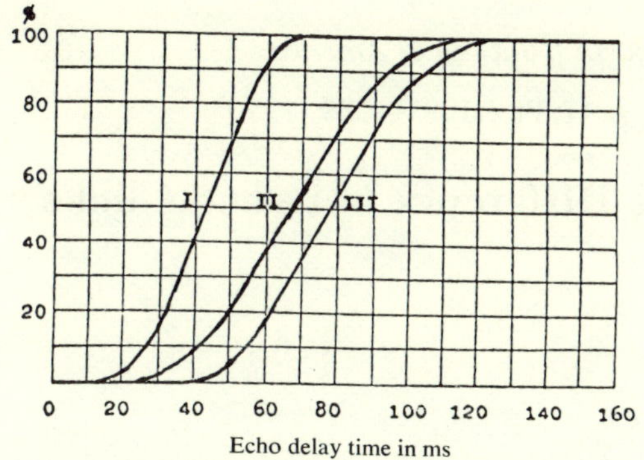

Echo delay time in ms

Fig. 15. Echo disturbance as a function of room reverberation time. Curve I—reverberation time 0 seconds; curve II —reverberation time approximately 0.8 second; curve III—reverberation time approximately 1.6 seconds.

apparatus is composed of a high-quality electroacoustic transmission installation and an endless-tape magnetophone equipment, from which the echo is obtained by a delayed pickup.

The measurements were made with a large number of observers under precisely specified conditions. Several suitable methods have been developed for the quantitative determination of the echo effects.

1) Tests with small echo delay differences between 1 and 30 ms showed an increase in loudness in agreement with the law of the addition of energies and a pleasant modification of the sound impression in the sense of a broadening of the primary sound source, while the echo source is not perceived acoustically. The magnitude of the auditory "suppression effect" for echoes with 1- to 30-ms difference was found to be 10 dB, i.e., the intensity of the echo must exceed that of the primary sound by 10 dB in order to make the echo separately perceptible in the said range of delay differences.

2) Echoes with greater delay differences above a rather marked threshold value cause the sound impression of speech to be disturbed, even to complete unintelligibility.

The conception of a "critical delay difference" is introduced as a mean of gauging the amount of disturbance, and of comparing measurements made under different circumstances.

a) Its value is approximately inversely proportional to the speed of speech in the range of 3.5 to 7.4 syllables per second.

b) The intensity of an echo exerts an important influence on the critical delay difference. An attenuation of the echo intensity by only 5 dB doubles the critical difference. Echo intensities more than 10 dB below that of the direct sound do not disturb at all the reproduction of continuous speech.

c) The high frequencies of the echoes determine the amount of the subjective disturbance. Their attenuation makes possible a considerable raising of the critical difference, with almost no noticeable reduction of the loudness of the echo.

d) The quantity of the echo disturbance does not depend on the loudness in the range belonging to speech.

e) The direction of incidence of the echo does not affect essentially the critical difference, provided that the direct sound is incident from the front.

f) A longer reverberation time in a room produces a greater critical delay difference.

REFERENCES

[1] Petzold, *Elementare Raumakustik* (Berlin, 1927), p. 8.

[2] H. Decker, "Eine Verzögerungsleitung für Messung und Vorführung von Laufzeitwirkungen in Fernmeldesystemen," (A delay conduit for measuring and demonstrating transit time effects in telecommunication systems), *Elek. Nachr. Tech.*, vol. 8, p. 516 (1931).

[3] H. Stumpp, "Experimentalbeitrag zur Raumakustik" (Experimental contribution to the acoustics of rooms), *Beihefte z. Ges. Ing.*, vol. 2, p. 17 (1936).

[4] W. Burk and H. Lichte, "Über die Schallfortpflanzung in Röhren" (The propagation of sound in tubes), *Akust. Z.*, vol. 3, p. 259 (1938).

[5] v. Bekesy, "Über das Richtungshören bei einer Zeitdifferenz oder Lautstärkeungleichheit" (On directional hearing in the case of a time difference or of unequal loudness), *Phys. Z.*, vol. 31, pp. 824, 857 (1930).

[6] M. Reich and H. Behrens, "Das Richtungsempfinden bei Tönen und Klängen" (Directional hearing of tones and sounds), *Z. Tech. Phys.*, vol. 14, p. 6 (1933).

[7] K. de Boer, "Plastische Klangwiedergabe" (Stereophonic sound reproduction), *Philips Tech. Rev.*, vol. 5, p. 108 (1940).

[8] H. Warncke, "Die Grundlagen der raumbezüglichen stereophonischen Übertragung im Tonfilm" (The fundamentals of stereophonic transmissions in the sound film with reference to rooms), *Akust. Z.*, vol. 6, p. 174 (1941).

[9] A. Lien, "Das Küchenmeister-Intervall und das Ultraphon," *Z. VDI*, vol. 70, p. 33 (1926).

[10] L. Cremer, *Geometrische Raumakustik* (Geometrical room acoustics), vol. 1 (1948), p. 126.

[11] v. Bekesy, "Zur Theorie des Hörens" (On the theory of hearing), *Phys. Z.*, vol. 30, p. 118 (1929).

[12] U. Steudel, "Über Empfindung und Messung der Lautstärke" (On the sensation of loudness and its measurements), *Z. Hochfreq. Tech. Elektrotech.*, vol. 41, p. 116 (1933).

[13] Bürk, Kotowski, and Lichte, "Die Lautstärke von Knacken, Geräuschen, und Tönen" (The loudness of clicks, noises, and tones), *Elek. Nachr. Tech.*, vol. 12, p. 278 (1935).

[14] F. Aigner and M. J. O. Strutt, "Über eine physiologische Wirkung mehrerer Schallquellen auf das Ohr und ihre Anwendung auf die Raumakustik" (On a physiological effect on the ear from several sound sources and its application to room acoustics), *Z. Tech. Phys.*, vol. 15, p. 355 (1934).

[15] E. Lübcke, "Über die Zunahme der Lautstärke bei mehreren Schallquellen" (On the increase in loudness obtained from several sound sources), *Z. Tech. Phys.*, vol. 15, p. 77 (1934).

[16] H. Barkhausen, "Ein neuer Schallmesser für die Praxis" (A new sound meter for practical use), *Z. Tech. Phys.*, vol. 7, p. 599 (1926).

[17] H. Panzerbieter and A. Rechten, "Subjective Bestimmung der Güte von Fernsprechverbindungen" (Subjective determination of the quality of telephone connections), *Arch. Tech. Messen*, vol. 3, p. 3719 (1942).

[18] CCI, "Recueil de Listes de Lagotoms," p. 2; also CCIF, White Book I, pp. 1-289.

[19] H. F. Mayer, "Verständlichkeitsmessungen an Telefonie-Übertragungssystemen" (Intelligibility measurements on telephone transmission systems), *Elek. Nachr. Tech.*, vol. 4, p. 184 (1927).

[20] H. Stenzel, "Über die Richtwirkung von Schallstrahlern" (On the directional effect of sound emitters), *Elek. Nachr. Tech.*, vol. 4, p. 239 (1927).

26

Reprinted from *Acoust. Soc. Am. J.* 47, Pt.2:1091–1099 (1970)

Monaural Detection of a Phase Difference between Clicks

DON A. RONKEN*

Department of Psychology, University of California, San Diego, La Jolla, California 92037

Pairs of very brief pulses can be arranged to produce transient signals having spectra that differ only in power, only in phase, or in both power and phase. Conventional intensity discrimination for such click pairs is obtained by using the signals that differ only in their power spectra. Some of the corresponding signals that differ only in their phase spectra are also readily discriminable. An attempt is made to assess the relative saliency of the power and phase variables by adding the phase cue as a distracting feature to the power-discrimination task. The presence of such an uncorrelated phase cue can lower the detectability of power differences.

INTRODUCTION

Contrary to von Helmholtz's original dictum (von Helmholtz, 1895), there now seems to be little doubt that the ear can perceive monaural phase cues contained in sustained, music-like sounds. Craig and Jeffress (1962) have presented a bibliography of work in this area, of which the best known is probably the study by Mathes and Miller (1947). There seems to have been no published work on an aspect of the problem Helmholtz originally avoided, namely, the existence of similar monaural phase effects for wide-band transient signals. Perhaps more important, there have been no attempts to compare the effectiveness of monaural phase cues with power, duration, or other well-established auditory cues. Thus, on one hand we have reports of the ear's sensitivity to phase in the Mathes and Miller sense, while on the other hand, experiments in speech analysis and synthesis (Flanagan, 1965) seem to indicate that phase information contributes very little to speech intelligibility.

The perception of monaural phase cues may also be of significance in evaluating some models of the auditory system based upon energy-detection schemes (Corliss, 1963; Jeffress, 1964; Green and Swets, 1966; McGill, 1967). An energy detector destroys all phase information in the signal by integrating over time, with the result that temporal aspects of stimulus events that occur within the time constant of the analyzing system are not preserved. As a consequence, transient signals with identical power spectra are indiscriminable to simple energy detectors, and pure phase detection for such stimuli should not exist.

A few studies have appeared indicating that monaural phase may be important for wide-band stimuli, but none have employed transient signals. Pfafflin and Mathews (1966) and Pfafflin (1968) obtained considerably different masking from short reproducible noise maskers that were constructed to have very similar power spectra. This result raises the question about the masking obtained with ordinary noise bursts. How much of the masking is contributed by the randomization over phase as compared to the randomization over amplitude? Bilsen (1967) listened to different wide-band continuous reproducible noise waveforms that had identical power spectra. He reported that phase changes are very evident in the qualitative nature of the sound produced.

The questions to be addressed here are twofold. *First*, can the auditory system respond to monaural phase cues contained in a transient signal so short that it falls within the nominal time constant of the ear? *Second*, how important are such cues relative to power or energy cues?

I. METHOD

Consider the usual intensity-discrimination experiment. The duration of the signal is held fixed, and the signal energy is varied by changing the signal amplitude. A more precise description of this experiment is to say that it involves the detection of a power difference. Such a description serves to emphasize the distinction to be made between power and phase variables.

To determine the relative strength of phase and power cues, we need a transient stimulus whose phase and

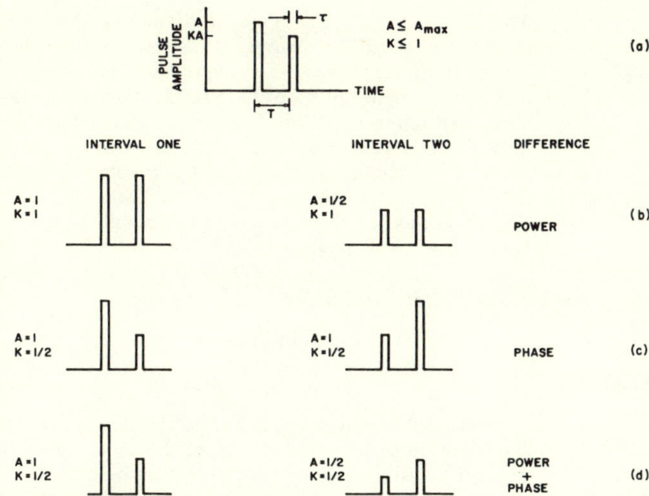

FIG. 1. Schematic representation of stimuli used in the power and phase discrimination experiments. The rectangular pulse pair, referred to as the "basic transient" in the text, is shown in (a). Sections (b), (c), and (d) diagram stimuli constructed from the basic transients that were used in Expts. 1, 2, and 3, respectively. In (b), the signals in the two observation intervals differ only in power. In (c), the two signals differ only in phase, while in (d), the two intervals contain signals differing in both power and phase.

power spectra can be independently varied. Such a stimulus was obtained by generating pairs of short-duration rectangular pulses with the parameters as illustrated in Fig. 1(a). For the work reported here, τ was held fixed at 250 μsec and T was a few milliseconds, so that the entire stimulus was a short-duration wide-band transient. Because these click pairs with various parameter values were used to construct the stimuli for all the experiments reported here, we refer to the click pair [(Fig. 1a)] as the basic transient. This basic transient was used to generate stimuli for three conditions, all using a two-interval same–different experimental design. The stimuli for the first experiment are illustrated in Fig. 1(b), where K was set equal to 1. By varying A between the two observation intervals, signals were obtained that differed only in their power spectra. For example, when $A=1$ in Interval 1, and $A=\frac{1}{2}$ in Interval 2, the signals have the same phase spectra but differ in power by 6 dB.

To generate stimuli that differ only in their phase spectra, we take advantage of two well-known facts: (1) the power spectrum of a transient is unaffected by a reversal of the time scale and (2) the transform representation is unique. If the transient is $f(t)$, then $f(-t)$ will have an identical power spectrum. From the uniqueness property of the transform, it follows that if $f(t)$ and $f(-t)$ are not in fact identical themselves, they will have different phase spectra. Figure 1(c) illustrates the kind of stimuli used in the second experiment. Now $A=1$ and $K=\frac{1}{2}$ in both observation intervals, but Interval 1 contains the basic transient as $f(t)$ and Interval 2 has its $f(-t)$ version. The value of K may be changed to vary the phase-spectrum differences that exist between the two intervals without disturbing the power spectrum equality.

Finally, a third experiment is obtained by combining the operations described above, namely, by the attenuation of one pulse in the basic transient and reversal in time, as illustrated in Fig. 1(d). Varying both A and K in this way produces signals in the two intervals that differ in both power and phase.

II. PROCEDURE

With this ensemble of stimuli available, we may approach the question of comparing the importance of power and phase sensitivity for transient signals. Using the arrangement of Fig. 1(c), we vary K until an observer can discriminate $f(t)$ from $f(-t)$ under same–different conditions. This experiment would provide the parameter value of K required for, say, 75% correct discrimination of the phase cue. By using the stimuli of Fig. 1(b), again in the same–different design, we can obtain the value of A corresponding to 75% correct discrimination of the power cue. In order to compare the relative salience of these cues, we can then repeat the power discrimination experiment but add the phase cue as a distracting feature. That is, we ask the observer to indicate whether the power is the same or different in both observation intervals [Fig. 1(d)] when there may be also be a phase difference between the two intervals that is discriminable by itself. To the extent that the presence of the irrelevant phase cue is distracting, we may expect to obtain some decrement in detection of the power cue. The magnitude of such a depression in power sensitivity would be some rough measure for the relative salience of the power and phase cues.

A PDP-8 computer was used to generate the stimuli and actively search for the observer's threshold using the PEST procedure (Taylor and Creelman, 1967). The threshold was defined as the point where the observer correctly identified the stimuli as being "same" or "different" on 75% of the trials. Feedback always followed responses, and the threshold search was ter-

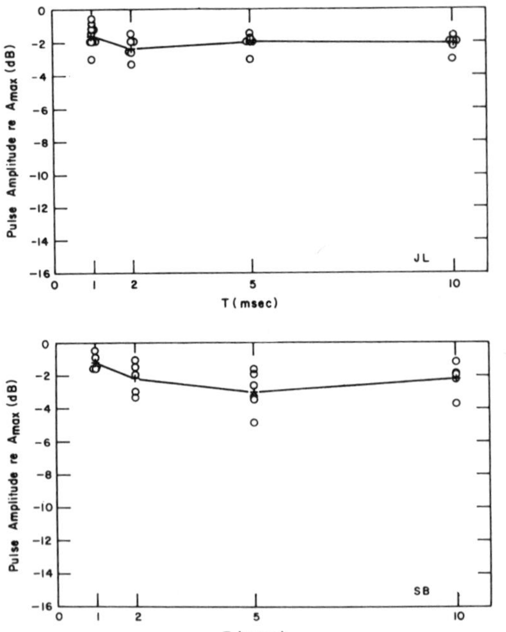

FIG. 2. Power-discrimination thresholds for the two observers obtained from Expt. 1. T is the basic transient parameter providing the delay between pulses [Fig. 1(a)]. The ordinate gives the attenuation of the lower power basic transient relative to A_{max} that was required for 75% correct responding. Each data point represents a separate PEST estimate. Mean values are indicated by plus signs and connected by solid lines.

minated when the step size would have been reduced to less than 0.4 dB on the next trial. This criterion required an average of about 55 trials to be reached.

The stimuli were presented in a continuous low-level masking noise background (N_0=2 dB spectrum level). The signals for Expt. 1 were 57 dB above the level corresponding to 75% correct detection for Observer JL and 56 dB for Observer SB. These detection measurements were made by a 2AFC (two-alternative forced-choice) search using PEST. The stimuli were presented over TDH-39 receivers driven binaurally in phase and mounted in Rudmose circumaural earmuffs.[1] A $\frac{1}{2}$-sec interval separated the observation intervals. The two paid observers practiced for some 63 threshold estimates before the data reported here were collected. The experimental conditions for T were alternated haphazardly from day to day.

III. EXPERIMENT 1

A. Power Discrimination

Sensitivity to power differences for the basic transient was determined by using stimuli of the type shown in Fig. 1(b). In one of the two observation intervals, the amplitude A was always equal to the maximum pulse amplitude, A_{max}. On each trial, the stimuli in the two intervals were the same, with probability one-half; when the power was different, the larger-power signal was presented first half of the time. PEST adjusted the amplitude of the smaller-power signal until the 75% correct point was found.

B. Results

Figure 2 provides the threshold estimates for the two observers under these conditions at T=1, 2, 5, and 10 msec. The ordinate provides the attenuation of the lower-amplitude pulse relative to A_{max} that was required for 75% correct discrimination. Each data point represents a separate PEST determination. Mean threshold values are indicated by plus signs and connected by solid lines. These data will serve as the basic reference condition for power discrimination and

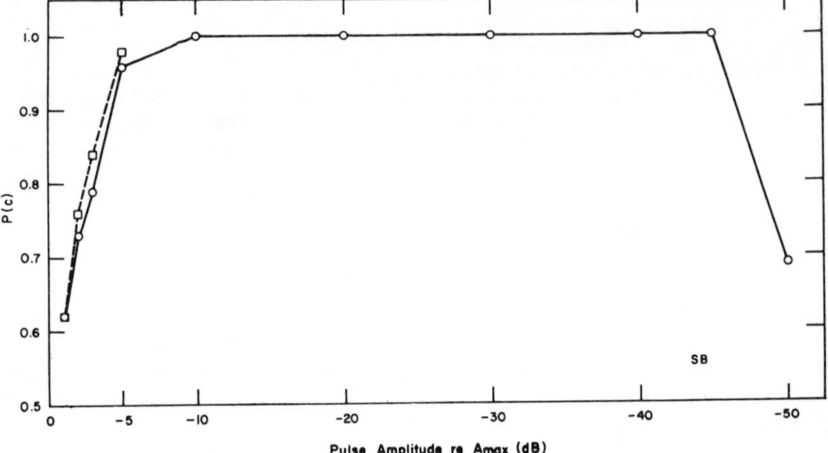

FIG. 3. Percentage of correct responses in a 2AFC pilot experiment using basic signals that differ only in phase [Fig. 1(c)]. The abscissa gives the value of K in terms of the attenuation relative to A_{max}. The pulse separation T equals 5 msec. Circles represent data obtained from rectangular pulses, squares are for pulses low-pass filtered at 600 Hz. Each point is based on 200 trials.

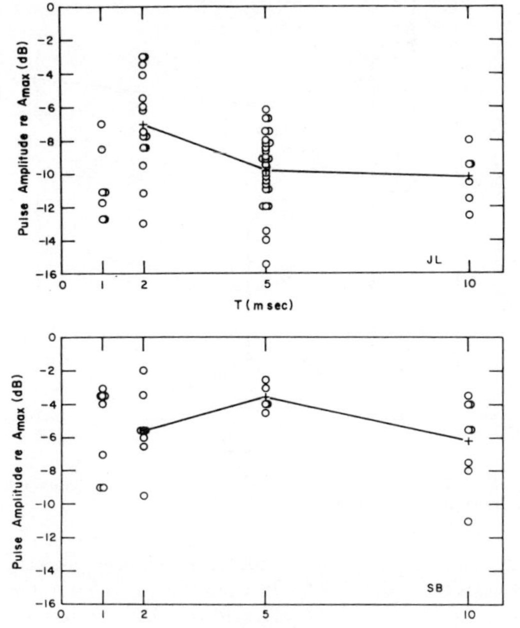

FIG. 4. Phase-discrimination thresholds for the two observers obtained from Expt. 2. The ordinate gives the value of K in terms of the attenuation relative to A_{max} for 75% correct [see Figs. 1(a) and 1(c) for definition of parameters]. Each data point represents a separate PEST estimate. Mean values indicated by plus signs and connected by solid lines.

provide an estimate for the over-all precision of the experimental technique.

IV. EXPERIMENT 2

A. Phase Discrimination

The stimuli used for the phase discrimination task are illustrated in Fig. 1(c), where K is varied to change the magnitude of the phase cue. It is clear that there are some values of K that cannot lead to discriminable stimuli. Thus, when $K=1$, the basic transient consists of two equal-amplitude pulses, as in Expt. 1, and reversal in time does not serve to distinguish between them. Likewise, when $K=0$, the signals are single pulses that remain unchanged when reversed in time. From pilot experiments, it was evident that there were values of K between 0 and 1 that lead to clearly discriminable signals.

The points plotted as open circles in Fig. 3 indicate a typical **U**-shaped psychometric function. These data were obtained at $T=5$ msec from Observer SB during pilot experimentation. When the two pulses are less than 1 dB apart, performance is near chance. All pulse differences greater than about 10 dB provided errorless performance until the attenuation is so large that the small pulse is made ineffective by the noise masker. The square points in Fig. 3 were obtained when the rectangular pulses were low-pass filtered at 600 Hz by an Allison 2ABR filter. Evidently, it is not essential to have high-frequency energy present in order to discriminate these signals.

These pilot data were collected in a 2AFC experiment where only one value of K was used for any given block of trials. The main experiments, on the other hand, used a same–different arrangement and the PEST procedure. The same–different method permitted simple instructions to be given to the observer for these somewhat unusual conditions where there is not a large vocabulary to describe what is a "signal" and what is a "noise." Also, using the same–different structure made it possible to investigate several minor variations, such as the eight possible types of trials for Expt. 3, during a single block of trials. Finally, it was anticipated that the efficiency of PEST would permit more experimental conditions to be investigated than would be practical with a strict use of 2AFC.

Experiment 2 used the basic signals $f(t)$ and $f(-t)$ in both possible temporal orders with equal probability, so that there were four types of trials. K was initially set to a value that would generate perfect performance,

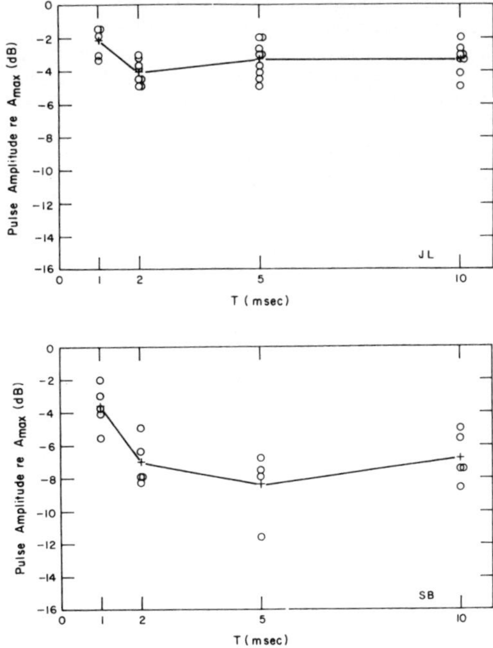

FIG. 5. Power-discrimination thresholds obtained in the presence of an irrelevant phase cue from the two observers (Expt. 3). Phase-cue parameter K set equivalent to 15 dB for Observer JL; 10 dB for Observer SB. Ordinate gives the attenuation of the lower power basic transient relative to A_{max} that was required for 75% correct. Each data point represents a separate PEST estimate. Mean values indicated by plus signs and connected by solid lines.

and PEST was to increase K and converge on the 75% point. A was held fixed at A_{max}.

B. Results

Figure 4 presents the resulting phase discrimination data for the same two observers.[2] Two points are apparent from these data. *First*, the variability of the threshold estimates is much greater than that obtained for the power discrimination task. *Second*, whereas the two observers were approximately equally sensitive to power differences for these transient signals, it appears that Observer SB is considerably more sensitive to phase differences than is Observer JL. This difference between observers was also evident from the amount of practice required before stable data were obtained, with Observer SB requiring far less practice.

The mean value for the thresholds at $T=1$ msec are not plotted on Fig. 4 because, on some occasions, the PEST routine failed to converge on the 75% correct point. On these runs, when the observer remained at less than 75% correct for a disproportionate number of trials, PEST would continue to adjust K to lower and lower values until, with continued incorrect responding, K could eventually reach zero. As mentioned before, when $K=0$, there is no difference between $f(t)$ and $f(-t)$, so the run was terminated. These instances of nonconvergence occurred only at $T=1$ msec and explain why no shorter values of T were used. Observer JL had six such instances of nonconvergence, while Observer SB had four.

For T greater than about 10 msec, the basic transients begin to sound like two successive clicks rather than a unitary event. Thus, for T very large, the phase task degenerates into one in which the observer hears two successive clicks, one louder than the other. To respond correctly under these conditions, the observer need only determine whether the loud click preceded or followed the soft click in both observation intervals. It was for this reason that no values of T greater than 10 msec were used.

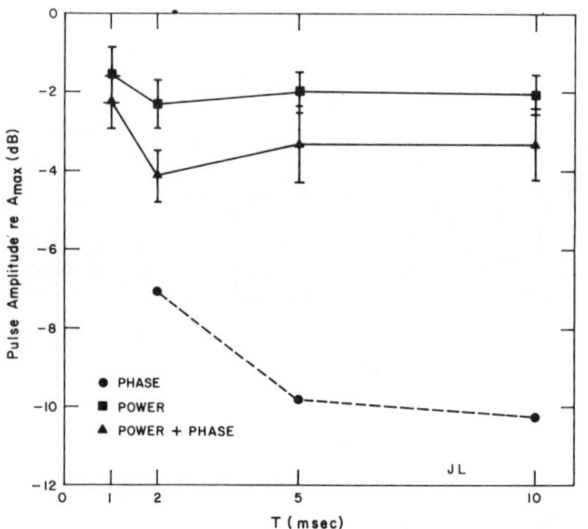

FIG. 6. Mean threshold data from Expts. 1, 2, and 3 for Observer JL. Ordinate gives attenuation required relative to A_{max} for 75% correct, as in Figs. 2, 4, and 5. *Squares*: Mean power-discrimination data of Expt. 1. *Circles*: Mean phase-discrimination data of Expt. 2. *Triangles*: mean power-discrimination data obtained in the presence of an irrelevant phase cue, Expt. 3.

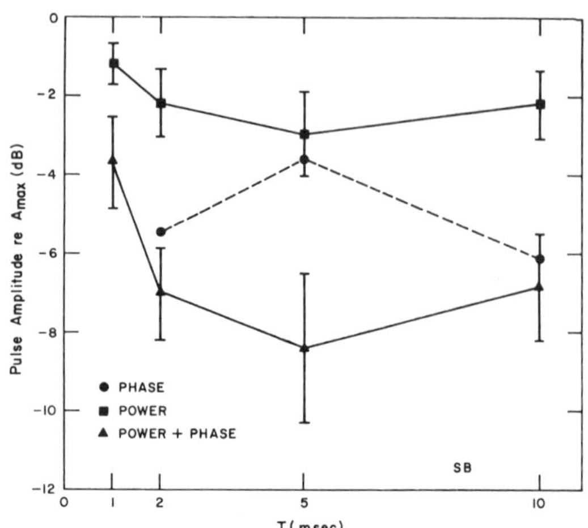

FIG. 7. Mean threshold data from Expts. 1, 2, and 3 for Observer SB. Axes same as Fig. 6.

V. EXPERIMENT 3

A. Power plus Phase Discrimination

From the data of Expt. 2 we now have estimates for values of K that lead to basic transients, that are discriminable solely on the basis of phase. Values of K corresponding to 15- and 10-dB attenuation were selected as producing a clearly detectable amount of phase cue for Observers JL and SB, respectively. These fixed K values were used, as outlined in Fig. 1(d), for the case where phase is added as an irrelevant cue to the power discrimination task.

There were eight possible types of trials in this experiment, selected with equal probability. These were generated by choosing the power variable to be the same or different in both intervals, the phase to be the same or different, and the waveform in the first observation interval to be either $f(t)$ or $f(-t)$. The feedback reflected the power difference, irrespective of the phase variable. The observers were informed of this situation, as they were about the conditions in all the other experiments.

B. Results

The power sensitivity under these conditions of the irrelevant phase cue is shown in Fig. 5. Since there were no interesting effects within the eight possible types of trials, the data for all possible pulse orders, etc., were combined. The variability of the individual threshold estimates appears to be slightly greater than that obtained for the straightforward power discrimination itself. Since these data are to be compared with data of the previous experiments, all the averaged thresholds are presented in Fig. 6 for Observer JL and in Fig. 7 for Observer SB. The vertical bars in these figures indicate ± 1 standard deviation of the individual estimates from the mean value. Comparing the power-discrimination thresholds (squares) to power discrimination in the presence of the irrelevant phase (triangles), we find it apparent that the phase cue served to depress the sensitivity to power differences. This effect is much more reliable for Observer SB, who was the more sensitive at phase discrimination. Also, the depression in power sensitivity is greatest for those values of T where phase discrimination is best, for both observers.

The same–different arrangement, in conjunction with PEST, treated the two-by-two confusion matrix in a symmetric fashion. Thus, either kind of success or failure resulted in the same action from PEST. Because the signals were the same or different with equal probability, the presence of a large response bias could result in PEST's overestimating the signal value required for the 75% correct point. Thus, in comparing Expts. 1 and 3, a dramatic increase in response bias for one condition relative to the other might lead PEST to produce spuriously different threshold values. To check on this possibility, the confusion matrix for each experimental condition was compiled, starting at the trial of the first error. The largest response bias observed by either observer for any experiment was 0.58. Using the psychometric function of Fig. 3, we estimated that the greatest error made in threshold estimation resulting from such response bias changes was about $\frac{1}{2}$ dB.

VI. DISCUSSION

It is not clear exactly what aspect of the stimulus is being used to perform the phase discrimination of the present experiment. One possible mechanism, based on the asymmetry between forward and backward masking, is considered briefly in Appendix B and rejected as implausible. The fact that low-pass filtering has no effect on the phase discrimination makes it unlikely that observers are listening through some high-frequency critical-band-type filter. (Such a filter would have a wide bandwidth and thus might be capable of following the amplitude fluctuations.)

Naturally, one can examine the details of the phase spectra for such obvious features as the rapidity of phase changes with frequency or the magnitude of the phase difference between $f(t)$ and $f(-t)$ at various frequencies, etc. But such an analysis is complicated in the present instance by the fact that as K is varied, ripples in the power spectrum occur in the vicinity of the phase transitions (see Eqs. A4–A6).

Some experimental procedures that are closely related to the techniques of the present experiments have been used in the studies on "sweep pitch" (Thurlow and Small, 1955), "time-separation pitch" (Small and McClellan, 1963) or "repetition pitch" (Bilsen, 1966). In these experiments, two periodic trains of signals are combined. The trains have the same fundamental repetition rate, but one train is delayed relative to the other. The findings are that a pitch exists that corresponds roughly to $1/T$, where T is the *shortest* interval *between any two signals.* Several of these studies have used rectangular pulse trains for the signals, corresponding to a periodic repetition of the basic transient with $K=1$. Typically, T is varied in these experiments in order to change the perceived pitch. This is complicated in the sense of the present experiments, for pulse trains with different T's differ in both power and phase spectra. However, Thurlow (1957) compared the detectability of a "time-difference pitch" for two periodic trains of pulses having different amplitudes corresponding to a periodic repetition of the basic transient with $K<1$. From listening to the transient stimuli of the present experiment, one would expect that these would lead to characteristically different-sounding trains, but Thurlow does not suggest that $f(t)$ type of trains have any different pitch than $f(-t)$ trains. Bilsen (1966) repeated signals formed from pulses aperiodically, some of which differed only in phase, and concluded that stimuli with identical power spectra have the same repetition pitch, independent of their phase spectra. Apparently, repetition per se is important in determining the processing of phase information, or the measure expressed by time delay pitches does not completely characterize these kinds of stimuli, as suggested by Jenkins (1961).

Investigations considerably more extensive than Expt. 2 would be necessary to discern the exact nature of the processing used to discriminate the signals that differ only in phase. Similarly, while Expt. 3 serves to indicate in a rough-and-ready way the interactions that can occur between the power and phase variables, it is far from being the quantitative comparison that would be desired.

VII. CONCLUSION

Observers can discriminate between very short wide-band signals that differ only in phase. This ability to detect phase differences is considerably more labile and subject to larger individual differences between observers than is the ability to detect power differences. The phase cue can, however, be salient enough to mask significantly detection of a power difference.

ACKNOWLEDGMENTS

Thanks are due to David M. Green for many helpful discussions as well as for a critical reading of an earlier draft of the manuscript. Barry H. Leshowitz first raised the forward–backward masking issue and was included, along with James H. Patterson and Roy D. Patterson, in several helpful discussions. G. Bruce Henning presented a very interesting point concerning a possible mechanism for phase discrimination in terms of effective duration. This issue will be considered in another paper.

Portions of this work were supported by grants from the National Institutes of Health, Public Health Service, U. S. Department of Health, Education, and Welfare. The author held an NIMH Postdoctoral Fellowship during this period.

Appendix A

The representation for the basic transient of Fig. 1(a) and the calculation of its power and phase spectra assume a mathematically tractable form for perfectly rectangular pulses. We must first consider how good an idealization of this perfect form was obtained in this experiment and how departures from this ideal might influcence the results. In fact, the signal was generated by a digital-to-analog converter which had a settling time on the order of 1.5 μsec. This is probably the least important variation from the ideal form, for other system components had much narrower bandwidths, although no filtering was done intentionally. The only effective filter was, therefore, the earphones themselves; and we assume that the earphones are a linear, time-invariant system. Calculations based on the retangular pulses should then be correct except for a linear transfer function imposed by the earphones.

The assumption regarding the power spectrum equivalence of $f(t)$ and $f(-t)$ was checked in the following ways. When the transients were played periodically, no differences were observed for the electrical waveforms on either a Ballantine 320A true rms voltmeter or a General Radio 1900 wave analyzer. Mathematical calculation of rms values and N_0 agreed with both the voltmeter and wave analyzer.

Since the more crucial comparison is between earphone outputs, measurements were also made according to the procedures suggested by Shaw and Thiessen (1963) for the calibration of circumaural earphones. The earphones were mounted on a flat plate coupler and the output measured by a General Radio 1551-C sound-level meter with a 1560-P5 microphone. Strip chart recordings of the acoustic output from 0 to 5000 Hz, using the 3-Hz bandwidth, were inspected, and no differences were observed that could not be attributed to the recording instrumentation itself. On the basis of this evidence and the compelling nature of the linearity assumption, it was concluded that the basic transients in their $f(t)$ and $f(-t)$ forms did in fact have the same power spectrum over the usable portion of the audio range.

Given rectangular pulses, the calculation of the power and phase spectra of $f(t)$ and $f(-t)$ is straightforward. Consider the basic transient as being composed of the sum of two pulses, one of height 1 centered about $t=0$, and another of height $K\leq 1$ centered about time T [i.e., set $A=1$ in Fig. 1(a)]. Call this pulse waveform $g(t)$ and its Fourier transform $G(\omega)$. Then, by the time-shift property of the Fourier transform, we obtain for $f(t)$ the transform

$$F(\omega)=G(\omega)+Ke^{-j\omega T}G(\omega), \tag{A1}$$

while for $f(-t)$ we have the transform

$$H(\omega)=KG(\omega)+e^{-j\omega T}G(\omega), \tag{A2}$$

where

$$G(\omega)=\tau\frac{\sin(\omega\tau/2)}{(\omega\tau/2)}. \tag{A3}$$

Thus,

$$F(\omega)=\tau\frac{\sin(\omega\tau/2)}{(\omega\tau/2)}(1+K\cos\omega T-jK\sin\omega T)$$

and

$$H(\omega)=\tau\frac{\sin(\omega\tau/2)}{(\omega\tau/2)}(K+\cos\omega T-j\sin\omega T).$$

The power spectra are

$$|F(\omega)|^2=|H(\omega)|^2=\tau^2\frac{\sin^2(\omega\tau/2)}{(\omega\tau/2)^2}\times(1+K^2+2K\cos\omega T), \tag{A4}$$

which is the $(\sin x/x)^2$ spectrum of the individual rectangular pulses multiplied by a periodic component, the frequency of which is determined by T. The corresponding phase spectra are

$$P(\omega)=\tan^{-1}[-K\sin\omega T/(1+K\cos\omega T)],\quad \text{for } f(t), \tag{A5}$$

and

$$Q(\omega)=\tan^{-1}[-\sin\omega T/(K+\cos\omega T)],\quad \text{for } f(-t). \tag{A6}$$

These nonlinear functions of ω become linear under certain special conditions, when $K=1$ or $K=0$.

DeBoer (1961) has formulated a monaural phase-distortion argument concisely for continuous signals. Referring to a system transfer function, he asserts that phase transformations that are shifts of a constant amount or are linear with frequency do not produce discriminably different stimuli. The comparison made in the present experiments between perception of $f(t)$ and $f(-t)$ is now seen to be a comparison between two phase spectra that are nonlinear with frequency. The comparison of a nonlinear spectrum ($K\neq 1$) to the linear ($K=1$) spectrum cannot be meaningfully made in this instance because the power spectra are also different in that case.

Appendix B

Since the issue under investigation here is perception of monaural phase effects, it perhaps would have been preferable to run all the conditions using just a single earphone rather than two earphones wired in phase at the two ears. As a partial check on the possible effect of using two ears, Observer SB (the observer most sensitive to the phase differences) was run through the phase discrimination conditions (Expt. 2) a second time, using a single earphone. The data obtained under these conditions are shown in Fig. B-1 and seen very similar

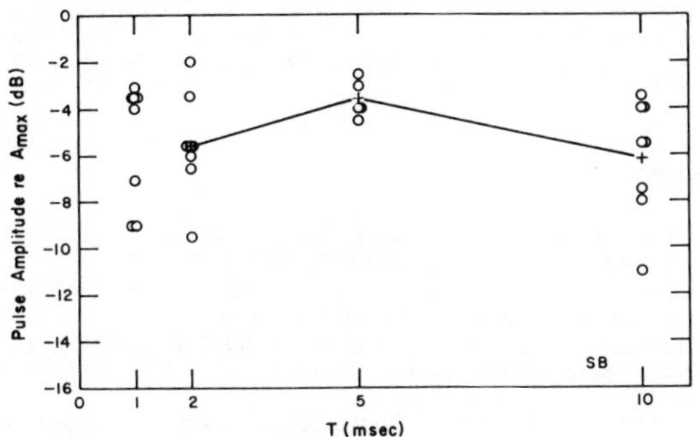

FIG. B-1. Phase discrimination thresholds for Observer SB under single-earphone conditions. Axes same as Fig. 4.

to the corresponding data of Fig. 4. From these results, it is concluded that the effects reported here are indeed monaural ones and do not depend on the use of two ears.

Another point of some concern was the nature of the phase discrimination itself. Experimentally, using the basic transient as a stimulus is very similar to the procedure used to investigate forward and backward masking of clicks (Chistovich and Ivanova, 1959; Raab, 1961). Thus one might try to "explain" the phase-discrimination performance by saying that the perception of $f(t)$ corresponds to the forward masking condition and $f(-t)$ results in a backward masking situation. In fact, such a proposal would have to postulate some additional assumptions—presumably, that the attenuated pulses of $f(t)$ and $f(-t)$ are at different levels above masked threshold and that these levels are discriminably different. Evidently, any asymmetry of the forward–backward masking curve would be crucial to this hypothesis. From the data of Chistovich and Ivanova and of Raab, it was difficult to determine whether or not there was an asymmetry in the masking curve at these short values of T. To pursue this possibility, forward–backward masking data for the basic transient were obtained from Observer JL.

The experimental setup for the forward–backward masking condition was identical to the previous experiments except that K was set equal to zero in order to create the masker stimulus that was always present in one observation interval. The other interval contained either the masker alone or masker plus the signal pulse, and PEST adjusted K to raise and lower the amplitude of the signal pulse. A less stringent convergence criterion of 1 dB was used for these masking conditions. The forward-masking condition was obtained by using the $f(t)$ version of the basic transient; the backward masking used the $f(-t)$ form.

Figure B-2 presents the individual threshold estimates for the masking data, with the mean values indicated by plus signs. Forward-masking conditions are indicated by positive values of T. The masking function appears approximately symmetrical around zero for $T=10$ msec and for $T=1$ msec. At $T=2$ msec, the asymmetry is about 5 dB, whereas at $T=5$ msec, it is around 8 dB, with the forward-masking condition producing the greater masking in both instances. From these data, the masking hypothesis would seem to predict that phase discrimination would be impossible or at best

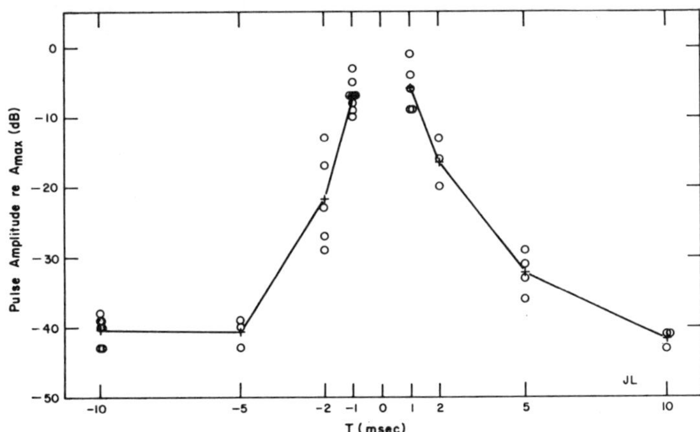

FIG. B-2. Forward–backward masked thresholds for Observer JL. Positive values of T obtained from $f(t)$ version of the basic transient, negative values from $f(-t)$. Ordinate gives attenuation of masked pulse relative to A_{max} for 75% correct detection. Each data point represents a separate PEST estimate. Mean values indicated by plus signs and connected by solid lines.

very difficult at 1 and 10 msec, better at 2 msec, and best at 5 msec. From the top half of Fig. 4, it appears that the phase-detection curve for this observer has quite a different form.

Some additional data that do not correspond to predictions of the masking hypothesis were obtained from Observer SB under the single-earphone phase-discrimination conditions. In this situation, the signal-to-noise ratio was reduced by setting A to lower and lower values until the phase discrimination could no longer be made. It was found that phase discrimination for $T=5$ msec remained essentially unchanged as long as the $f(t)$ stimulus was about 14 dB above threshold. Since, by the time $T=5$ msec, the masking is 30 or 40 dB down, it seems unlikely that such low levels could serve as a reliable reference.

The masking hypothesis also seems implausible on intuitive grounds, for the subjective impression of the observer listening to the $f(t)$ basic transient as compared to $f(-t)$ is that they are qualitatively quite different. A description agreed to by the observers is that one sounds like "tick," while the other sounds like "tock."

* Present address: Central Institute for the Deaf, 818 South Euclid, St. Louis, Missouri 63110.

[1] Some assumptions and measurements regarding the stimuli are presented in Appendix A, together with the calculation of their power and phase spectra.

[2] Data from a supplementary condition using a single earphone are given in Appendix B. Also presented in this Appendix are some additional data that were collected in the process of evaluating a hypothesis about the mechanism responsible for the phase discrimination performance.

REFERENCES

Bilsen, F. A. (1966). "Repetition Pitch: Monaural Interaction of a Sound with Repetition of the Same, but Phase Shifted, Sound," Acustica *17*, 295–300.

Bilsen, F. A. (1967). "Phase Sensitivity and (or?) Short Time Analysis of the Hearing Organ," Acustica *18*, 182 (L).

deBoer, E. (1961). "A Note on Phase Distortion and Hearing," Acustica *11*, 182–184.

Chistovich, L. A., and Ivanova, V. A. (1959). "Mutual Masking of Short Sound Pulses," Biophysics *4*, 46–57.

Corliss, E. L. R. (1963). "Resolution Limits of Analyzers and Oscillatory Systems," J. Res. Nat. Bur. Stand. *67A*, 461–474.

Craig, J. H., and Jeffress, L. A. (1962). "Effect of Phase on the Quality of a Two-Component Tone," J. Acoust. Soc. Amer. *34*, 1752–1760.

Flanagan, J. L. (1965). *Speech Analysis, Synthesis and Perception* (Springer-Verlag, Berlin).

Green, D. M., and Swets, J. A. (1966). *Signal Detection Theory and Psychophysics* (John Wiley & Sons, Inc., New York).

von Helmholtz, H. (1895). *On the Sensations of Tone* (Reprinted by Dover Publications, Inc., New York, 1954).

Jeffress, L. A. (1964). "Stimulus-Oriented Approach to Detection," J. Acoust. Soc. Amer. *36*, 766–774.

Jenkins, R. A. (1961). "Perception of Pitch, Timbre, and Loudness," J. Acoust. Soc. Amer. *33*, 1550–1557.

McGill, W. J. (1967). "Neural Counting Mechanisms and Energy Detection in Audition," J. Math. Psychol. *4*, 351–376.

Mathes, R. C., and Miller, R. L. (1947). "Phase Effects in Monaural Perception," J. Acoust. Soc. Amer. *19*, 780–797.

Pfafflin, S. M. (1968). "Detection of Auditory Signal in Restricted Sets of Reproducible Noise," J. Acoust. Soc. Amer. *43*, 487–490.

Pfafflin, S. M., and Mathews, M. V. (1966). "Detection of Auditory Signals in Reproducible Noise," J. Acoust. Soc. Amer. *39*, 340–345.

Raab, D. H. (1961). "Forward and Backward Masking between Acoustic Clicks," J. Acoust. Soc. Amer. *33*, 137–139.

Shaw, E. A. G., and Thiessen, G. J. (1962). "Acoustics of Circumaural Earphones," J. Acoust. Soc. Amer. *34*, 1233–1246.

Small, A. M., Jr., and McClellan, M. E. (1963). "Pitch Associated with Time Delay between Two Pulse Trains," J. Acoust. Soc. Amer. *35*, 1246–1255.

Taylor, M. M., and Creelman, C. D. (1967). "PEST: Efficient Estimates on Probability Functions," J. Acoust. Soc. Amer. *41*, 782–787.

Thurlow, W. R. (1957). "Further Observation of Pitch Associated with a Time Difference between Two Pulse Trains," J. Acoust. Soc. Amer. *29*, 1310–1311.

Thurlow, W. R., and Small, A. M. (1955). "Pitch Perception for Certain Periodic Auditory Stimuli," J. Acoust. Soc. Amer. *27*. 132–137.

27

Reprinted from *Acoust. Soc. Am. J.* **19**:798–807 (1947)

Masking Effect of Periodically Pulsed Tones as a Function of Time and Frequency

R. L. MILLER
Bell Telephone Laboratories, Inc., New York, New York

(Received July 11, 1947)

IN the course of the experimental work on the effects of phase and of envelope waves on perceived sound, which is described in a companion paper,[1] it was observed that there was a close correlation between the general raucousness or roughness of a sound, and the degree that the envelope wave periodically reduces to zero or low values. In order to investigate this effect, especially with regard to the possibility of fatigue, some experiments were undertaken in which the masking effect of a repeated pulse of a single-frequency tone on a second similar pulse was measured when the latter was varied in time with respect to the first. While the results of the tests show some evidence of the originally looked-for fatigue effect, some of the other results obtained would appear to be of even greater general interest. The results are here summarized:

SUMMARY OF RESULTS

1. If repeated pulses of two different frequencies occur at equal rates, then the masking of one upon the other increases, in general, as they occur more closely together in time.
2. There is an optimum point of masking which generally occurs when the weaker pulse slightly leads the stronger pulse. (1 to 2 milliseconds.)
3. The amount of this time difference is independent of the pulse repetition rate over the range measured of 30–100 c.p.s.
4. This time difference is a function of the frequencies involved under the pulsed envelope wave.
5. While the degree of masking varies considerably between individuals, the pulse time difference for optimum masking remains fairly constant.
6. There is appreciable masking in regions where the pulses are non-overlapping, the amount of masking decreasing towards threshold as the pulse separation becomes large.
7. There is evidence of a fatigue effect in the degree of masking obtained subsequent to a pulse.

While a number of hypotheses have been considered as to a possible cause of the time difference required for optimum masking, there does not appear to be any clear-cut explanation for it from information at present available to the author. However, it does seem definite that it cannot be explained by considering the ear as a simple mechanical resonance system alone, since time differences obtained by this consideration are actually in the wrong direction from that required. The most likely source appears to be in the nerve stimulation and transmission processes.

EXPERIMENTAL SYSTEM AND TECHNIQUE

An over-all block, schematic of the circuit which was used in making the experiments, is shown in Fig. 1. This circuit is substantially the same as used in the previously mentioned experimental work on phase and envelope waves. Since all of the individual elements which go to make up the circuit are quite well known, they will not be described in detail. The over-all circuit is made up essentially of two modulator branches which are quite similar to each other. In the top modulator branch the carrier frequency is divided into two branches, one branch being

[1] R. C. Mathes and R. L. Miller, *Phase Effects in Monaural Perception*, J. Acous. Soc. Am. **19**, 780 (1947).

passed through an attenuator while the other is applied to a double-balanced (ring) modulator.[2] The double-balanced modulator is so arranged that only the upper and lower sidebands are obtained in the output, both the carrier and the signal frequencies being essentially balanced out. The outputs of both the attenuator branch and the modulator are combined by a hybrid arrangement and passed on to the listening point through a variable low pass filter and a second hybrid. In order to produce the pulsed-type envelope wave which is used in most of the experiments, a half-wave rectifier with variable bias is placed in the signal frequency branch at point A. When pulsed waves are produced in this manner the carrier, which is normally resupplied through the attenuator branch, is reduced to zero. The lower modulator branch is much the same as the top branch except that a phase shifter[3,4] has been included in the signal frequency branch. This phase shifter allows the position of the pulsed wave, derived in the bottom branch, to be shifted in phase or time with respect to that originated in the top branch. The variable low-pass filters which appear in both the top and bottom branches are necessary to remove the sidebands associated with the higher harmonics of the carrier frequency. The main disturbing higher harmonic components are centered around the third harmonic although small amounts may appear around the second harmonic because of residual unbalances.

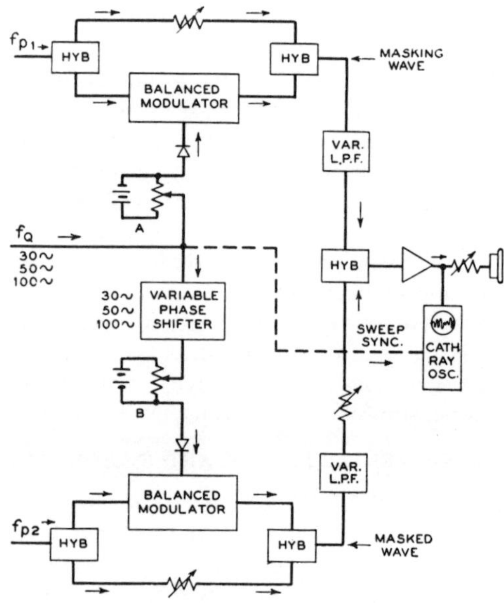

FIG. 1. Block diagram of modulation system used for producing pulsed waves.

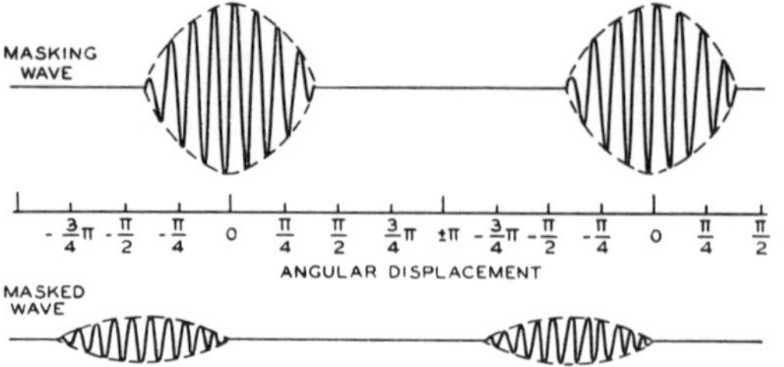

FIG. 2. Illustration of typical pulsed tones used in masking tests. Frequency of tone under the envelope wave may be varied for either the masking or masked wave.

The form of wave which is utilized in a majority of the tests is illustrated in Fig. 2. The top or masking wave is produced in the top main branch of the modulation system. The envelope wave which is shown by the broken line is controlled by varying the ratio of the d.c. bias to the amplitude of the applied signal frequency. Having fixed the shape of the envelope wave by this procedure, the carrier frequency can then be changed as desired, without affecting the envelope shape. Although the carrier by-passed around the modulator is reduced to zero there is still carrier present in such a pulsed wave, since one of the components produced by the rectification process is d.c. The bottom wave, or masked wave, is normally adjusted to have the same envelope shape as the masking wave. The amplitude ratio of the masked wave to the masking wave is determined by the adjustment of the variable attenuator in the branch of the masked wave. Before making any masking tests the over-all adjustment and calibration are checked by observing, with a cathode-ray oscilloscope, the wave which is connected across the listening receivers. Having selected the desired carrier and signal frequencies, the amplitude and shape of the envelope waves are adjusted to be exactly the same with the attenuator of the

[2] R. S. Caruthers, "Copper oxide modulators in carrier telephone systems," Bell Sys. Tech. J. **18**, 315 (1939).
[3] U.S. Patent No. 2,004,613.
[4] H. T. Friis and C. B. Feldman, "A multiple unit steerable antenna for short wave reception," Proc. I.R.E. **25**, 841 (1937).

masked wave set at zero. The setting of the phase shifter associated with the envelope frequency of the masked wave is determined such that the peaks of the two envelope waves exactly coincide in time.

In making the masking measurements, the observer is placed in a quiet booth. By means of a push-button signaling system, he can indicate to the operator whenever the masked tone is observed along with the masking tone. The procedure which is followed is for the operator to apply the masked signal to the masking signal at irregular intervals and at the same time gradually reduce its level. In this way the ability of the observer to synchronize his signaling with the actual application of the masked tone is very apparent. In making the test the level of the masked tone is first reduced to a point where the observer can no longer follow it and then increased until he picks it up again. This process is repeated several times until the operator is satisfied that the lowest observed point remains consistent. By removing the masking tone, the actual threshold of the masked tone can be determined in the same manner. From experience obtained in these tests, the average region of uncertainty was indicated to be approximately 2 db. This figure varies some for different observers and also for different conditions. In general, when the threshold shift was great, (small difference of relative levels) the uncertain region was small, some observers being able to determine the presence of a masked tone within 1 db. When the threshold shift was small (large difference of relative levels) the uncertain region increased to the order of 4 db for some observers In testing an observer for the several angular displacements of a condition, the general policy was followed of interleaving the points so that readings were obtained in a given region at different parts of the test.

In plotting the data obtained from the various tests two alternatives present themselves: (1) the relative level of the masking to the masked wave may be plotted directly or (2) the difference in relative levels may be subtracted from the threshold value to obtain the amount of masking or threshold shift. Since the threshold value will vary between observers as well as between conditions, the two values cannot be plotted accurately on the same chart. When the masking is high, the relative level of the masking to the masked tone for the "just perceptible" condition become fairly independent of the listening level, while near threshold, it is very nearly a direct function of it. Thus when the masking is high the reading of relative values is the most accurate indication, since it involves the error of only one reading, and that reading is obtained in a region when the uncertainty is least. When threshold shift is used it reflects not only the error of the relative levels but also the measurement of threshold, which is itself measured in the region of greater uncertainty. Since most of the values plotted are for large threshold shifts, the actual values have usually been plotted against the scale of relative levels. The scale "approximate threshold shift" has been included for convenience of visualizing in terms of masking. Actually the greatest correction required to change to actual threshold shift is not greater than 3 db for the main sets of curves. Where the approach to threshold is thought to be of special importance the correction has been applied and the relative level scale omitted.

In order to be sure that some of the effects observed were not due to abnormal hearing, audiograms were made of all of the observers on the Western Electric No. 6 Audiometer. With but one minor exception none of the observers had any particular abnormality in hearing, most of them being above average in the frequency regions which apply to the tests. The observer *A* had a sharp loss in hearing in the left ear beginning at approximately 3500 c.p.s.

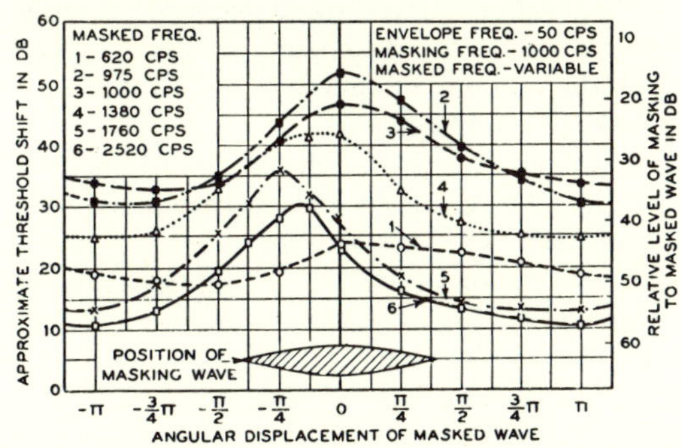

FIG. 3. Masking curves obtained by averaging the results of a number of observers.

RESULTS OF EXPERIMENTS

The first series of tests were made with a masking frequency of 1000 c.p.s. and a pulse repetition rate of 50 c.p.s. (20 millisecond intervals), the pulse being on for 0.4 (8 ms.) of a cycle and off for 0.6 (12 ms.). The results of these tests are shown on Fig. 3, the parameters of the various curves being the different masked frequencies. These curves indicate that the masking increases by the order of 20 db when the two pulses are near coincidence and when the masked frequencies are higher than the masking frequency. When the masked frequency lies appreciably below the masking frequency, the masking is poor, and the change near coincidence is small, being only about 6 db. There is a consistent shift of the point of maximum masking as the masked frequency is increased up to approximately 1760 c.p.s. Above 1760 c.p.s. the shift is reversed, but to a lesser extent. The shift in the point of maximum masking is such that the low level or masked wave leads the masking wave in angular displacement of time. At 1760 cycles the amount of this is equal to 0.25π (50 c.p.s.) or 2.5 milliseconds.

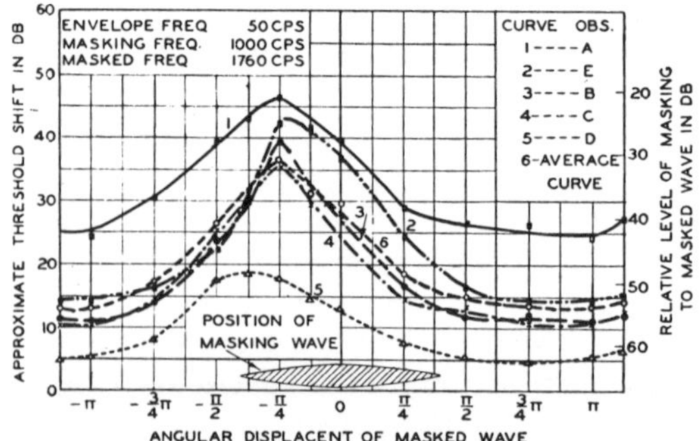

FIG. 4. Masking curves of individual observers obtained for a typical condition.

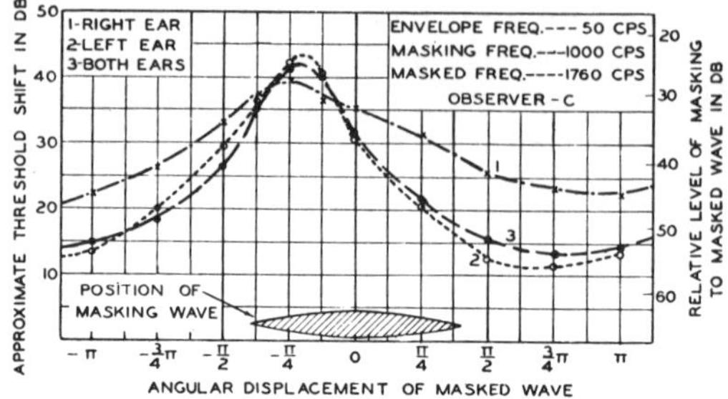

FIG. 5. Masking curves obtained from right, left, and combined ears of an individual observer.

The above curves have been obtained by averaging the results of five observers. In order to show the type and degree of variations between various observers, their individual curves are shown on Fig. 4 for the condition of 1760 cycles masked frequency. While there is a large variation in over-all masking between observers, the general shapes of the curves are quite consistent, as are also the points of maximum masking. It is interesting to note in this connection, that the measured thresholds of the masked tone for the different observers under this condition, varied by only 3 db as compared to the approximately 20 db threshold shift variation shown by the above curves.

Also of interest concerning individual observers are the results obtained for the right and left ears separately as well as for the combined result. The curves obtained for one observer are shown on Fig. 5. The indications from these curves and from results on other observers are that individual ears differ to about the same extent that individuals themselves differ. The other characteristic noticed is that if a person has one ear which is much more sensitive than the other, then the curve for both ears will tend to follow the curve of the more sensitive one. The curves shown in Fig. 5 are a good illustration of the latter characteristic.

In order to obtain further information as to what the effect is that requires the masked wave to lead the masking wave, similar experiments were conducted in which the time spacing between pulses was varied. The results of these tests are shown on Fig. 6. In plotting up the results, the angular displacement of the various pulse rates has been converted to time, so that the different curves can be compared more easily on this basis. In one condition for each of the three rates (30, 50 and 100 c.p.s.) the length and shape of the pulses were adjusted to be as nearly the same as possible on a time basis. For the 100 c.p.s. rate (10 ms. interval) a 100 percent amplitude modulated wave was considered to give a very close approximation to the pulse shape used for the other rates.

Inspection of the curves shows that the time

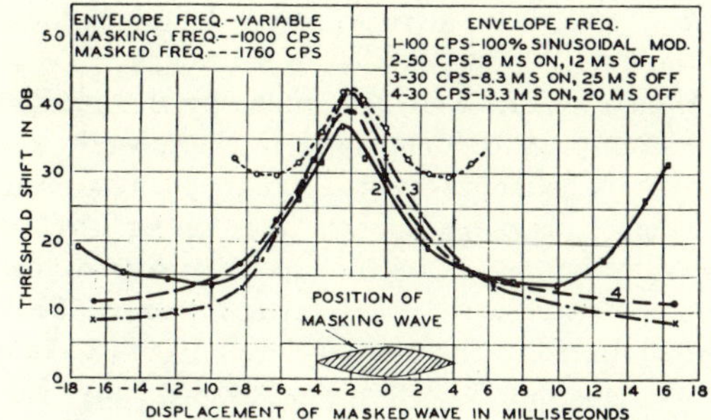

FIG. 6. Average masking curves for several pulse repetition rates plotted on an absolute time scale to illustrate constant time difference for point of optimum masking.

displacement of the point of optimum masking is almost exactly the same for the different pulse spacings. The shape of the curves in the region where the pulses overlap is also very much the same. It was felt that in these curves the degree to which each approached threshold as the spacing increased would be of considerable interest. For this reason threshold corrections were applied to each individual curve so that they would be as nearly correct as possible in the neighborhood of threshold. The result here is consistent with what might be expected, in that the approach to threshold is closer the greater the spacing between pulses. In order to see if there was any significant change in the shape of the curve with a change in the width of the pulses, the width of the pulse for the 30 c.p.s. rate was increased to 13.3 ms. as compared to 8.3 ms. The displacement of the curve remained the same as before. Two minor changes do appear to take place which are consistent with the change in pulse width. One of these is that the curve does not approach threshold quite as closely as the narrower pulse, and the other is that the rate of increase in masking is less sharp in the region of overlap.

In order to show the data on the point of maximum masking a little more clearly, it has been replotted in (a) of Fig. 7, not only for the average curves but also for different individuals. These curves show that the time lead required by the masked wave tends to stay constant not only for the averages, but also for the various individuals.

The time of maximum masking plotted as a function of the masked frequency, both for individuals and for the average curves, is shown in Fig 7 (b). It should be noted that the curve obtained from the average curves of Fig. 3 is not quite the same as if the points of the individuals themselves were averaged. This apparent inconsistency is due to the fact that in drawing a particular masking curve, the best estimated curve does not always pass through the experimental points. Except for the observer A the curves show the same general shape in that they rise to a maximum at approximately 1760 cycles and then fall more slowly thereafter.

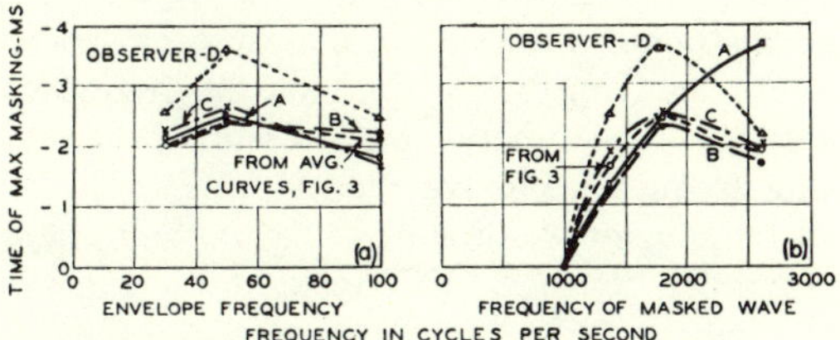

FIG. 7. The time of optimum masking for both individual observers and average curves (Fig. 6). Masking frequency under the envelope is 1000 c.p.s. (a) As a function of envelope repetition rate when the masked frequency is 1760 c.p.s. (b) As a function of the masked frequency when the masking frequency under the envelope is 1000 c.p.s. and repetition rate 50 c.p.s.

In order to investigate a little more fully what happens to the point of maximum masking for different pulsing rates and for higher masked frequencies, a different experimental technique was applied. This method, although not as accurate, gives a much more rapid means of obtaining the point of maximum masking. The technique consisted of setting the relative levels of the masking and masked waves such, that the level of the masked wave was slightly above threshold at the approximate point of maximum masking, and then, by turning the pulse frequency phase shifter, the masked tone could be made to fade out and then increase as the maximum masking point was traversed. By reading the phase shifter for equal loudness of the masked tone on either side a good approximation could be obtained of the desired point. For the lower pulse rate this method was least accurate because the movement of the phase shifter dial required for estimating becomes large compared to the time intervals measured.

The results obtained by this method are shown in Figs. 8(a) and 8(b). Figure 8(a) shows the same general information as that given by Fig. 7(b) except that the frequency range has been extended and curves are also given for different pulse rates. (b) gives curves which were obtained for several masking frequencies other than 1000 c.p.s. The pulse rate remained fixed at 50 c.p.s. for these latter curves. The indications are that the maximum time lead of the masked wave becomes larger for lower masking frequencies; likewise it occurs for a masked frequency more closely spaced to the masking frequency. It is interesting to note that for higher masking frequencies (2000 c.p.s.) it is possible to find the point of maximum masking for masked frequencies lying below the masking frequency. In this case the direction of time shift is the same as for frequencies above the masking frequency and the magnitude of shift is about the same.

In order to check this latter finding actual

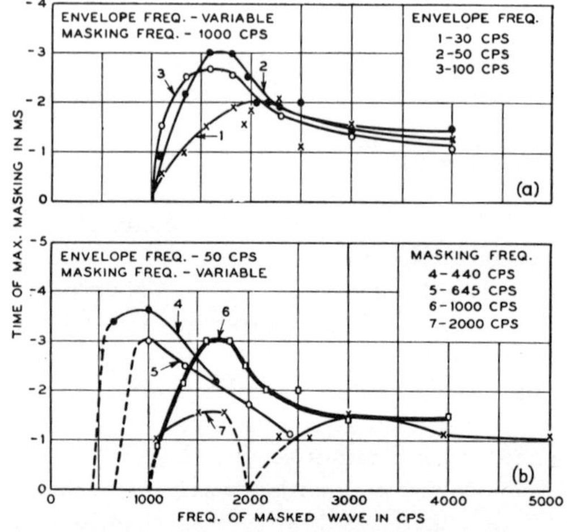

FIG. 8. Time of optimum masking obtained as a function of masked frequency by method of estimating. (a) Repetition rate as a parameter, masking frequency 1000 c.p.s. (b) Masking frequency as a parameter, repetition rate 50 c.p.s.

masking curves were made for the same observers used in previous tests. The average curve obtained in this manner is given on Fig. 9. The shift in time of the point of maximum masking checks quite closely the figure obtained by the method of estimating. This curve also shows that there is about twice the range in masking as the pulse positions were varied compared to the condition of 1000 c.p.s. masking frequency and 620 c.p.s. masked frequency which was shown on Fig. 3. This is the reason that the effect could be detected by the method of estimating.

Measurements were also made, by the method of estimating, to determine if there were any significant changes in the point of maximum masking caused by changes in listening level of the masking wave itself. The intensity of the masking wave was varied by as much as 15 db and 20 db below the usual listening level (67.5 db above threshold) without observing any significant changes in the point of maximum masking. Observations were made with masked frequencies of 1380, 1760 and 2520 c.p.s., the masking frequency remaining at 1000 c.p.s. and the repetition rate to 50 c.p.s.

DISCUSSION OF RESULTS

In order that a clearer picture may be obtained as to the significance of the application of a pulse frequency to the ear, it is desirable to analyze the wave into its various components. A convenient and well-known method of representing such a wave is to consider it as having the frequency of the carrier and an amplitude coefficient which is variable with time or

$$e_p = f(qt)\cos pt. \tag{1}$$

Since the variable amplitude coefficient or envelope wave is a repeated function with time, it can be readily represented by means of a Fourier series. The series for the type of envelope wave most generally used (0.4 on, 0.6 off) is given by the expression

$$\begin{aligned} f(qt) = \frac{Em}{\pi}[0.85 &+ 1.23\cos(qt+\phi) \\ &+ 0.83\cos(2qt+2\phi) \\ &+ 0.25\cos(3qt+3\phi) - 0.07\cos(4qt+4\phi) \\ &- 0.12\cos(5qt+5\phi) \\ &- 0.02\cos(6qt+6\phi)\cdots]. \end{aligned} \tag{2}$$

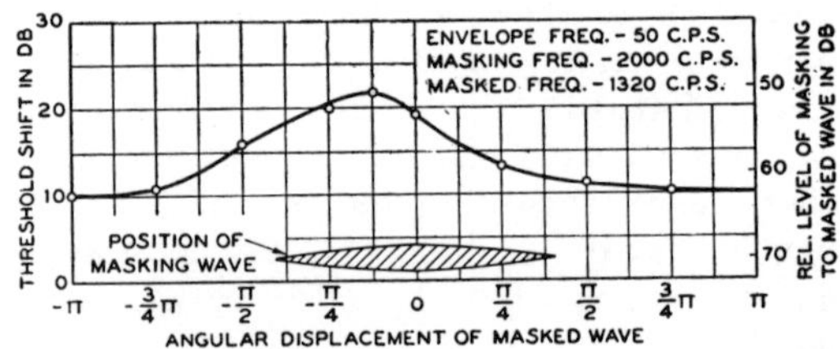

FIG. 9. Average masking curve obtained with the masking frequency (2000 c.p.s.) higher than the masked frequency (1320 c.p.s.).

Where Em is the maximum amplitude of the envelope, q is the pulse rate and ϕ may be the angular displacement of the pulse. If (2) is substituted into (1), assuming for simplicity that the angular displacement is zero, then we obtain

$$e_p=\frac{Em}{\pi}[0.85\cos pt+0.61\cos(p\pm q)t +0.41\cos(p\pm 2q)t+0.12\cos(p\pm 3q)t -0.035\cos(p\pm 4q)t-0.06\cos(p\pm 5q)t -0.01\cos(p\pm 6q)t+\cdots].$$

This expression indicates that on a steady state basis, the pulse of frequency may be viewed as a carrier wave, corresponding to the d.c. term of the envelope wave, and sets of upper and lower sidebands, corresponding to the various harmonics. A plot of these amplitudes is shown in Fig. 10(a). In order to check that the waves, which were being used in the tests, were in substantial agreement with the theoretical ones, the various components were measured with a wave analyzer. These values are shown in Fig. 10(b). It was also determined by means of the analyzer that other extraneous frequency components present in the experimental wave due to higher modulation products, unbalances and inadequate filtering were substantially smaller than any of the components shown. It should be noted that a major part (98 percent) of the energy is accounted for by the carrier and sidebands corresponding to the first and second harmonics.

If we view the application of the pulse more in the light of expression (1), (i.e., the application of a disturbance centering about the carrier frequency but varying with time) then it seems reasonable that if the masking and masked pulses are coincident in time, the masking effect should approximate that of the corresponding steady frequencies. If the values of maximum threshold shift given by Fig. 3 are checked with published masking curves,[5] it will be found that a good degree of correspondence exists. In making this comparison the question arises as to whether the values taken should correspond to those for zero displacement or those corresponding to the maximum point of masking. The use of the maximum point of masking gives the best agreement, and it seems logical to use these values if it is assumed that some delay phenomenon is entering into the effective position of the two pulses.

By means of the steady state analysis, it is possible to obtain a fairly clear picture of what happens for the special case in which the two carriers are the same (1000 c.p.s.). Since the two carriers of the two pulses were adjusted to add in phase, then it is convenient to treat the addition of the masked wave simply as a change in the over-all envelope wave, which is modulating the carrier. When the two envelope waves are lined up, then the components are all in phase and what a person hears is simply a change in amplitude. The value given by the curve represents a 10 percent change in amplitude, which is consistent with published data on differential amplitude sensitivity.

As the masked wave is displaced from the masking wave, the frequency components of the combined envelope wave change amplitudes with respect to each other. This is due to the fact that the phase of the nth harmonic is n times the displacement as measured in terms of the fundamental. For example, if the masked wave is displaced by π, then the expression for it corresponding to that of (2) above would become

$$e_2=\frac{Em_2}{\pi}[0.85-1.23\cos qt+0.83\cos 2qt -0.25\cos 3qt-0.07\cos 4qt +0.12\cos 5qt-0.02\cos 6qt\cdots]. \quad (4)$$

It will be noticed, that for this condition, the odd harmonics have a negative sign compared to expression (2), so that when the masking and masked waves are added together, the odd harmonics oppose each other, while the even harmonics add in phase. This change in quality results in conditions being more readily differentiated than if it were just a change in amplitude.

For masked frequencies lying close to and above 1000 c.p.s., the trend of the curves is much the same as that for 1000 c.p.s., except for the peculiar effect of the peak appearing earlier in time. We can no longer analyze so simply what happens to the perceived wave, since the carrier

[5] Harvey Fletcher, *Speech and Hearing* (D. Van Nostrand Company, Inc., New York, 1929).

frequencies shaped by the envelope waves differ and affect different regions of the basilar membrane; although, if we assumed that the stimulus to the brain was proportional to the envelope wave, in each case, we might get an analogous effect.

It is probably just as well to consider the change in masking from the viewpoint that the damping of the ear is quite high and can follow the amplitude variations to a great extent. Thus, as the two pulses are separated, the ear can more readily differentiate the masking and masked waves. If the curves for the masking of frequencies lying above the masking wave are compared to those lying below, it will be noticed that there is a much greater variation in masking as the pulses are shifted with respect to each other. The variation for 620 c.p.s. masked frequency is 6 db while for 2520 c.p.s. it is 20 db. Also, if the curve shown on Fig. 9 for a masking frequency of 2000 and masked frequency of 1320 c.p.s. is compared to the curve for a masking frequency of 1000 c.p.s. and masked frequency of 1760 c.p.s. in Fig. 3, it will be found that there is only a 12 db range for the former compared to 23 db for the latter, even though the frequencies and their spacings are very nearly the same in the two cases, the essential difference being that the relative frequency positions of the masking and masked wave have been interchanged. It is probable that this effect is interrelated with the fact that stimulation patterns of low frequencies tend to overlap high frequency regions on the basilar membrane more effectively than for the reverse condition.[6]

There is some evidence of the originally looked-for effect of fatigue, taking place subsequent to the application of the pulse. This is indicated by the fact that a majority of the curves show that the increase in masking is more rapid as the position of the masked pulse approaches the point of maximum masking from in front, than the decrease in masking subsequent to this point. It is also evidenced by the fact that the low point in masking for curves of the 50 c.p.s. pulse rate usually occurs at a point $\frac{3}{4}\pi$

[6] George von Bekesy, "On the resonance curve and dying-out time of various points of the septum cochlea," Akustiche Zeits. **8** (March 1943).

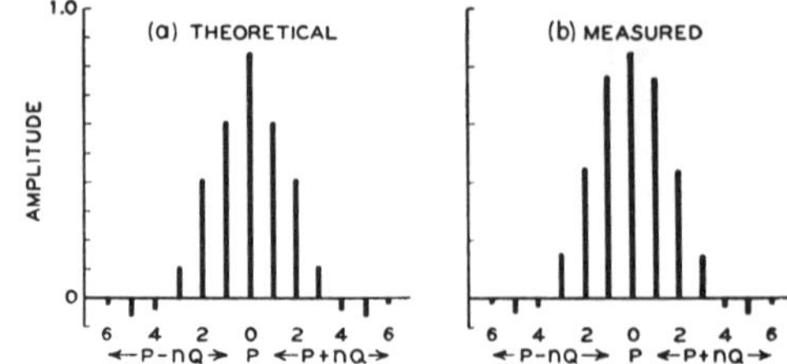

FIG. 10. Spectrum analysis of a typical pulsed wave used in masking tests in terms of a carrier (P) and sidebands ($\pm nQ$). (a) Computed and (b) measured.

in front of the peak, while the subsequent decrease occupies $1\frac{1}{4}\pi$ of this interval.

One of the most interesting results of these masking experiments is the fact that when the masked frequency departs from the masking frequency, the envelope must be made to lead it by substantial times in order to obtain maximum masking. The fact that the amount of time involved remains essentially constant regardless of pulse rates or shapes (as indicated in (a) of Fig. 7), would seem to indicate that it is a time-delay effect. Since there does not seem to be any basis for action of an anticipatory nature, the effect would appear to be due to a difference in the time required for perception between the masking and masked wave when compared at the point where the masking takes place. Since the effect requires that the masked wave lead the masking wave, then this would require that the time interval for perception of the masked wave be longer than for the masking wave.

The first point at which some delay might be expected, would be that of the receiver, since the comparisons of time are made on the wave applied to the receiver. The type of receiver used was the Western Electric HA-2, which is very highly damped. Response characteristics of this receiver taken when it is coupled to a volume of air equivalent to that of the ear show that it is extremely flat between 200 and 2800 c.p.s. Check measurements on the test equipment, which were made by coupling the receiver to a high quality microphone and thence to an oscilloscope, also showed that there were no appreciable delay differences over the range used in the tests. Transmission of the pressure wave from the outer ear and through the middle ear is extremely rapid in terms of the time intervals in which we are interested. The fact that the ear responds to frequencies of over 10,000 c.p.s. and also that there are normally no sharp variations in over-all responses such as indicated by threshold curves, implies that there are little variations of delay in this part of the ear. Measurements by Derbyshire and Davis[7] on cochlea response potentials indicate that they appear 0.1 millisecond or less after the application of the pressure wave to the eardrum.

The first point at which it appears possible to obtain delays of appreciable magnitude is that of the resonant member of which the basilar membrane is an important part. In order to determine what order of delays is possible, it is necessary to know the sharpness of the resonance or the damping decrement. At present there appears to be an unanswered disparity between the rather broad resonant response as given by Bekesy[6] for the motion of the basilar membrane, and the relatively sharp stimulation patterns obtained from masking data[8] or responses of single nerve fibers.[9] However, there is general agreement that the widths of the response curves are approximately constant when plotted on a logarithmic frequency scale. This means that in terms of absolute band-width the high frequency elements are much wider than for low frequencies, and consequently can build up much more rapidly. The fact that the part of the basilar membrane which responds to high frequencies lies nearest to the oval window, also means that the time required for a wave to reach this region is less than for the regions stimulated by lower frequencies. This has been demonstrated by Bekesy in his measurements of "transit time" described in the article referred to above.[6] Thus we see that delay differences obtained by these considerations are actually in the wrong direction to explain the effect which is being obtained, so that we must look further on or else consider more complex relations involving the basilar membrane.

It may well be that the difference in delays takes place in the nerves and nerve-stimulation system associated with the cochlea. One clue to a source of delay, which might explain the effects obtained, is given in the paper by Derbyshire and Davis referred to before.[7] They show that when a click is applied to the ear of a cat, a train of three action potentials having different degrees of delay will characteristically appear in the auditory nerve. These have been labelled the *F*, *G* and *H* waves in the order of increasing lateness. When the intensity of the click is increased from threshold it is the latter two (*G*, *H*) action potentials which make their appearance first. The delay of these potentials decreases as the intensity increases above threshold. The greatest delays given for these waves (*H*) were 2.6 milliseconds, whereas for high levels, the first action potentials (*F*) could occur with as little delay as 0.5 to 0.6 millisecond. The implications of these results as applied to the present experiments would be that the masking wave produces nerve impulses which appear very quickly, while those produced by the masked wave being near threshold appear later in time, and in order to obtain the maximum masking, the applied masked wave would have to be shifted ahead of the masking wave.

Another effect in nerve stimulation which must be considered is that when a pulse of frequency is applied to an ear, the initial response rate of an auditory-nerve fiber is very rapid, but decreases asymptotically thereafter. This effect has been demonstrated by Galambos and Davis[9] in the paper mentioned previously. In the present experiment, this might mean that the peak of response by the nerve fiber could effectively lead the peak of the applied pulse. If the masked wave were not similarly affected, then delays of the required type could be obtained. Two things seem to rule against obtaining the delays in this manner: one, the pulse time intervals are short compared to the time intervals shown for the decrease in nerve pulse-rate and two, increasing the width of the pulse as was done under the condition of a 30 c.p.s. pulse rate did not affect the time of delay appreciably.

There are several significant details given by the curves shown on (a) and (b) of Fig. 8 which would appear to have a bearing on the final answer as to what is causing the time differences.

---

[7] A. J. Derbyshire and H. Davis, "The action potentials of the auditory nerve," Am. J. Physiol. **113**, 476 (1935).

[8] H. Fletcher, "A space-time pattern theory of hearing," J. Acous. Soc. Am. **1**, 311 (1939).

[9] Robert Galambos and Hallowell Davis, "The response of single auditory-nerve fibers to acoustic stimulation," J. Neuro-Physiol. **6**, 39–58 (1943).

One is the fact shown by (b) that the direction of time difference can be the same regardless of whether the masked frequency is above or below the masking frequency. A system having a uniform trend in time intervals as a function of frequency, would require that the direction of the time difference reverse. Also of significance are the indications that the ratio of the masking frequency to the masked frequency having the maximum time difference on the higher side, tends to stay constant for different masking frequencies (ratio is approximately 0.66); and, that the amount of the maximum time difference tends to increase for lower masking frequencies. These latter two results would seem to be an indication that the sharpness of resonance of the ear is entering into the delay effect in some complex manner. It may also be observed, that for masked frequencies considerably above the masking frequency, the trend of the curves is such as might be explained by the change in delays associated with the increasing band widths of the response curves. Thus several different factors might ultimately be found to underlie the characteristics observed.

It is interesting to note that while most of the discussion has been in terms of time intervals, the experiments could also be viewed as actual measurements of some of the effects of phase on audible perception.

28

Reprinted from *Acoust. Soc. Am. J.* 34:1116–1117 (1962)

Backward and Forward Masking of Probe Tones of Different Frequencies*

LOIS L. ELLIOTT
Ear, Nose, and Throat Branch, School of Aerospace Medicine, Aerospace Medical Division (AFSC), Brooks Air Force Base, Texas

ALTHOUGH Samoilova[1] investigated the masking effect of pure tones on pure tones in the monotic situation, the masking effect of white noise on various frequencies of pure tones in dichotic as well as monotic listening conditions has not been previously explored. A previous experiment which studied backward and forward masking of one pure tone (1000 cps) demonstrated the existence of masking in the dichotic situation, where the probe is presented to one ear while the masking noise is presented to the other ear.[2] Sherrick and Albernaz[3] investigated the masking effect of noise pulses on *simultaneously* pulsed tones of different frequencies under both monotic and dichotic listening conditions. Their results indicated considerable frequency differences with 4000 cps showing the greatest amount of masking for both monotic and dichotic conditions. The present study was designed to investigate masking effects on three different probe frequencies under both monotic and dichotic listening conditions. It was expected that obtained results would resemble the findings of Sherrick and Albernaz in showing greater masking for higher frequencies.

The stimulus sequence for the backward masking condition was identical to that used in the previous study.[2] A ready light signaled to the subject that the next stimulus sequence was about to begin. After a ready interval lasting 0.6 sec, the standard, or comparison, masking stimulus was presented. This standard was identical to the second masking stimulus except that it was never associated with a probe tone. The interval between the end of the standard masking signal and the probe tone was 1 sec. The time between the end of the probe tone and the beginning of the second masking stimulus was designated as the masking interval and varied from 0–100 msec. White noise at 90 dB SPL *re* 0.0002 dyn/sec^2 was used as masking; probe tones of 500, 1000, and 4000 cps were employed. Signal durations were 50 msec for the masking and 7 msec for the probe. Rise–fall times were 1 msec for the probe tone and 10 μsec for the masking. The situation for forward masking was analogous to this except that the probe tone always followed the second masking signal. The subject controlled intensity of the probe tone, varying it until he could just discriminate a difference between the combined probe-and-masking and the standard masking. This difference was perceived not as a difference in loudness but as a difference in associated pitch. Each judgment was repeated at least twice. Attenuation was introduced in the experimenter's console so that the subject had no fixed reference for making threshold adjustments.

Equipment used to produce this stimulus series was the same as that described in the previous report.[2] Six subjects with normal hearing started daily practice sessions for the experiment, but only three completed the one-month training period. Results, therefore, are based on responses of three highly experienced listeners who were tested for each treatment combination on at least three different days spread over a six-week period of daily testing.

Results for the monotic listening condition are shown in Fig. 1, which plots masking interval on the

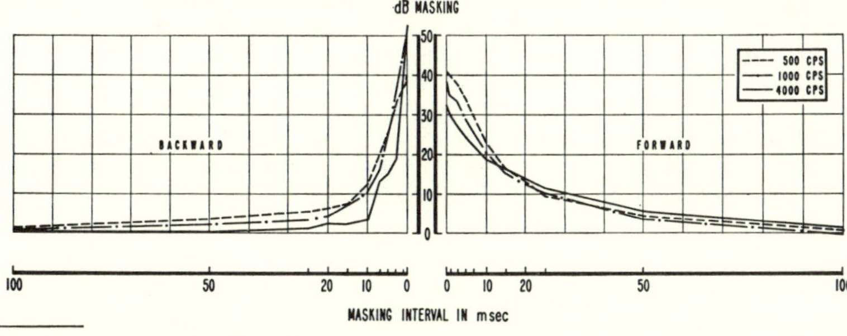

FIG. 1. Results of monotic backward and forward masking (At 0 backward masking interval the points are 50-dB masking for 1000 cps and 53.5-dB masking for 4000 cps.)

* A modified version of this paper was presented at the meetings of the Acoustical Society in May 1962.
[1] I. K. Samoilova, Biophysics 4, 44–52 (1959).
[2] L. L. Elliott, J. Acoust. Soc. Am. **34**, 1108 (1962); also School of Aerospace Medicine Tech. Rept. 62–76.
[3] C. E. Sherrick and P. L. M. Albernaz, J. Acoust. Soc. Am. **33**, 1381–1385 (1961).

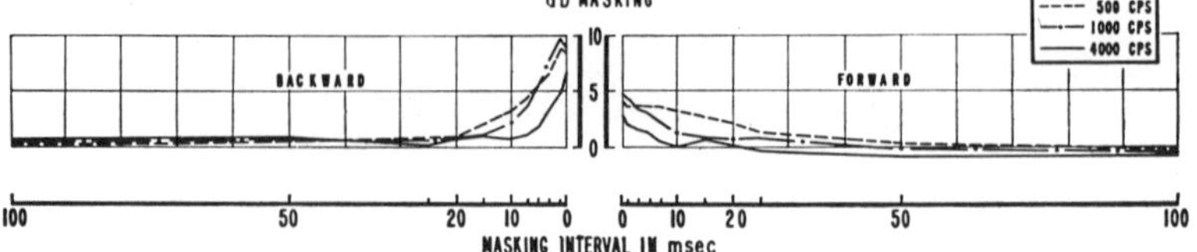

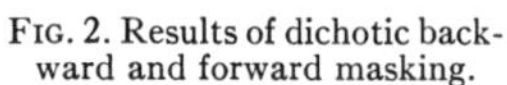
FIG. 2. Results of dichotic backward and forward masking.

abscissa while the ordinate represents amount of masking obtained (i.e., the difference between the masked and unmasked thresholds). At the zero masking interval of the backward condition results for the three probe frequencies line up as would be expected from the results of Sherrick and Albernaz; 4000 cps shows greatest masking and 500 cps shows least masking. However, this order of frequencies is not maintained for longer masking intervals; at 3 msec 4000 cps shows the least amount of masking—a position which is held through the 100-msec masking interval. Although differences between the frequencies are not large, at longer masking intervals they are consistent with frequencies maintaining their relative positions from 5–100 msec masking intervals.

In considering the forward monotic condition, there is less masking of 4000 and 1000 cps at short masking intervals than occurs in backward masking. This agrees with previous findings. The third frequency of 500 cps, however, does not follow this pattern and shows slightly more forward than backward masking. At masking intervals from 0 to 10 msec, 500 cps shows the greatest amount of forward masking and 4000 the least. From 20 to 100 msec, 4000 cps shows the greatest amount of masking while the other two frequencies fall slightly below. The most parsimonious conclusion which can be drawn for monotic listening is that the order of masking of frequencies as seen at the 0-msec masking interval of the backward condition and also in the simultaneous masking data of Sherrick and Albernaz is not representative of longer masking intervals. (It should be noted that stimuli of Sherrick and Albernaz were of longer duration than those used here.)

In previous research using only 1000-cps probe tones it was noted that a major change in the slope of the backward masking curve occurred at about 15-msec masking interval. This change again appears for 1000 as well as for 500 cps; however, 4000 cps changes slope at 10 msec. As before, no abrupt slope changes occur for forward masking.

Figure 2 presents results for dichotic listening. In both forward and backward conditions 1000 cps shows greatest and 4000 cps least masking at zero masking intervals. At 5 msec for backward masking and 3 msec for forward masking the two lower frequencies reverse positions, while at longer masking intervals there are essentially no differences between frequencies.

For the dichotic condition there is less forward than backward masking at all three frequencies. The backward masking curves show rather abrupt changes in slope which occur at approximately the same masking intervals as occurred in the monotic condition. Finally, one must conclude for the dichotic condition that observed results do not order frequencies as would have been anticipated from work on simultaneous pulsed dichotic masking.

During the experiment subjects were also required to judge the temporal relationship of the tone and masking signals. They reported the probe as a tone distinctly separate from the masking noise and occurring either before or after the masking, as a tone combined with masking but associated with either the beginning or termination of masking, and as occurring simultaneously with masking. Analysis of these results indicated that transition from one category of response to another —for example, from hearing a distinctly separate tone to hearing the tone associated with the beginning of masking—was not clearly related to any change in the slopes of the curves.

These results are more easily described than explained. Several possible explanations for backward masking in general were discussed in the previous paper.[2] It has been noted that the acoustic reflex more readily affects lower frequencies than higher ones. However, it is difficult to see how the acoustic reflex could be involved in backward masking where the probe tone precedes the masking signal. Also, this possibility could not explain the change in the 4000-cps curve which occurs at brief masking intervals in the backward monotic condition. It seems very likely that whatever mechanisms produce increased backward masking at very short masking intervals are also responsible for the increased masking of the 4000-cps probe tone at this point. Undoubtedly this is dependent upon the magnitude, location, and time relationships among bursts of neural firings.

29

Reprinted from *Acoust. Soc. Am. J.* **36**:277–282 (1964)

Rate of Decay of Auditory Sensation

R. Plomp

Institute for Perception RVO–TNO, Soesterberg, The Netherlands

(Received 10 October 1963)

The rate of decay of auditory sensation was investigated by measuring the minimum silent interval that must be introduced between two noise pulses to be perceived. The value of this critical time Δt was determined for different intensity levels of both the first and the second pulse. It is shown that in this case the sensation level of the second pulse may be considered as a very good approximation of the level of auditory sensation after Δt, due to the first pulse. From the experiments, we may conclude (1) expressed in dB as a function of log t, the decay of sensation is represented by a straight line; (2) independent of the sensation level of the stimulating sound, the hearing threshold is reached at the same time of about 200–300 msec. These results are compared with other experiments and the differences are discussed.

As EARLY as thirty years ago, von Békésy[1] determined the slowest rate of an exponential decay of a tone that gives the same impression as a tone ending abruptly. Assuming that this rate is equal to the rate of decay of sensation itself, Stevens and Davis[2] concluded from these experiments that, regardless of the initial intensity, a disrupted tone of 800 cps reaches the value of auditory threshold in approximately 140 msec.

These experiments were repeated by Miller,[3] using white noise instead of tones as the stimulus. The results confirmed the conclusion that the time needed for the sensation to reach threshold is independent of intensity. Miller found critical durations somewhat shorter than for tonal decay, varying between 50 and 80 msec for different observers.

Both experiments suggest that, plotting sensation in dB relative to a linear time scale, the decay is represented by a straight line that reaches hearing threshold after about 140 msec for tones and 50–80 msec for white noise. The intensity of the sound would affect only the slope of this line.

It is of interest that Miller, before following von Békésy's method, first tried another way to study the decay of sensation. He determined the intensity level of noise just detectable during interruptions of a white noise. Finding still a 20-dB threshold shift 330 msec after the interruption of a white noise of 80 dB sensation level, he concluded that this method did not give an adequate estimate of the decay of sensation and abandoned the method.

In Fig. 1, Miller's data for a single listener are reproduced, using a logarithmic time scale instead of the linear scale of the original diagram. As we see, the points can be fit rather well by straight converging lines reaching threshold for times of 600–1200 msec.

This relation between masking and interruption time was confirmed by experiments on the masking of noise and tones by periodic noise bursts.[4–7] So Dubout's data show by extrapolation that poststimulatory threshold shifts occurred until about 700 msec, independent of the intensity of the stimulus.

Several investigators have studied poststimulatory masking with single sound pulses for both the stimulus and the test pulse. In some of these experiments, pure

[1] G. von Békésy, "Über die Hörsamkeit der Ein- und Ausschwingvorgänge mit Berücksichtigung der Raumakustik," Ann. Physik **16**, 844–860 (1933). Also G. von Békésy, *Experiments in Hearing* (McGraw-Hill Book Co., Inc., New York, 1960), pp. 321–332.

[2] S. S. Stevens and H. Davis, *Hearing* (John Wiley & Sons, Inc., New York, 1938), pp. 220–224.

[3] G. A. Miller, "The Perception of Short Bursts of Noise," J. Acoust. Soc. Am. **20**, 160–170 (1948).

[4] G. A. Miller and W. R. Garner, "The Masking of Tones by Repeated Bursts of Noise," J. Acoust. Soc. Am. **20**, 691–696 (1948).

[5] I. Pollack, "Sensitivity to Differences in Intensity between Repeated Bursts of Noise," J. Acoust. Soc. Am. **23**, 650–653 (1951).

[6] I. Pollack, "Masking by a Periodically Interrupted Noise," J. Acoust. Soc. Am. **27**, 353–355 (1955).

[7] P. Dubout, "Observations of Persistence of Post-Stimulus Masking," Acustica **9**, 353–358 (1959).

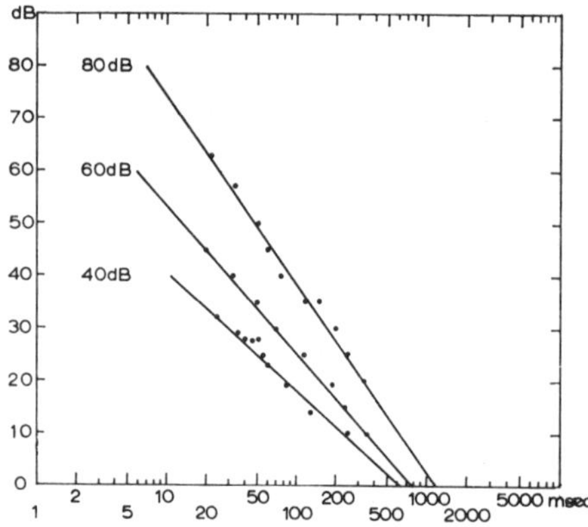

FIG. 1. Sensation level of noise that was just detectable during interruption of a white noise as a function of interruption time. [After Miller.[3]] The sensation level of the white-noise bursts is indicated.

tones were used for both pulses[8–14] in others noise was used either for the stimulus[11,15,16] or for both pulses.[17,18] Also, the mutual masking of clicks was investigated.[19–21]

However, these experiments have not given a conclusive answer about the rate of decay of sensation. Lüscher and Zwislocki[8] and Rawnsley and Harris[10] found poststimulatory threshold-shift values, plotted in dB as a function of t (linear), which varied between a more linear course for sensation levels above 50 dB of the stimulating tone pulse and a more exponential course for lower sensation levels. Also, the data of Samoilova[13] and Elliott[15,16] point to a rate of decay inconsistent with a straight line on a linear, as well as on a logarithmic, time scale. On the contrary, Stein's[17] results agreed very well with a linear course as a function of log t, all curves reaching threshold for about 300 msec, independent of the intensity level of the stimulus.

In order to contribute to the solution of this problem, the present author planned a series of experiments with a different method of approach. Not the poststimulatory masking of a sound pulse was measured, but the minimum silent interval that must be introduced between two sound pulses to be perceived. The value of this critical time was investigated for different intensity levels of both the first and the second pulses.

Figure 2 illustrates the basic idea of these experiments. At a time interval Δt after a first sound pulse, a second one is given with the same or a lower intensity level. In the lower part of the graph, the level of subjective sensation is plotted as a function of time. We take the durations of the sound pulses for so long that the sensations reach their end values. Most recently, Port[22] has shown that loudness of short pulses of white noise does not increase for durations above 70 msec, so it is likely that after that this end value is reached. We may assume that starting a second sound pulse at $t=t_3$ affects the decay curve of the first one in a way as plotted. This representation has some resemblance with the description of the threshold for periodic tone pulses proposed by the author before.[23]

It is reasonable to suppose that the interruption between the two pulses can be perceived only for ΔS values exceeding a critical amount. It is reasonable, too, that this just-noticeable ΔS may be identified with the difference limen of intensity. Above a sensation level

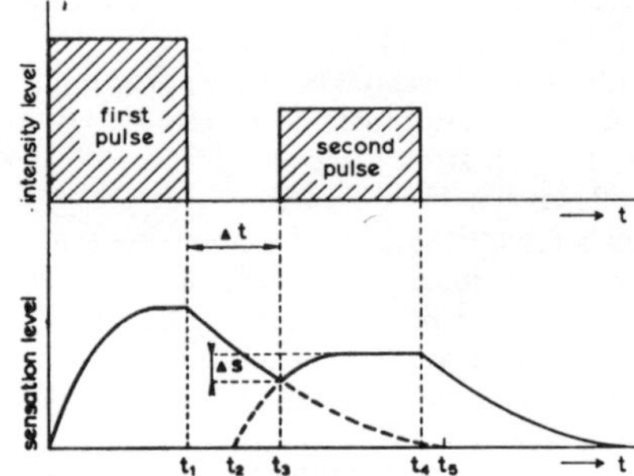

FIG. 2. Illustration of the basic idea of the experiments: the time interval Δt between two sound pulses is adjusted so that the interruption is just noticeable.

[8] E. Lüscher and J. Zwislocki, "The Decay of Sensation and the Remainder of Adaptation after Short Pure-Tone Impulses on the Ear," Acta Oto-Laryngol. **35**, 428–445 (1947).

[9] E. Lüscher and J. Zwislocki, "Adaptation of the Ear to Sound Stimuli," J. Acoust. Soc. Am. **21**, 135–139 (1949).

[10] A. I. Rawnsley and J. D. Harris, "Studies in Short-Duration Auditory Fatigue: II. Recovery Time," J. Exptl. Psychol. **43**, 138–142 (1952).

[11] J. Zwislocki, E. Pirodda, and H. Rubin, "On Some Poststimulatory Effects at the Threshold of Audibility," J. Acoust. Soc. Am. **31**, 9–14 (1959).

[12] C. M. Harris, "Residual Masking at Low Frequencies," J. Acoust. Soc. Am. **31**, 1110–1115 (1959).

[13] I. K. Samoilova, Biofizika **4**, 550–558 (1959) [English transl.: "Masking of Short Tone Signals as a Function of the Time Interval between Masked and Masking Sounds," Biophysics **4**, No. 5, 44–52 (1959) and summary in *Proceedings of the Third International Congress on Acoustics*, edited by L. Cremer (Elsevier Publishing Co., Amsterdam, 1961), Vol. 1, pp. 139–141].

[14] H. Rubin, "Auditory Facilitation following Stimulation at Low Intensities," J. Acoust. Soc. Am. **32**, 670–681 (1960).

[15] L. L. Elliott, "Backward Masking: Monotic and Dichotic Conditions," J. Acoust. Soc. Am. **34**, 1108–1115 (1962).

[16] L. L. Elliott, "Backward and Forward Masking of Probe Tones of Different Frequencies," J. Acoust. Soc. Am. **34**, 1116–1117 (1962).

[17] H. J. Stein, "Das Absinken der Mithörschwelle nach dem Abschalten von weissem Rauschen," Acustica **10**, 116–119 (1960).

[18] W. Burgtorf, "Untersuchungen zur Wahrnehmbarkeit verzögerter Schallsignale," Acustica **11**, 97–111 (1961).

[19] L. A. Chistovich and V. A. Ivanova, Biofizika **4**, No. 2, 170–180 (1959) [English transl.: "Mutual Masking of Short Sound Pulses," Biophysics **4**, No. 2, 46–57 (1959)].

[20] L. A. Chistovich, "Mutual Masking of Clicks following in Rapid Succession and Their Loudness Discrimination," in *Proceedings of the Third International Congress on Acoustics*, edited by L. Cremer (Elsevier Publishing Co., Amsterdam, 1961), Vol. 1, pp. 137–138.

[21] D. H. Raab, "Forward and Backward Masking between Acoustic Clicks," J. Acoust. Soc. Am. **33**, 137–139 (1961).

[22] E. Port, "Über die Lautstärke einzelner kurzer Schallimpulse," Acustica **13**, Akust. Beih. **1**, 212–223 (1963).

[23] R. Plomp, "Hearing Threshold for Periodic Tone Pulses," J. Acoust. Soc. Am. **33**, 1561–1569 (1961).

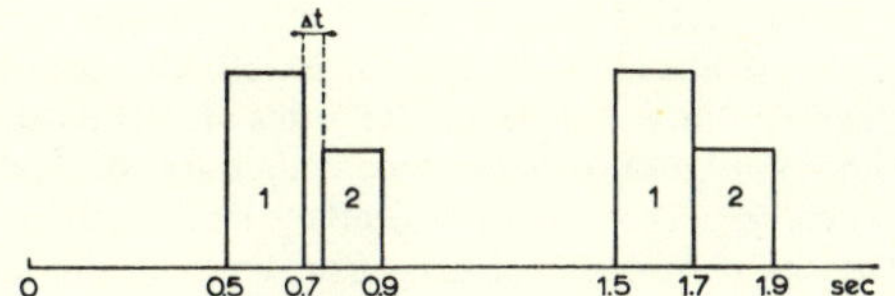

FIG. 3. Order of sound pulses during the experiments. The time interval Δt was introduced at random in the first or the second presentation of the two pulses.

of 20 dB, this difference limen is very small (about 0.4 dB for white noise[24]). This involves that, determining the minimum interval time Δt that can be heard, the sensation level of the second sound pulse represents very accurately the poststimulatory sensation level after Δt due to the first pulse. So, Δt as a function of the sensation level of the second sound pulse will give us the course of decay as a function of time.

Along these lines, a series of experiments was carried out, which are presented in this paper.

PROCEDURE AND EQUIPMENT

Preliminary tests showed that is it a rather difficult task to perceive a time interval between two sound pulses of different intensity levels. Therefore, a two-alternative forced-choice procedure was used.

Figure 3 illustrates this procedure. At $t=0$, a short, visual, warning signal was given, followed by two equal sound pulses after 0.5 and 1.5 sec, respectively. The pulse duration (200 msec) was sufficiently long to reach a stable sensation level. At an adjustable time interval (variable in steps of 0.1 msec) after one of these pulses, another pulse started. In the other case, this pulse started without a time interval. In both cases, the secondary pulses stopped 200 msec after the end of the leading pulses. So the only difference between the two presentations was that in one case the start of the second pulse was delayed by a time Δt. This interruption was given at random in the first or the second presentation, and the observer had to decide in which case the gap was introduced. These presentations were repeated with a repetition time of 5 sec, so the observer always had about 3 sec to give his response. To avoid any effects of transients, white noise was used for both sound pulses.

Figure 4 shows a block diagram of the equipment. The output of a white-noise generator is connected to a switch, as well as to two electronic gates. These gates are opened and closed by electronic spikes produced by a 5-decade preset counter excitated by a 10-kcps oscillator. This counter has a rather complicated switching program. A total of 4 spikes can be taken off, each variable in steps of 0.1 msec relative to a zero moment. The repetation time of these spikes is alternately 1 and 4 sec, so the order of sound pulses of Fig. 3 can be produced and repeated each 5 sec. By way of the noise-operated switch in each pair of two presentations, one time the start of the second noise pulse is controlled by the spike that stops the first noise pulse, instead of by its appropriate spike.

The two noise pulses are amplified and attenuated separately and their intensity levels can be varied in steps of 1 dB. The outputs of both attenuators are led to a matching box that is connected to the headphone (Permoflux PDR-10). The observers listened monaurally.

The observer has two pushbuttons at his disposal. He presses the left one if he perceives the time interval Δt in the first presentation of the noise pulses, and the right one in the other case. The observer is always forced to press one of these buttons. By means of magnetic relays, the result of the observer's response is automatically recorded by two electromechanical counters. One of them records the total number of responses, the other one the number of correct responses. The pushbuttons and the counters are combined in one "response box," so the observer knows immediately after his response whether he has made a correct choice. This is very convenient to maintain the rather difficult criterion of perceiving a time interval between two noise pulses of different intensity levels.

With this equipment, the observer could determine the just-noticeable time interval Δt without the assistance of others. After adjusting the intensity levels of the first and the second noise pulse, the observer in a typical test session adjusted the minimum Δt for which 100% correct responses were obtained. From that value on, Δt was diminished in steps of about 10% and for each value 50 decisions were made. After about 6 steps, Δt was usually so short that the decisions were made at random, resulting in about 50% correct responses. With this time interval, 100 responses were recorded and from this value on Δt was increased, using the same intervals as before, each time also giving 50 presentations.

In this way, at about 6 time intervals 100 responses were obtained, varying from 100% to about 50% cor-

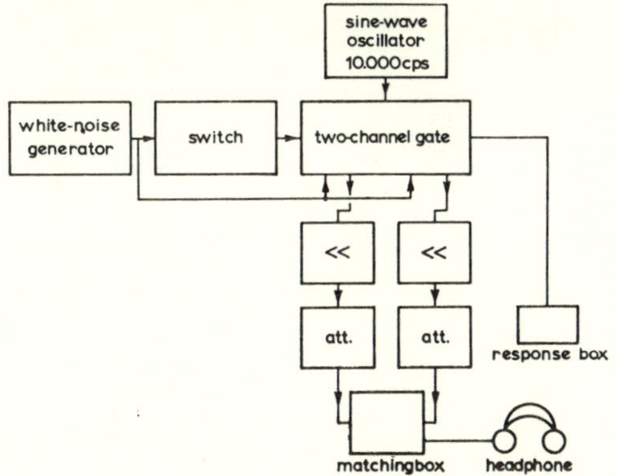

FIG. 4. Block diagram of the equipment.

[24] G. A. Miller, "Sensitivity to Changes in the Intensity of White Noise and Its Relation to Masking and Loudness," J. Acoust. Soc. Am. 19, 609–619 (1947).

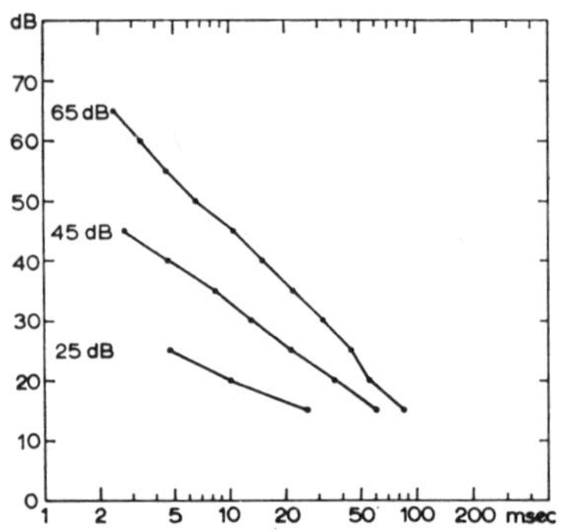

Fig. 5. Just-noticeable time interval between two noise pulses as a function of the sensation level of the second pulse. The sensation level of the first pulse is indicated (observer 1).

rect responses. The percentages were plotted as a function of Δt and the best-fit curve was drawn. Always, the 75% value was taken as the critical-interval duration. So each data point is based on about 600 decisions. One test session lasted about one hour. The observer usually took part in only one session a day.

Two observers were used in the experiments, both having much experience in hearing experiments. They were given a long training in order to get very accurate results.

EXPERIMENTAL RESULTS

In the first part of the experiments, the just-noticeable time interval was measured with a constant-intensity level of the first noise pulse and different levels of the second pulse. Table I represents the results of these

Table I. Duration in msec of just-noticeable time interval between two noise pulses.

Sensation level second noise pulse (dB)	Sensation level first noise pulse (dB) Observer 1			Observer 2		
	65	45	25	65	45	25
65	2.4			2.8		
60	3.3			3.6		
55	4.5			5.0		
50	6.5			6.5		
45	10.5	2.7		9.5	2.7	
40	14.8	4.6		12.7	4.3	
35	21.7	8.3		17.3	6.4	
30	31	13.0		24	11.5	
25	44	21	4.7	37	18.8	4.0
20	55	36	10	48	30	7.6
15	83	60	26	73	48	17.5
10				102	70	36

experiments. The intensity levels are given relative to the hearing threshold of a noise pulse of 200 msec duration, so they are sensation levels. In three series of experiments, the sensation levels of the first pulse were 65, 45, and 25 dB, respectively. The sensation level of the second noise pulse was varied in steps of 5 dB. The order of this level at the successive test sessions was, for instance, 45, 35, 25, 15, 20, 30, 40 dB to avoid any systematic influence of the order on the data.

Figures 5 and 6 reproduce the data of Table I graphically. The just-noticeable time interval is plotted as a function of sensation level of the second noise pulse, with the sensation level of the first pulse as a parameter.

In further experiments, Δt was measured with equal sensation levels of the two noise pulses. These values are given in Table II and are plotted as a function of sensation level in Fig. 7.

Table II. Duration in msec of just-noticeable time interval between two noise pulses.

Sensation level of the two noise pulses (dB)	Observer 1	Observer 2
75	3.2	3.7
70	2.8	3.2
65	2.4	2.8
60	2.5	2.8
55	2.3	2.9
50	2.4	2.7
45	2.7	2.7
40	2.8	3.1
35	3.2	3.1
30	3.8	3.5
25	4.7	4.0
20	6.0	4.4
15	12.5	7.2
10	25	14
5	...	31

Already, a first glance at Figs. 5 and 6 shows that on a logarithmic time scale the relation of just-noticeable time interval to sensation level of the second pulse can be approximated very well by a straight line. The slope of this line depends on the sensation level of the first noise pulse, being flatter for lower levels.

To examine these relations more thoroughly, the best-fit straight lines through the data points that give the smallest sum of the squares of deviations from the line

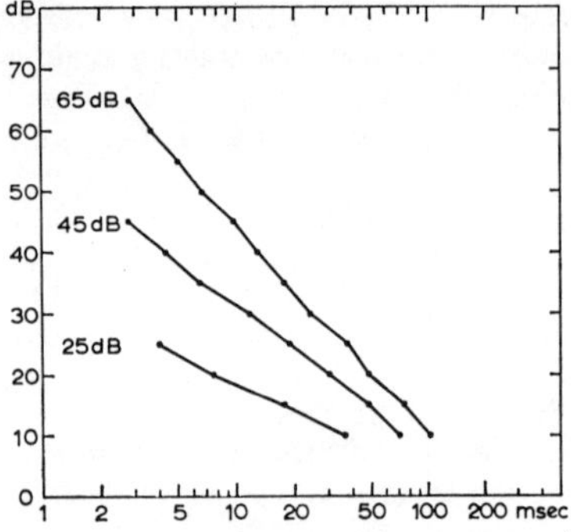

Fig. 6. Just-noticeable time interval between two noise pulses as a function of the sensation level of the second pulse. The sensation level of the first pulse is indicated (observer 2).

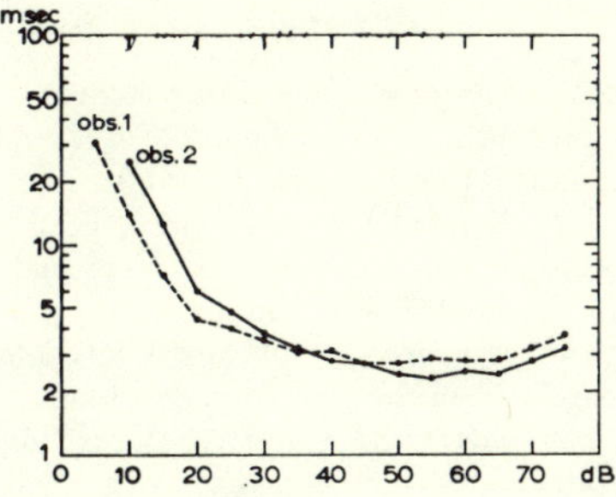

Fig. 7. Just-noticeable time interval between two noise pulses as a function of sensation level (both pulses same intensity).

were calculated. From the equations of these lines, the points where they intersect the zero sensation level (hearing threshold) were derived. These points are represented in Table III. For both observers, the differ-

Table III. Times in msec for which the best-fit straight lines through the data points of Figs. 5 and 6 intersect hearing threshold.

	Sensation level first noise pulse (dB)		
	65	45	25
Observer 1	260	280	310
Observer 2	190	190	160

ences between these time durations are so small that they may be considered as insignificant. This means that the data points of Figs. 5 and 6 can be fitted by straight lines converging to one point at zero sensation level.

In Fig. 8, the mean values for the two observers are plotted and approximated by straight converging lines. These lines agree very well with the experimental points, the largest deviation being about 1 dB.

In the same diagram also the mean values of just-noticeable Δt at equal sensation levels of the two noise pulses are reproduced. The dashed line connects these points.

The solid lines may be considered as drawn between a point of the dashed line to a point on the abscissa, corresponding with a time interval of 225 msec. In the same way, other lines can be drawn representing the just-noticeable Δt between a first pulse of a sensation level, given by the point on the dashed line, and a second pulse of a varying sensation level, given by the ordinate. As all these lines intersect the abscissa at $t=225$ msec, it implies that the dashed line must also reach zero level at this time value, as is drawn.

DISCUSSION

In the introduction, it was stated as reasonable that, for Δt as the minimum noticeable time interval between a first noise pulse and a second one of lower sensation level, this level will be a very good approximation of the level of auditory sensation after Δt due to the first pulse. So, the curves of Fig. 8 may demonstrate how the poststimulatory sensation of a noise pulse decays as a function of time.

Now, we may compare our results with the results of some other investigators, mentioned in the introduction.

At first, we see that our data, showing a linear relation between sensation level in dB and the logarithm of time, strongly disagree with an exponential decay suggested by Stevens and Davis[2] and by Miller.[3] However, we must remember that their conclusions were based on experiments that are in fact inadequate to decide on the course of the decay function.

On the contrary, the data of Miller,[3] Pollack,[5,6] and Dubout[7] on the masking of an interrupted white noise can be described satisfactorily by straight lines as a function of log t. The most important difference with our results is the larger time duration before hearing threshold is reached (600–1200 msec; see Fig. 1). This discrepancy can be explained by the fact that, in the experiments of the investigators mentioned, each interruption was followed by a noise burst. As is shown by Elliott[15] and others, this will induce "backward masking," resulting in higher sound levels during interruption or longer interruption times to detect this sound. As this effect increases with growing difference between the intensity level of the noise bursts and the level during the interruptions, it can account for the large time durations over which poststimulatory masking exists according to the experiments using interrupted noise.

As is mentioned in the introduction, several investigators have studied poststimulatory masking with single sound pulses for both the stimulus and the test pulse. In this way, the influence of backward masking is cancelled. This manifests itself in the fact that in these experiments the masking effects are limited to times better in agreement with our results.

However, this does not mean that these investigations all point to a similar masking versus time function. Whereas the data of Stein[17] and Burgtorf[18] can be described very well by straight converging lines as a func-

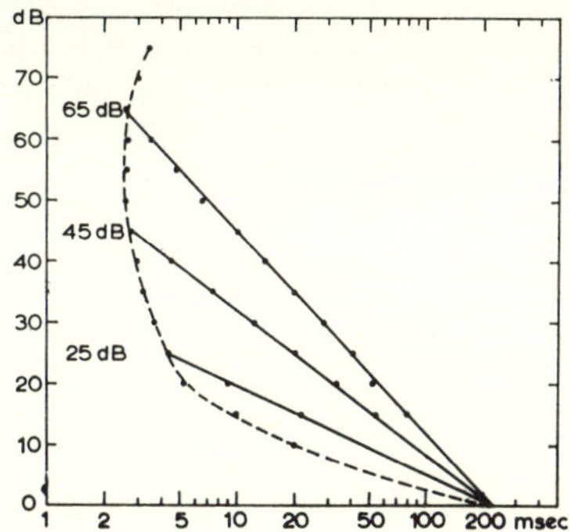

Fig. 8. Just-noticeable time interval between two noise pulses as a function of the sensation level of the second pulse (solid lines) and sensation level of both pulses (dashed line), respectively. The data points give the average for the two observers.

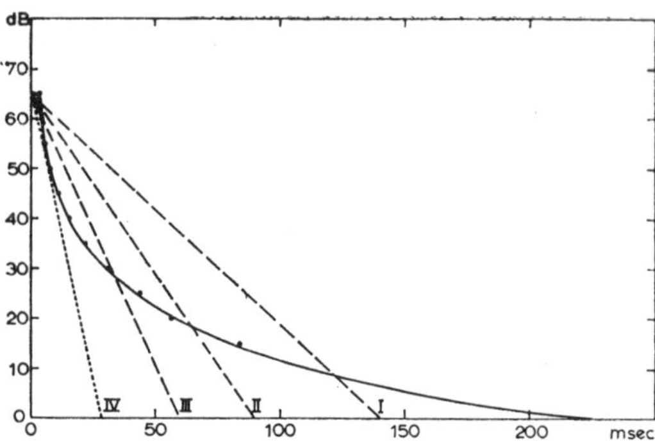

Fig. 9. Rate of decay of sensation on a linear time scale (solid line). The dashed lines I, II, and III correspond to the artificial decays used by Miller,[3] being well-audible, just-audible, and inaudible, respectively. The dotted line (IV) represents the acoustical decay of an anechoic room required for studying poststimulatory effects, using loudspeakers. For a room of 5×5×5 m³, this decay corresponds with a sound-absorption coefficient of the walls of about 99.5%.

tion of log t, the results of Lüscher and Zwislocki,[8] Rawnsley and Harris,[10] Samoilova,[13] and Elliot[15,16] do not agree with this behavior. An analysis of the methods used by these investigators strongly supports the suggestion that the discrepancies are caused by the time interval used to plot the data. As is stated by Lüscher and Zwislocki,[9] the masking of a test pulse by a preceding sound is not determined by the beginning but by the end of the pulse—so the masking has to be plotted as a function of the time between the end of the masking pulse and the end of the test pulse. Burgtorf, indeed, plotted his data in this way, whereas Stein used very short test pulses (30 μsec) so that, for his results, the problem in question is not relevant. On the contrary, the other investigators mentioned presented their masking values as a function of the time interval between the end of the stimulus and the beginning of the test pulse, so we may expect deviations for times comparable in length or shorter than the duration of the test pulse. Replotting their data as a function of the correct time interval resulted, in each case, in a much better agreement with straight lines on a log t scale than the original figures show.

These considerations indicate that the divergences between the results of experiments in which the poststimulatory masking was investigated can be explained by the different experimental methods and inadequate interpretations of the data. This taken into account, we may conclude that these investigations confirm our results.

CONCLUSIONS

From our experiments, we may conclude:

(1) Expressed in dB as a function of log t, the decay of sensation is represented by a straight line.

(2) Independent of the sensation level of the stimulating sound, the hearing threshold is reached at the same time of about 200–300 msec.

Though these results are obtained with noise pulses, we may expect from the masking experiments with tones referred to in the last section that the conclusions also hold for pure tones.

It is interesting that the threshold for single and periodic tone pulses as a function of duration and repetition time is also controlled by a time constant of 200–300 msec.[23,25] This strengthens the evidence that interactions between successive sounds always extend over a time interval of about this value. The fact that the difference of critical decay time for the two observers (Table III) agrees with a similar difference of time constant of the same observers (see Fig. 19 of Ref. 25) may be an indication that the two phenomena are closely related.

In Fig. 9, the data points of Fig. 8 representing the decay of a 65-dB stimulus are reproduced on a linear time scale. The dashed lines represent the artificial decays used by Miller,[3] corresponding with an exponential relation between time and intensity. As we see, the sensation decreases much faster for small times than the lines of Miller would predict. This indicates that the ear is capable of following rapid fluctuations in sound levels much better than would have been the case for an exponential rate of decay.

This fact must be realized when studying poststimulatory effects with loudspeakers in a sound-treated room. The sound-absorption coefficient of the walls has to be so high that the acoustical decay will be more rapid than the decay of the ear. This means that, after a sound of 65 dB sensation level, the threshold of hearing must be reached within about 25 msec (dotted line of Fig. 9). For a room of 5×5×5 m³, this can be obtained only with a sound-absorption coefficient of the walls of about 99.5%, so we see that for this type of experiment an anechoic room of a high quality is required.

ACKNOWLEDGMENT

The author thanks A. M. Mimpen for his assistance in building the equipment and participating in the experiments.

[25] R. Plomp and M. A. Bouman, "Relation between Hearing Threshold and Duration for Tone Pulses," J. Acoust. Soc. Am. **31**, 749–758 (1959).

30

Reprinted from *Acoust. Soc. Am. J.* **34**:1752-1760 (1962)

Effect of Phase on the Quality of a Two-Component Tone*†

JAMES H. CRAIG AND LLOYD A. JEFFRESS
Defense Research Laboratory and *Department of Psychology, The University of Texas, Austin 12, Texas*
(Received August 6, 1962)

AUDITORY theory does not readily account for monaural phase effects (MPE's). Helmholtz's theory certainly did not, but he avoided the difficulty by denying their existence. He classified an admittedly heard phase-determined auditory effect (the faint beats produced by a tone and its mistuned octave) as only an *apparent* exception to his phase rule. For the greater part of a century his dictum that ". . . *differences in musical quality of tone depend solely upon the presence and strength of partial tones, and in no respect on the differences in phase under which these partials enter into combination*"[1] has colored the interpretations of those experiments which it did not preclude.

The history of the controversy that has been waged over the phase rule is reported in detail elsewhere.[2] In brief, Koenig first pointed out the semantic problem posed by the "apparent exception" principle and then demonstrated credible MPE's with a wave siren of his own design.[3] Beasley,[4] Chapin and Firestone,[5] Lewis and Larsen,[6] Trimmer and Firestone,[7] Schouten,[8] Mathes and Miller,[9] Egan and Klumpp,[10] de Boer,[11] Lawrence and Yantis,[12] Licklider,[13] and most recently, Schroeder[14] have all demonstrated monaurally detectable changes which are related to phase changes in tonal stimuli. Although the existence of MPE's is clearly no longer in doubt, the integration of them into auditory theory is still far from being realized.

With two exceptions[10,12] the recent studies tend to use complicated stimuli which, although eliciting striking MPE's, increase the difficulty of finding a physiological explanation. In the present experiment, the stimulus employed was the simplest which can elicit MPE's. Its parameters were systematically varied to determine whether there are corresponding changes in the subject's sensory experience.

The current investigation took its direction from the informal discovery of a new MPE by Charles L. Wood[15] at the Defense Research Laboratory during 1957. He used as a signal a sinusoid partially clipped during half of each cycle [see Fig. 1(A)]. The resulting sound had a different timbre when the flat-topped portion was presented to the ear as a rarefaction than it did when the phone leads were reversed and the flat-topped portion was presented as a compression. The attempt to explore

* Based in part on JHC's unpublished doctoral dissertation (The University of Texas, 1961).

† A brief version of this report was presented at the 58th Meeting of the Acoustical Society of America, Cleveland, Ohio, October 1959, under the title, "The Effect of Phase on the Quality of a Two-Component Unsymmetrical, Complex Tone." The abstract appears in J. Acoust. Soc. Am. **31**, 1584 (1959).

[1] H. Helmholtz, *On the Sensation of Tone*, translated by A. J. Ellis (Longmans, Green and Company, Inc., London, 1885), p. 127c (italics his). Helmholtz excepts from ". . . this important law" such unmusical components as "jarring, scratching, whizzing, hissing," which "are either not to be considered as periodic at all . . . or form strident dissonances." These he was unable to embrace in his experiments with phase, and so left the importance of their phase relations doubtful.

[2] J. H. Craig, unpublished doctoral dissertation (The University of Texas, 1961).

[3] A. J. Ellis (editor and translator), in reference 1, p. 537.

[4] W. Beasley, "The Monaural Phase Effect with Pure Binary Harmonics," J. Acoust. Soc. Am. **1**, 385–402 (1930).

[5] E. K. Chapin and F. A. Firestone, "The Influence of Phase on Tone Quality and Loudness; The Interference of Subjective Harmonics," J. Acoust. Soc. Am. **5**, 173–180 (1934).

[6] D. Lewis and M. J. Larsen, "The Cancellation, Reinforcement, and Measurement of Subjective Tones," Proc. Natl. Acad. Sci. U. S. **23**, 415–421 (1937).

[7] J. D. Trimmer and F. A. Firestone, "An Investigation of Subjective Tones by Means of the Steady Tone Phase Effect," J. Acoust. Soc. Am. **9**, 24–29 (1937).

[8] J. F. Schouten, "Synthetic Sound," Philips Tech. Rev. **4**, 167–173 (1939).

[9] R. C. Mathes and R. L. Miller, "Phase Effects in Monaural Perception," J. Acoust. Soc. Am. **19**, 780–797 (1947).

[10] J. P. Egan and R. G. Klumpp, "The Error Due to Masking in the Measurement of Aural Harmonics by the Method of Best Beats," J. Acoust. Soc. Am. **23**, 275–286 (1951).

[11] E. de Boer, *On the 'Residue' in Hearing*, Doctoral dissertation, University of Amsterdam (Excelsior Publishers, 'S–Gravenhage, The Netherlands, 1956).

[12] M. Lawrence and P. A. Yantis, "Onset and Growth of Aural Harmonics in the Overloaded Ear," J. Acoust. Soc. Am. **28**, 852–858 (1956).

[13] J. C. R. Licklider, "Effects of Changes in the Phase Pattern upon the Sound of a 16–Harmonic Tone," J. Acoust. Soc. Am. **29**, 780 (A) (1957).

[14] M. R. Schroeder, "New Results Concerning Monaural Phase Sensitivity," J. Acoust. Soc. Am. **31**, 1579 (A) (1959).

[15] Now with the General Electric Company, Syracuse, New York.

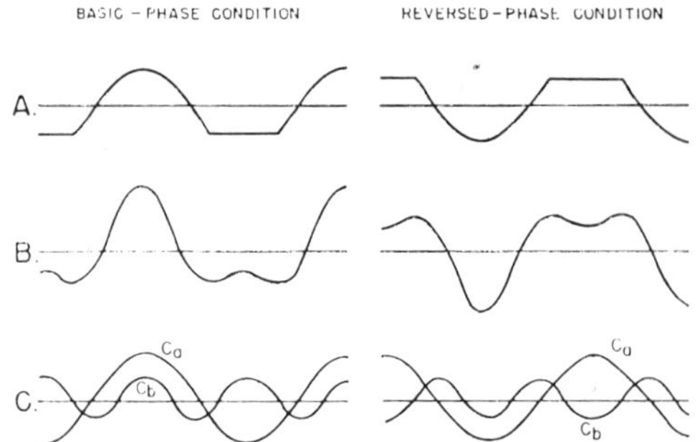

FIG. 1. Changes in the waveforms due to phase reversals. (A) The stimulus used by Wood. (B) The simplified two-component stimulus used in the present study. (C). The two components making up the complex waveform of Fig. 1(B).

the Wood effect more thoroughly led to the simplified stimulus and to the parameter variation used in the present study.

EXPERIMENTAL PROCEDURE

The experimental work was carried out in the audition laboratory[16] of the Department of Psychology at The University of Texas. The experimenter and most of the apparatus were in an anteroom from which the signals were led to an earphone worn by the observer sitting comfortably in an adjoining darkened, quiet room.

Subjects

The two subjects employed in the formal portion of this study had reasonably normal hearing. For the frequencies used, their absolute thresholds were: 250 cps, both 14 dB SPL[17]; 500 cps, JHC—7 dB SPL, RHW—13 dB SPL. Both subjects were experienced in the task and familiar with the apparatus and procedure, since both had participated in an earlier pilot study. They did not, however, know the program being followed at any given moment.

Stimuli

The stimuli used, while preserving the asymmetry and general configuration of the half-clipped sinusoid used by Wood [see Figs. 1(A) and 1(B)], represent a great reduction in complexity. Each stimulus consisted of a carefully filtered 250-cps fundamental component C_a and its 500-cps second harmonic C_b [see Fig. 1(C)]. C_a was presented at 40, 50, 60, 70, 80, and 84 dB SPL. C_b was varied between 3 and 73 dB SPL in 10-dB steps. The stimuli were presented in four basic phase conditions: 0° and 90° were used at all levels, and 45° and 135° were added at the 60-dB level of C_a (see Fig. 2 for

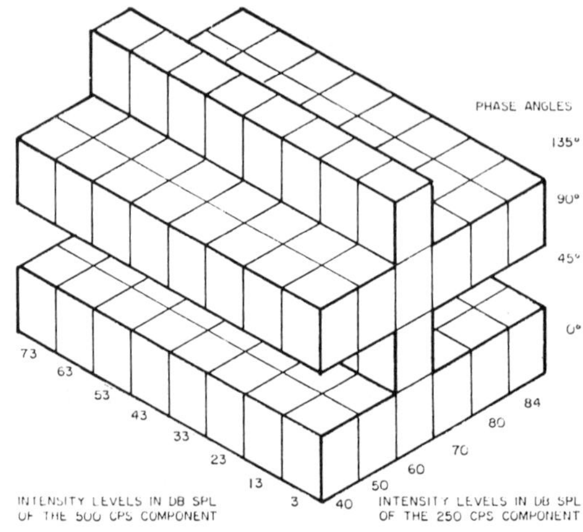

FIG. 2. Stimulus conditions used in the experiment. Each cell represents 60 stimulus presentations to the right ear of each of the two subjects.

the complete array of conditions used). The basic phase conditions are specified by the cosine phase φ of C_b relative to C_a (see Fig. 3). The stimulus may be specified as

$$p = \pm[A \cos\omega t + B \cos(2\omega t + \varphi)],$$

the plus-or-minus sign indicating whether a given half-cycle is a condensation or a rarefaction. It was the sub-

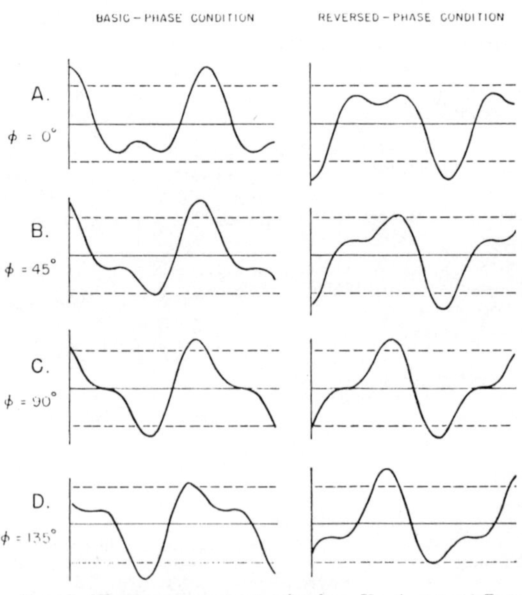

FIG. 3. The two-component stimulus, $Y = A \cos\omega t + B \cos(2\omega t + \varphi)$, for the four phase conditions used in this study (drawn with an arbitrarily selected component-amplitude ratio, $A = 2B$). Positive values indicate inward displacements of the eardrum.

[16] For a description of the auditory suite, see K. M. Dallenbach, "The Psychology Laboratory of The University of Texas," Am. J. Psychol. **66**, 90–104 (1953).

[17] All thresholds and stimulus levels are given in sound-pressure evel (SPL) *re* 0.0002 μbars.

1. Audio Signal Generator
2. Audio Amplifier
3. Variable Phase Shifter
4. Frequency Doubler
5. Narrow, Band-pass Filter
6. Matching Transformer
7. Electronic Timer
8. Electronic Switch, 2-channel
9. and 10. Attenuators
11. and 12. Filters
13. Mixing Transformer
14. Program Drum
15. Relay
16. Impedance-matching Transformer
17. and 18. PDR-10 Phones
19. Calibrated Microphone and Coupler
20. Microphone Base and Preamplifier
21. Microphone Power Supply
22. Amplifier
23. Harmonic Wave Analyzer
24. RMS Voltmeter
25. Cathode Ray Oscillograph

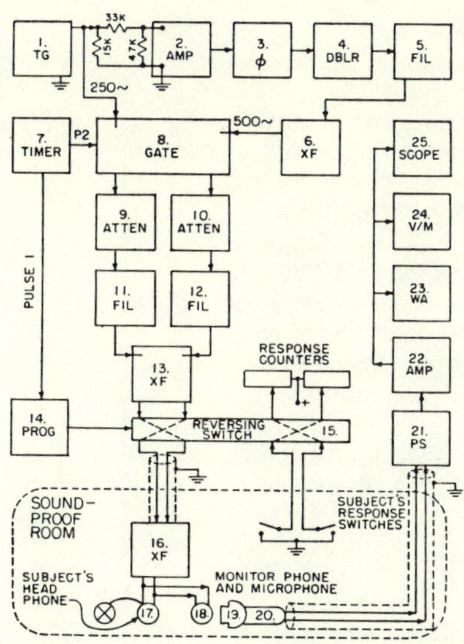

FIG. 4. Block diagram of apparatus and list of principal components.

ject's task, in effect, to decide whether this sign was plus or minus during a given stimulus presentation.[18]

Apparatus

Figure 4 gives a block diagram of the equipment. Both stimulus components had their source in a single 250-cps tone generator. Part of the output led directly into the 250-cps channel, the rest was amplified and passed through a variable phase-shifter, a frequency doubler, and a narrow-bandpass filter adjusted to peak at 500 cps. A two-channel electronic gate, with rise and fall times of 25 msec, gave transient-free on-and-off switching. An IBM program drum provided the sequence of stimuli used. Each of the frequency channels included a separate attenuator and an additional filter before terminating in a mixing transformer. The transformer output led to two PDR-10 earphones which had been carefully matched for phase as well as for amplitude of response. One of the phones was mounted in the listener's headset; the other, serving as a monitor source, was coupled to a calibrated microphone whose output was fed back into the anteroom. Here an oscilloscope, a vacuum-tube voltmeter, and a harmonic wave analyzer served to monitor the phase relations, levels, and purities of the signal components. Distortion products were kept at least 50 dB below the levels of the signal components as measured at the amplified microphone output.

Procedure

An experimental session consisted of 8 different series of 20 presentations each, all at the same C_a level and phase condition, but with each series of 20 presented at a different C_b level.

Each series was composed of 20 randomly ordered presentations, 10 in the "basic" phase condition and 10 with the earphone connections reversed. These correspond to the plus and the minus signs of the equation for the stimulus. To each of the stimuli the subject responded, making an "absolute" judgment. If he judged the stimulus to be "plus," he pressed a key to the right; if "minus," a key to the left. Each stimulus was presented for one second, followed by one second of silence.

The subject's choice of responses was made on the basis of any personal criterion he could establish for identifying the two different stimuli—a difference of pitch, of loudness, of roughness, of timbre, or of any other characteristic which he could discriminate and remember. If he pressed the right-hand key when the stimulus was in its "basic" phase (see Fig. 3), his response registered on a counter, the "yes" counter; if he pressed the left-hand key, the response registered on the "no" counter. When the phase of the signal was reversed (right-hand portion of Fig. 3), the connection from the keys to the counters were also reversed, so pressing the left-hand key registered on the "yes" counter. If the subject was consistent in his judgments and responses, all of the responses would be registered on the same counter. If his personal criterion coincided with the stimulus designation, all of his responses would be registered on the "yes" counter, otherwise, on the "no."

Each session of eight series of 20 stimuli was administered to the subject three times, usually on different days, one to six sessions in any one day. Each stimulus condition, therefore, evoked 60 responses.

[18] The phase reversal was actually accomplished by reversing the connections to the earphone, but the same stimulus would have resulted from reversing the phase of the 500-cps component, or by shifting it 180° in phase.

RESULTS

The results are presented for each subject separately in Figs. 5, 7, and 8 as a series of graphs having as abscissa, b, the SPL of C_b, and as ordinate the number of "yes" responses made in the course of the 60 judgments under the specified conditions. Thirty "yes" responses would indicate a chance level of responding. Sixty "yes" responses would indicate perfectly consistent sorting of the phase conditions, as would 60 "no's," but the categories would be reversed in the latter case. As many as 40 "yes" or 40 "no" responses out of any group of 60 represents a deviation from chance at the 1% level of significance. These levels are indicated on each graph.

Figure 5(A) shows the subjects' responses, with a, the SPL of C_a, constant at 60 dB, and with the phase φ constant at 0°. At $b=3$ dB, only chance responses occurred. Both subjects reach a significant level of discrimination when b is increased to 23 dB, with JHC considerably better than RHW. With further increases of b, both subjects' responses drop back to chance, and with still further increase of b, become significant again but in the reverse sense. Here RHW's discriminations reach nearly 100% with JHC's somewhat inferior. Finally, at $b=73$ dB, both subjects' responses deteriorate.

The remainder of Fig. 5 bears out the reality of this unexpected reversal. An expected response pattern would have started at chance for low levels of b and would have advanced monotonically toward either 60 or 0 with increasing C_b levels, or perhaps would have resembled the solid curve of Fig. 5(C) if the increasingly intense C_b began to mask the MPE. The response

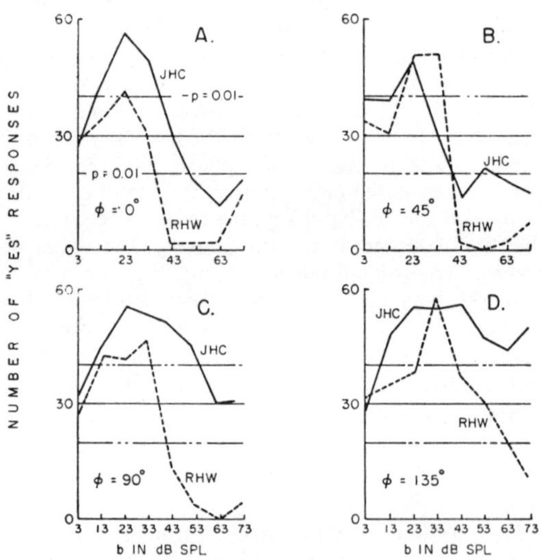

FIG. 5. ($a=60$ dB SPL) Discriminatory responses of subjects JHC and RHW as a function of b, the level of the 2nd harmonic component of the stimulus, for four values of φ.

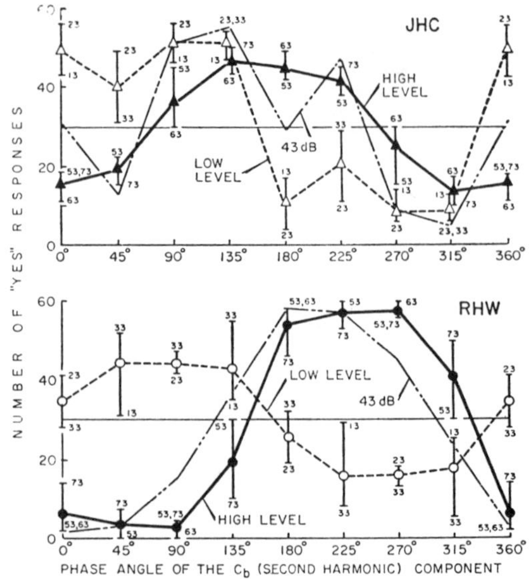

FIG. 6. Phase- and level-related response patterns. Responses of RHW and JHC at the 60-dB level of C_a. Open symbols indicate, for each phase angle, the mean number of "yes" responses at the 13-, 23-, and 33-dB levels of C_b; filled symbols, the means for 53, 63, and 73 dB. The 43-dB transition-level responses are indicated by points connected by dot-dash lines.

patterns actually obtained, with their reversals and nulls, point to a dual mechanism of phase detection: one part operating at low levels and the other adding its effect or replacing the first at higher levels. The particular differences found between subjects give additional support to such a concept. Although JHC shows greater sensitivity to phase reversal at the lower levels of C_b, there the differences in response patterns are otherwise slight. However, at the higher levels, RHW is generally the more sensitive. At $\varphi=90°$ and 135°, large *pattern* differences appear as well.

To explore the dual-aspect concept further, the number of "yes" responses at $b=13$, 23, and 33 dB were averaged to obtain a low-level response pattern; those at 53, 63, and 73 dB were averaged for the high-level pattern. The responses at 43 dB, which fell within RHW's high-level pattern, but within neither of JHC's response patterns, were treated separately. In this way, the data of Fig. 5 were grouped and replotted as Fig. 6, where now φ is used as abscissa. To provide better visualization of the phase-related changes in the patterns, the data were extended to 360° by simply adding 180° to the φ of each set of conditions and reversing the sign of the responses for those altered conditions. Thus, 54 "yes" responses at 45° can be expressed equally well as $60-54=6$ "no" responses, or as 6 "yes" responses at 225° (see footnote 18). The range of points making up each plotted mean is indicated by the vertical bar through the point. As constructed, Fig. 6 brings out the new information that the low-level response patterns

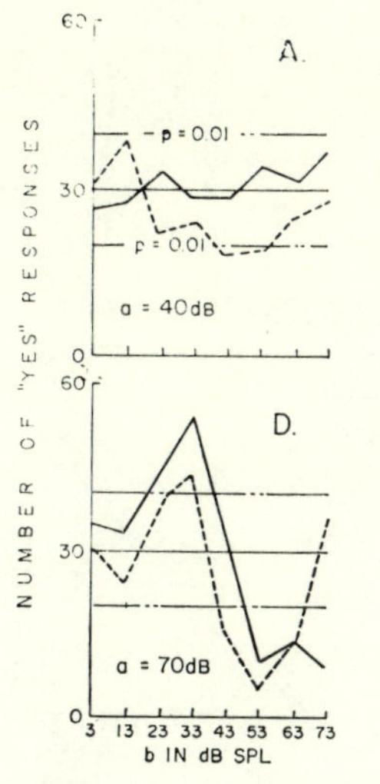

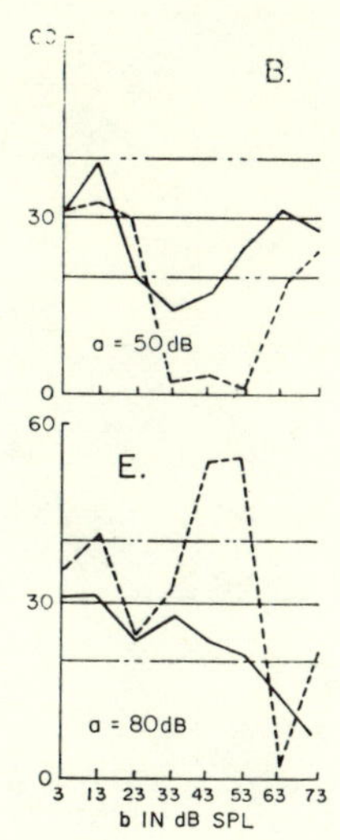

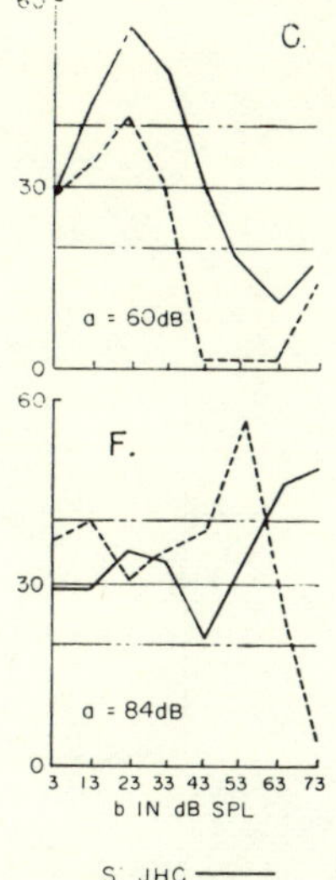

FIG. 7. ($\varphi=0°$) Discriminatory responses of S's JHC (solid line) and RHW (dashed line) as a function of b, the level of the 2nd harmonic component, when $\varphi=0°$ for six levels of a.

for the two S's, though differing in amplitude, have just about the same "phase." The high-level response patterns, however, in addition to their amplitude differences, differ in "phase" by about 90° between S's: a problem of intersubject differences which will be discussed later.

Figure 7 presents the responses elicited at the $\varphi=0°$ condition. The C_a level is the parameter, and once again b, the SPL of C_b, is the abscissa. In the same fashion, Fig. 8 presents the responses for the $\varphi=90°$ conditions. These figures show that the response *patterns* for the 0°-phase conditions are different from those for 90°, although the over-all number of significant responses does not differ appreciably.

In both Figs. 7 and 8 discriminatory responses appear at $a=40$ dB, are well established at $a=50$ dB, and continue to show up at the highest C_a levels used. Also, the response patterns seen at $a=50$ dB, after developing smoothly into the patterns seen at 60 and 70 dB, are disrupted at $a=80$ and 84 dB. Associated with this break in the progression of response patterns is a change in the phase-related differences of sensation. Below a C_a level of about 75 dB most of the discriminations had been made on the basis of pitch or timbre differences. At $a=80$ and 84 dB, both subjects experienced a loudness difference which they used in making many of their highest-level discriminations. This is the second level-related change of pattern observed. The first occurred when C_b exceeded about 40 dB SPL.

Throughout the experiment, whenever a subject was producing significantly consistent responses, the fact not only indicated that the difference in phase was being detected, but also, that each response carried the meaning, "This tone seems slightly higher (or lower, louder, softer, purer, less pure, etc.) than the other." Without being so instructed, the two S's had associated a higher pitch (or pitch-like) quality, a greater purity, and a greater loudness with the right-hand response switch, producing "yes" responses.

DISCUSSION

Experimental Findings

The most obvious results of this study are its confirmation of Beasley's finding[4,19] of monaural phase effects at low levels of stimulation, its denial of Pierce's conclusion[20] that more than two components are necessary for the production of MPE's, and its demonstration (in contrast to Békésy's findings[21] with respect to a fundamental tone slowly beating with its octave) that listeners can consistently assign different sensory qualities to different phase relations.

Three Classes of Monaural Phase Effect

The results suggest that, within the range of stimulus variables sampled, MPE's can usefully be separated into three classes on the basis of whether one or both of the stimulus components exceed certain experimentally determined "critical levels"—about 75 dB SPL for C_a and about 40 dB SPL for C_b. The following scheme will be used in referring to the three classes: low-MPE, that which appears when both C_a and C_b are below their critical levels; mid-MPE, that which appears when C_b

[19] W. Beasley, "Differential Responses to Cyclic Phase Variations in Compound Sounds," J. Gen. Psychol. **5**, 329–351 (1931).

[20] J. R. Pierce, "Some Work on Hearing," Am. Scientist **48**, 40–45 (1960).

[21] G. von Békésy, "Sensations on the Skin Similar to Directional Hearing, Beats, and Harmonics of the Ear," J. Acoust. Soc. Am. **29**, 489–501 (1957).

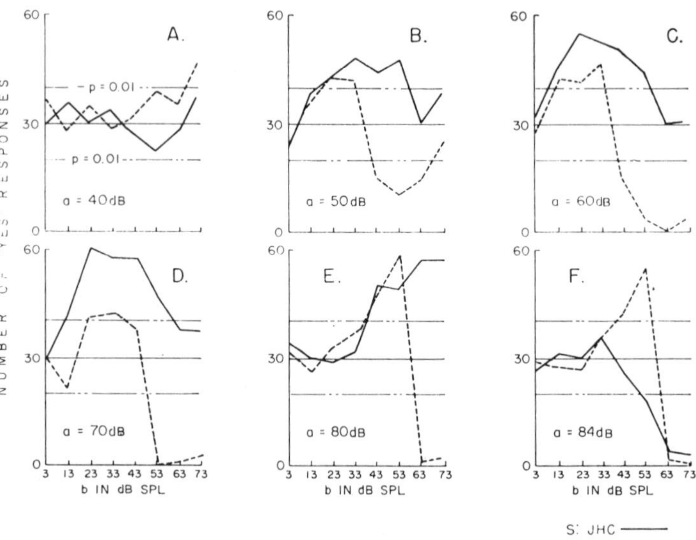

FIG. 8. ($\varphi=90°$) Discriminatory responses of S's JHC (solid line) and RHW (dashed line) as a function of b, the level of the 2nd harmonic component of the stimulus, when $\varphi=90°$ for six levels of a.

is above and C_a is below its critical level (the reverse combination showed nothing unusual); and high-MPE, that which arises when both C_a and C_b are above their critical levels. The phase-related sensation differences characteristic of both low- and mid-MPE's are slight changes in pitch and/or timbre. Phase-related loudness differences appear as the predominant characteristic of the high-MPE.

High-MPE

A finding implicit in the results of earlier work is the change in the phase-related sensation difference when C_a is increased beyond a critical level. Egan and Klumpp,[10] working with a 350 cps C_a and its mistuned octave C_b, found at low levels that the resulting beats seemed to involve C_b only. However, when the fundamental was increased in level to 80 dB or more, both C_b and C_a seemed to become involved in a complex interaction. At the same levels where Egan and Klumpp reported changed sensations and increased difficulty of judgments, the subjects of the present study reported a change in discriminatory sensation. At these levels, an abrupt change disrupted the rather regular evolution of response pattern which had accompanied the increases of C_a up to the 70-dB SPL level (see Figs. 7 and 8).

Low- and Mid-MPE's

Another finding, apparently *not* implicit in any earlier work, was the change in response pattern, without a concurrent change in the character of the sensations, which appeared when a low-level C_b was increased to above its critical level. The two features of the results (seen in Fig. 6) which lead to this finding are: (1) the "phase" difference between the high-level and the low-level response patterns, and (2) the consequent nulls in discriminatory response which sometimes developed as C_b passed through its critical level while the phase condition was held constant.

Experimenters working with complex tones having constantly shifting phase relations, such as Egan and Klumpp[10] and Lawrence and Yantis,[12] would have had no opportunity to make such observations. Neither would experimenters who worked exclusively at low stimulus levels, such as Beasley[4,19]; nor those who worked exclusively at high stimulus levels, such as Lewis and Larsen,[6] Chapin and Firestone,[5] and Trimmer and Firestone.[7]

Intersubject Differences

A surprising finding of this study is that certain combinations of phase and level in complex waveforms produce a tone which, when reversed in phase, sounds higher pitched, louder, or purer to some listeners, and lower pitched, softer, or less pure to others.

This finding, however, was implicit in the results of the study by Lewis and Larsen.[6] They showed that the phase of a "difference tone" heard as loudest by their subject A led by some 120° the phase of the same "difference tone" heard as loudest by their subject B. Consequently, the phase angle that made the "difference tone" loudest for A was only 60° from the phase angle that made it softest for B. At some intermediate angle, subject A, no doubt, would hear the tone at nearly its loudest, while B would be hearing it at its weakest. A phase reversal of the complex tone would reverse the subjects' judgments, but would leave them still in disagreement.

Similarly, Trimmer and Firestone[7] added a C_b with an adjustable phase angle to a C_a. Not only did their sub-

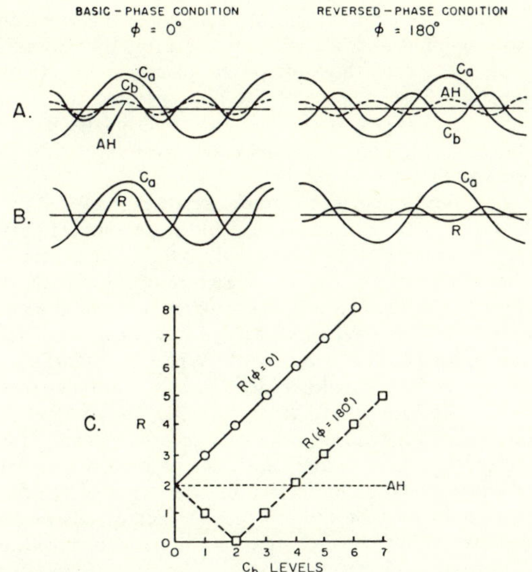

FIG. 9. Hypothetical role of AH in phase effects. The fundamental component C_a is assumed to generate its 2nd aural harmonic AH, which in turn is assumed to interfere directly with the 2nd harmonic component C_b of the stimulus to produce a single component R, of the common frequency. The size of R depends upon the amplitude and φ of C_b. Note that $R_{(\varphi=180°)}$ can never become larger than $R_{(\varphi=0°)}$.

jects differ by as much as 140° about the phase which provided the loudest combination, but one subject's ears differed by 110° of phase for the same judgment. It would have been possible for the two ears of this particular S to disagree as to which of two tones was the louder, just as A and B did in the experiment cited above. When Trimmer and Firestone's five S's each selected the φ which provided the minimum roughness, the range of phase angles extended over 90°. After an audiometric examination of these 10 ears, the experimenters concluded that the phase angles selected for optimum roughness or loudness could not be correlated with any known characteristic of the ears, and that "probably differences in φ are related to more subtle or less familiar features of the hearing organs" (p. 27). The results of the present study support the findings just outlined, and likewise the state of our ignorance concerning the reasons for them.

Theoretical Interpretations

Aural–Harmonic Explanation of MPE's

Ever since the time of Helmholtz, the interaction of aural harmonics (AH's) and other "subjective" tones with the physical components of the acoustic stimulus has frequently been thought to provide the basis for MPE's, particularly for the beats of mistuned consonances. The support given such a concept by the ready detection of cochlear microphonics of appropriate frequencies in the ears of laboratory animals, while persuasive,[22] is nevertheless inconclusive. Let us see just how well the AH explanation fits the results of the present study.

Figures 9(A) and 9(B) illustrate the effective stimulus furnished by the two-component tone used in this study, under the assumption that an AH is generated by C_a—and that the effect of this AH is to combine with C_b, either constructively or destructively. The resultant R equals (AH$+C_b$) when $\varphi=0°$, and R$=$(AH$-C_b$) when $\varphi=180°$. In theory R effectively replaces C_b in the cochlear activity leading to neural stimulation. As shown in Fig. 9(C), the initial increases of C_b from below threshold would serve to decrease R when $\varphi=180°$, and would serve to increase R when $\varphi=0°$. Thus the early increases of C_b would increase the difference between the stimuli at the two phase conditions. However, once C_b became equal to AH, further increases of C_b, regardless of φ, would serve only to increase R and would no longer increase the difference between the basic and phase-reversed neural stimulation. Although different pairs of φ conditions would change the straight-line plots of R in Fig. 9(C) into curved lines, in no instance would they ever cross each other.

On the basis of this model we would have predicted that, with increases of C_b, MPE would become more and more noticeable until $C_b=$AH. Any further increases of C_b would then be expected to leave detectibility unchanged, or to lead to reduced discrimination as C_b became relatively larger and larger than AH. A consideration of higher-order AH's and of combination tones would lead to the same sort of model and to the same prediction. In no case could we have reason to expect response reversals. It is thus evident that the simple AH paradigm does not provide us with an explanation for the patterns of response observed in this study.

The AH paradigm might be saved by postulating that when C_b reaches its critical level, a difference tone or another distortion product begins to make its appearance. This new component then interacts with C_a to produce the observed response reversals. Such an *ad hoc* explanation, however, has little merit since, on the one hand, there is no independent evidence of its validity; and on the other hand, subjective-tone explanations have failed in the case of the best-known MPE, the "residue."[23] In addition, Békésy[21] has recently shown that "best beats" can be accounted for without the help of any subjective tones. Although none of the foregoing should be taken as a direct denial of the validity of the

[22] E. G. Wever, C. W. Bray, and M. Lawrence, "The Locus of Distortion in the Ear," J. Acoust. Soc. Am. **9**, 427 (1940); "A Quantitative Study of Combination Tones," J. Exptl. Psychol. **27**, 469 (1940).

[23] J. F. Schouten, "The Perception of Pitch," Philips Tech. Rev. **5**, 286 (1940); J. C. R. Licklider, "'Periodicity' Pitch and 'Place' Pitch," J. Acoust. Soc. Am. **26**, 945 (1954); "Three Auditory Theories," in *Psychology: A Study of a Science*, edited by S. Koch (McGraw–Hill Book Company, Inc., New York, 1959).

AH hypothesis, it seems advisable, at least for the low- and mid-MPE's, to provide an explanation which does not depend upon distortion products, although, very possibly, they are involved in the case of the high-MPE.

Rectifier Aspect of Neural Excitation

It has been fairly well established that the neural responses of the cochlea originate during that half of each cycle of the cochlear microphonic which is associated with the outward movement of the eardrum.[24,25] Thus, the nerve fibers in contact with the cochlear hair cells are, in effect, excited by a half-wave-rectified aspect of the stimulus at that place. Whether or not such rectification occurs would be immaterial according to a strict cochlear-place theory, which sees the cochlea as a perfect frequency analyzer distributing each frequency component to that place along the cochlea which responds maximally to its frequency.

In such an idealized situation, reversing the phase of even a very unsymmetrical stimulus, whose components are rectified during the process of neural excitation, would not lead to any change in the neural response. However, Rosenblith and Rosenzweig[26] found that reversing the phase of a click stimulus did change the neural response. This implies that either the neural response at the place associated with one component is contaminated by some effect resulting from the other components, or that there exists a common area in the cochlea where the components act together. Békésy[21] and Tonndorf[27] provide us with evidence for the first of these departures from the idealized situation; Tasaki[28] for the other.

Spatial–Pattern Explanation of MPE's

Békésy[21] used the combination of a fundamental and its mistuned octave to drive his enlarged model of the human cochlea which uses the skin of the arm as its organ of Corti. He observed that during each beat cycle the sensation on his arm shifted back and forth over nearly the entire distance between the points stimulated by either of the primaries independently applied. When he paid close attention to either end of the model and disregarded the place shift, he noted a waxing and waning of the sensation at that place. When, during the cycle of phase changes, the flattened portion of the waveform was directed toward the arm [see the bottom of Fig. 3(A)], the sensation was located toward the "high pitch" or basal end of the model; and when the more pointed end was toward the arm, the sensation occurred toward the "low pitch" or apical end. In the light of the subtleness of the phase-related pitch and loudness changes of the present experiment, we can only conclude that the model vastly overemphasizes the pitch shift.

Tonndorf,[27] using a much smaller model, found definite but very small changes in the patterns of particle movement within the "cochlear fluid" of the model when the phase relation of the two-component tone was altered. The change was particularly noticeable in the vicinity of the maximum of amplitude associated with the higher-pitched component. While Tonndorf's observations do not make it clear what sensation changes should be predicted, they suggest, in contrast to Békésy's, that the sensation change will be small. If we accept the phase-related behavior of Békésy's greatly enlarged model as indicative of the effect of the tiny changes of particle motion seen in Tonndorf's model, then we would predict that a pitch change will be associated with phase reversal. However, a response reversal following increases of C_b would not be predicted with respect to pitch. If the listener were merely responding to the loudness of the predominate component, C_a, when C_b was still at low levels, and C_b, after its level had been somewhat increased, we then would predict response reversal.

This explanation fits the objective responses although it does not agree very well with listener's subjective reports. It still accounts for no more than two of the three MPE's, and is limited to waveforms showing unsymmetrical amplitudes. It would not predict discriminations in the case of the $\varphi=90°$ condition [see Fig. 3(C)]. There, not the amplitudes, but rather the waveform must provide the cues of phase discrimination. The stimulating wavefront is much steeper in the reversed-phase than in the basic-phase condition. Hence, it may well be that, contrary to Békésy's conclusion (footnote 21, p. 498), the change in the first derivative of the waveform does provide a cue for discrimination. Békésy himself, investigating beats between an electric square wave and a sinusoid, found a more intense sensation associated with the steeper wavefront. If both of these ideas are accepted, a sensation change would be expected following either a phase-related cochlear shift of the point of maximum excitation or a phase-related change in the sharpness of onset.

Temporal–Pattern Explanations of MPE's

The preceding explanations all fell within the scope of cochlear place theory. Another possibility is that MPE's are in part due to phase-related changes in the temporal patterns of neural stimulation. Instead of merely considering shifts in the place of maximal stimulation along the cochlea and changes in the relative amplitudes, let us consider interaction of the neural

[24] H. Davis, "The Electrical Phenomena of the Cochlea and the Auditory Nerve," J. Acoust. Soc. Am. **6**, 205 (1935).

[25] R. Galambos and H. Davis, "Response of Single Auditory–Nerve Fibers to Acoustic Stimulation," J. Neurophysiol. **6**, 39 (1943).

[26] W. A. Rosenblith and M. R. Rosenzweig, "Electrical Responses to Acoustic Clicks," J. Acoust. Soc. Am. **23**, 583 (1951).

[27] J. Tonndorf, "Beats in Cochlear Models," J. Acoust. Soc. Am. **31**, 608 (1959).

[28] I. Tasaki, "Nerve Impulses in Individual Auditory Nerve Fibers of Guinea Pig," J. Neurophysiol. **17**, 97 (1954).

events originating at the two cochlear loci associated with the two components of the tone. Spiral fibers may provide the means for the interaction between the two involved cochlear loci. When the phase relations are favorable for summation, the probability of firing the spiral fiber would be greater than for other phases.

If the spiral fiber cannot behave in the manner outlined, the neural interaction may occur further up the auditory system. Neural firing in the auditory nerve follows very closely the periodicity of low-frequency stimulus tones[25] such as those used in the present study. Thus temporal representation of the phase relations of the stimulus appears in the higher auditory centers. The evidence from studies of localization and lateralization of tones[29] indicates that such central interaction is likely.

However, in an unreported part of the present study, when C_a was presented to one ear and C_b to the other, phase discrimination did not occur at those lower stimulus levels which produced good phase discrimination with monaurally presented signals. Only when the signal intensity had been raised so much that sound could have been leaking through the head and producing MPE's at one or both ears did phase discrimination begin to appear. Thus, if a neural-interaction mechanism for MPE's does exist, it differs at least in part from that which mediates binaural phase effects, and probably lies below the level in the auditory system where neurons from the two ears begin to form functional connections.

A third possible place where changed phase relations of a complex stimulus could be reflected in changed patterns of neural response is suggested by the work of Tasaki.[28] He found that although nerve fibers from the apical end of the cochlea respond only to low tones, in accordance with traditional auditory place-theory, the fibers from the basal end respond to tones of *all* frequencies. He thereby indicated that "in the basal turn . . . any mixture of tones can act without being separated into its components" (p. 120). With *amplitude* (maximum displacement) of the complex wave as stimulus, many 180° phase shifts would distinctively change the neural response; with *steepness* (the first derivative of the waveform) as the stimulus, every substantial phase shift would do so.

[29] G. Moushegian and L. A. Jeffress, "Role of Interaural Time and Intensity Differences in the Lateralization of Low-Frequency Tones," J. Acoust. Soc. Am. **31**, 1441 (1959); R. H. Whitworth and L. A. Jeffress, "Time vs Intensity in the Localization of Tones," *ibid.* **33**, 925–929 (1961).

Only those waveforms which have envelopes characterized by large amplitude variations exhibit the "residue" effect. For such waveforms, it is reasonable to assume that basal-turn fibers will fire in bursts related to the time of maximal amplitude. In doing so these fibers, though located in the high-frequency part of the cochlea, will be providing low-frequency information. Such a correlation device as that suggested by Jeffress[30] or Licklider[31] could serve as an "envelope reader" and provide the basis for hearing a low-pitched tone. The low frequency responsible is a low frequency of the envelope—it would not be found as a spectral element of the physical sound.

Sources of MPE's

In summary, it can be observed that no single explanation for MPE's can account for the subjects' response patterns. It appears evident that two or more of several possible mechanisms are involved. While none of the proposed explanations is completely untenable, none is clearly superior. The three best supported by outside evidence and which fit the present results are: (1) the phase-related shift of the cochlear locus of maximal stimulation; (2) the "envelope-reader" connected with the basal turn; and (3) the traditional explanation: phase-determined interaction of distortion products with the primary components of the stimulus. It seems probable that one of the first two of these mechanisms produces the low MPE's. As stimulus level increases, one (or both) of the other mechanisms makes its contribution to the differences of sensation.

ACKNOWLEDGMENT

This research was supported under Contract NObsr-72627 with the Bureau of Ships.

[30] L. A. Jeffress, "Interaural Phase Difference and Pitch Variation; Day-to-Day Changes," Am. J. Psychol. **62**, 1 (1949).

[31] J. C. R. Licklider, "A Duplex Theory of Pitch Perception," Experientia **7**, 128 (1951).

31

Reprinted from *Acoust. Soc. Am. J.* **31**:759–767 (1959)

Auditory Perception of Temporal Order*

IRA J. HIRSH
Central Institute for the Deaf, St. Louis, Missouri
(Received January 28, 1959)

INTRODUCTION

THE study of auditory perception has been characterized by an overwhelming concern for the attributes of single sounds. We know fairly well the rules concerning the limits of discrimination with respect to pitch, loudness, and quality. We know less about discrimination of durations and certain other single-sound dimensions because they have not been studied so extensively. The perception of speech has required that we consider other dimensions, like formant structures, transitional properties relative to foci of frequency, etc., but even in this case the auditory studies have been concerned with single sounds.

We propose to examine auditory perception at a more complex level. The discrimination among and identification of single sounds, which we shall refer to as acoustic *events*, is undoubtedly an important part of the perceptual process, but perhaps more important are the rules by which we distinguish and identify sequences of acoustic events. Auditory psychophysics has been concerned with the acoustic characteristics of the sequence-parts, the events; but we need to know more about the ways in which the parts combine to form patterns which, since they are generated in time, we may call *sequences*.

Temporal Order

If we examine all of the ways in which acoustic patterns are generated as a function of time, we find that we can point to different kinds of pattern description in order to specify the ways in which these patterns may sound different to listeners. Some of the different ways of talking about temporal patterns will be pointed out in the Discussion section so that a theoretical framework may be evolved into which we can place the problem of temporal order. The problem for experimental investigation here concerns the ability of listeners to tell in what order two sounds occur. It turns out that there are a number of examples in everyday listening which seem to require that such a judgment be made for ordinary perceptual recognition to take place. Two examples will suffice—one from music and the other from speech.

The perception of a melodic line involves not only the discrimination of different frequencies but also the ordering of these frequencies in time. The simplest case that we can discuss involves a melody consisting of only two frequencies. Suppose, for example, that one depresses the keys on a piano corresponding to C and E. If the two keys are depressed simultaneously, one hears only a simple chord; but if one key is depressed before the other, then the beginning of a melody is heard. The judgment concerning whether this melodic segment is moving upward or downward depends upon the listener's perceiving which of the two tones came first.

In the perception of speech, we find several cases in which speech sounds must not only be discriminated from one another, but also must be judged with respect to order. Consider the following word pairs: boots-boost, mitts-mist, axe-ask, leech-leashed. In all of these cases, the listener must distinguish one from the other member of a pair primarily on the basis of the order in which the last two sounds occur. In the case of "mitts" and "mist," we have perhaps the clearest example because the tongue is in approximately the same position for /*s*/ as it is for /*t*/ and, therefore, we would assume that the spectra would be similar. These two speech sounds are distinguished from each other primarily on the basis of duration. However, in distinguishing between the two words, the listener must not only be able to discriminate the two speech sounds themselves, but further must be able to perceive their order of occurrence.

There are other examples but these two general ones will serve to emphasize the fact that there are perceptual tasks in everyday hearing that require a judgment based upon temporal order. Several questions concerning this judgment emerge. First, how much time must intervene between the onsets of two sounds for their order to be reported correctly? Second, does this minimum time depend upon the frequency of tones involved or upon other acoustical characteristics of more complex sounds? Third, are the small times, of about a few milliseconds, that permit a listener to identify two sounds as opposed

* These experiments were initiated under a grant (B-243) to the Central Institute for the Deaf from the National Institutes of Neurological Diseases and Blindness and were continued under a grant (NSF G-4457) from the National Science Foundation.

to one, sufficient also to permit him to identify correctly their order of occurrence?

EXPERIMENTS

I. Continuous Sounds of Different Pitch

The example given above, concerning which of two tones from the piano came first, may serve as a model for the questions asked in this first experiment. We wished to know how great a temporal interval must intervene between the onsets of two pure tones of different frequency in order for a listener to be able to report correctly which of the two tones came first.

Five pairs of tones were used, the two tones of each pair being separated by an interval roughly corresponding to a musical minor third or this interval plus two or four octaves. The frequency pairs used were 250–300, 250–1200, 250–4800, 1000–1200, and 1000–4800 cps. The lower tone of each pair was 250 cps for the first three cases and 1000 cps for the second two. The minimum separation was 50 cps while the maximum separation was 4550 cps. The tones lasted approximately 0.5 sec and recurred once every 1.8 sec. The temporal interval between the onset times of the lower and higher frequency was varied between -60 and $+60$ msec. Both tones were terminated simultaneously.

This procedure was finally adopted after some preliminary work in which we found that if the durations of the two tones were equal, then there appeared to be as much information about order in the times at which the tones ceased as in the times at which they began. We decided, therefore, to vary the onset times of the two tones independently but to turn them off simultaneously. At first we permitted the listeners to choose between saying that one or the other came first or that they appeared to start simultaneously. The middle or doubtful category contained too many judgments to permit meaningful results to be obtained. Also in this preliminary work, we set the frequencies of the two tones one octave apart. The confusion was considerable and it was found that almost any other interval would yield more consistent judgments.

Apparatus

The two tones were turned on by two separate channels (A and B) of an electronic switch. The rise and fall times were approximately 20 msec. Each of the two channels of the electronic switch was triggered independently by a 45-v dc step delivered by a battery connected in series with one of three microswitches, two of which turned on channels A and B, respectively, while the third turned off both channels simultaneously. These microswitches were engaged by three brass cylinders mounted on the periphery of a large, broadcast-type turntable operating at $33\frac{1}{3}$ rpm. A large 360-deg protractor was centered on the turntable. The second and third of the three brass cylinders were fixed 100 deg apart, while the first was mounted on a movable arm that could be placed at any angle relative to the second. Now, a turntable moving at $33\frac{1}{3}$ rpm has a radial velocity of 200 deg/sec. Therefore, the two fixed cylinders, 100 deg apart, produced a time interval of 500 msec and were used to turn on and off, respectively, channel B. The duration of the tone keyed by channel A was determined by the distance between the movable first cylinder and the third (fixed) cylinder. The duration varied between 440 and 560 msec because the relation between the movable first cylinder and the fixed second cylinder was varied between ± 60 msec. After suitable amplification and control attenuation, the tones were delivered monaurally through earphones to five listeners.

Procedure

A panel of five listeners was presented a series of tone pairs for each value of onset-time differences until all the listeners had signified that they could make a judgment. They wrote down either "lower" or "higher", depending upon which frequency they thought came first. The choice between these two alternatives was forced; they could not respond "simultaneous" or "doubtful."

Each experimental session was restricted to a single pair of frequencies. The method of constant stimuli that was used involved ten trials at each of the fixed values of temporal separation between the onsets of the two tones. A first session included temporal separations between lower and higher frequencies of -60, -40, -20, 0, 20, 40, and 60 msec, and a later session included interpolated settings of -50, -30, -10, 10, 30, and 50 msec.

In addition to the five pairs of tones mentioned above, the experiment was repeated for a low-pitched (center frequency 440 cps) and a high-pitched (center frequency 4000 cps) narrow band of noise. For this experiment temporal separations from -60 to $+60$, in multiples of 20 msec only, were used.

Results

For each of the five subjects, the number of times out of ten trials that he reported the "higher first" was recorded. Then the average percentage of judgments that were "higher first" for all subjects was converted to the corresponding value in standard deviations according to the normal-probability table, on the assumption that the function relating the probability that a subject would say "higher first" to the temporal interval by which the higher preceded the lower frequency would be a normal ogive. These converted values are presented in Fig. 1, where each point represents the mean normalized proportion of judgments "higher first" among ten trials on five observers.

The abscissa of Fig. 1 shows the temporal interval that separates the two tones. Negative values indicate that the lower tone precedes the higher while the positive values indicate that the higher precedes the lower. The assumption that the relation between response probability and temporal separation would be a normal ogive appears tenable because the distributions for the five different frequency pairs and the noise-band pair appear to fall reasonably well on a straight line. The broken lines represent straight-line fits by eye to the data for each condition. The solid line, the same for each of the six conditions, represents a hypothetical function, the hypothesis for which will be dealt with in the following.

Three main conclusions stand out: first, a temporal separation of a little less than 20 msec will afford reasonably correct (75% or a normal probability value of 0.67) judgments of the order in which two tones or two bands of noise of different pitch occur; second, there is no constant error; that is, the point at which "higher-first" and "lower-first" judgments are given with equal frequency corresponds to physical simultaneity or no temporal difference between the onsets of the two sounds; third, the relation does not appear to depend greatly on the amount of frequency separation between the two tones nor upon whether the low- and high-pitched sounds are tones or bands of noise. A possible exception to this last point may be seen at the left where the frequency separation is small, i.e., corresponds to a minor third. Particularly for the pair 1000-1200 cps, it appears that the judgments become either inconsistent or, for some reason, stabilized when the lower precedes the higher over a fairly sizeable range of onset-time differences. There is only a suggestion of a similar effect for the pair 250–300.

Since the difference between the frequencies of the two tones used in this experiment did not appear to be crucial for this judgment of temporal order, it was of considerable interest to know whether differences in intensity would make a difference. This question was not explored fully in the present experiment but some variation in intensity was introduced for the frequency pair 250–1200 cps. The results shown in the middle graph of the upper row in Fig. 1 hold for the condition in which both tones had a loudness level of 80 phons. Two subsequent experimental sessions were carried out in which the loudness level of the 1200-cps tone was maintained at 80 phons while the loudness level for 250 cps was set at 70 or 60 phons. Within this relatively small range of variation in level, the functions produced, not shown in Fig. 1, were not very different from that given for the equal-loudness case. The role of level will be dealt with more fully in Experiment IV.

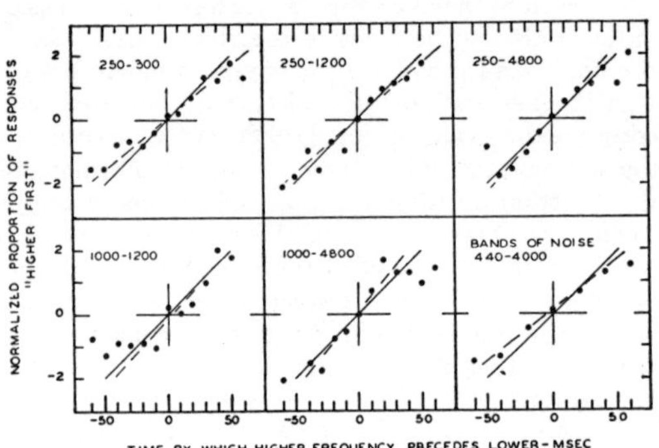

FIG. 1. Probability that the higher pitched of two sounds will be judged to have occurred first as a function of the temporal interval separating the onsets of the two sounds. The ordinate is percentage of response converted to normal values while the abscissa shows the amount by which the higher frequency precedes the lower. The six graphs are for six different pairs of sounds.

II. Continuous Sounds of Different Quality

For a listener to judge which of two sounds came first, the two sounds must be discriminably different so that he can identify them separately. In the first experiment the sounds were different with respect to frequency. In this second experiment we still asked the listener to tell which of two continuous sounds started first, but now the sounds were made different with respect to quality. One was a tone while the other was a wide-band noise.

Procedure

The apparatus and listening procedure were the same as that described for Experiment I except that the output of a noise generator was fed to channel B of the electronic switch instead of a second tone. Three tonal frequencies were employed: 250, 1000, and 4000 cps. Both tone and noise were turned on with rise-times of approximately 20 msec. All tones were set at a loudness level of 80 phons and the noise voltage was adjusted so that the noise would be equally loud according to the results of Pollack.[1]

Results

The top row of Fig. 2 shows the results for two different groups of observers. The open circles represent the normalized proportions of judgments "tone first" based

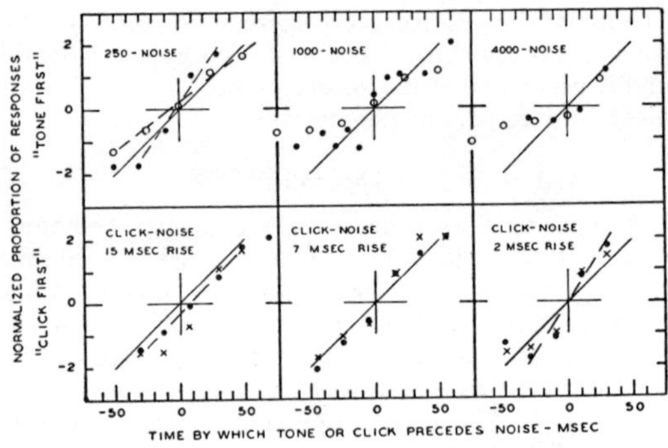

FIG. 2. Probability that a click or a tone will be judged to have occurred earlier than a noise as a function of the interval between tone or click and noise. In the top line the open and the filled circles represent data for the same conditions on two different groups of observers. In the bottom line the filled circles show results for low-frequency noise, while the X's show results for high-frequency noise.

[1] I. Pollack, J. Acoust. Soc. Am. 23, 654–657 (1951).

on ten trials for four observers with temporal intervals between the onsets of tone and noise at ±75, 50, 25, and 0 msec. The closed circles represent results for a different group of five observers with the temporal intervals set at ±50, 30, and 10 msec for 250 cps; ±60, 50, 40, 30, 20, 10, and 0 msec for 1000 cps; and ±30 and 10 msec for 4000 cps. Where points are omitted at the extremes, the percentage judgment was 0 or 100%.

The two groups of observers appear to give somewhat different results for the 250-cps tone but similar results for the two higher frequencies. In the case of the two higher frequencies, and especially 4000 cps, we observe a situation very much like that seen for the tone pair 1000–1200 cps in Fig. 1, namely, that when the noise precedes the high-frequency tone, the orderly relation between response probability and temporal interval is replaced by a confusion in which the observers report that the tone comes first between 10 and 20% of the time over a substantial range of temporal intervals. This finding was initially so different from that for other pairs of sounds, that a repetition with a second group of observers seemed advisable. Perhaps here, as well as in Fig. 1 where the frequency interval was small, a masking effect of the sound that comes first interferes with the judgments. The broken lines in the graph for 250 cps represent linear fits by eye, but no similar attempt has been made for the data of 1000 and 4000 cps. The solid line is the same hypothetical line that was used in Fig. 1.

III. Click and Noise

In the first two experiments both sounds, whose order was to be judged, were continuous and they were made different with respect either to frequency (I) or spectrum (II). Another way in which two acoustic events may be made different involves duration. If a listener hears a brief click and a longer noise, how much time must intervene between the occurrence of the click and the onset of the noise in order for the listener to report correctly which of the two sounds came first? This may be the experimental analog of the practical problem suggested earlier with respect to the distinction between "mitts" and "mist," where the listener must be able to judge correctly the order of the plosive and fricative sounds.

With a click that could serve as a perceptual time marker, two parameters of the noise were investigated: rise-time and spectrum.

Apparatus

Two pulse generators were driven by a single wave form generator in such a way that the temporal interval between the two pulses could be controlled precisely (to the nearest microsecond as monitored by a Berkeley Counter Timer). One of these pulses was amplified and passed through a 2400-cps low-pass filter so that the electrical wave form was known to represent the acoustical wave form produced by the earphone in a 6-cc coupler. The other pulse was used to trigger one channel of the electronic switch that turned on the noise. Originally the temporal intervals between these two pulses were set at ±50, 30, and 10 msec, but subsequent examination of the components of the apparatus revealed that the time of the trigger pulse did not correspond precisely to the opening of the electronic switch, and further that this time relation between the trigger pulse and the onset of the noise changed with the rise-time that was set in the switch. Appropriate corrections were introduced for the results to be presented.

Three different rise-times for the noise were used: 15, 7, and 2 msec. Futhermore, in one-half of the experiments the noise was passed through a high-frequency octave-band filter (2400–4800 cps), while in the other half the noise was passed through a low-frequency octave band (300–600 cps).

The level of the noise was 70-db sound pressure level while that of the click was set so that the first half-wave of the filtered click was equal in peak amplitude to a pure tone whose rms sound pressure level was 96 db.

Procedure

The listening procedure was carried out in the same way as in the first two experiments. The click-noise pair was repeated every 1.5 sec and the listeners were permitted to hear as many pairs as they wished before rendering judgment as to which sound came first. Instead of ten trials per temporal interval, twenty trials were used with five observers.

Results

The results of this experiment are shown in the bottom row of Fig. 2 where the abscissa represents the time by which the click preceded the onset of the noise. The odd values of the abscissa over which points are placed result from the error discussed above. For the 15-msec rise, the points correspond to the click preceding the noise by −32, −12, 8, 28, 48, and 68 msec. For the 7-msec rise, the time by which the click preceded the noise was set at −44, −24, −4, 16, 36, and 56 msec. For the 2-msec rise, the values corresponded to the original interpulse interval of ±50, 30, and 10 msec.

The filled circles represent the results for the low-frequency noise while the X's represent the results for the high-frequency noise, with the click the same throughout.

A broken line has been used to fit the data by eye except for the case of the 7-msec rise where a fit by eye could do no better that the same hypothetical line that has been used throughout. No attempt has been made to draw separate broken lines for the data of the high-frequency and low-frequency noises because the differences do not appear to be substantial. Except for the shortest rise time (2 msec), the slope of the function that relates response probability for "click first" to the temporal interval between the click and the onset of

TABLE I. Durations of tone (msec).

Rise-time (msec)	Level of tone (SPL) 50	90
7	50	20, 50
15	50	50, 100

the noise does not appear to be different from those already reported for pairs of tones or for pairs of sounds, one of which is a tone and the other a noise. There is some suggestion for a constant error in the data for the 15-msec rise. It appears that the judgments "click first" and "noise first" are about equally probable when the click precedes the onset of the noise by about 10 msec. This is the first instance in which reasonable evidence for a difference between the point of subjective simultaneity and the point of objective simultaneity is found. Data for the 2-msec rise also constitute the first instance in which there may be a significantly steeper slope, which would correspond to greater sensitivity to differences in onset times as reflected in a judgement of temporal order.

IV. Click and Tone

In the preceding experiment, the two sounds, whose order was judged, differed with respect to duration but both had considerable band width. The next complication to be introduced was an experimental analog for the situation in which the conductor of an orchestra brings his baton down and notices a discrepancy between the starting time of his trumpeter and his drummer. Which of them started too soon or too late? Here we propose to use the same low-pass click as a time marker relative to the onset time of a 1000-cps tone. Three parameters of the tone are varied: rise-time, duration, and level.

Procedure

The listening procedure and apparatus was the same as those described for the preceding experiment. Tone-click pairs were repeated every 1.5 sec and after a sufficient number of them had occurred for all five listeners to render a judgment, the next temporal interval was set. The click level was maintained at a peak equivalent rms sound pressure level of 80 db. The tone was varied in level, rise-time, and duration according to the arrangement shown in Table I.

Results

The upper left graph in Fig. 3 shows the relation between the normalized proportion of responses "click first" and the time by which the click preceded the tone. In this upper left graph the tone had a rise-time of 15 msec and a duration of 50 msec. The filled circles represent results for a tone level of 90 db SPL, while the X's represent a tone level of 50 db SPL. Each point is the mean normalized proportion of judgments for 5 listeners on 20 trials. Again broken lines represent an attempt to fit the two groups of data by eye. The lower left graph in Fig. 3 shows the same relations between symbols and tone level for a rise-time of 7 msec and a duration of 50 msec. For the faster rise-time, there is some evidence that the higher-level tone appears to begin sooner than the lower-level tone because the click must precede the higher-level tone by about 10 msec for the judgments to be divided equally between "click first" and "tone first."

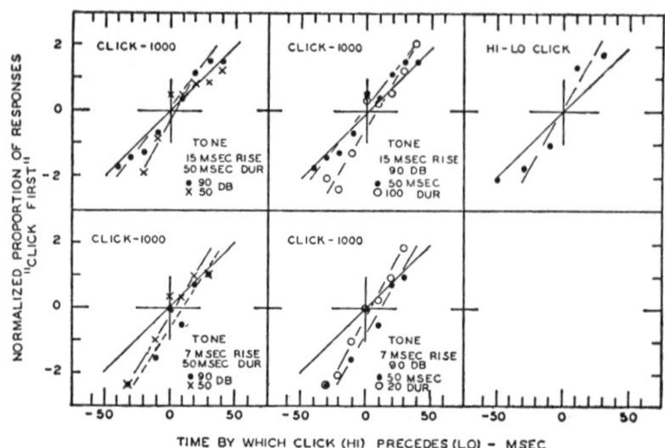

FIG. 3. Probability that a click will be judged to have occurred before a tone as a function of the temporal interval between a click and the onset of a tone. The legends within the four first graphs show the effects of varying rise time, duration, and level of the tone. The graph at the upper right shows the relation between the probability of judging that a high-pitched click has preceded a low-pitched click as a function of the temporal interval between the two clicks.

The middle two graphs of Fig. 3 show the effect of duration of the tone for rise-times at 15 msec (upper) and 7 msec (lower). Tone level was maintained at 90 db SPL. For the slower rise-time (15 msec, upper) the slopes of the two broken lines may be different and also it seems that the 100-msec tone appears to begin earlier than the 50-msec tone. Similarly for the shorter rise-time (7 msec, lower), the 50-msec tone appears to begin earlier than the 20-msec tone.

We may summarize the effects of these changes in parameters of the tone in the following way. When the tone level is 90 db, a faster rise time makes the tone appear to begin earlier, but when the level is only 50 db, this difference no longer holds. With a 7-msec rise time, a 90-db tone appears to begin earlier than a 50-db tone, but with a slower 15-msec rise-time this dependence on level no longer holds. At 90 db, a tone appears to start earlier as its duration is increased, for both a short (7 msec) and a long (15 msec) rise-time.

These effects are less important, however, than the general agreement between these data and the same hypothetical line that has been entered here in Fig. 3 as a solid line, as will be shown in the following.

V. Two Clicks

One further experiment fills out certain combinations of duration and band width as stimulus dimensions. In the first two experiments, we asked the listeners to judge the order of two continuous sounds that differed with respect to pitch or quality. In the third and fourth experiments, we saw that brevity, both in the form of a click as such or a fast rise-time at the beginning of a continuous sound, might steepen the relation between probability of response and temporal interval. In Experiment V we asked the listener to report the order of two brief sounds that differed with respect to pitch. To continue our analogies, this represents the situation in which the same orchestral conductor observes a discrepancy in time between the beats of his snare drum and kettle drum and he must judge which of them preceded the other.

Procedure

The two pulse generators that were used in Experiment III were utilized here, but in this instance both pulses were amplified and passed through filters, one at 1000-cps low pass and the other at 4000-cps band pass. The clicks were clearly discriminable on the basis of pitch. The two clicks were set at a peak equivalent rms sound pressure level of 80 db for the first half-wave of the electrical response after filtering. Temporal intervals between the two clicks were set at ±50, 30, and 10 msec. The listeners were asked to report whether the "higher" or "lower" came first.

Results

The results of this brief experiment are shown in the upper right graph of Fig. 3. Each point is based on 5 listeners and 20 trials. It is difficult to interpret what appears to be an ogival shape on a normal probability ordinate, and the necessity for such interpretation has been avoided by attempting a straight-line fit by eye as represented by the broken line. The slope of the function appears to be steeper than those of previous experiments but not very much so, as will be seen presently in the discussion. Here the listener demands a greater temporal interval for the judgment of order than the 2 msec or so that is required for these same two differently pitched clicks to be judged as separate. These clicks were also used in an informal study to ascertain how much time must intervene between two dissimilar clicks if they are to be judged as two rather than one. The time does not appear to be different from that required for two similar brief clicks.[2]

DISCUSSION

In the preceding experiments we have attempted to examine one important component of auditory perception, namely, the judgment of temporal order. Experiment I indicated that the ability of listeners to report correctly the order in which two tones of different frequency occurred as a function of the temporal interval between their onsets did not vary as the difference in frequency between the two tones was varied. The same result was obtained when the two sounds were not tones but high and low-frequency bands of noise. Experiment II gave similar functions even when one of the two sounds was a tone and the other a noise. In the third and fourth experiments a click was compared with a noise or tone, respectively, and again similar functions were obtained. Finally, in the fifth experiment a similar function resulted from the use of two clicks, one high-pitched and one low-pitched. These five experiments sampled various kinds of stimulus pairs representing combinations of sounds that differ in frequency, band width, and duration. The samplings are summarized in Table II.

The minimum temporal interval separating the onsets of two sounds that is required for a correct judgment of temporal order might be independent of the acoustical nature of the sounds. This possibility led to the formulation of an empirical hypothesis, based on averaging across all experimental conditions. The results of this averaging are shown in Fig. 4. The open circles represent the averages of all of the average points in the five tone-pair graphs of Fig. 1. The filled circles show the relation for high- and low-pitched noise in the lower right corner of Fig. 1. The X's average the two groups of observers shown in the upper left corner of Fig. 2, for a sound pair consisting of a 250-cps tone and noise. (The other two frequencies were not used because of the possibility that the masking effect mentioned earlier contaminated the results.) Finally, the $+s$ average the data in the two left-hand columns of Fig. 3 for clicks paired with tones of various rise-times, durations, and levels. (The data for click paired with noise have not been put into Fig. 4 because of the complication mentioned earlier that the three conditions shown in the bottom half of Fig. 2 did not involve the same temporal intervals.) On this normal probability ordinate, we have drawn a straight line by eye attempting to fit points that fall between about 20 and 90%. This line constitutes our tentative hypothesis. It relates the probability that a subject will judge correctly the order in which the two sounds occurred to the temporal interval between their onsets, independent of what the two sounds are. It is the solid line that has been drawn through all of the previous graphs and it shows a

TABLE II. Combinations of sounds used.

Experiment	Sounds	Band width	Duration	Different with respect to:
I	Tones, noise bands	Both narrow	Both long	Frequency
II	Tones *vs* noise	One narrow One wide	Both long	Quality
III	Click *vs* noise	Both wide	One short One long	Duration
IV	Click *vs* tone	One wide and One narrow and	short long	Duration, quality
V	Hi click *vs* lo click	Both narrow	Both short	Frequency

[2] Wallach, Newman, and Rosenzweig, Am. J. Psychol. **62**, 315–335 (1949).

75% correct judgment (probable error) at 17 msec, or a standard deviation of 25 msec.

Not all of the points fall on this line but our hypothesis is that those points that do not fall on the line represent either random deviations or less important systematic effects. By random deviations we mean those deviations of single points that do not appear to be members of another single function that is different from the hypothesized function. The two chief sources of what we may consider to be the less important systematic effects involve masking and the temporal characteristics of certain sounds. We have already referred to the possibility that a 1000-cps tone might mask a 1200-cps tone and that this masking would account for an apparent systematic deviation of points representing conditions in which the lower frequency precedes the higher frequency as shown in the lower left graph of Fig. 1. This explanation may similarly account for the systematic deviation of points from the hypothetical line in the two right-hand graphs in the upper row of Fig. 2 where noise precedes tones of 1000 or 4000 cps.

The second source of possible systematic deviation requires further study. The graphs in the lower half of Fig. 2 suggest that a slope steeper than the hypothesized slope is obtained when the rise-time of noise is very short. When the noise is turned on more slowly, for example in 7 or 15 msec, this increase in slope does not appear. A similar increase in slope is seen for several of the functions in Fig. 3. When the tone is turned on quickly (7 msec), steeper functions result than when it is turned on more slowly (15 msec). In addition to a change in slope, there may be a constant error; that is the judgments "click first" and "tone first" appear equally often in most cases where there is physical simultaneity, but in the bottom row we see that they occur equally often when the click precedes a 90-db tone by about 10 msec. The click must also precede slightly to be perceived as simultanous as the duration of the tone is made longer. These observations, however, suggest parameters to be investigated further. When we call these possible effects "less important," we mean that the deviations are small and unimpressive in comparison to the general agreement among the experimental results as a whole over a wide range of conditions.

TIME IN AUDITORY PERCEPTION

These experiments were undertaken within a theoretical framework that holds that time is the dimension within which patterns are articulated for hearing in a manner analogous to the way in which space is the patterning dimension for vision.[3] Just as some theorists in vision have been concerned with the "grain" of visual space, so we are interested here in gradients of acoustic changes in time. Change appears to be the essence of auditory temporal perception and we are examining what kinds of physical changes are necessary in order that there be perceived changes. Troland[4] has suggested that a perceived change requires that the physical change be large enough and slow enough. The limits that define "large enough" have comprised the traditional study of differential sensitivity or difference limens. The limits that define "slow enough" have been called by Troland "psychophysical inertia." The problem of stating the conditions for psychophysical inertia is complicated by the fact that there seem to be several levels at which temporal discrimination can be discussed.

Attributes of the Steady State

Time plays a role even within a single acoustic event that may be characterized as a steady-state pattern. This level may be trivial in that the kinds of cues included can better be expressed in terms of frequency and phase. We could say, for example, that the pitch of a tone increases as the time between successive sinewaves decreases. We could also say that the quality of a tone depends upon the temporal relations among the harmonics. Both of these examples, however, exemplify temporal relations that stay put, so to speak, for as long as the sound is produced. The temporal relations among the components of a steady-state sound comprise the bulk of the classical psychophysics of pure and complex tones. We know, in summary, that the temporal differences involved are very small indeed when we consider the limits of frequency discrimination for pure tones and also the limits for quality discrimination among complex tones.

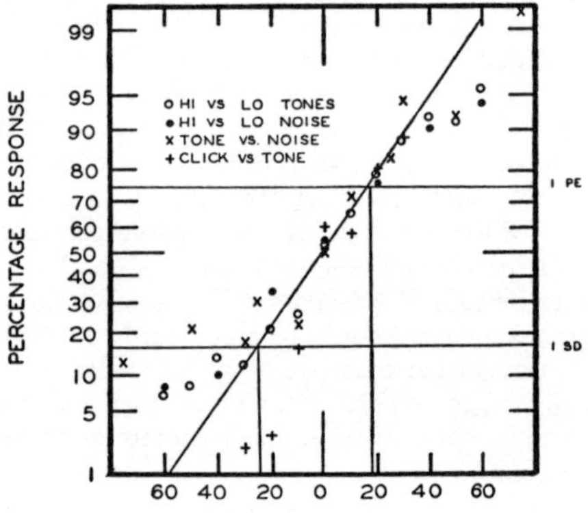

FIG. 4. Probability of judgment concerning which of two sounds came first as a function of the temporal separation between sounds. The open circles represent an average through the first five conditions of Fig. 1. The closed circles are the data from the sixth graph of Fig. 1. The X's result from averaging the two groups of data in the upper left graph of Fig. 2. The +s represent averages for all conditions of the tone in Fig. 3. Points corresponding to one probable error (75% judgment) and one standard deviation (16% judgment) are shown.

[3] I. J. Hirsh, Science, **116**, 523(A) (1952).

[4] L. T. Troland, *Psychophysiology* (D. Van Nostrand Company, Inc., Princeton, New Jersey, 1929), p. 398.

Nonsteady-State Quality

There are other, brief acoustic events that may be differentiated from each other in terms of their internal temporal structure. The pitch of a click that has passed through a filter will change, depending upon the resonance and decay characteristics of the filter. This is very much like the relation already stated for the pitch of a sustained tone. In addition, however, there are cases in which two acoustic events give rise to one auditory event and, further, the temporal separation between the two acoustic events is responsible for a change in the quality of the single auditory event. If two brief clicks are delivered to one ear and are separated by less than 2 msec,[2] they will be heard as one sound and, further, the quality of that sound, whether "dull" or "sharp," will be determined by the amount of separation between the two acoustic clicks. Another example in which the temporal relation between two acoustic events changes the nature of a single perceived event is the special case in which each of two clicks is presented to a separate ear, in which case very small differences between the times of arrival at the two ears will produce changes in the apparent location in space of the single perceived click. When the components of a brief, single sound are clicks and the two clicks are delivered to separate ears, we know that temporal differences as small as 10 μsec will effect a shift in the apparent localization.[5]

Fusion

So far we have been dealing in *microtime*, where temporal relations among the components of a single sound change its quality. As we increase the temporal interval between two clicks delivered to the same ear, however, a listener begins to report that there is no longer just one sound but rather two. The two acoustic events are now separated by enough time so that there are two corresponding auditory events.This question has been studied for a long time,[6] but only recently have stimuli been well enough controlled for decisive answers. When the two clicks are delivered to the same ear, a single sound will be heard so long as the temporal difference between them is no more than 2 msec.[2] These experiments have to do with only pairs of clicks. It is likely that other experiments, in which a whole series of clicks or bursts of noise was presented and the listener was asked to judge whether there was a fused tone-like sound or a series of discrete sounds, are probably also related. According to Boring,[7] Exner in 1875 reported that if the clicks generated by the spokes of a Savart wheel were separated by as much as 2 msec, the observer reported a succession of discrete sounds. This value is not far from the middle of the range of values given by Miller and Taylor for a series of bursts of noise.[8]

Qualitative Differences between Two Events

A different kind of response, and possibly a different magnitude of temporal difference, is involved when we ask a listener not only to detect the presence of two as opposed to one sound, but also to judge whether or not the two sounds are the same or are different. This particular judgment has not been investigated sufficiently for us to know whether it is really different from the previous one, but the kind of judgment involved is sufficiently different so that we must leave room for it to emerge as a possibly separate level. If a temporal separation of 2 msec is sufficient to give rise to the perception of two as opposed to one sound, then is this same time also sufficient to permit a listener to say whether the two separated sounds are different in quality? No evidence on this point has come to our attention, but some preliminary experiments of our own indicate that the necessary time is no different if one uses, for example, two clicks like those of Experiment V whose pitches are made different by different filters. There are other ways to create differences between the two events that are to be judged fused or separate, e.g., intensity, duration, etc., but they have not been investigated.

Order between Successive, Different Sounds

Finally, we ask a listener to tell us not only that there are two separate sounds, and not only that they are different from each other in some respect, but also to tell us in what order the sounds are perceived. Actually this question of temporal order has not been separated from questions regarding successiveness. A clear example of the equating of these two questions is provided by Pieron.[9]

> "We receive an impression of simultaneity for two events perceived, when these two events belong to the same mental present and are not able to be placed in order of time. The events may be very brief, or be the onset of lasting ones. Temporal acuity corresponds to the discriminative power in the time dimension, just as spatial acuities represent discriminative powers in the dimensions of space. A certain minimum separation between two events is necessary in order that their succession may be perceived and their order of appearance determined. The reciprocal of this separation can be taken as a measure of temporal acuity."

His implication is that "their succession" and "their order of appearance" come to the same thing. But our experiments clearly indicate that two sounds that are separated just enough to be heard as two cannot be

[5] E. M. von Hornbostel and M. Wertheimer, Sitzber. deut. Akad. Wiss. Berlin, **15**, 388–396 (1920).

[6] G. T. Ladd and R. S. Woodworth, *Elements of Physiological Psychology* (Charles Scribner's Sons, New York, 1911), p. 475.

[7] E. G. Boring, *Sensation and Perception in the History of Experimental Psychology* (Appleton-Century, Crofts, New York, 1942), p. 363.

[8] G. A. Miller and W. G. Taylor, J. Acoust. Soc. Am. **20**, 171–182 (1948).

[9] H. Pieron, *The Sensations* (Frederick Muller, London, 1952), p. 294.

placed in correct order until the temporal separation is increased about tenfold.

We have suggested five levels or ways in which perceptual differences are brought about by temporal cues. These include changes in the quality of single sounds, either prolonged or transient, changes from singleness to two separate sounds, changes from merely two sounds to two perceptually different sounds, and finally the order of occurrence of two perceptually different sounds. These five levels of temporal cues describe some very fundamental aspects of temporal grain. We have not dealt at all with the kinds of temporal cues that give rise to such complex auditory patterns as rhythmic structure, etc.

When the temporal grain for auditory perception can be described in such small units as microseconds or milliseconds, as is the case for spatial localization and mere successiveness, then it seems probable that we can think about its mechanism in terms of the peripheral auditory system where differences as small as a few milliseconds have some physiological meaning; but when we discover a temporal interval as large as 15 or 20 msec that must be exceeded for auditory perception, as in this case of temporal order, then we must look to more central structures for the anatomical and physiological correlates of such a judgment.

CONCLUSIONS

Whereas a temporal interval of about 2 msec between two brief sounds appears to be sufficient to enable a listener to report that there are two sounds, and not one, a considerably greater interval must elapse if the listener is to report correctly the *order* in which the sounds occurred. This greater temporal interval appears to be about ten times larger, or about 17 msec for the judgments to be 75% correct.

This minimum time that is required for a correct judgment of temporal order between two sounds appears to be independent of their difference in frequency when the sounds are of different pitch. It is the same when one of the sounds is a tone and the other is a noise and when one of the sounds is a click and the other is a noise.

Combinations of clicks with noises or tones that begin abruptly seem to result in greater sensitivity to small temporal differences but these changes, within the range of conditions studied, are small relative to the general agreement among all experimental conditions.

Because the judgment of temporal order requires temporal separations of as much as 20 msec, we conclude that more of the perceptual system is involved than merely the ear itself. Therefore, the judgment of temporal order will not be closely related to the factors that have been shown to be important for the peripheral auditory system.

Part VI

ADVANTAGES OF THE BINAURAL SYSTEM

Editor's Comments on Papers 32 Through 36

32 STEVENS and NEWMAN
The Localization of Actual Sources of Sound

33 WALLACH, NEWMAN, and ROSENZWEIG
Excerpts from *The Precedence Effect in Sound Localization*

34 JEFFRESS et al.
Masking of Tonal Signals

35 KOCK
Binaural Localization Localization and Masking

36 LEVITT and RABINER
Binaural Release from Masking for Speech and Gain in Intelligibility

A listener with normal vision has no occasion to realize the full potential of the binaural system. It is apparently more nearly taxed to its limit when conjunctive visual cues are absent. The fascinating story of the search for the cues used by expert blind "travelers" related by Griffin (1960), as well as the more data-oriented account by the experimenters themselves (Supa, Cotzin, and Dallenbach, 1944) reveals more of the ultimate versatility of the system than most of us have occasion to realize and is one of the most engrossing episodes in the history of research. Here, apparently, the binaural system's capability is—or can be—exploited to the limit. It would be unkind to dull the excitement with a prosaic summary. I would rather urge the interested reader who has not followed the story to read at least chapter 6 of Griffin's book. Attempts to furnish an auxiliary echo-locating system for blind individuals, taking advantage of the short wavelengths of an ultrasonic source and translating the reflected information down to the audible range, have also been at least partly successful (Kay and Do, 1977).

The function of the two ears in localizing sound sources has been known for many years. An excellent brief history is contained in Paper

32 by Stevens and Newman. Much of the prior work seeking to identify the factors that contribute to localization had no option but to use sound-conducting tubes to control the variables at the two ears, and therefore presumably was investigating what we now call lateralization rather than localization.

This is the group Stevens and Newman refer to as the dichotic school, and it profited by considerable aid from outside the field of psychology. Both G. W. Stewart and Lord Rayleigh, whose activities were primarily focused on objective physics, performed listening experiments designed to resolve the question of the role of intensity and phase in sound localization.

In reporting such an experiment in 1907, Lord Rayleigh remarked that he had been interested in this particular problem for thirty years.* Using himself and Lady Rayleigh as listeners, he employed slowly beating tones to create the desired phase difference between ears. The separate tones were led to the two ears through rubber tubes. During appropriate phases of the beating cycle, the image moved from one side of the head to the other. Lord Rayleigh concluded from the responses at various frequencies that for low-frequency tones, the phase difference was the controlling factor and that, as the frequency rose and the ratio of wavelength to head size vitiated the phase clue, the interaural intensity ratio gradually furnished a more reliable indication of direction.

Stewart and his students also performed listening experiments in the early 1900s and reached the same conclusion about the relative role of interaural differences in phase and intensity. By 1920 they were using earphones to control interaural differences (Stewart, 1920). Thus the Stevens and Newman experiment on localization of an actual sound source was a timely contribution in an area of great interest. It has been necessary, even in subsequent years, to remind workers in binaural hearing to heed the distinction between localization and lateralization.

In connection with these studies on binaural processing of sounds, there were early indications of the extreme time-difference sensitivity of the binaural system (see Woodworth, 1938). Klemm's (1920) discovery that one of his observers could sense a deviation from the median plane equivalent to a difference of two microseconds not only was a great surprise to him but still elicited some incredulity a couple of decades later (see Boring, 1942). By now, however, the fact that the auditory system is sensitive to interaural differences of a few microseconds in impinging signals is no longer surprising, and it appears that

*For an earlier paper, see *Acoustics: Historical and Philosophical Development*, ed. R. B. Lindsay (Stroudsburg, Pennsylvania: Dowden, Hutchinson & Ross, 1973), p. 399.

under some conditions, disparities of a fraction of a microsecond may be useful (Nordmark, 1976). Probably this extraordinary time sensitivity is a major factor in permitting the binaural system to accomplish the signal-processing tasks it performs in reverberant conditions and with competing signals frequently present. By comparison, localization of single sources in the absence of reflection becomes almost a matter of simple geometry.

One of the most notable contributions to binaural literature came from the Harvard psychoacoustic laboratory during an especially productive period in the late 1940s. I refer to the study of the precedence effect by Wallach, Newman, and Rosenzweig (Paper 33). Though this paper appears in print later than two important contemporary ones, the work began earlier, must have helped to spark heightened interest in the binaural system, and hastened the realization that the system performs more complex processing than was formerly realized.

The particular effect being studied had been noted before by Békésy (1930) and Langmuir et al. (1944), but this is the first systematic introduction and exploration of the concept. More importantly, it was the first widely available description of the kind of specific mechanism that enables the binaural system to do much more than simply provide for location of the sound source in an uncomplicated nonreverberant sound field.

Students of psychological acoustics should remain aware of the fact that part of this remarkable accomplishment of the binaural system comes about because of its interaction with other sensory domains. In the binaural realm, this kind of synergy was convincingly demonstrated by Wallach (1940) with his experimental work on, and his excellent discussion of, the role of head movements and vestibular and visual cues in sound localization.

But the other two papers mentioned earlier really introduced the notion that the localization of sound sources is definitely not the only advantage of having two inputs to the auditory processing system. Previous discussions of binaural hearing had concerned themselves mostly with localization and binaural beats, as Hirsh (1948a) pointed out in reviewing the history of binaural summation. That situation changed dramatically in the few ensuing years, an exceedingly rich period for binaural discoveries.

First of all, Licklider (1948) showed that under extremely difficult listening conditions (low signal-to-noise ratio), the binaural system apparently processed speech differently when polarities (and presumably other phase relations) of signal and noise differed interaurally. He was able to demonstrate as much as 20 percent improvement in word intelligibility scores when speech and interfering noise were switched from both being in phase at the two ears (homophasic) to the condition where one or the other was out of phase interaurally (antiphasic). This triggered not only a search for an explanation but also for the way to apply this finding in practical listening situations. The first has resulted in the equalization-cancellation theory of binaural processing by Durlach (1963). The second was pursued vigorously for a time by those concerned with communication in noisy aircraft and by workers aiding the hearing impaired, but it is essentially still unsuccessful at this point.

In the meantime in the same laboratory, Hirsh was investigating the changes in audibility of a tone mixed with an interfering noise under these same interaural conditions. This particular branch of the resurgent binaural investigation got off to a running start, but unfortunately in not quite the right direction. Hirsh (1948b) presented measurements that convinced auditory psychologists that under certain conditions, interaural inhibition influenced auditory thresholds,—that is, that binaural thresholds were sometimes poorer than monaural. The paper is cited frequently and, except for a small error in the selection of the reference interaural condition, is an excellent demonstration that thresholds differ appreciably for the several different interaural conditions. But the emphasis was unmistakably on the surprising finding of binaural conditions with higher thresholds than monaural and the consequent belief that inhibition was operating. Following Hirsh's account of the manner of variation of the effect with frequency, Webster (1951) used the critical band concept to show how it could be understood as a differing interaural phase relation in two filter outputs, and Hirsh and Webster (1949) explored the effect of various changes in the waveform of the signal and masker. It was not until eight years later that Jeffress and his coworkers furnished the key to the puzzle in an article that is included here because it is an excellent exposition of the fundamental principles of the masking of tonal signals by noise (Paper 34). These authors pointed out clearly that the idea of interaural inhibition arose because Hirsh's various conditions did not include a truly monaural condition against which to compare binaural performance (see p. 417). As a matter of fact, we now know that the homophasic condition—with no difference in the signal-noise configuration at the two ears (one of Hirsh's binaural conditions)—yields the same detection performance as the monaural condition (Egan, 1965). An important proviso is that the noise employed must be sufficiently above ambient and physiological noise so that it is the controlling masker. We have already noted the effect that a mixture of physiological and ambient noise may have on auditory sensitivity measurement when both ears receive the signal (see Paper 4).

The Jeffress et al. paper does much more than correct the notion about interaural inhibition; it is a complete assessment (as of 1956) of the nature of the masking level difference, that difference in signal-to-noise ratio at which the same signal is just detectable under the monaural (or homophasic) and various binaural conditions. It is also a commendably concise account of its historical antecendents, placing the masking-level-difference concept into the auditory perspective of the time. It is an indispensable background for psychoacousticians.

Not all of the early work was confined to the effect of interaural conditions on the detectability of pure tones in random noise. We know, indeed, a number of useful things about the ways in which binaural detection of a signal in noise depends on the various interaural relations, on the properties of the signal, and on the nature of the interfering noise. With the speech signal in phase at the two ears, Licklider (1948) demonstrated that decreasing the interaural correlation of the masking noise increased intelligibility, a technique later shown by Robinson and Jeffress (1963) to have a systematic effect on tonal signals also. Hirsh (1950) verified that the speech enhancement held for loudspeaker listening when the speech and noise come from different directions. The increase in speech intelligibility also holds for a single-valued delay between ears for speech signals and for delays longer than those normally encountered in sound field listening (Schubert, 1956). McFadden suggested recently (1973) that the latter capability may be developed because such delays occur while listening in reverberant environments. In such settings, of course, comparable delays occur monaurally as well. Is the increase exclusively binaural?

That these effects have their efficacy outside the laboratory in a wide variety of acoustic environments was implied in a brief note by Koenig (1950), who described a simple technique for contrasting monaural and binaural listening. A more complete description by Kock is included here as Paper 35.

These reports offered a convincing demonstration that the perceptual contrast was not limited to threshold-level signals, to tonal signals in random noise, or to conditions in the laboratory. This contrast came to be known as the *cocktail part effect:* a fleeting but comforting assurance that auditory researchers range outside the laboratory in pursuit of knowledge.

On the question of a binaural advantage for complex sounds other than speech, Flanagan and Watson (1966) used periodic pulse trains. They investigated the masking level difference both for polarity reversal at the two ears and as a function of time delay between ears. The effect is maximum for 1.5msec delay and for the 300Hz component of the pulse trains, an interesting corroboration and extension of Hirsh's (1948b) estimate of the maximum effect occuring at 250Hz for pure tones.

Blodgett et al. (1958) showed that the hierarchy of masking level differences established in the Jeffress et al. study (Paper 34) holds for short signals and that all these interaural conditions show approximately the same rate of energy integration for threshold.

One cause for excitement when the simultaneous work by Hirsh and Licklider appeared in 1948 was the hope that under proper circumstances, the masking level difference (MLD) for speech could be put to good practical use. However, whereas MLDs for tones in noise ran as high as 14dB, and as much as 20dB for the highest contrast in Flanagan and Watson's complex signals, attempts to employ the phenomenon for gain in speech intelligibility, both in the laboratory and in hearing-aid use, yielded equivalent gains no more than 3–5dB. To a great degree, that puzzle was solved by Levitt and Rabiner (Paper 36), who measured and compared the binaural advantage for both detection and intelligibility of speech signals.

But the question implied by the Levitt and Rabiner work should be framed more broadly: Is the masking level difference solely a detection phenomenon? Does it give no benefit in the "above-threshold" processing of signals? We do not yet really know the answer. Townsend and Goldstein (1972) compared loudness growth for signals under the two contrasting conditions and found that the initial advantage for the binaurally favorable condition had nearly disappeared by 20dB above the poorer (homophasic) threshold. Cohen (1974) took cognizance of the fact that the auditory system exhibits greater precision as measured by just noticeable differences for intensity, frequency, and interaural time discrimination as signals get further above threshold. She asked whether precision as thus measured improved at the same rate with a given increase above the antiphasic threshold as above the homophasic and found that it did not. Gebhardt et al. (1972) also found that for signals 10dB above their respective thresholds (homophasic and antiphasic), binaural jnd's for frequency were poorer. Goldstein and Stephens (1975) made an attempt to determine how the MLD is related to other auditory measures by testing individuals with partial hearing loss but found no simple relations that would help to clarify the nature of the MLD mechanism. But none of these represents a strong case against the general usefulness of the binaural MLD. We probably have yet to run the appropriate above-threshold experiments.

Between 1956 and 1976 the binaural MLD was a thoroughly searched area. Even with the papers included here, I have furnished only sketchy coverage. Good brief expositions are available by McFadden (1975) and Green (1976). For a complete and sophisticated account, the chapters by Durlach and Colburn (1977) in *Handbook of Perception* are recommended.

Having two matched inputs to a system one wishes to analyze can be a distinct advantage. One useful technique consists of placing the two inputs in competition with each other, presumably to deduce how they behave when working cooperatively. Perhaps the earliest such use for the auditory system was the time/intensity trade attempted by Shaxby and Gage (1932; see Woodworth, 1938, pp. 529-530). They purported to show that a given interaural time disparity could be offset by an opposing intensity disparity. I say "could" because I take the later experiments of Whitworth and Jeffress (1961) to indicate that when the adaptive system discerns that the inputs are no longer complementary, it may no longer behave in its accustomed fashion. On repeated exposure to these interaurally opposed signals, some of their subjects, perceived two separate images—one apparently responsive to the time relation and the other to intensity differences.

But the independent manipulation of two usually cooperative inputs is not to be decried. Dichotic listening can undoubtedly tell us a great deal about truly binaural behavior or even about monaural processing as Gutman, van Bergeijk and David showed in 1960 in their investigation of monaural masking using binaural indexes. Even more applicable is the agreement between Flanagan's results on lateralization of clicks and Nordmark's pitch of separated pulses (see Nordmark, 1963).

During the last decade, this competition method has been used in a much more ambitious undertaking: the attempt to understand the division of labor in the brain hemispheres in processing language or language-like messages. This quickly moves outside the boundary of psychological acoustics, but the same precaution is highly recommended.

I began this prospectus of the important papers in psychological acoustics with an admonition that we must not underestimate the complexity of this intricate, highly adaptive system. It seems fitting that I exit "by the same door wherein I went."

REFERENCES

Békésy, G. V. 1930. Zur theorie des Hörens. Über das richtungshören bei einer zeitdifferenz oder lautstarkenungleichheit der beiderseitigen schallein wirkungen. *Phys. Z.* 31, 824-835; 857-868.

Blodgett, H. C., L. A. Jeffress, and R. W. Taylor. 1958. Relation of masked threshold to signal-duration for various interaural phase-combinations. *Am. J. Psychol.* **71**:283-290.

Boring, E. G. 1942. *Sensation and perception in the history of experimental psychology.* New York: D. Appleton-Century.

Cohen, M. F. 1974. Functional significance of the binaural masking level difference. Ph.D. dissertation, Stanford University.

Durlach, N. I. 1963. Equalization and cancellation theory of binaural masking level differences. *Acoust. Sco. Am. J.* **35**:1206-1218.

Durlach, N. I., and H. S. Colburn. 1977. The binaural system. in *Handbook of perception,* vol. IV ed. E. Carterette and M. Friedman. New York: Academic Press.

Egan, J. P. 1965. Masking-level differences as a function of interaural disparities in intensity of signal and of noise. *Acoust. Soc. Am. J.* **38**:1043-1049.

Flanagan, J. L., and B. J. Watson, 1966. Binaural unmasking of complex signals. *Acoust. Soc. Am. J.* **40**:456-468.

Gebhardt, C. J., D. P. Goldstein, and R. M. Robertson. 1972. Frequency discrimination and the MLD. *Acoust. Soc. Am. J.* **51**:1228-1232.

Goldstein, D. P., and S. D. G. Stephens, 1975. Masking level differences as a measure of auditory processing capability. *Audiology* **14**:354-367.

Green, D. M. 1976. *An introduction to hearing.* New York: Wiley.

Griffin, D. R. 1959. *Echoes of bats and men.* Garden City, New York: Doubleday Anchor.

Guttman, N., W. A. van Bergeijk, and E. E. David, Jr. 1960. Monaural temporal masking investigated by binaural interaction. *Acoust. Soc. Am. J.* **32**:1329-1336.

Hirsh, I. J. 1948a. Binaural summation—A century of investigation. *Psychol. Bull.* **45**:193-206.

Hirsh, I. J. 1948b. The influence of interaural phase on interaural summation and inhibition. *Acoust. Soc. Am. J.* **20**:536-544.

Hirsh, I. J. 1950. The relation between localization and intelligibility. *Acoust. Soc. Am. J.* **22**:196-200.

Hirsh, I. J., and Webster, F. A. 1949. Some determinants of interaural phase effects. *Acoust. Soc. Am. J.* **21**:496-501.

Kay, L., and M. A. Do, 1977. An artifically generated multiple object auditory space for use where vision is imparied. *Acustica* **36**:1-8.

Klemm, O. 1920. Über de einflüss des binauralen zeitunterschiedes auf die localisation. *Arch. gesamte psychol.* **40**:117-146.

Koenig, W. 1950. Subjective effects in binaural hearing. *Acoust. Soc. Am. J.* **22**: 61-62.

Licklider, J. C. R. 1948. The influence of interaural phase relations upon the masking of speech by white noise. *Acoust. Soc. Am. J.* **20**:150-159.

Langmuir, I., V. J. Schaefer, C. F. Ferguson, and E. F. Hennelly, 1944. A study of binaural perception of the direction of a sound source. *OSRD Rep. 4079,* PB 31014, U.S. Dept. of Commerce

McFadden, D. 1973. Precedence effects and auditory cells with long characteristic delays. *Acoust. Soc. Am. J.* **54**:528-530.

McFadden, D. 1975. Masking and the binaural system. In *Human communication and its disorders,* ed. E. Eagles, pp. 137-146. New York: Raven Press.

Nordmark, J. O. 1963. Some analogies between pitch and laterilization phenomena. *Acoust. Soc. Am. J.* **35**:1544-1547.

Nordmark, J. O. 1976. Binaural time discrimination. *Acoust. Soc. Am. J.* **60**:870-880.

Rayleigh, Lord. 1907. On our perception of sound direction. *Phil. Mag.* **13,** 6th ser.:214-232.

Robinson, D. E., and L. A. Jeffress. 1963. Effect of varying the interaural noise correlation on the detectability of tonal signals. *Acoust. Soc. Am. J.* **35**:1947-1952.

Schubert, E. D. 1956. Some preliminary experiments on binaural time delay and intelligibility. *Acoust. Soc. Am. J.* **28**:895-901.

Shaxby, J. H., and F. H. Gage, 1932. Studies in the localization of sound. *Med. Res. Council Spec. Rep. No. 166,* 32p.

Stewart, G. W. 1920. The function of intensity and phase in the binaural localization of pure tones. *Phil. Mag.* **15,** ser. 2:425-445.

Supa, M., M. Cotzin, and K. M. Dallenbach. 1944. Facial vision: The perception of obstacles by the blind. *Am. J. Psychol.* **57**:133-183.

Townsend, T. H., and D. P. Goldstein, 1972. *Suprathreshold binaural unmasking. Acoust. Soc. Am. J.* **51**:621-624.

Wallach, H. 1940. The role of head movements and vestibular and visual cues in sound localization. *J. Exp. Psychol.* **27**:339-368.

Webster, F. A. 1951. The influence of interaural phase on masked thresholds: I. The role of interaural time deviation. *Acoust. Soc. Am. J.* **23**:452-461.

Whitworth, R. H., and L. A. Jeffress, 1961. Time versus intensity in the localization of tones. *Acoust. Soc. Am. J.* **33**:925-929.

Woodworth, R. S. 1938. *Experimental psychology*. New York: Holt.

32

Reprinted from *Am. J. Psychol.* **48**:297-306 (1936)

THE LOCALIZATION OF ACTUAL SOURCES OF SOUND

By S. S. STEVENS and E. B. NEWMAN, Harvard University

Quantitative information relative to the ability of an *O* to localize actual sources of sound in free space is prerequisite to the formulation of an adequate theory of localization. The acquisition of such information depends upon the possibility of generating pure tones for a wide range of frequencies and of presenting them to an *O* in such a way that no reflected waves reach the ears. The present study attempts to satisfy these two conditions.

ANTECEDENTS

The earliest systematic investigations of localization were conducted by what might be called the 'sound-cage school.' Their results were limited by the fact that, owing to the absence of electrical generating apparatus, they were forced for the most part to use clicks and noises as stimuli. Another limiting factor was their custom of experimenting in closed rooms whose walls were not sound-absorbent. In spite of these drawbacks, certain facts were established.[1] *Os* are able (1) to locate noises better than tones and (2) to distinguish right from left. However, they tend (3) to confuse the location of sounds lying in the median plane and (4) to locate sounds at the sides with the least accuracy. The greater inaccuracy of localization at the sides is exactly what one would expect on the basis of recent measurements[2] of the variation of the difference in loudness at the two ears of a speech-source rotated in a horizontal plane around the head. Throughout an angle of about 70° on either side the difference in loudness at the two ears remains virtually constant. In the face of this constancy it is obvious that within the 70°-angle there could be no intensive cues for exact localization. An area of inexact localization at the sides is also indicated as the effect of the difference of phase at the two ears,[3] when the stimulus is a tone of low frequency.

From the sound-cage attention turned to the matter of the presentation of sounds which differ at the two ears in respect of intensity, phase, time of arrival, or a combination of these factors. In this way there arose the 'dichotic school,' whose problem it was to determine the relative merits of the intensity-theory, the phase-theory, and the time-theory.[4] Each of the differential factors—intensity, phase and time—influences localization, each has been nominated by one or more experimenters as the most

* Accepted for publication October 1, 1934.

[1] A. H. Pierce, *Studies in Auditory and Visual Space Perception,* 1901, 52.

[2] J. C. Steinberg and W. B. Snow, Physical factors in auditory perspective, *Bell System Tech. J.,* 13, 1934, 247-260.

[3] G. W. Stewart, Phase relations in the acoustic shadows of rigid sphere, *Phys. Rev.,* 4, 1914, 252-258; R. V. L. Hartley, Function of phase difference in binaural localization of pure tones, *ibid.,* 13, 1919, 373-385.

[4] O. C. Trimble, The theory of sound localization: A restatement, *Psychol. Rev.,* 35, 1928, 515-523.

important factor in localization, and each has also been reduced in theory to one of the others. The facts established by this school are (1) that localization is towards the side of greatest intensity, (2) that in the case of low tones lateral localization can be got by advancing the phase at one ear, and (3) that localization is towards the side of the sound which leads in time. Presumably phase-difference is but a special case of time-difference[5] so that in reality there are just two factors available as cues

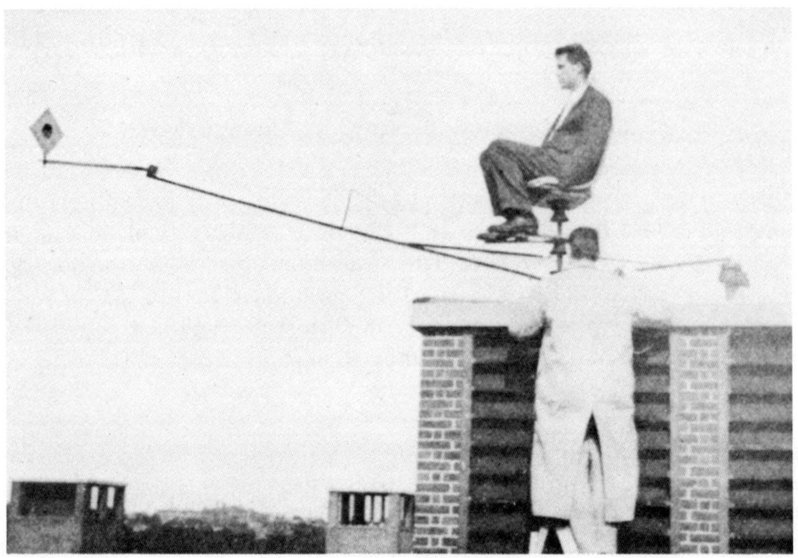

FIG. 1. THE EXPERIMENTAL SET-UP
Note the absence of vertical reflecting surfaces at the level of the observer.

for the localization of pure tones. A final answer as to the rôle of these two factors could not be given, however, since it has not been known to what extent actual sounds can be localized.

A novel attack on the problem of localization, only recently initiated, is the investigation of auditory perspective: the stereophonic effect of multiple sources of sound.[6] Sounds picked up in one room by three microphones spaced several feet apart and broadcast through three correspondingly placed loud speakers in another room can be localized with considerable accuracy. The localization is what would be expected on the basis of the intensitive difference at the ears of the *O* as calculated

---

[5] E. M. von Hornbostel and M. Wertheimer, Über die Wahrnehmung der Schallrichtung, *Sitzber. d. preuss. Akad. d. Wissensch.*, 1920, 388-396; E. G. Boring, Auditory theory with special reference to intensity, volume, and localization, this JOURNAL, 37, 1926, 157-188.

[6] H. Fletcher et al., Auditory perspective: A symposium, *Bell System Tech. J.*, 13, 1934, 239-310. The essential facts of perspective with two-channel transmission were demonstrated in the Harvard Psychological Laboratory in 1929; cf. unpublished affidavit by M. Upton and W. D. Turner.

from measurements[7] of the effect of the sound-shadow cast by the head. Up to the present time, however, such studies have dealt only with complex sounds.

Apparatus

The present experiments were conducted entirely in the open air (Fig. 1). In order to avoid possible reflecting surfaces a tall swivel chair was erected on top of a ventilator which rises 9 ft. above the roof of the new Biological Laboratories at Harvard University. *O* was thus placed in a position where there were no vertical reflecting surfaces on any side of him, and the nearest horizontal surface on the side toward the source of the sound was approximately 12 ft. below him. At the present time this procedure appears to be the only practicable means of avoiding errors due to the reflection of sound.

The source of the sound was mounted on the end of a 12-ft. arm attached to the pedestal of the chair. When properly counterbalanced, it could be moved noiselessly in a complete circle in a horizontal plane on the level of *O*'s ears.

For the larger portion of the experiments a small 4-in. magnetic speaker, mounted in a 12-in. baffle, served to generate the tones. Only in the case of the lowest frequency (60 cycles) was it necessary to use a large Western Electric type-560 cone speaker in order to obtain sufficient power. This speaker was mounted on the same arm at a distance at 6 ft. from *O*.

A beat-frequency oscillator, which could be adjusted to the desired frequency, supplied ample power to the loud speaker. The voltage was adjusted by means of a 7000-ohm potentiometer, while a further shunting resistance was used to turn the tone on and off without producing clicks. The elimination of clicks in the loud speaker is, indeed, an important consideration. The tones were made reasonably pure by the use of suitable filters: tones of 2200 cycles and above passed through a high-pass section with a cut-off frequency of 2500 cycles; tones 3000 cycles and below passed through suitable low-pass sections which reduced the partials other than the fundamental by at least 30 db. The 60-cycle voltage was obtained directly from the lighting circuit. Two check experiments with unfiltered power at frequencies of 400 and 1000 cycles showed that slightly more accurate localizations could be expected with these less pure tones.

Comparative results for two noises were obtained by the use of a click and a hiss. The click was produced by applying 45 volts from a battery to the loud speaker for a brief instant. It was heard by *O* as a single sharp click which possessed the high frequency characteristic of the speaker. The hiss was produced by blowing air through a small brass tube, the end of which had been cut and pinched. The brass tube was attached to the end of the swinging arm and was blown through a long rubber tube by *E*. The sound produced contained a perceptible high-pitched whistle with a frequency of about 7000 cycles. The remaining energy was probably distributed over a wide band of frequencies.

The sensation level of the tones used in this experiment was determined approximately by comparison of the voltages used with threshold voltages determined under comparable conditions in a soundproof and sound-deadened room. Comparison of the sensation levels thus determined with standard audibility curves shows that tones of the middle range from 400 to 4000 cycles had a loudness level of 50 to 60 db. Tones

[7] L. J. Sivian and S. D. White, Minimal audible sound fields, *J. Acous. Soc. Amer.*, 4, 1933, 288-321.

in the extreme ranges, although they were of moderately high intensity, reached a loudness level of about 30 db.

The apparent intensity of the tones was reduced in the experimental situation by the presence of a constant background of sound consisting of distant traffic noises. The level of this noise was determined by a comparison of the thresholds obtained in the soundproof room with those obtained on the roof. The masking effect is measured by the rise in threshold for the various tones. The average rise in threshold for five frequencies between 400 and 7000 cycles, the region in which the effect was greatest, was 28.0 db.

Procedure

In the present experiment each of the two authors acted alternately as *O* and *E*. The tones were presented at certain definite positions in the horizontal plane of the *O*'s head. The *O*'s task was to name the position of the source of sound in this plane. We found in some preliminary experiments conducted in the spring of 1933 that reversals of right and left practically never occurred. Therefore, in the main series of observations which were made during the summer of 1934, the sounds were presented at 13 different positions on the right side of the *O*. These positions were spaced 15° apart from 0° directly in front to 180° directly behind. Ten observations were made at each position by each *O*.

The *O* tried, of course, to distinguish sounds in front from sounds behind, but his success, as will be shown later, depended upon what sound was being used. Since front-back reversals were frequent, we decided that the fairest measure of localizability could be obtained only if such reversals were not counted as errors. Therefore, the size of the error in the localization of a given sound was obtained by taking the difference between the reported position and either the actual position or the corresponding position in the other quadrant, depending upon which was the smaller. Thus, when the source was at 0° the localization was considered correct if it were either 0° or 180°; if the source was at 30°, both 30° and 150° were considered correct responses. This procedure is equivalent to the assumption that dichotic differences of phase or intensity provide a basis for lateral localization alone.

Localization As a Function of Frequency

The average of the errors made by both *O*s at each of the frequencies used is shown in Fig. 2. The errors, computed by the method described above, are relatively constant at low frequencies, but become larger as the frequency approaches 3000 cycles. This change accords with the general findings of the 'dichotic school.' However, above 4000 cycles localization improves again and is fully as accurate at 10,000 as at 1000 cycles. This result, as far as we know, has not been anticipated by previous experimenters. In fact, it has been suggested[8] on several occasions that high tones can not be localized at all—for no better reason, it would seem, than that no one had really tried to localize high tones.

The explanation of the shape of the curve in Fig. 2 must concern us.

[8] H. M. Halverson, The upper limit of auditory localization, this JOURNAL, 38, 1927, 97-106, esp. p. 97.

The inexact localization of tones between 2000 and 4000 cycles is precisely what we should expect from a consideration of the effects of the two localizing factors, difference in phase and in intensity. Owing to the size and shape of the head, there are certain theoretical limits to the possible effectiveness of each of these factors. The limits are shown graphically in Fig. 3. It is well established that differential phase is most effective in determining the localization of low tones, and that above about 600 cycles its effectiveness decreases with increasing frequency. In Fig. 3 are shown the results (dotted line) obtained by Halverson[9] for the maximal lateral shift in localization obtainable with 180° phase-difference as a function of frequency and also the results to be expected theoretically. The theoretical curve (solid line) is a first approximation and was obtained by considering the difference in the distance a sound-wave would have to travel to reach the two ears. If the radius of the head is taken as 8.75 cm. the difference in distance is given by

$$d = 8.75 (\sin\Theta + \Theta).$$

Since our method of treating front-back reversals reduces the problem to a consideration of the phase-effect within a single quadrant, we should not expect confusions to arise until the frequency is so high that two or more positions within a quadrant would give rise to the same phase-difference at the ears of the *O*. The frequency at which this first occurs is that whose wave-length is equal to the maximum value of d, or 1520 cycles.

Fig. 3 also shows the difference in intensity at the two ears for tones of different frequency originating at the side of the *O* (dot-dash line). This curve is due to Steinberg and Snow[10] and shows that the difference at the two ears tends to increase with frequency, as one would expect in view of the sharper sound-shadows obtained with high frequencies.

It is obvious from Fig. 3 that at low frequencies the phase-effect is ample to account for localization, and that at high frequencies the intensity-effect is sufficiently marked to afford good cues. Furthermore, in the region of 3000 cycles neither phase nor intensity is available as a differential cue. Hence the sharp maximum in the curve in Fig. 2 at about this frequency. In general, then, we can conclude that at low frequencies the localization of pure tones is made on the basis of phase-differences, at high frequencies it is made on the basis of intensitive differences, and that in a region near 3000 cycles localization is poor, because of the absence of both types of differences.

Additional reason for believing that differences in intensity alone are

---

[9] Halverson, *loc. cit.*

[10] Steinberg and Snow, *loc. cit.*

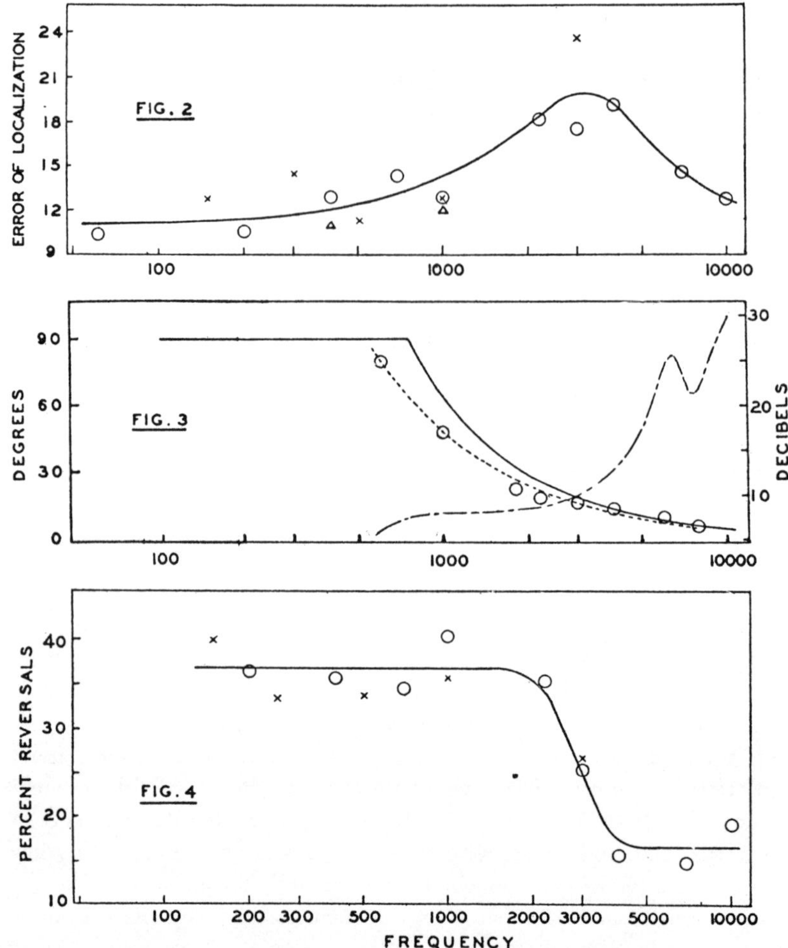

FIG. 2. DEPENDENCE OF LOCALIZATION ON FREQUENCY

The ordinate represents the average of the errors in degrees made by both *O*s. The crosses are for the shorter series of judgments made in 1933. The circles represent the results obtained in 1934. The triangles represent the results obtained with unfiltered tones. Note the critical region at about 3000 cycles.

FIG. 3. ABSENCE OF PHASE-EFFECT AT HIGH FREQUENCIES AND OF INTENSITY-EFFECT AT LOW FREQUENCIES

The solid curve represents theoretically the maximum angle by which a tone can be displaced by 180° change in phase. The circles on the dotted curve are the observed maxima of displacement (Halverson). The dot-dash curve represents the observed difference in intensity at the two ears of tones originating at the side of the observer (Sivian and White).

FIG. 4. PERCENTAGE REVERSALS OF THE FRONT-BACK QUADRANTS

The crosses are for the data obtained in 1933, the circles for 1934. The critical region is at about 3000 cycles; cf. Fig. 2.

operative at high frequencies is afforded by the fact that at about 2800 cycles the action currents in the auditory nerve cease to be synchronized with the stimulus.[11] This fact suggests that although below 2800 cycles phase-differences might well be effective since they could be transmitted as such to the brain, whereas above 2800 cycles any discrimination in terms of the phase-effect should be impossible. On the other hand, Halverson's results show at this frequency no sharp break which could be associated with a breakdown of synchronization. However, Halverson reports that marked changes of intensity occurred as the phase of the high-frequency tones was altered. It may be that his results were due to changes in intensity rather than phase.

Localization as a Function of Position

Since the work of Bloch[12] in 1893, it has been generally recognized without serious contradiction, that the localization of sounds in the horizontal plane is most accurate in the region directly in front or behind the *O*.

The average results for the fourteen main series of our experiment are shown in the following table.

Position in degrees from median plane	0°	15°	30°	45°	60°	75°	90°
Average error in degrees	4.6°	13.0°	15.6°	16.3°	16.2°	15.6°	16.0°

The values for 60° and 75° are weighted means. The weights were assigned in proportion as the errors due to reversals exceeded those expected on the basis of a normal distribution of errors. In order to determine these values the mean average deviation of the distribution was used: it is 15.8°. Using this value the number of reversals to be expected when the stimulus was at a given position could be determined from a table of the probability integral. The 'weighted mean' is thus a mean which includes those errors of localization in the other quadrant which would be expected as errors and which considers the remaining errors in the other quadrant as true reversals.

The results for individual frequencies show considerable variability because of the limited number of cases involved in each average. With the exception, however, of the three critical frequencies, 2200, 3000, and 4000 cycles, they are in substantial agreement with the table presented above.

---

[11] H. Davis, A. Forbes and A. J. Derbyshire, The recovery period of the auditory nerve and its significance for the theory of hearing, *Science*, 78, 1933, 552.

[12] E. Bloch, Das binaurale Hören, *Zsch. f. Augenheilkunde*, 24, 1893, 25-86.

Since localization at low frequencies is based on the phase-effect, we should expect the errors of localization to be inversely proportional to the rate of change of phase-difference as a function of azimuth, or equal to $k/(\cos\Theta + 1)$. The errors made by *N* at low frequencies agree fairly well with this expectation, but those made by *S* are too large at the 15° and 30° positions. We have reason to suspect a systematic error at these positions.

In general, the shape of the function relating errors and position is what might be expected upon theoretical grounds.[13] The fact that the function is essentially the same at the very high frequencies, however, requires explanation. The greater effectiveness of differential intensity near the median plane is not, as early investigators supposed, an example of Weber's Law. On the contrary, the effect can be predicted from the way in which the relative intensity at the two ears depends upon the azimuth of the sound. Both the theoretical values of Hartley and Fry[14] and the experimental determinations of thresholds by Sivian and White[15] indicate that a relatively large displacement of the source is necessary at the side of the *O* to produce a given change of intensity. It is to be expected, therefore, that localization would be best near the median plane and poorest at the extreme lateral positions.

Somewhat more striking in our experiments was the ability of the *O* to distinguish between front and back. The relative frequency of reversals has been taken as a measure of front-back discrimination. In Fig. 4 are presented the average results of both *O*s plotted against frequency. The individual curves agreed closely in form with the average curve. One function (for *N*) was displaced upward and slightly to the left of the other (for *S*).

It is apparent at once that the total range of frequencies is divided into two distinct regions separated by a narrow critical range at about 3000 cycles. For tones below 2000 cycles, where localization is based on phase-differences, discrimination between the front and back quadrants is only a little better than chance. Above 4000 cycles the number of reversals is but one-third of those expected by chance. Taken in connection with the other data presented in this paper, these results offer striking confirmation of the double mechanism (differential phase and intensity) involved in normal localization. The ability of the *O* to distinguish front from back in the case of tones of high frequency is very largely a function of the

[13] Stewart and Hartley, *loc. cit.*

[14] R. V. L. Hartley and T. C. Fry, The binaural localization of pure tones, *Phys. Rev.*, 18, 1921, 431-442.

[15] Sivian and White, *loc. cit.*

difference in intensity between sounds in front and behind.

A number of checks were made in order to demonstrate the validity of this hypothesis. A continuous tone of high frequency, when swung about the *O* decreased very markedly in loudness from front to back. A number of tests were made in which intensity was varied from trial to trial in chance order; and the percentage of reversals, for six series at 3000 to 7000 cycles, was found to increase from 18.6% with the usual procedure to 47% with this test procedure. It appears that the *O* had formed a subjective standard of intensity in the main series after a very few trials. After this the tones in back "seemed weak" while those in front were loud and close. Sound-shadows from the pinna are probably sufficient to account for this effect.

Localization as a Function of Complexity

The experimental series in which the click and the hiss were used confirm the fact that complex sounds are more easily localized than pure tones. The localization of the hiss in particular was very definite, almost as definite as though one were looking at the source! The average of the errors of localization was only 8.0° for the click and 5.6° for the hiss. Thus it may be remarked that the fact that the click was much better localized than any of the pure tones shows the importance of eliminating all of the clicks and extraneous noises which are present if the onset of a pure tone is too abrupt. In the case of the hiss neither *O* was aware of any intensitive or qualitative difference at the different positions during the test series; but careful observation afterwards revealed noticeable differences of both kinds. When in front the hiss was more *shh* and less *sss* and was louder than when behind. The qualitative differences were due, of course, to the differential effect of the shadow of the head upon the frequencies composing the hiss.

In view of findings of the present experiment relative to the ease with which high tones can be localized, it is not surprising that noises with high-frequency components are very easily localized. Noises in general have both high and low frequencies present. The low frequencies provide sufficient phase-differences and the high frequencies sufficient intensitive differences for localization. The two types of cue render each other mutual support, and the result is an accuracy of localization greater than that obtainable with pure tones.

Conclusions

(1) The ability to localize tones varies markedly with frequency. It is approximately constant below 1000 cycles, drops rapidly to a minimum

between 2000 and 4000 cycles, and rises again to its former level at higher frequencies. See Fig. 2.

(2) The error of localization is smallest for tones located near the median plane and increases as the tone is moved toward the side of the *O*. The relation between the azimuth of the tone and the error of localization is approximately the same for both high and low frequencies.

(3) The confusion of positions lying in the quadrant in front of the *O* with those in the quadrant behind him is very frequent. Below 3000 cycles the frequency of such reversals was about that which should be given by chance. Above 3000 cycles it was only about one third of the chance value.

(4) Noises (a click and a hiss) were localized more readily than any of the tones. Differences of quality and intensity were discernible between different positions of the noises.

(5) All of the above facts are consistent with the hypothesis that the localization of low tones is made on the basis of phase-differences at the two ears, and that the localization of high tones is made on the basis of intensitive differences. There is a band of intermediate frequencies near 3000 cycles in which neither phase nor intensity is very effective and in which localization is poorest.

33

Reprinted from pages 315-316 and 324-336 of *Am. J. Psychol.*
62:315-336 (1949)

THE PRECEDENCE EFFECT IN SOUND LOCALIZATION

By HANS WALLACH, Swarthmore College, EDWIN B. NEWMAN and MARK R. ROSENZWEIG, Harvard University

To anyone who is familiar with our modern knowledge of room acoustics, one of the most puzzling questions must be how it is that sounds can be localized at all in a reverberant room, let alone heard in the rather precise positions that are often reported. Most psychologists know, for instance, that fairly good results were obtained with the 'sound cage,' a cumbersome instrument that stood in the corner of every well-equipped laboratory forty years ago. With the sound cage many of the basic factors in localization were demonstrated, even though the experiments were repeatedly performed in highly reverberant rooms in which every sound must have been reflected over a hundred times before it could no longer be heard. Each of these hundred reflections should have given rise to a different and confusing set of cues, and the experiment would seem to be doomed to failure. Such experiments were not failures, and everyday observation told their authors, as it tells us today, that localization within a reverberant room is both common and useful. The problem of how this is possible remains, however, unsolved.

There is actually a second problem that the existence of reverberation raises, a problem that is so closely related to the first one that it must be mentioned here. This problem is to explain why, in a reverberant room, we hear only a single sound and not the long sequence of separate, successive sounds that would be suggested by physical considerations. The fact is that the repetition of essentially the same stimulus in quick sequence leads to a single auditory experience that is qualitatively not very different from the experience resulting from a single stimulus alone. This fact underlies the work we wish to report, but it is not separately considered here. Our

---

* Accepted for publication March 30, 1949. The Harvard part of this research was carried out under Contract N5ori-76 between the Psycho-Acoustic Laboratory, Harvard University, and the Office of Naval Research, U. S. Navy (Project NR147-201, Report PNR-69). Reproduction for any purpose by the U. S. Government is permitted.

observations suggest certain limitations of the range of such fusion but they are too incomplete to describe it adequately.

The present paper is a combined report of several experiments that bear on the selective mechanism underlying the localization of sounds in reverberant surroundings. Actually three steps in this study have been brought together here for the reader's benefit. The first experiments, which were done by one of us (*HW*) some years ago, used actual sources of sound and an *S* located in a well-treated but not perfectly deadened room. Based on these studies, a second one of us (*EBN*) projected an analytic study that used clicks of short duration generated by an electronic timer and delivered separately to the two ears by earphones. The actual experimental work was carried out by the third author (*MRR*) who has since carried certain aspects of this problem well beyond the limits of this report.

[*Editor's Note:* Material has been omitted at this point.]

III. Analytical Study of the Precedence Effect

In the preceding sections of this paper we have been able to show two separate instances in which the precedence effect plays an important part in the localization of sounds in free space. It seemed rather desirable to establish some of the contributing factors under circumstances that would permit their separate control. We set out, therefore, to synthesize an apparent localization of a click, making use of a sequence of stimuli corresponding roughly to the series shown in Fig. 3 A.

It will be useful to point out the main points of difference between this experiment and those reported in Section I. They are as follows.

(1) The present series delivered clicks to *S* through earphones. By careful matching of the phones and other controls, we achieved better control of the intensity of the sound than was possible in the open field.

(2) The fusion of the successive clicks or transients is almost certainly influenced by the kind of 'filling' that exists in the interval between the first and last click. This 'filling' cannot be controlled in the experiments in reverberant rooms. It is totally eliminated in the synthetic experiment. The two experiments offer extremes, then, in the control of this factor.

(3) As is well known, the synthetic procedure does not produce tangible, 'out-there' localization of sounds. The present experiment is not an exception. The ex-

periments in Section I have all the good and bad features that produce these distant localizations: head movements are permitted, the sight of the loudspeakers suggests an external source of the sound, and there are doubtless subtle intensive and qualitative cues to the distance. The earphones exclude such secondary cues and suggest localization near the head. The result is a certain difficulty in comparing the quantitative data of the two experiments.

(4) The synthetic experiment furnishes more complete numerical data. It gives answers to some questions that the other experiments leave open, such as what effect if any the second suggested localization has on the complex experience. Is the

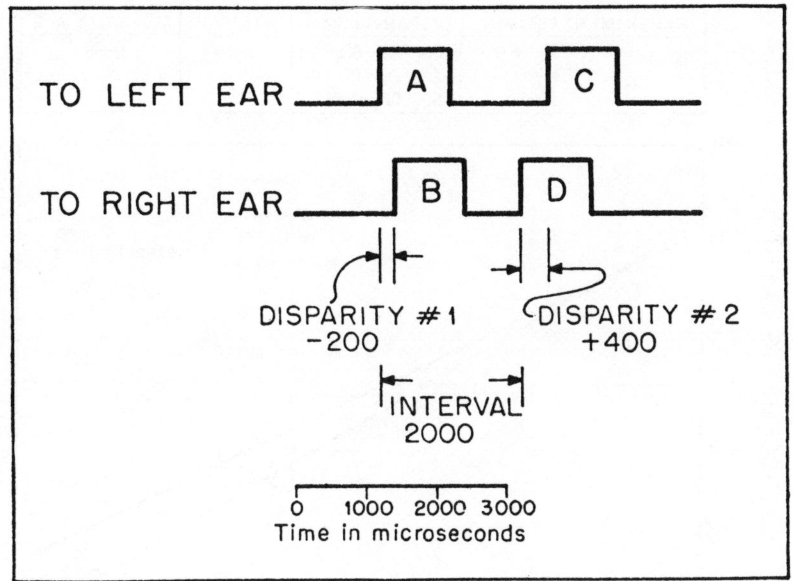

Fig. 5. Voltages Delivered to the Right and Left Earphones
Diagram shows the four separate clicks and the three time-intervals (Disparity #1, Interval, and Disparity #2) which could be manipulated by *E*.

precedence effect an all-or-none affair, or is there some degree of interaction?

Apparatus and procedure. The technical details of this series of experiments may be described quite simply. A pulse generator, built by Mr. Paul Dippolito, delivered brief electrical pulses separately to each of two earphones. All of the pulses were of the same length, 1.0 m.sec., and they produced substantial clicks in the carefully matched pairs of moving-coil earphones (Permoflux PDR-10's) worn by *S*. The actual acoustical output delivered to the ear was checked by mounting each of the phones on an acoustic coupler and by then examining the click with a condenser microphone and oscilloscope. The result looked as much like a square wave as we could hope.

At each trial, the generator delivered four pulses, two to each of the earphones. *E* controlled the timing of the four pulses through electronic 'flip-flop' circuits. The four pulses were arranged in two pairs, as Fig. 5 shows. Each pair (A-B and C-D) consisted of a single pulse to each ear, and a pair represented a click from some direction out in space. The first pair (A-B) was thus the counterpart of the initial sound in Wallach's experiment, and the second pair (C-D) represented the later sound or some reverberation in the room.

The *S*s were so seated in the experimental room that they could not see each other's record. In a preliminary training session given to each *S* individually, pulses were presented with various disparities between the members of the pair A-B so that *S* heard a click having various apparent localizations. Every *S* perceived the clicks

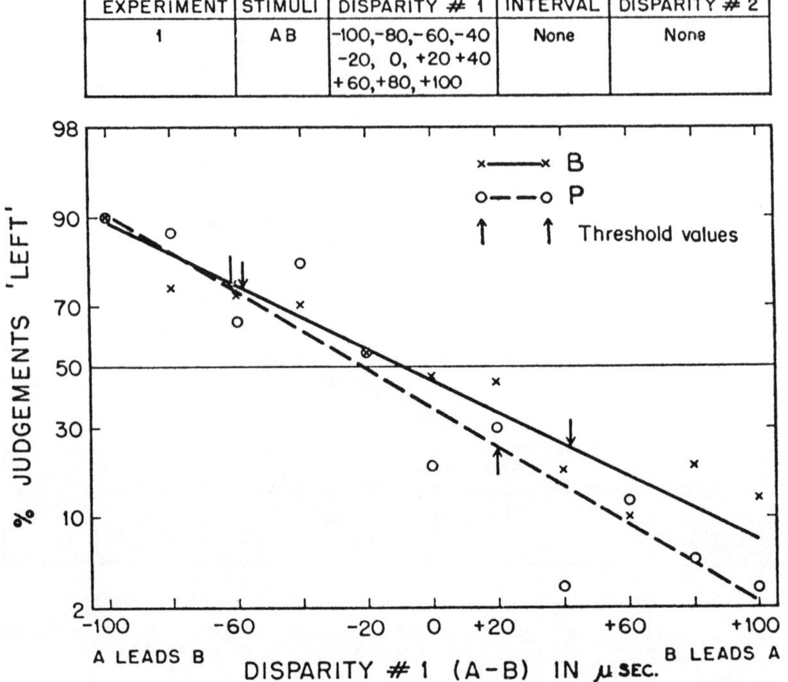

EXPERIMENT	STIMULI	DISPARITY # 1	INTERVAL	DISPARITY # 2
1	AB	-100,-80,-60,-40 -20, 0, +20 +40 +60,+80,+100	None	None

FIG. 6. ABILITY OF *B* AND *P* TO DISTINGUISH 'RIGHT' FROM 'LEFT'
Percentage of reports 'left' when a single pair of clicks was presented with the disparities indicated by values along the abscissa. Every point represents 40 observations.

as being close to his head; locations were reported along an arc from ear to ear. For some the arc crossed the top of the head; for others, it travelled around the back. In reporting, *S* was asked to divide the arc from ear to ear into six sectors, three on either side. Clicks lying between 90° and 60° on the right were recorded as 3 R, from 60° to 30° as 2 R, and from 30° to the center as 1 R. In the same way, they might record 3 L, 2 L, and 1 L. Actually, only Rs and Ls were used in the computations that follow. Successive trials followed each other every 7 sec.

It was desirable that the entire set of four clicks be heard as one sound. To insure this we made a preliminary determination of what interval between successive clicks would make them sound double. Only stimuli A and C in Fig. 5 were used for this purpose and the threshold was determined by the method of limits. In an ascending series it was found that an interval of 6000 μ sec. was required for a clearly 'double' sound; in the descending series an interval of 3000 μ sec. gave a single sound. The intervals used in the remaining experiments were all *below* this lower threshold.

Experiment 1. The first synthetic experiment was done to determine the basic threshold for localization. We measured the least perceptible displacement of the sound image from the center, using only a single pair of

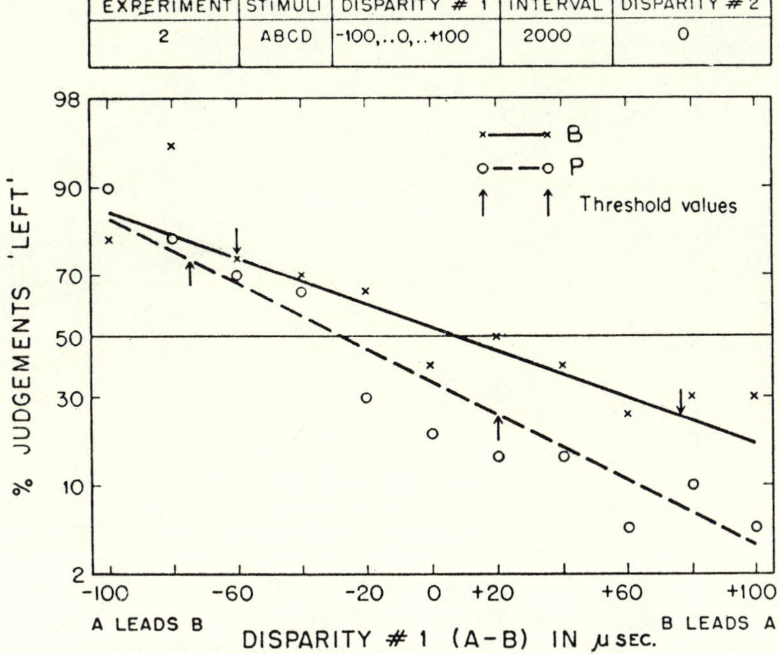

EXPERIMENT	STIMULI	DISPARITY # 1	INTERVAL	DISPARITY # 2
2	ABCD	-100,..0,..+100	2000	0

FIG. 7. LOSS OF PRECISION IN DISTINGUISHING 'RIGHT' FROM 'LEFT' WHEN FIRST PAIR OF DISPARATE CLICKS IS FOLLOWED AFTER 2 M.SEC. BY A SECOND SIMULTANEOUS PAIR

Every point represents 20 observations.

stimuli, A-B. The various intervals used are shown in the table above Fig. 6, and the results for two *Ss*, *B* and *P*, are shown separately in the accompanying graph.

Two points are worthy of note in these results. The first is that both *B* and *P* showed some constant error. They judged a pair of clicks delivered simultaneously to the two ears as right more often than left. In making further comparisons we must keep this constant error in mind. The second point is that the thresholds reported here are relatively low. They are 45 μ sec. for B and 40 μ sec. for *P*. These correspond to a displacement of an actual sound by about 5° from center, roughly one and one-half times the best reported threshold for sounds in open air.

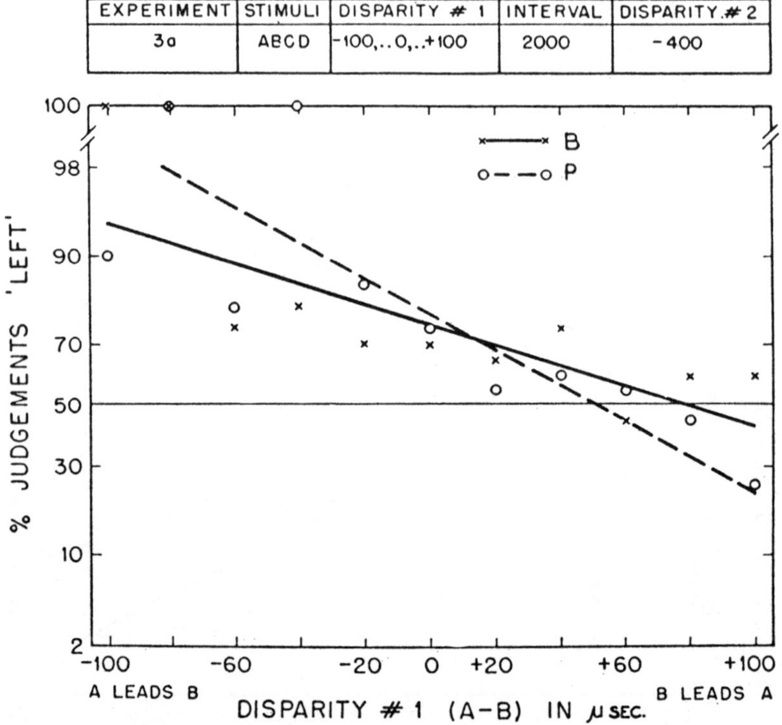

FIG. 8. ADVANCING CLICK TO LEFT EAR BY 400 μ SEC. IN THE SECOND PAIR PRODUCES A SMALL INCREASE IN ALL PERCENTAGES OF REPORTS 'LEFT'
Every point represents 20 observations.

Experiment 2. In the second experiment, we approximated the conditions of the precedence effect. The second pair of clicks, C-D, given with no disparity, suggested a localization in the center. The first pair, A-B, was given with the same range of disparity as those given in Experiment 1. The plan of the experiment and the results are given in Fig. 7.

Comparison of Figs. 6 and 7 makes it evident that the disparity in the first pair alone is sufficient to produce a lateral localization. Measured in terms of the threshold, there is some effect of the second pair; the threshold is larger in this experiment than it was in the previous one. *B* now requires 70 as against 45 μ sec.; and *P* requires 46 in place of 40 μ sec. The existence of the precedence effect seems to be confirmed qualitatively, but from these results we should conclude that the effect is relative and not absolute. The second pair has a small effect since a larger disparity is now required, but

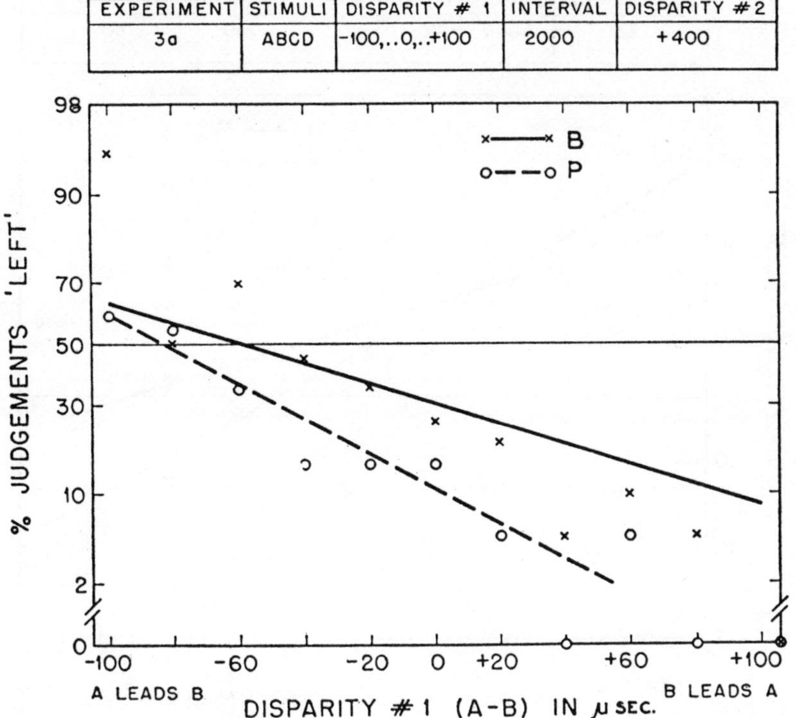

EXPERIMENT	STIMULI	DISPARITY # 1	INTERVAL	DISPARITY #2
3a	ABCD	-100,..0,..+100	2000	+400

Fig. 9. Retarding Click to Left Ear by 400 μ Sec. in the Second Pair Produces a Small Decrease in All Percentages of Reports 'Left'
Every point represents 20 observations.

its effect is less than that of the first pair, depending perhaps on the interval between the first and second pair.

Experiment 3a. Since it appeared that the second pair had some effect on the localization of the fused sound, this series and the next were run to discover more clearly how great was that effect. In this series, for instance, the second pair, C-D, was separated by the relatively large disparity of 400 μ sec. This disparity was presented with C leading in half of the trials and D leading in the remainder, the two arrangements occurring in irregular order. Had the second pair occurred alone, they would have sounded far to the right and to the left. In the whole sequence, ABCD, the two orders of C and D were combined with the 11 disparities of the first pair used in Experiments 1 and 2. The resulting psychometric functions are shown in Figs. 8 and 9 in which judgments of left are plotted against the disparity

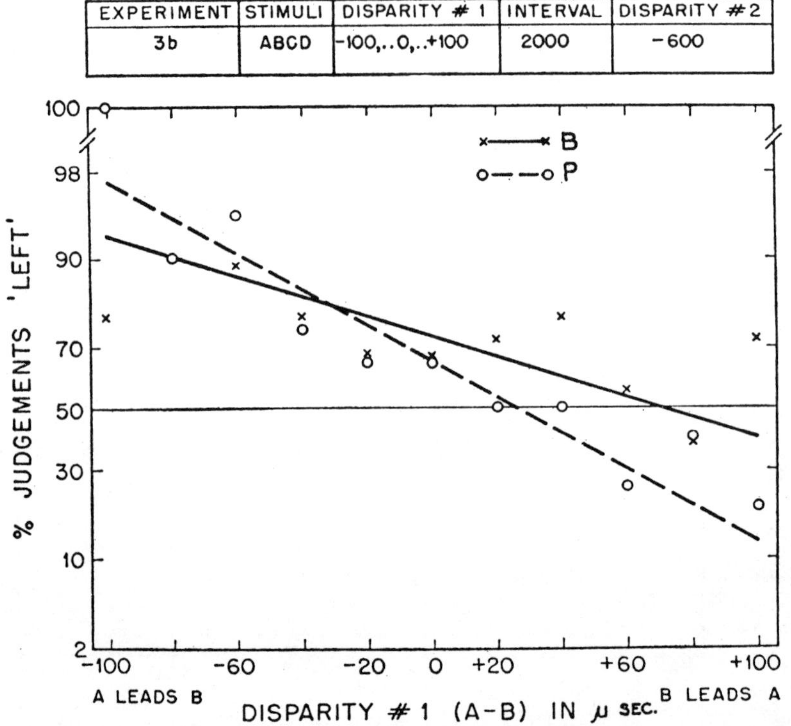

FIG. 10. ADVANCING CLICK TO LEFT EAR BY 600 μ SEC. IN THE SECOND PAIR PRODUCES A SMALLER INCREASE IN PERCENTAGES OF REPORTS 'LEFT' THAN DID 400 μ SEC. (FIG. 8)

Every point represents 20 observations.

of the first pair. The fit of the curve to the individual points is somewhat less good than in the earlier series.[8] The result is quite clear, however. With C in the left ear leading, there are many more judgments 'left'; with D leading, there are more judgments 'right.'

Experiment 3b. This experiment was like Experiment 3a except for the

[8] The actual procedure used was to determine separately for each *S* the average slope in the five series of Experiments 2, 3a and 3b and then, using this slope, to find the mean intercept with the 50% line. Equal weight was given to all points except the 0% and 100% values indicated as lying off the graph.

fact that the disparity between the second pair, C-D, was increased to 600 μ sec. The results are shown in the curves of Figs. 10 and 11. Again the same general conclusion can be drawn: if the second pair favors a localization to the right, the body of judgments is shifted this way, and conversely,

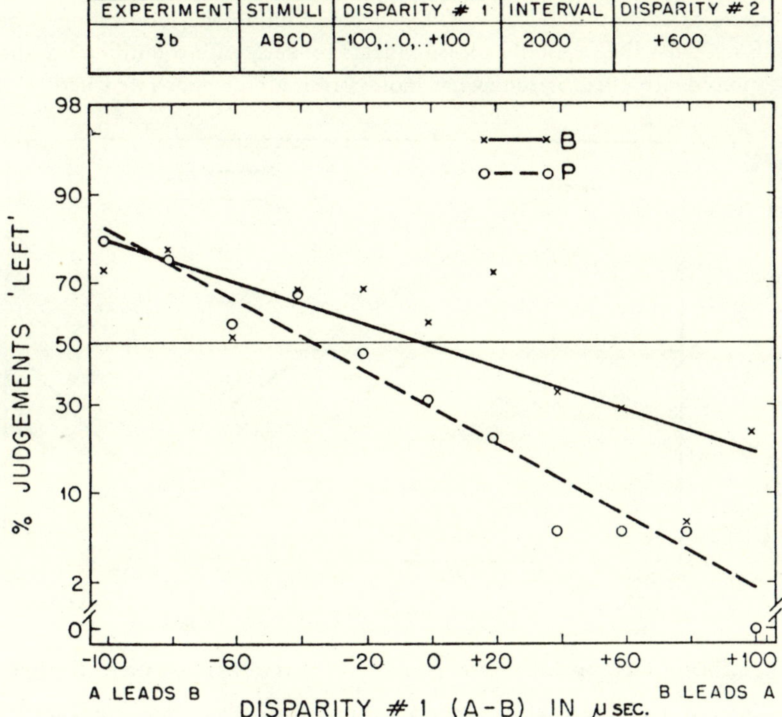

EXPERIMENT	STIMULI	DISPARITY # 1	INTERVAL	DISPARITY # 2
3b	ABCD	-100,..0,..+100	2000	+600

Fig. 11. Retarding Click to Left Ear by 600 μ Sec. in the Second Pair Produces a Smaller Decrease in Percentages of Reports 'Left' than Did 400 μ Sec. (Fig. 9)

Every point represents 20 observations.

if, by itself, it is heard to the left, the entire sound shifts slightly that way.

It is now possible to make an important comparison. By noting the point where each of these curves passes through the 50% point, we have a measure of the degree of disparity of the first pair that just offsets the disparity of the second pair. Obviously the two disparities will be in the opposite direction, that is to say, we shall note how much the right ear must lead in the first pair just to compensate for a lead of the left ear in the second pair. This gives us some estimate of the relative effectiveness of the two pairs in determining the localization of the total sound.

The results of this comparison are plotted in Fig. 12. The two center points have been taken from Experiment 2. It is quite remarkable how similar the results are for the two *Ss*, *B* and *P*. The slope of the curves through the middle portions shows that the initial pair, A-B, is about 6 times as effective as is the second pair, C-D, in determining the localization. This confirms what the threshold measurements told us, with the difference that the precedence effect is somewhat more strikingly demonstrated here.

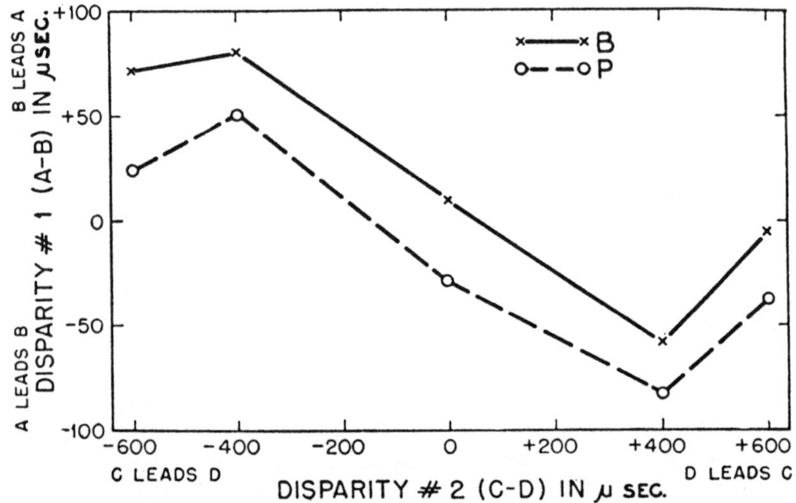

FIG. 12. DISPARITY OF FIRST PAIR (ORDINATE) THAT JUST BALANCES DISPARITY OF SECOND PAIR (ABSCISSA)

Results are plotted separately for *B* and *P*, and represent intercepts with 50% line in Figs. 7-11.

More interesting, and quite unexpected, is the fact that these curves turn over at the ends. Had the comparison of first pair with second pair been made in terms of Experiment 3b, *i.e.*, with a 600-μ. sec. disparity between the second pair, the first pair would have come off far stronger. The ratio of effectiveness of first to second is now of the order of 16 or 20 to 1. The next experiment investigates this curious reversal more fully.

Experiment 4. The previous experiments furnished such striking evidence of a reversal in the effect of disparity in the second pair as the size of the disparity was increased that it seemed wise to test this relation directly. To do this, the first pair was held constant in the center, *i.e.* zero disparity, while the disparity of the second pair was varied from −1000 μ. sec. to +1000 μ. sec. in 200 μ. sec. steps.

The results confirm completely the previous finding. They are shown in Fig. 13. For the smaller values the total sound is displaced to the side of the leading ear but with increasingly large values the effect weakens and, in three of four cases, the total sound returns to the center line. These

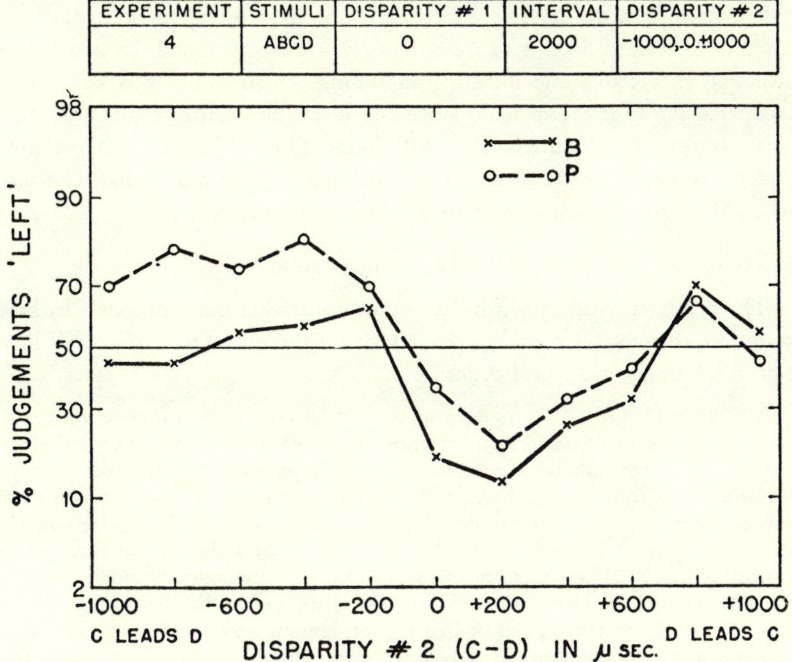

EXPERIMENT	STIMULI	DISPARITY # 1	INTERVAL	DISPARITY # 2
4	ABCD	0	2000	-1000,.0.+1000

FIG. 13. THE EFFECT OF DISPARITY IN THE SECOND PAIR WHEN THE FIRST PAIR IS PRESENTED SIMULTANEOUSLY

Note that increasing disparity gives an increasing percentage of judgments 'left' (or 'right') until maximum is reached, beyond which greater disparity gives decreasing percentage. Every point represents 40 observations.

results are the more striking when note is taken of how large are the time differences used. Were the second pair presented alone, 600 to 1000 μ. sec. would be sufficient to produce localizations completely on one side or the other. Yet *S*, trying to hear the least possible displacement, reports the fused sound in the center line. No such reports ever occur with a single pair of clicks, or when the initial pair has this large disparity.

Experiment 5. A final experiment was run in which the interval between the first and second pair was increased from 2 to 10 m.sec. (2000 to

10,000 μ sec.), sufficient to separate clearly the two sounds. This series was not run until after the other series had been completed because we did not wish *S* to know that there was potentially a 'double' click present. Various temporal disparities were introduced between both the first and second pairs. At first the *S*s complained that they could not follow the instructions to report localization because there were two sounds present and they often had different positions. One *S*, of his own accord, tried to report both localizations, so this instruction was given to both of them. They were able to do this fairly accurately, reporting sounds in two places, although they had some difficulty in telling which sound was heard first. No extensive tests were made since the direction of the results was quite clear. It remains to remark that with these single clicks the interval over which fusion can be obtained is much less than the 35 m.sec. that we found when the sounds were music in a reverberant room.

IV. Related Studies

The precedence effect can be delimited somewhat more precisely by brief reference to two other studies that touch on these findings. We shall mention them in chronological order.

Békésy reported in 1930 a number of observations made when four separate clicks were led to the two ears in arrangements not unlike those of our analytical study.[9] His procedure was usually to produce two clearly separated localizations, as in our Experiment 5, and then to decrease the interval until the two pairs were roughly simultaneous, or the pairs were intermingled so that the order (using the terminology of Fig. 5) was ADCB or BCDA. His principal interest lay in the fact that the pairing AB and CD was often maintained in these intermingled or ambiguous combinations, especially when aided by qualitative differences between clicks AB and CD. These observations point to pairing or grouping as a result of *S*'s 'set,' a factor that goes beyond any we have investigated. Békésy reports, at the same time, the existence of a precedence effect. For instance, under conditions very much like our Experiment 2, he says "das mittlere Bild verhältnismässig spät eintrifft, so dass es von den seitlichen verdeckt wird." Thus he speaks of a suppression or concealment of the sound image which arrives later.[10]

It is possible from Békésy's results to draw a rough line between two alternatives. If the interval between two pairs of stimuli is greater than about 1 m.sec., there is suppression of the second pair. This is our precedence effect. If the interval is shorter than 1 m.sec., there is usually some combination or compromise in the indicated localization. The nature of some of these compromises is explored in Békésy's study.

The existence of the precedence effect and the added fact that it can be overcome

---

[9] G. v. Békésy, Zur Theorie des Hörens, Ueber das Richtungshören bei einer Zeitdifferenz oder Lautstärkenungleichheit der beiderseitigen Schalleinwirkungen, *Physikal. Zsch.*, 31, 1930, 824-35; 857-868.

[10] G. v. Békésy, *op. cit.*, 858-859.

by making the second sound enough more intense than the first sound were both reported by Langmuir and his associates in the course of wartime research on underwater listening equipment.[11] The peculiar feature of this equipment was the use of a compensating circuit by which the delay in transmission from a remote source to one hydrophone could be offset by a complementary delay in the listening equipment.

The precedence effect was demonstrated in a trainer in which two sounds were brought, almost simultaneously, to *S*'s ears. As in Békésy's experiments, these two sounds had different apparent localizations, a difference which it was the task of *E* to minimize. When the same source was used for both sounds, there was a 'first-arrival effect' such that "a necessary condition for sharp binaural shift of the directional sound [was] that it should not arrive at the receivers later than the non-directional sound." In one test, the directional sound was delayed 2.2 m.sec. "Binaural shift of directional sound then became so confused as to be worthless when directional and background sounds were held at equal intensities. . . . To restore perception of binaural shift the delayed . . . sound had to be raised about 15 db. above background . . . a delay in the directional sound as short as 0.6 m.sec. confused the binaural shift detection."

Langmuir and his associates conclude, referring to the first-arrival effect: "This effect, like others discussed in this report, is one closely associated with our instinctive use of the binaural sense. It is illustrated in a simple way by the common experience that in a room or hall where echoes and reverberations are present a listener can pay attention to the voice of the speaker and locate its direction. . . . We have formed the habit of paying attention only to that sound which arrives at our ears first, and to ignore the same sound, though louder, arriving a fraction of a second later" (p. 43). The present writers would certainly agree with these observations but would prefer to depend on something more secure than an educated faculty of attention for an explanation.

SUMMARY

This paper has been concerned with what an *S* hears when two nearly identical sounds reach his ears from different directions and one follows the other after a slight delay. Our conclusions can be stated in terms of two rather general propositions and five corollaries.

(1) Two brief sounds that reach *S*'s ears in close succession will be heard as a single sound if the interval between them is sufficiently short. The fact of fusion is not new, but it has a special interest here because it is a necessary condition of the precedence effect. The interval over which fusion takes place is not the same for all kinds of sounds. The upper limit of the interval was found to be about 5 m.sec. for single clicks and is apparently much longer, perhaps as much as 40 m.sec., for sounds of a complex character.

[11] I. Langmuir, V. J. Schaefer, C. V. Ferguson, and E. F. Hennelly, A study of binaural perception of the direction of a sound source, OSRD Report 4079, June, 1944, PB No. 31014 (available through the Office of Technical Services, U. S. Department of Commerce, Washington 25, D.C.).

(2) If two brief sounds are heard as fused into a single sound, the localization of the total sound is determined largely by the location of the first sound. We have called this a *precedence effect* in sound localization. While it is not indispensable to the theory, the precedence effect can be described most readily if it is assumed that the underlying localization is based on time differences between the two ears.

The following are specifications or limitations of the precedence effect.

(a) The precedence effect can be demonstrated best when the sounds have some discontinuous or transient character. Steady tones or continuous and uniform noises are obviously not suitable because there is no way to define precedence. Clicks, on the other hand, work quite well, and speech or piano music are reasonably satisfactory.

(b) Under proper conditions the second sound can be shown to have a quite small yet demonstrable effect. If the second sound departs more and more from the location of the first sound, it will pull the total sound along with it up to a maximal amount (perhaps 7°) and then it becomes progressively less effective.

(c) If the interval between the arrival of the two sounds is so short that the time cues to the two ears are ambiguous, some average or compromise localization will be heard (Békésy). In other words, the precedence effect describes what takes place between some lower limit, 1 m.sec. or less, and an upper limit, the limit of fusion.

(d) The foregoing description has been of two sounds that are somewhere nearly equal in intensity. If the second sound is made sufficiently intense (more than 15 db. louder than the first sound) it overrides the precedence factor (Langmuir *et al.*). We may suppose that, if the second sound is less intense than the first, the precedence effect will be aided.

(e) It is presumed that the fusion of two sounds and, correspondingly, the precedence effect in localization are favored when the two sounds are qualitatively quite similar. Békésy reports, for instance, that qualitatively *dissimilar* sounds are better able to maintain their separate locations under the ambiguous conditions of nearly simultaneous arrival at the *S*'s ears. In all our experiments we have assumed the converse proposition, that very similar sounds would help to give a single localization.

The existence of the precedence effect helps us to understand our ability to localize sounds under many natural circumstances. In particular, it is of the first importance in explaining our ability to locate sounds in reverberant surroundings. Furthermore, it makes much more intelligible the success of stereophonic sound systems in which sound is picked up and reproduced through two channels, effectively recreating the illusion of sound coming from more than one direction.

34

Reprinted from *Acoust. Soc. Am. J.* **28**:416-426 (1956)

Masking of Tonal Signals*

LLOYD A. JEFFRESS, HUGH C. BLODGETT, THOMAS T. SANDEL,† AND CHARLES L. WOOD, III
Defense Research Laboratory and Department of Psychology, The University of Tesas, Austin, Texas
(Received August 29, 1955)

1. MONAURAL PHENOMENA

THE equivalence of the masked threshold and the difference limen for intensity has been shown by Miller.[1] From his discussion we are led to the conclusion that the simplest example of masking is the masking of a tone by itself—the intensity-difference limen for pure tone. Let us therefore consider this first.

1.1. Difference Limen for Pure Tones

Riesz[2] has presented data on the DL (difference limen) for pure tones. His technique consisted of beating two tones, one of them three cycles per second different from the other (the signal) and adjusting the signal intensity until the beats were just audible. He had previously discovered that a rate of three beats per second is optimal for this purpose. He found that the DL for intensity is a function of both intensity and frequency, and expressed the relation in an equation.

1.2. Masking of One Tone by Another

Many texts in discussing masking present the curve of Wegel and Lane[3] on the masking of one tone by another. The curve is characterized by a rapid rise in masking as the two tones approach each other in frequency, followed by a sharp drop or notch as they approach still closer. This notch is also shown in the curves published by Egan and Hake[4] for tonal maskers. Munson and Gardner[5] show, however, that the notch is an artifact of the method and that if beats between the masker and the signal are avoided the masking curve resembles the response of a narrow filter. Munson and Gardner employed residual masking in their work. The present writers in an unpublished study used a 25-msec signal to avoid beats and obtained a similar curve.

1.3. Masking of a Tone by Noise

Workers at the Bell Telephone Laboratories pioneered in studies of the masking of tones by noise, and developed the concept of critical bands. Fletcher[6] and Fletcher and Munson[7] discuss the concept, and French and Steinberg[8] present curves showing the magnitude of the critical band as a function of frequency, for both monaural and binaural listening. They reported about a 1.5-db advantage for binaural listening. The basic finding which led to the concept was that a long signal is detectible in the presence of noise about 50% of the time, when its energy equals the energy in that part of the noise lying within a certain range of frequency.

More recent studies have refined the concept considerably. Egan and Hake[4] used tones and bands of noise of different widths, and Schafer, Gales, Shewmaker, and Thompson[9] made estimates of the Q of the filter for different frequencies.

1.4. Effect of Signal Duration upon the Masked Threshold

Garner and Miller[10] investigated the effect of signal duration upon the masked threshold for tone. They

* This work was performed under Bureau of Ships Research and Development Contract NObsr-52267.

† Now at Research Laboratory of Electronics, Massachusetts Institute of Technology.

[1] G. A. Miller, J. Acoust. Soc. Am. 19, 609–619 (1947).

[2] R. R. Riesz, Phys. Rev. 31, 867–875 (1928).

[3] R. L. Wegel and C. E. Lane, Phys. Rev. 23, 266–285 (1924).

[4] J. P. Egan and H. W. Hake, J. Acoust. Soc. Am. 22, 622–630 (1950).

[5] W. A. Munson and M. B. Gardner, J. Acoust. Soc. Am. 22, 177–190 (1950).

[6] H. Fletcher, Revs. Modern Phys. 12, 47–65 (1940).

[7] H. Fletcher and W. A. Munson, J. Acoust. Soc. Am. 9, 1–10 (1937).

[8] N. R. French and J. C. Steinberg, J. Acoust. Soc. Am. 19, 90–119 (1947).

[9] Schafer, Gales, Shewmaker, and Thompson, J. Acoust. Soc. Am. 22, 490–496 (1950).

[10] W. R. Garner and G. A. Miller, J. Exptl. Psychol. 37, 293–303 (1947).

found that within wide limits the threshold is determined by the energy in the signal, following the law, $I\cdot t=c$. Gales and Wilcott[11] extended the principle to include signal pulses having a variety of envelope shapes.

2. BINAURAL PHENOMENA

2.1. Binaural *vs* Monaural Critical Bands

As has already been mentioned, French and Steinberg found the critical band for binaural listening to be about 1.5 db narrower than that for monaural listening —a fact that makes their concept of critical bands seem a little fuzzy, but is really only saying that two ears are slightly better than one for simple discriminations. Recent work by Wilcott and Gales[12] suggests that the two values are nearly equal.

2.2. Binaural "Summation" and "Inhibition"

During the war, the Harvard Psycho-acoustic Laboratory conducted many experiments on masking, particularly of speech, and discovered that if either the masking noise or the signal (speech) is reversed in phase at one ear, a substantial improvement in hearing results. This work was first described by Licklider[13] who referred to the case where either the noise or the signal is reversed in its interaural phase as *antiphasic*, and the case where neither is reversed or where both are reversed as *homophasic*. This terminology is convenient and will be employed in the course of the present paper.

Hirsh[14] presented a series of studies in which he employed tonal signals of various frequencies. He found that for a tone of 200 cps or 500 cps reversing phase of either the signal or the noise—the antiphasic condition—produces an improvement (a masking level difference or MLD, in the terminology employed by Hirsh and Webster[15] amounting to 10 or 12 db over the homophasic condition.

Hirsh unfortunately regarded the condition where the signal was presented to one ear and the noise to both as "monaural." This led him to conclude that when the signal was also presented to both ears, and the masked threshold was higher, he was dealing with binaural "inhibition." He therefore found binaural inhibition for the two homophasic conditions and binaural summation for the two antiphasic conditions. Had he seen the relevance of French and Steinberg's binaural critical band widths to his work, he would have realized that his worst conditions, the homophasic, are still slightly better than the truly monaural condition, and that therefore all binaural stimulus conditions produce "summation," that there is no binaural inhibition.

[11] R. S. Gales and R. C. Wilcott, J. Acoust. Soc. Am. 26, 944(A) (1954).
[12] Private communication.
[13] J. C. R. Licklider, J. Acoust. Soc. Am. **20**, 150–159 (1948).
[14] I. J. Hirsh, J. Acoust. Soc. Am. **20**, 536–554 (1948).
[15] I. J. Hirsh and F. A. Webster, J. Acoust. Soc. Am. **21**, 496–501 (1949).

This fact can be illustrated by the following demonstration. We start with both signal and noise presented to one earphone, say, the left, and adjust the level of the signal, which is occurring periodically, until it is a few decibels below threshold and we can no longer hear it. This is the monaural condition. Now as we bring up the noise in the right earphone we find that the signal becomes clearly audible. When the noise levels in the two phones are equal we have Hirsh's "monaural" condition. Now we add the signal gradually to the noise in the right earphone. By the time its level has reached that in the left phone the signal has again become inaudible, and we have the homophasic, binaural condition.

2.3. Hirsh Hierarchy of Masking Level Differences

When we add the truly monaural condition, Hirsh's sequence of MLD's, beginning with zero for the monaural case, is, for most frequencies, as follows: N_m-S_m, $N_\pi-S_\pi$, N_0-S_0, $N_\pi-S_m$, N_0-S_m, $N_\pi-S_0$, N_0-S_π, where the symbols have the following meanings: N_0= noise in phase at the two ears, N_π= noise reversed in phase at one ear relative to the other, N_m= noise presented monaurally, S_0= signal in phase at the two ears, S_π= signal reversed in phase at one ear relative to the other, S_m= signal presented monaurally, to which let us add for completeness and later reference, N_u= noise uncorrelated at the two ears, i.e., two independent noise sources.

2.4. Effects of Other Phase Changes

Hirsh[14] also reported the effects of shifting a 200-cps signal in interaural phase through steps of 30°, and Jeffress, Blodgett, and Deatherage,[16] using a 500-cps signal, shifted both it and the 500-cps component of the noise through all combinations of 36° steps. They also shifted the noise in interaural time by means of a delay mechanism. Both sets of experiments found a rapid drop in masking as the signal and the noise are shifted apart. Jeffress, Blodgett, and Deatherage also found that the greatest MLD's (masking level difference) occur when the difference between the shift for the signal and the shift for the noise is 180°, e.g., if the 500-cps masking component of the noise is shifted 36° to the right, the greatest masking occurs when the signal is also shifted 36° to the right, and the least masking, when the signal is shifted 144° to the left.

2.5. Variation of the MLD's with Frequency

Hirsh's experiments were performed at several frequencies and showed great variation with frequency. He obtained the largest MLD's at 200 cps, with much smaller values at 100 cps and above 1000 cps. Jeffress,

[16] Jeffress, Blodgett, and Deatherage, J. Acoust. Soc. Am. **24**, 523–527 (1952).

Blodgett, and Deatherage,[17] using a 167-cps signal, reversed it and the noise in phase, and also shifted the noise in time through various amounts up to a half-period. They found an MLD of 11 db for the N_0-S_π condition, of 4.4 db for $N_\pi-S_0$, and MLD's associated with interaural time shifts for the noise, ranging from 1 db for 0.3 msec, and 3.6 db for 0.6 msec to about 4.5 db for 3 msec. The curve relating MLD and time shift is essentially flat for delays beyond 0.6 msec.

2.6. Effects of Phase-Reversal with Tonal Masker

Hirsh and Webster reported Licklider as saying that he found little change in the masked threshold using a tonal masker and reversing the phase of either it or the signal tone, and Jeffress, Blodgett, and Deatherage in an unpublished study found the same. Using a 499-cps masker and a 500-cps signal and various phase combinations they found no systematic differences among them, and no differences larger than 2 db.

2.7. Effects of Interaural Correlation

Licklider,[13] using speech as his signal, showed that reducing the interaural correlation for the noise by adding uncorrelated noise at the two ears reduces the advantage of reversing the noise or signal in interaural phase. Jeffress, Blodgett, and Deatherage[18] employing a similar technique with a 500-cps signal found that the advantage of reversing either the noise or tone is gradually reduced as the correlation for the noise is reduced by adding uncorrelated noise at the two ears. They erroneously concluded that using completely uncorrelated noises at the two ears will eliminate the MLD found for correlated noise under the N_0-S_π condition. Work described in a later section shows that for short signals a considerable MLD can be obtained.

2.8. Sensitivity to Interaural Time Difference

Klumpp[19] found that subjects can respond to sudden changes in the interaural time difference for tone signals and noise signals of the order of 10 to 15 μsec, although they can hear no change for tones above about 1500 cps. The greatest sensitivity for tone is in the range near 1000 cps. Jeffress, Blodgett, Deatherage, and Musik,[20] using a delay line to adjust the interaural time for a noise mixed with uncorrelated noise at the two ears, reported standard deviations of the order of 30 to 60 μsec in the settings subjects made while attempting to center the correlated part of the noise.

Wilcott[21] obtained thresholds for interaural movement. He employed a simulated movement produced by changing the interaural time delay for a wide-band noise. The noise was intially presented either with no delay, corresponding to a position in the median plane, or with a 792-μsec delay, corresponding to an extreme, lateral position. He studied the effect of various velocities upon the subjects' thresholds for the detection of the movement. At moderate velocities he obtained thresholds of the order of 50 to 60 μsec for movements from the median position, and of 150 to 160 μsec, for movements from the lateral position.

2.9. Effect of Signal Duration

Jeffress, Blodgett, and Deatherage[16] in their work at 500 cps found a substantially greater MLD for the N_0-S_π condition than Hirsh did. They attributed this to the difference in signal duration, and argued that while a short signal is masked inversely as its energy (duration) for the N_0-S_0 condition, it is not so adversely affected in the N_0-S_π condition. Recent unpublished work by the present writers shows this to be true. For a 500-cps tone the masked threshold for a 500-msec signal is 75 db for N_0-S_0 and 62 db for N_0-S_π, a masking-level difference of 13 db, while for a 25-msec signal the thresholds are 91 db and 75 db—a MLD of 16 db (all levels relative to 0.0002 dynes/cm^2 for a spectrum level for the noise of 58 db).

3. HYPOTHESIS FOR MONAURAL PHENOMENA

All of the monaural phenomena we have discussed can be understood through the use of a simple model—a narrow filter followed by an elementary detector. The detector needs to be sensitive only to changes in over-all level and to have a certain time characteristic. To illustrate this let us assume that we are listening to a "noise" made up of two beating tones. If the beats are very slow, we can hear a change when a very small signal of nearby frequency is suddenly added to the complex. If the beats are faster, five or ten per second, the added signal cannot be distinguished unless it is sufficient to change the level considerably. If the beats are still faster, fast enough to sound smooth, a small signal is again sufficient. The same type of detector behavior is exhibited by a simple voltmeter. If the beats are very slow, the momentary signal is seen as a small, quick deflection of the slowly swinging pointer. If the beats are faster, the pointer oscillates rapidly, and we can no longer distinguish the displacements due to the signal. If the beats are still faster so that the pointer cannot follow them, the pointer will be steady and will again show small deflections when the signal is added. For specialized signals, a more sophisticated detector (the moving-target indicator of radar, for example) can achieve a substantially better signal-to-noise ratio, but apparently the ear is fairly simple.

When we listen to a pure-tone signal in the presence of a wide-band noise, we hear the signal as a tone even near threshold levels. We seem, therefore, to be behav-

[17] Jeffress, Blodgett, and Deatherage, J. Acoust. Soc. Am. 25, 190(A) (1953).

[18] Jeffress, Blodgett, and Deatherage, J. Acoust. Soc. Am. 25, 832(A) (1953).

[19] R. G. Klumpp, J. Acoust. Soc. Am. 25, 823(A) (1953).

[20] Jeffress, Blodgett, Deatherage, and Musick, J. Acoust. Soc. Am. 26, 141(A) (1954).

[21] R. C. Wilcott, J. Exptl. Psychol. 49, 68–72 (1955).

ing as a sophisticated detector, we are picking the tone out of the noise. But if we measure the threshold signal-to-noise ratio and compare it with what we get when we are listening to a tone in a narrow-band noise, we find little or no difference. In the latter case we no longer hear the tone as different in quality from the noise, it merely increases the level. The detector is essentially simple.

For such detectors the performance has been expressed by Lawson and Uhlenbeck[22] roughly in the equation $(\langle S+N\rangle_{Av}-\bar{N})/\sigma_n=k$, where σ_n is the standard deviation of the envelope of the band of noise, and the barred quantities are the average levels of the signal plus noise, and of the noise, and k is a constant equal approximately to unity for simple detectors. To be complete, the equation would need some expression for the time properties of the detector, and for the duration of the signal.

3.1. Predictions from Monaural Hypothesis

3.1(a) DL for Pure Tones

If we attempt to apply the equation of the preceding section to the case where the masker is a pure tone, we find that we are lacking a standard deviation for the masker. The tone has a constant level. If, however, we think of the subject as having a certain amount of "system noise," we can proceed. Such a noise was suggested by the equations of Riesz who included a residual constant which is a function of frequency only, along with his second term which is a function of both frequency and level. Since the only noise present is attributable to the subject, we should find large individual differences in their difference limens for pure tone, and we do.

3.1(b). Masking of One Tone by Another

When we add one tone, the signal, to another of different frequency, the masker, the situation is very different from the preceding case. Because our signal is sometimes in phase, sometimes in phase opposition, and sometimes in quadrature with the masker, the vector resultant will be louder, less loud, or relatively unchanged in amplitude. Since the resultant can differ in size when the signal is added, from not-at-all, to masker-plus-signal, or to masker-minus-signal, the variation in the resultant now becomes important in determining whether the subject will hear the change or not.

3.1(c). Effects of Signal Duration and Phase

When we add a 500-cps signal to a 500-cps masker, there will be a transient period during which the filter is adjusting to the new level. If the signal is in phase with the masker, there will be simply an increase of output achieved at a rate which is a function of the Q of the filter. If the signal is added out of phase with the masker, there will be a momentary drop in the output either during the onset of the signal or after it is turned off. The extent of the drop will depend upon the size and duration of the signal, the size of the phase difference, how abruptly the signal is added, and when in the cycle the addition is made. The effect of these factors on the output may be noticed as a momentary drop in level followed by a rise (if the signal is on long enough), and as a shift of phase of the output relative to the phase that had preceded the addition of the signal. These phenomena appearing in the output from the filter should affect the subject's threshold observably.

For the case where the signal is in phase with the masker, the only expected change will be an increase in level for the duration of the signal. We should therefore find that long signals are more easily detected than short. This proves to be true, as we will see later.

For the case where the signal is out of phase with the masker, we may possibly hear a short signal as readily as a longer one, we may hear it better, or we may hear it less readily depending upon the response of the filter to the sequence and spacing of the changes. If the signal is fairly strong, we may be able to hear it even if the phase is adjusted so that there is no increase in the resultant amplitude of the input to the filter. If we do, it will be because there is a momentary change in level as the phase is changing in the filter. These effects are testable experimentally and will be discussed in a later section.

3.1(d). Noise Masking

When the masking sound is a tone differing in frequency from the signal, the important variable determining the S/N ratio for detection is the phase relation between the signal and the masker. In the case of a thermal-noise masker we have an additional variable in the fluctuation of amplitude. We should therefore expect that a much larger signal will be required for detection, and that individual differences will be small compared with the variations in the signal.

3.1(e). Experimental Test of Predictions

We have made several predictions from our model. One, that the curve for pure-tone masking will resemble a filter-response curve without a deep notch near the signal-frequency, has been verified. The other predictions will be considered in detail in Sec. 4.3 where we deal with a series of closely related experiments.

4. HYPOTHESIS FOR BINAURAL PHENOMENA

The spectacular phenomena of binaural interaction require a mechanism in addition to our monaural one. It must take the outputs of the detectors for the two ears and compare them for time difference. Such a

[22] J. L. Lawson and G. E. Uhlenbeck, editor, *Threshold Signals* (McGraw-Hill Book Company, Inc., New York, 1950).

device was proposed by Jeffress[23] to explain localization of sound. It is about as simple as possible, is not altogether improbable physiologically, and satisfies the Huggins and Licklider principle of sloppy workmanship.[24] This mechanism receives impulses from corresponding filter sections of the two ears and delays them progressively by small increments, either by means of fine nerve tissue with a slow conduction rate or by a series of synapses. The delay nets are in opposition, so that undelayed impulses from one side meet delayed impulses from the other. A time delay in the stimulus to one ear can therefore be matched by an equal delay in the neural channel from the other. A series of detectors, in the form of synapses requiring coincident impulses from both ears in order to respond, completes the mechanism. As is usual in such models, the device achieves precision statistically by the use of large numbers of elements.

Evidence from localization of sound experiments and from direct measurements such as those of Klumpp[19] and Wilcott[21] indicate that the binaural mechanism is sensitive to interaural time shifts which for some subjects may be as small as 10 μsec when the shift is compared with a zero interaural time difference. When a difference of several hundred microseconds is already present, as for a sound to one side of the head, a considerably larger time shift is needed for detection. At the other extreme, Wilbanks, Blodgett, and Jeffress[25] have shown that subjects can still detect sidedness in a noise when it has been delayed in its path to one ear by as much as 20 msec. The mechanism must therefore be capable of delays of this order of magnitude.

We picture, therefore, a system of delay nets with a finely graded series of delays in the region corresponding to the median plane, and coarser and coarser delay steps as the total delay becomes larger. The longer delays are probably provided by chains of synapses. We picture also a considerable mass of nerve tissue in the region representing the median plane and greater sparsity of tissue as the delays become longer. Thus a 500-cps tone reaching the left ear 100 μsec earlier than the right would be represented by groups of impulses every 2 msec (once per cycle) in both channels, but the impulses in the left channel would lead the corresponding ones in the right by 100 μsec. A 100-μsec neural delay in the left channel would therefore be required to achieve coincidence. A delay of 2100 μsec in the left channel would also achieve coincidence and so would a 1900-μsec delay in the right channel, since in these cases the impulse from one side would coincide with the previous or the succeeding impulse from the other. Thus we might well have multiple regions of neural coincidence, but since we assume the greatest mass of tissue in the region of small delay, it would be the dominant region.

If we now reverse the phase of our 500-cps tone or displace it in time by 1 msec, we will achieve a dual and symmetrical condition. There will be no coincidence in the region representing the median plane, but undelayed impulses from one side will meet impulses from the other which have been delayed 1 msec and so in step. We will therefore hear the sound as coming from both sides at once. Reversing the phase at one ear for a wide-band noise will achieve a similar effect for each frequency component of the noise up to the limit of the nervous system's ability to follow, (approximately 1500 cps for binaural interaction). Thus, the high-frequency components of the noise should be localized near the median plane, but on both sides of it. The low-frequency components should be localized much farther to the sides, since they will require much longer neural delays for coincidence. Thus, we should hear the noise as filling the head, and this is the figure employed by Licklider to illustrate the N_π condition.

4.1. Webster's Hypothesis

Webster[26] proposed a hypothesis to account for the improvement in signal audibility which occurs under antiphasic conditions. The hypothesis is this: The narrow-band, tone-like noise of the ear's filter can, for short intervals, be considered a tone to which the signal-tone is added in random phase. The resultant will generally be different in phase from the noise. When the interaural conditions are homophasic, the phase change at each ear will be in the same direction and no interaural phase shift will result. However, if we reverse the interaural phase of the signal, adding it will advance the phase of the resultant at one ear and retard it at the other. This will cause a difference in the time of the neural signals from the two ears—a difference which can be detected by some central mechanism.

Webster assumes that the randomness of the noise plays an important part in the process but does not explain just what. He points to Licklider's failure to obtain MLD's using pure-tone maskers as evidence for the importance of randomness. He also cites work by Hirsh and Webster,[15] where the signal is a narrow band of noise and where a still larger MLD is obtained than with a tonal signal, as further evidence for the importance of randomness. Except for the lack of an explanation of the role of randomness, Webster's hypothesis is very satisfactory, and will be used, along with our model, as the basis for the present attempt to explain the binaural phenomena of masking.

4.2. Role of Randomness in Binaural Phenomena

Until we can explain the failure of pure-tone maskers to show appreciable MLD's under antiphasic conditions,

[23] L. A. Jeffress, J. Comp. Physiol. Psychol. **41**, 35–39 (1948).

[24] W. H. Huggins and J. C. R. Licklider, J. Acoust. Soc. Am. **23**, 290–299 (1951).

[25] Wilbanks, Blodgett, and Jeffress, J. Acoust. Soc. Am. **26**, 945(A) (1954).

[26] F. A. Webster, J. Acoust. Soc. Am. **23**, 452–462 (1951).

we will not have a very clear understanding of binaural masking phenomena. This is equivalent to saying that we must discover the means by which the randomness of noise produces the large MLD's commonly found.

The most striking difference between masking by noise and by tones, apart from the MLD's is the large difference in the monaural masked thresholds. The noise requires a much larger signal for detection. Since Webster has shown that the cause of the reduction of masking under antiphasic conditions is the interaural phase shift (time shift) produced by the signal, and since the size of this shift is dependent upon the intensity of the signal, we should expect that increasing the signal-intensity would increase the MLD. That is, any condition which requires a large signal for monaural detection has the potentiality for a substantial MLD under antiphasic conditions. If this is so, the role of the randomness of the noise is simply to create a monaural condition which requires a large signal for detection. Any other masker which requires a large signal should provide an MLD of comparable size. There are at least two ways of requiring a large signal with pure-tone masking. One is to employ a short signal which will require for detection a considerable increase in level. The other is to use as the masker a tone of the same frequency as the signal, and to add the signal 90° out of phase with it.

4.3. Experiments Employing Various Maskers

In Sec. 3.1 we made a number of predictions about monaural phenomena which should result from the properties of a narrow filter. Let us combine an experimental test of these predictions with a study of the binaural phenomena suggested in the preceding section. We will accordingly employ short signals, and use a variety of maskers under both homophasic and antiphasic stimulus conditions. Table I presents the results of these experiments.

Table I presents $S-N$'s, and where appropriate, MLD's, for three subjects under a variety of conditions.[27]

Table I. $S-N$ differences and masking level differences for various maskers under various phase conditions.

				Averages	
	Masker	[a]	[b]	100 msec	25 msec
	500~	0	0	−23.3	−18.7
	500~	π	0	−29.6	−22.4
	500~	0	π	−22.1	−18.1
Predicted[c]	500~	$\pi/2$	0	−8.5	−5.7
Observed	500~	$\pi/2$	0	−9.7	−10.0
	500~	$\pi/2$	π	−20.5	−19.6
	499~	R	0	−22.0	−14.7
	499~	R	π	−21.7	−19.0
	Noise	R	0	+4.5	+11.1
	Noise	R	π	−11.0	−5.4
Uncorrelated	Noise	R	0	−0.2	+5.0
Uncorrelated	Noise	R	π	−1.1	+6.1
	Masking level differences[d]				
	500~	$\pi/2$	$0-\pi$	10.8	9.6
	499~	R	$0-\pi$	−0.3	4.3
	Noise	R	$0-\pi$	15.5	16.5
Uncorrelated	Noise	R	$0-\pi$	0.9	−1.1
Uncorrelated	Noise	R	-0[e]	4.7	6.1

[a] Phase relation between signal and masker, R indicates random phase.
[b] Interaural phase for signal, π indicates reversed phase at one ear.
[c] The predicted values were based on the observed values for $\alpha=\beta=0$.
[d] A negative sign indicates that making is greater for S_π than for S_0.
[e] MLD was the comparison between N_0-S_0 and N_u-S_0.

Two signal durations were employed, 100 msec and 25 msec, and several different maskers, 500-cps tones, 499-cps tones, and noise, both correlated at the two ears, and uncorrelated. The table shows the resulting averages. Let us examine them systematically.

4.3(a). DL *for Intensity Increase*

The first row of the table presents the $S-N$'s for a 500-cps masker where the signal is added to it in phase. We have employed the symbol a to refer to the phase between the signal and masker, and b to refer to the interaural phase of the signal. In our present case $a=b=0$. Adding the signal in phase will simply increase the intensity of the 500-cps tone. Our $S-N$, therefore, is a measure of the DL for intensity.

For the 100-msec signal, $S-N=-23.3$ db, and for the 25-msec signal, −18.7 db. Expressed as S/N these become 0.068 and 0.116, respectively. These quantities are also, of course, the values of $\Delta I/I$, the usual way of expressing a DL for intensity.‡ We see that the shorter signal requires a considerably higher level for detection.

4.3(b). DL *for Intensity Decrease*

By reversing the phase of the signal relative to the steady 500-cps masker we will subtract the signal from the masker instead of adding it as in the previous section. Again we obtain $\Delta I/I$, but this time for an

[27] In the masking experiments described in the present paper an electronic switch was employed for presenting the signal. When the masker was a noise, the rise time and fall time of the switch was set at 0.5 msec. This was found to produce a slight, audible transient when the lower signal levels for pure-tone masking were used, and therefore a time of 10 msec was employed for tones. The switch was actuated by a counter which turned it off after a preset number of cycles. For short signals the 10 msec rise time and fall time becomes an appreciable part of the duration. In the case of the 25 msec signal used with pure-tone maskers the signal was above half its maximal amplitude for 25 msec. It was at approximately its maximal amplitude for 15 msec.

Threshold measurements were made using the constant method. Two-hundred stimuli were presented automatically at seven different levels, 2 db apart, including 60 "blanks" where no signal occurred. The subject responded by pressing a button when he heard the signal, and his response registered on a counter associated with the level. The 50% threshold was computed by the method described in reference 16. In most of the results reported here a threshold value is based upon 400 judgments from each of three subjects, in some cases more judgments were used.

Of the several possible methods of reporting thresholds we shall employ the signal-to-noise-ratio, based on the effective level of the noise, the spectral level plus the critical band width in db, for monaural listing. Where we express the signal-to-noise ratio in db, we will abbreviate $S-N$ and where we are referring to the actual ratio, we will employ S/N.

‡ In $S-N$, S and N are considered to be expressed in decibels. In S/N, S and N are considered to be sound pressure amplitudes. Also, ΔI and I are pressures, not powers or energies.

intensity decrease. The results are shown in the second row of the table. It will be seen that the thresholds are much smaller. Expressed as $S-N$ they are -29.6 db for the 100-msec signal and -22.4 db for the 25-msec. The corresponding S/N or $\Delta I/I$ values are 0.033 and 0.076, respectively. Apparently subjects can detect a sudden drop in level more readily than a sudden rise. As we will see, this fact plays a considerable role in other masking phenomena.

4.3(c). *Effect of Increasing Intensity at One Ear and Decreasing It at the Other*

By reversing the interaural phase for the signal, i.e., by making $b=\pi$, we will add the signal to the masker at one ear and subtract it from the masker at the other. The third row of the table shows the results for this condition. Here $S-N=-22.1$ db for the 100-msec signal and -18.1 db for the 25-msec. These levels are somewhat higher than either of the preceding. The momentary interaural intensity difference resulting here is apparently of no help to the subject in detecting the signal.

4.3(d). *Effect of a* 90° *Monaural Phase Shift*

Let us predict the threshold for a 90° phase difference between masker and signal. We will assume, since a signal at 90° will produce an increase of level while it is on, that we are concerned here solely with the DL for this increase. We will employ the data from Sec. 4.3(a) and determine the length of signal vector required to produce the indicated ΔI. These values are given in the fourth row of the table, and are followed in the fifth row by the values actually observed in the experiment. It will be seen that in every case the observed value is smaller. Our subjects are detecting something other than the ΔI which results from the signal addition. Apparently they are hearing the transients produced by the filter in response to the sudden phase change. This is as predicted, and is supported by our findings in Sec. 4.3(b). There we found that subjects could hear a drop in intensity more readily than an increase. The transient response of a filter to a phase change usually involves a momentary drop, either at the onset of the change or at its termination, and it is this drop which is responsible for the lower thresholds.

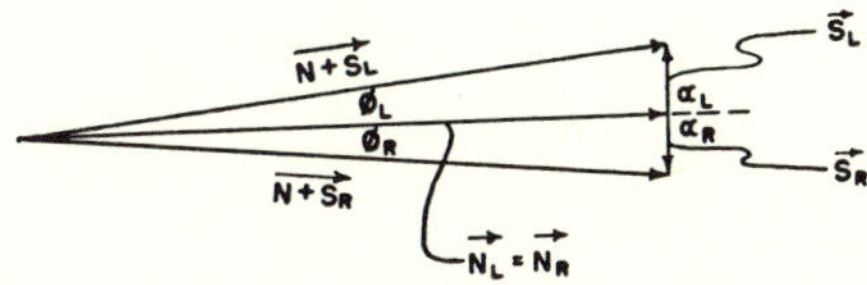

FIG. 1. Phase diagram for 500-cps pure-tone masker. Signal is added at +90° for left ear and −90° for right ear. **N** is noise vector (500-cps tone, in the present case) **S** is a signal vector, **N+S** is resultant vector, α is angle between masker and signal, ϕ is angle between masker and resultant, θ is interaural phase shift owing to the presence of the signal, subscripts L and R refer to left and right ears.

Our second prediction based on filter transients was that the transient effects of a short signal might be sufficient to overcome the advantage ordinarily associated with a longer one. A comparison of the differences between the $S-N$ for 25 msec and for 100 msec shows this to be true. For the in-phase condition the 100-msec signal showed a 4.6-db advantage over the 25-msec. For the 90° phase-difference between masker and signal the difference is 0.3 db in the opposite direction. Two of the three subjects showed an advantage in favor of the shorter signal.

4.3(e). MLD's *for Tonal Maskers*

We predicted that a monaural condition which requires a large increase in the signal vector for detection would also increase the possible MLD to be found with a reversal of the interaural phase of the signal. Specifically we predicted that the N_0-S_π condition, for the case where the signal was added at 90° to the 500-cps masker, would show a substantial MLD. The sixth row of the table shows the results for this condition. It will be seen that there is an MLD of 10.8 db for the 100-msec signal and of 9.6 db for the 25-msec, really substantial values.

Let us discover what interaural phase shift (time shift) is responsible for this MLD. We have added the signal at 90° to the masker, +90° at one ear, and −90° at the other. The S/N for the 100-msec signal is 0.094. Let us draw the appropriate vector diagram for determining the resultant phases. Figure 1 shows the construction. The signal vector for the left ear is drawn +90° from the masker, and the signal vector for the right ear is drawn −90° from the masker. Since the masker is in phase at the two ears, the two "noise" vectors, $\bar{N}_L$ and $\bar{N}_R$ are drawn in coincidence and of magnitude 1.000. The two resultants $\mathbf{N}+\mathbf{S}_L$ and $\mathbf{N}+\mathbf{S}_R$ indicate both the magnitude and phase of the sounds at the left and the right ears. Computation shows that the new magnitudes are 1.0045, giving $\Delta I=0.0045$, a value much too small to be detected as a difference of level. The monaural phase angles ϕ_L and ϕ_R are 5.4° and the interaural phase angle θ, therefore, is 10.8°. At 500 cps this corresponds to an interaural time difference of 60 μsec. This is, therefore the threshold of our localization center under the present conditions. The corresponding figure for the 25-msec signal is 67 μsec.

We predicted that the increase required in the signal vector when we employ a 25-msec signal in connection with a 499-cps masker would also provide a substantial MLD. Here, again, our prediction is borne out. The seventh and eighth rows of the table show $S-N$ for the N_0-S_0 and for the N_0-S_π conditions for a 499-cps masker and a 25-msec and a 100-msec signal. Here, as predicted, there is only a small MLD for the longer signal (1.4 db) and a considerably larger MLD (4.3 db) for the shorter.

Let us again construct the appropriate vector diagram. Here we are dealing with a signal which can make any angle with the masker. For small angles there will be little interaural phase shift, for large angles the phase shift will be large. Since detection is based on the 50% threshold, and since the detectibility of the phase shift depends upon its size, we should determine the shift on the basis of the phase angle which will be exceeded 50% of the time, namely ±45° and ±135°. If we therefore draw the signal vector for one ear at +45° and for the other ear, which is 180° out of phase with it, at −135°, we shall have the condition for 50% detection providing the amplitude of the signal is that for the 50% threshold. Figure 2 shows the construction for the 25-msec signal, where $S-N=-19.0$ db and $S/N=0.112$.

Here $\phi_L=4.2°$, $\phi_R=4.9°$ and consequently $\theta=9.1°$. This corresponds to an interaural time difference, Δt, at this frequency of 50 μsec. This is considerably smaller than the 67 μsec we found in the previous case for a 25-msec signal. Does this mean that the threshold for a time shift is smaller for the random phases encountered with the 499-cps masker than for the steady conditions found with the 500-cps masker? This does not seem very likely. A more reasonable explanation is that we are sometimes hearing a change of *level*, and that this is helping to reduce the magnitude of the required signal vector. Our signal in this case was 0.112. In Sec. 4.3(c) where we also had an S_π phase condition, our S/N was 0.105 which is smaller than our present value. This means that at moments when the phase angle between the signal and masker is small enough so that **S+N** is greater than 0.105, we should be able to hear the change of level, and when the phase angle is large we will hear the interaural phase shift. Our threshold of 50 μsec is therefore too small, because our binaural detection is being contaminated by monaural detection of level changes. This sort of contamination will always occur when the MLD's are small enough to permit the magnitude of the signal vector to produce changes of level sufficient for monaural detection. Only when the **S+N** vector, even for $\alpha=0$, is too small to yield a ΔI large enough for monaural detection, will we obtain an uncontaminated value for Δt. The values we obtained in the previous example, $\Delta t=60$ μsec for 100 msec and 67 μsec for 25 msec, were satisfactory, since here ΔI was too small to be detected monaurally under any phase condition.

4.3(f). MLD's for Uncorrelated Noise

When the masking noise at the two ears is uncorrelated, previous experiments have found that there is no advantage in binaural listening. Here again we find that the use of a short signal, with its required increase

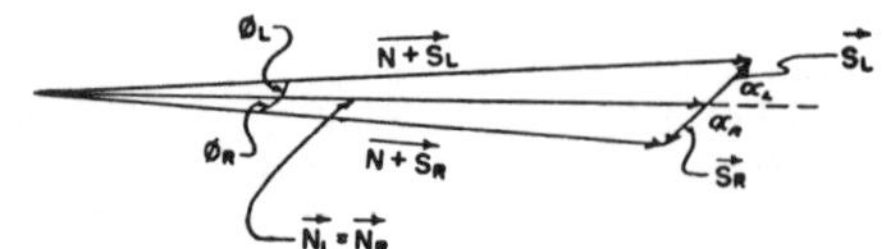

FIG. 2. Phase diagram for a 499-cps pure-tone masker. Signal is added in random phase, the angle shown is the median value. See Fig. 1 for meaning of symbols.

of level, yields a substantial MLD. The eleventh row of the table presents the $S-N$ values for a 100-msec and a 25-msec signal. It will be seen that these values are somewhat below the corresponding ones for the N_0-S_0 condition presented in the ninth row. The MLD's are presented in the last row of the table. For a 25-msec signal the MLD is 6.1 db. As predicted this is somewhat greater than the MLD for 100 msec, 4.7 db, and, of course, much greater than the negligible ones obtained previously with long signals. A discussion of the mechanism for this release from masking will be given later.

The next-to-the-last row of the table presents the MLD's for the N_u-S_0 *vs* the N_u-S_π conditions. They are of negligible magnitude, a fact that will also be discussed later.

4.4. Narrow-Band Noise

Before proceeding to other masking phenomena, let us consider in somewhat more detail the features of thermal noise which are relevant to our problem. According to Rice[28] we may think of thermal noise which has been passed through a narrow band-pass filter as being a sinusoid which varies in amplitude and in frequency (phase). The possible rates of variation of these two quantities are determined by the characteristics of the filter.

For simplicity let us assume that at 500 cps we are dealing, in the ear, with an ideal filter 50 cps in width. Using Rice's equations we can predict the extent of both the amplitude variation and the phase variation.

If we take the rms amplitude of the noise, $\sqrt{\psi_0}$ in Rice's equations, as unity, we find that 25% of the time the amplitude of the envelope of our pseudo-tone will be less than 0.76, that 50% of the time it will be less than 1.17, and that 75% of the time it will be less than 1.67. If we use in reckoning phase or frequency variation the interval between successive axis crossings, we find that 50% of the times this interval will lie between 1.014 and 0.986 msec.

Since we are concerned with adding a signal to this fluctuating quantity, and will be interested sometimes in the increase or decrease in the resultant vector-magnitude, and sometimes in the change of phase, let

[28] S. O. Rice, Bell System Tech. J. **23**, 282–332 (1944) and **24**, (1945). Reprinted in *Noise and Stochastic Processes* (Dover Publications, New York, 1954), pp. 133–294. A convenient secondary reference is L. L. Beranek, *Acoustical Measurements* (John Wiley and Sons, Inc., New York, 1949), pp. 446–456.

us examine this question in some detail. Rice (reference 28, p. 214) has shown that the probability density for the envelope, R, of a narrow-band noise is given by $(R/\psi_0)\exp(-R^2/2\psi_0)$ where $\sqrt{\psi_0}$ is the rms voltage (current, in Rice's demonstration) for the band of noise.

This expression is also the probability density for a circular normal distribution where $R^2=x^2+y^2$, $\sigma_x=\sigma_y=\sqrt{\psi_0}$, $\bar{x}=\bar{y}=0$. With this familiar distribution we may determine the x, y coordinates of n points in the plane, each associated with $1/n$th of the total volume under the probability surface. A line from the origin to one of these points will therefore represent one of the n equally probable noise vectors in amplitude and in direction.

Representing our signal as a vector in this plane, we will draw it as a line of appropriate length to the origin from a fixed point in the plane. We will draw the resultant from the tail of the signal vector to the head of the noise vector. There will be n such resultants. If we now order them in magnitude, we may determine the upper and lower quartile values. These quartiles will represent approximately the 50% threshold values of the stimulus. The lower quartile will represent the stimulus value, below which the difference will be detectible as a decrease in level. The upper quartile will be the value for the resultant, above which the difference will be detectible as an increase in level. The 25% below the lower quartile and the 25% above the upper quartile make up the 50% of detectible signal additions. (This is not strictly true, since the 50% of detectible signals will not be distributed exactly evenly. In Sec. 4.3 we discovered that subjects hear a drop in intensity more readily than an increase.)

It can be shown that the same quartile values can be obtained in another, much simpler, way. If we employ as our noise vector the median amplitude of the noise envelope (1.17) and draw it in a 45° phase direction relative to the signal, we will obtain the upper quartile of the resultant. If we use the same magnitude and draw the vector at 135°, we obtain the lower quartile value.

A similar procedure can be employed in determining the median interaural phase angle for the N_0-S_π condition. Here again the median value can be obtained by the simpler method of drawing the noise vector as having the median magnitude and a phase angle of 45° for one ear and −135° for the other.

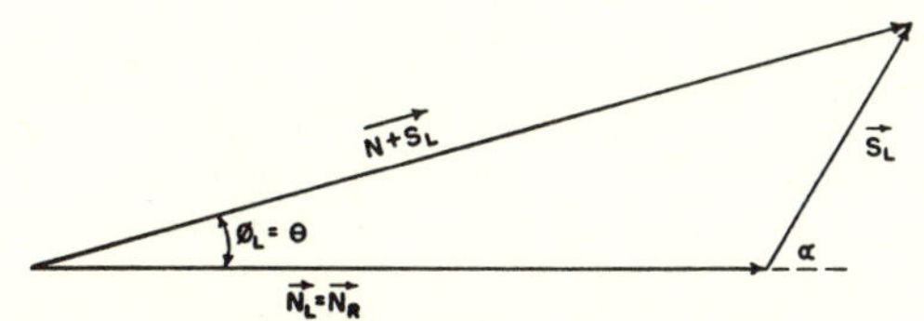

Fig. 3. Phase diagram for noise masker, N_0-S_m interaural phase condition. $\alpha=60°$ here for reasons given in text. See Fig. 1 for meaning of symbols.

If, however, we attempt the same procedure in determining the median phase angle between the noise and the resultant (interaural phase angle for the N_0-S_m case), we find that no general solution is possible. We must employ a signal vector of appropriate length and compute the median phase angle anew for each new value of the signal vector. Employing the median amplitude of the noise envelope and a phase angle of 60° gives a rough approximation which will be employed later for illustrative purposes.

4.5. Hirsh's Hierarchy of MLD's

Let us now attempt to explain the hierarchy of MLD's found by Hirsh and by ourselves and Deatherage, in various experiments employing a 500-cps signal and a noise masker. We will use Hirsh's data, supplemented by our own where necessary. Let us begin with the conditions where the noise is in phase at the two ears. Hirsh used a noise having a spectral level of 59.1 db. This corresponds at 500 cps to an effective level of 76.2 db. In our future constructions, we will represent the rms value corresponding to this effective level for the noise as unity.

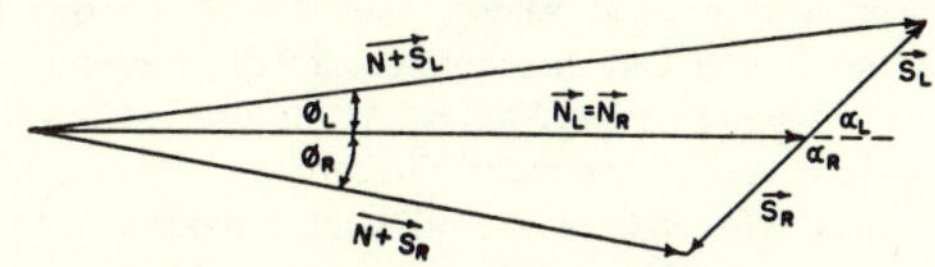

Fig. 4. Phase diagram for noise masker, N_0-S_π interaural phase condition. See Fig. 1 for meaning of symbols.

Let us consider first the case of a binaural noise and monaural signal, N_0-S_m. Hirsh found the masked threshold to be 69.3 db, *SPL*. This corresponds to $S-N=-6.9$ db and $S/N=0.45$. Under these conditions the monaural phase-shift ϕ_L will equal the interaural phase shift θ since the noise at the right ear will remain unaltered by the signal. Figure 3 shows an illustrative vector diagram. We have employed a noise vector, common to the two ears, of 1.17 in magnitude, corresponding to the median value of the noise envelope. We have drawn the signal vector, of magnitude 0.45, at an angle of 60° for the reason given earlier. To find the value of ϕ_L, we must compute it by the method described in Sec. 4.4, since the diagram in Fig. 4 is merely illustrative. The value proves to be 14.5°, which corresponds to an interaural time-shift, Δt, of 81 μsec. This value is probably too small because of contamination with monaural-intensity factors. The MLD here is not quite large enough to eliminate such monaural detection for small phase angles between the noise and the signal.

Let us now consider the N_0-S_π condition. Here Hirsh found a threshold of 64.1 db, corresponding to $S-N=-12.1$ db and $S/N=0.25$. Let us determine Δt. Here again we draw the median value of the noise envelope as our noise-vector, which is common for the two ears. The signal vector, magnitude 0.25, will make an angle of $+45°$ for the left ear and $-135°$ for the right. Figure 4 shows the diagram, and we find that $\theta=\phi_L+\phi_R=17.4°$. This corresponds to an interaural time shift, $\Delta t=97$ μsec. This is slightly larger than the value we previously obtained for the N_0-S_m condition, and agrees with our conclusion that the value was somewhat too small due to contamination by detectible intensity-changes. In the present case our signal vector is too short to produce an appreciable change of intensity, so we may take the value of Δt as correct for the conditions of the experiment.

Comparable figures from our present experiments can be obtained using the data of Table I. They prove to be $\Delta t=110$ μsec for the 100-msec signal and 220 μsec for the 25-msec signal. In both cases the MLD's were larger than 15 db, so we are safely below the signal levels where intensity changes can contaminate our results. Apparently our localization-center detector, as well as our monaural detectors, is sensitive to the duration of a tonal signal.

Let us consider next the case where the noise is reversed in interaural phase, the $N_\pi-S_0$ condition. Hirsh found a masked threshold of 65.9 db, corresponding to $S-N=-10.3$ and $S/N=0.31$. Figure 5 shows the appropriate vector diagram. The noise is reversed in direction at the right ear, and is shown at an angle differing slightly from 180° to remind us that we are dealing with a noise which can vary slightly in phase from one half-cycle to the next. The magnitude of this variation is negligible here, but becomes of some importance at low frequencies. The interaural phase shift when the signal is added is from approximately 180° to approximately 159°, an interaural phase shift of 22°. This corresponds to a time shift, Δt of 120 μsec, somewhat more than is required under the N_0-S_π condition.

The case where the noise is reversed in phase, $N_\pi-S_0$, presents a very different task to our localization center from that where the noise is in phase and the signal reversed, N_0-S_π. In the latter case, the noise is mainly represented in the median region where accuracy is greatest and where we are sensitive to the smallest changes. In the former case, the noise will be doubly represented, with some fluctuation in position as the frequency (in the band we are considering) fluctuates slightly. The fluctuation will result in a movement inward on both sides as the frequency increases with a consequent reduction in the delays required for coincidence, and an outward movement as the frequency decreases. These movements should be nearly symmetrical since the time intervals between successive axis crossings for the narrow band of noise will be nearly equal.

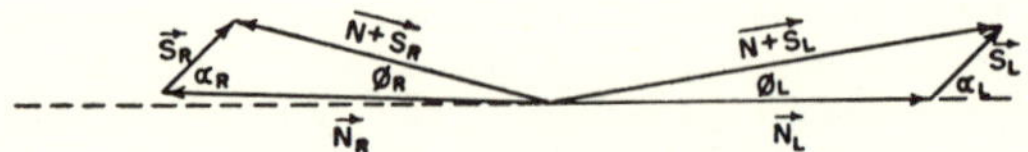

FIG. 5. Phase diagram for noise masker, $N_\pi-S_0$ interaural phase condition. See Fig. 1 for meaning of symbols.

4.6. Variation of MLD's with Frequency

As we go down in frequency, we should expect the MLD's for the $N_\pi-S_0$ condition to decrease because of the increased neural delays required for the N_π case. The increased delays will be accompanied by a decrease in precision and a correspondingly increased threshold for interaural time shift. This is borne out by Hirsh's results. At 200 cps his MLD for the N_0-S_π condition relative to N_0-S_0 is 13.6 db, while that for the $N_\pi-S_0$ condition is 7.6 db. The corresponding figures for 500 cps are more nearly equal, 10.8 db and 9.0 db, respectively.

4.7. Effect of an Interaural Time Delay for the Noise

If we introduce into the noise channel to one ear a time delay of a millisecond, at 500 cps we shall have a condition similar to that achieved by reversing the interaural phase of the noise. The vector diagrams for the two cases will be the same, but the effects on the localization center will be somewhat different. Since we have delayed the sound to, say, the right ear by 1 msec, a neural delay of 1 msec will restore coindidence. That is, each impulse from the right will match the neurally delayed impulse from the left. However, the case will be different for the other side. Impulse 1 from the right, when delayed neurally an additional millisecond, will match impulse 2 from the left, and so on, but these delays will need to vary somewhat because of the fluctuations in the period of the noise. Thus, we shall have a steady localization on one side and a varying localization on the other, and this variation will be about twice the magnitude of the variation in the N_π case, since there we were matching half-periods rather than whole periods. If we delay the noise by 3 msec, the variability will be still greater and will now occur on both sides. On one side we will be matching impulse 3 with a delayed impulse 1, and on the other side we will be matching impulse 1 with a delayed impulse 2. Since there is a longer interval for frequency change, the fluctuations in this case should be larger than in the previous case. This is borne out by the findings of Jeffress, Blodgett, and Deatherage[16] who obtained for a 150-msec 500-cps signal, MLD's of 12.5 db for the $N_\pi-S_0$ condition, 10.5 db for a 1-msec delay, and 8.5 db for a 3-msec delay in the noise channel to one ear.

4.8. Masking and Localization

It has frequently been assumed that the release from masking that accompanies changes in interaural phase is owing to the separation of the noise and the signal in phenomenal space. That this is not a sufficient explanation has been pointed out by several writers who have shown that phase conditions which produce the greatest spatial separations are not those which produce the greatest MLD's. A subject often cannot tell without careful comparison whether a signal by itself is being presented with an interaural phase reversal or not, yet reversing the phase of the signal leads to the greatest release from masking. Our hypothesis makes it clear why this is so. What we hear is not the signal in one place and the noise in another: we hear the *noise plus signal* move from where the noise has been.

SUMMARY AND CONCLUSIONS

This paper examines many of the phenomena of masking in relation to two models, one concerned with monaural, and one with binaural listening. The monaural model is the familar narrow band-pass filter followed by a detector responsive to changes in output level. The binaural model is a series of coincidence detectors associated with a delay network capable of matching a delay in the stimulus with a delay in the neural path. The two models have proved helpful in understanding the phenomena of pure-tone masking, and have led to a number of predictions which were subsequently verified by experiment. Among the new experimental findings were the following.

(1) Subjects are more sensitive to a decrease in the level of a pure tone than in an increase. This fact, taken with the fact that subjects are sensitive to a sudden change of phase of a tone, plays a significant role in monaural masking phenomena.

(2) The transient responses of a narrow filter are paralleled in subjects' responses to short signals.

(3) A large masking-level-difference (MLD) results from reversing the phase of a signal tone when it is added 90° out of phase with a tone of the same frequency.

(4) Substantial MLD's are found with pure-tone maskers when the interaural phase of the signal is reversed, provided the signal is short. The previous negative results were owing to the use of long signals.

(5) Substantial MLD's are found for the case where a binaural signal is employed with uncorrelated noise at the two ears, providing the signal is short.

(6) The increased MLD's found for short signals are owing to the fact that a different mechanism is responsible for binaural detection than for monaural, and this mechanism is not so adversely affected by a short signal duration.

(7) The absence of marked individual differences in the threshold for tones masked by noise, an often-noted fact, is owing to the large variation in the stimulus. When the noise plus signal is large, all subjects hear it, when it is small, none do. The variability of the subjects' thresholds is small in comparison.

(8) The threshold for the binaural detection of a change in the masker when a signal is added antiphasically, is about 100 μsec for a noise masker, and about 60 μsec for a pure tone.

In addition to the foregoing specific findings a few general conclusions can be drawn.

(1) There appears to be no evidence for "binaural inhibition." When the MLD associated with a monaural signal and binaural noise is recognized as a binaural phenomenon, the other masking level differences all favor binaural listening. The most unfavorable binaural condition is no worse than the monaural condition.

(2) There appears to be no evidence requiring the assumption of a "sophisticated" detector to explain monaural or binaural masking phenomena. We do not "pick the signal out of the noise," we hear a change of level when the signal is added, or we hear a movement. Under binaural conditions, when the masked threshold is lower, it is lower because we hear the sound move when the signal is added to the noise, not because we hear the signal in one place and the noise in another. This experience does occur, but only for strong signals, not for signals near threshold.

35

Reprinted from *Acoust. Soc. Am. J.* **22**:801–804 (1950)

Binaural Localization and Masking

W. E. Kock
Bell Telephone Laboratories, Inc., Murray Hill, New Jersey
(Received August 10, 1950)

INTRODUCTION

BINAURAL hearing is a subject which has occupied the attention of experimenters in acoustics for over a century. The ability of the two ears to yield directional perception has probably been best explained as being due to the difference in time of arrival of sounds at the two ears.* Recently, W. Koenig of the Bell Telephone Laboratories conducted certain binaural experiments which pointed up an additional interesting property of the two ears, namely their ability to "squelch" reverberation and background noises.[1] He compared two conditions: (1) a single microphone in a reverberant room connected to receivers on both ears and (2) two microphones individually connected to separate earphones on each ear. He observed that with the second arrangement reverberation and background noises (which were very evident in the first case) were effectively squelched. Even with an appreciable amount of background noise in the room such as street noise, electric fans, people walking nearby, etc., the listener could concentrate very easily on a desired signal coming from a particular direction. His experiments also showed that forward and rearward directional perception (normally lost in a binaural circuit) could be regained when a mechanical system was supplied which rotated the microphone pair whenever the listener rotated his head. Both of these phenomena appeared difficult to explain by existing binaural theories; the experiments described in this paper were therefore made in an attempt to gain a better understanding of the binaural mechanism.

EXPERIMENTAL

Figure 1 shows a photograph of "Oscar," the dummy used in some of the early binaural experiments conducted at the Bell Laboratories. Microphones were placed in the approximate position of the dummy's ear and connected through amplifiers to individual earphones. In these experiments, the talker seemed to be confined to the azimuth semicircle behind the listener; he could never be imagined in front of the listener. Figure 2 shows the mechanical link employed by Koenig which caused the microphone pair to be rotated whenever the listener rotated his head. With this system it was found possible to locate the position of the talker and make the dummy face him almost exactly, regardless of his initial position. Our preliminary experiments employed the arrangement shown in Fig. 3; we observed both results reported by Koenig; namely, the ability to differentiate front and rear, and the ability to squelch background noises which were very evident under monaural conditions.†

An interesting psychological effect was produced in this set-up by crossing the connections; that is, connecting the left-hand microphone to the right-hand ear and vice versa. Talkers on one's right then sounded as if they were on one's left; talkers who were behind sounded as if they were in front, etc.

A brain mechanism which could account for binaural localization and reverberation squelching was thought

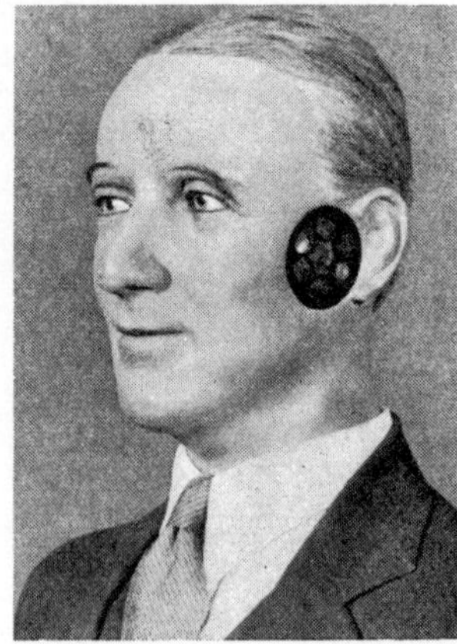

Fig. 1. "Oscar," the dummy used in some early binaural experiments.

* An excellent discussion on the localization of sound in space has appeared recently [Herbert Klensch, Naturwiss. (May, 1949)] in which both the directional properties of the single ear and the directional effect due to binaural hearing are considered.

[1] W. Koenig, J. Acous. Soc. Am. 22, 61 (1950).

† This second effect can readily be observed by anyone in a noisy surrounding such as a restaurant by closing one ear; nearby conversation easily heard binaurally often becomes submerged in the noise.

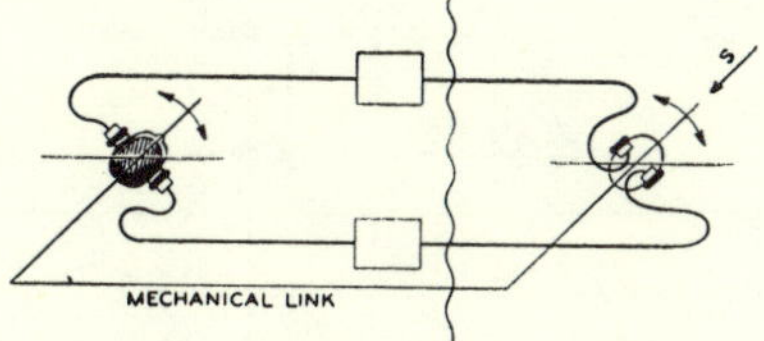

Fig. 2. The mechanical link employed by Koenig to rotate the pick-up microphones with the listener's head rotation.

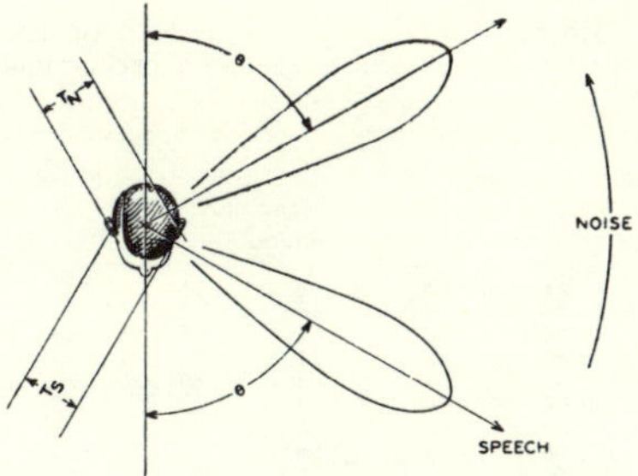

Fig. 4. An observer concentrating on speech arriving at an angle θ in the forward quadrant discriminates (by a factor of about 10 db) against noise arriving from other directions, except at the equal angle θ in the rearward quadrant where the arrival time difference for the speech (T_S) is the same as for the noise (T_N).

to be the following: If the brain could introduce, at will, a time delay in either of the nerve paths connecting each ear to the brain, the directional pattern of the two ears as a combination could be "steered" so that maximum response could be "aimed" in a given direction.‡ Aiming the directional pattern could favor sounds coming from a given direction over those coming from other directions. This "direction finder" effect could be made considerably more sensitive if the brain were able furthermore to subtract the signals in the two ears. For no phase delay in either channel this would produce a directional pattern consisting of a null or minimum straight head and by varying the amounts of time delay, this null could be pointed in different directions.§ The minimum in such a system has a very narrow angular width and a high degree of angular discrimination can thus result.

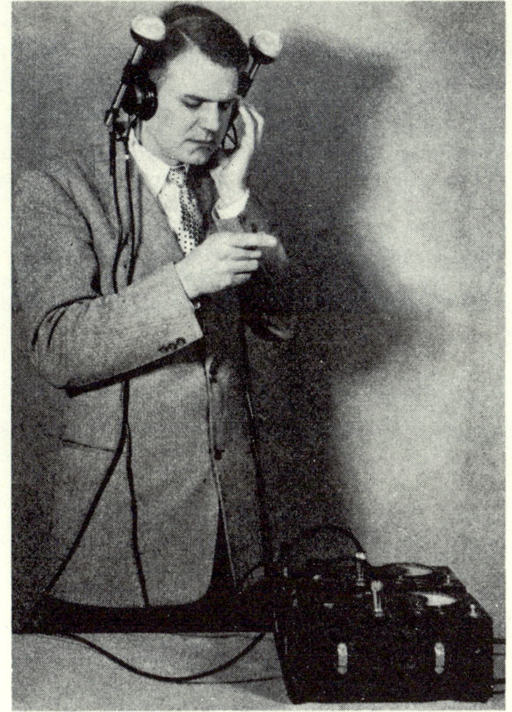

Fig. 3. The author's binaural arrangement to cause rotation of the pick-up microphones.

‡ A time delay insertion is only one possible mechanism for shifting the directional perception pattern; the fundamental requirement is that the brain be able to recognize and evaluate relative time delays in each of the two ear circuits.

Such a proposed mechanism leads, however, to a consequence which can be explained with the help of Fig. 4: a delay inserted in one ear path will cause the null to move in the direction of that ear but there will also be a null in the rearward direction which will also move toward the same ear. This would mean that if a person is concentrating on a talker located at 45° in the forward right-hand quadrant he would also be concentrating in a rearward direction at 45° in the rear right quadrant. More specifically, the directions of concentration would lie on the surface of a half-cone whose axis lies along the line joining the two ears, its apex midway between the two ears and its generating line making an angle of 45° with the axis.

To test this hypothesis, it was decided to measure, in the Murray Hill free-space room of the Bell Laboratories, the ability of the ears to detect and understand one talker when a single noise source was also present in

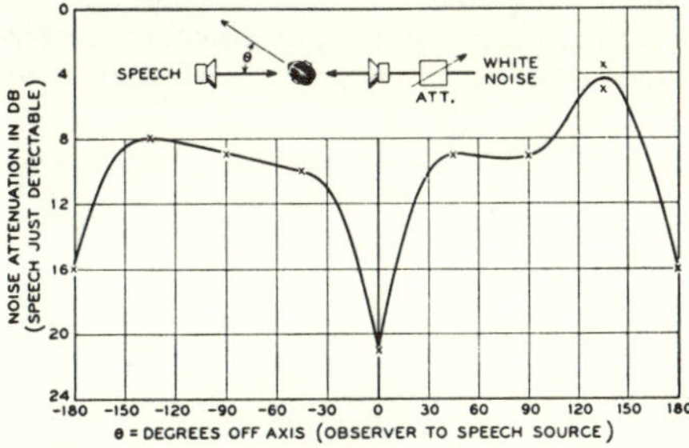

Fig. 5. Effect of angular position on binaural discrimination. The relative values shown here at 180°, 0°, and −90° compare favorably with the values (**BF**, **FB**, and **RL**) in Hirsh's table (see Table I).

§ Such direction finding principles are commonly employed in both sonar and radar equipment for increasing the bearing accuracy.

TABLE I. Human head listening: Threshold (in db *SPL*) of intelligibility of speech presented against a background of noise (at 80-db *SPL*).

Position of		Anechoic chamber Head moving		Reverberant room Head moving		Head fixed	
Speech	Noise	Binaural	Monaural	Binaural	Monaural	Binaural	Monaural
F	*F*	61	63	68	68	67	67
L	*F*	56	59	66	65	63	65
B	**F**	**64**	60	67	65	69	66
R	*R*	66	66	71	69	68	67
F	*R*	60	61	68	69	69	71
B	*B*	60	59	69	68	67	68
R	*B*	59	59	64	66	63	66
F	**B**	**66**	65	69	71	67	67
B	*L*	59	60	67	67	67	66
R	**L**	**57**	59	66	67	64	66
Average		61	61	67	67	66	67
Variance		10.4	7.5	3.7	3.4	4.6	2.5

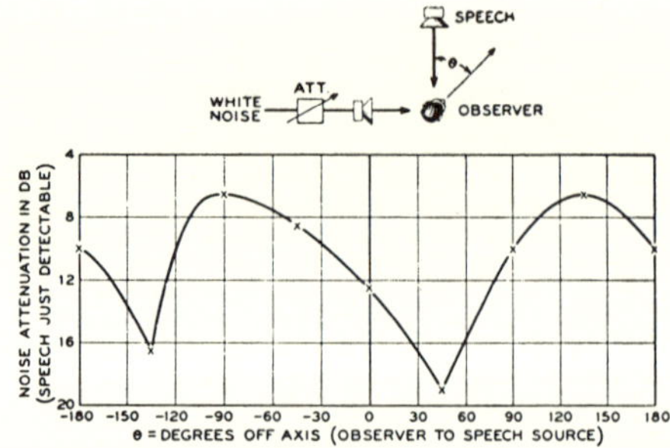

FIG. 7. Effect of angular position on binaural discrimination for a third arrangement.

the room. The arrangement is shown in the top sketch of Fig. 5. The speech signal consisted of a recording of a standard sentence repeated over and over at constant level. The disturbing noise consisted of thermal noise whose intensity could be adjusted by the listener. When the listener assumed a head position such that the same relative delay was obtained at the ears for both speech and noise then binaural discrimination was expected to be impaired. The curve at the bottom of Fig. 5 shows this to be the case for $\theta=0$ or 180°. Between 10 and 15 db attenuation had to be inserted in the noise circuit for the speech to be as perceptible as for those angles where the relative time delay for speech and noise was different. It is interesting to observe that similar conclusions can be drawn from results reported by Hirsh[2] shown in Table I. Only three of the results shown in the chart are applicable; these have been set in boldfaced type in Table I. Comparing the two bottom boldfaced results, it is seen that Hirsh reports a 9 db improvement in intelligibility as against the 12 db shown in our Fig. 5. Similar results were obtained for other positions of the speech and noise sources as shown in Figs. 6 and 7. In Fig. 6 the speech source has been moved around 90°. Under this condition equal time delays to the two ears for speech and noise occur when the observer positions his head at $-45°$ and at $+135°$. Again the drop in ability to concentrate on the speech signal is observed at these angles. Figure 7 shows a similar situation for the noise coming from the left as shown. Here equal time delays occur at $+45°$ and $-135°$.

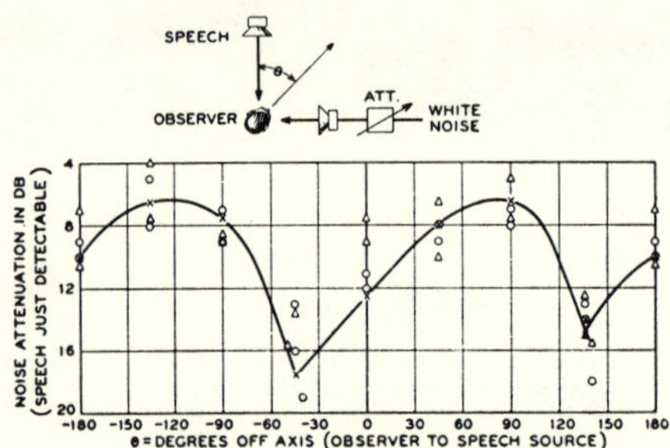

FIG. 6. Effect of angular position on binaural discrimination for a second arrangement.

[2] I. J. Hirsh, J. Acous. Soc. Am. **22**, 199 (1950).

Similar results were obtained when the observer was supplied with earphones which were individually connected by separate lines to two microphones as shown in Fig. 8. The discrimination ability again drops when the delays are equal. In this condition two microphones are seen to be no better than one single microphone.

Finally, an experiment was performed in which two separate sources of white noise were led independently to each ear, whereas the desired signal was led to both earphones. The ability of the ear to detect the desired signal under these conditions was compared with its ability to detect the same desired signal when the noise fed to the two ears came from the same noise source in phase. In the first case the desired signal was in phase so that it sounded as though it were coming from straight ahead or directly back. The noise, however, coming from two independent noise sources, sounded like noise coming from all directions, the effect being very similar to the sound of rain falling on a tin roof. In the second case, on the other hand, both the signal and the noise were identical at both ears so that no binaural benefit would be expected. Between 5 and 10 db improvement was observed in the ability of the ear to detect the signal in the first case as against the second case. These results are similar to those obtained by Licklider[3] in which he

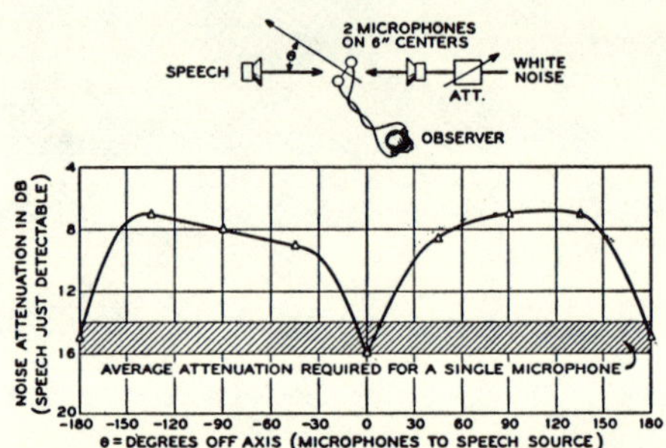

FIG. 8. Effect of angular position on binaural discrimination using a two-channel system of microphones.

[3] J. C. R. Licklider, J. Acous. Soc. Am. **20**, 150 (1948).

showed a higher percentage word articulation for case 1 than for case 2. He has given the term "heterophasal" to the condition where independent noise sources are conducted to each ear.

CONCLUSION

The above experiments suggest that the brain preserves and evaluates time delays (perhaps by the mechanism of delay insertion in one or the other of the nerve paths between the ear and the brain) to achieve not only the directional localization of sound but also the observed discrimination against reverberation and background noise. When the disturbing sound and the desired sound arrive at the two ears with the same relative time delay, this discrimination fails. Also, the time delay hypothesis explains how two ears (or Koenig's mechanical arrangement) permit one to decide whether a sound source is in front or behind by a twisting motion of the head. If the talker is in front and the head is rotated, a delay must be added in one ear path in order to retrieve the original situation; if, however, the speaker is behind the listener, the delay must be added in the other path. Twisting the head thus gives immediate information as to the forward or backward hemisphere.

ACKNOWLEDGMENT

The author wishes to acknowledge the cooperation of Messrs. B. P. Bogert, R. L. Hanson, F. K. Harvey, and G. Raisbeck in this work.

36

Reprinted from *Acoust. Soc. Am. J.* **42**:601–608 (1967)

Binaural Release From Masking for Speech and Gain in Intelligibility

H. Levitt and L. R. Rabiner

Bell Telephone Laboratories, Incorporated, Murray Hill, New Jersey 07971

Relative importance of different frequency regions in binaural release from masking (for detection) and binaural gain in intelligibility was investigated. Experiments showed that the release from masking ($S\pi N0$ case) for single words in high-level, broad-band Gaussian noise is roughly 13 dB and is determined primarily by interaural phase opposition in the low-frequency (<500 Hz) region. The binaural gain in intelligibility at the 50% level was on the order of 6 dB and only partly dependent on interaural phase opposition in the low-frequency region. Interaural amplitude differences were not considered in the investigation. Subjecting the speech to a large interaural time dealy with the noise binaurally in phase resulted in a relatively constant masking level difference approaching 13 dB over the measured range from 0.5 to 10 msec. The corresponding binaural gain in intelligibility at the 50% level was on the order of 3 dB.

INTRODUCTION

Research in hearing is characterized by a marked dichotomy between experiments involving speech and experiments involving mathematically well defined stimuli such as tones or pulses. The reasons for the dichotomy are obvious; the problem is to find valid and useful relationships between the two bodies of data. Research into binaural release from masking provides a compelling example of the lack of interaction between the two areas of interest. Although binaural unmasking (for detection) and binaural gain in intelligibility were first demonstrated at roughly the same time[1,2] there have been few attempts at relating the two effects.

The investigation reported here represents a modest attempt at bridging this gap. The purpose of the experiment was twofold:

(1) The primary aim was to determine whether binaural release from masking for detection of speech (single words) in broad-band Gaussian noise is dependent on factors similar to those for tones and pulses. Flanagan and Watson[3] have shown that the release from masking for periodic pulsive stimuli in high-level broad-band Gaussian noise is dependent primarily on interaural phase differences between signal and noise in the region of 300 Hz. As these authors point out, "in regard to spectral structure, periodic pulses bear a useful similarity to voiced speech sounds." It was, therefore, of interest to determine whether release from masking for the detection of speech in broad-band Gaussian noise is similarly dependent on low-frequency interaural phase information. Interaural amplitude differences were not considered in this investigation.

(2) A secondary aim was to investigate the relationship between release from masking for detection and the corresponding gain in intelligibility. In particular, it was of interest to compare the relative importance of different frequency regions in binaural unmasking and in improving intelligibility.

Some work along these lines has been reported by Schubert[4] and by Schubert and Schultz[5] who measured the binaural gain in intelligibility of bandlimited speech in broad-band Gaussian noise. The speech was restricted to one of three contiguous bands symmetrically placed about a frequency of 1630 Hz. The width of each band was chosen so as to provide an articulation index of 0.5 under conditions of quiet. The results showed that

[1] I. J. Hirsh, "The Influence of Interaural Phase on Interaural Summation and Inhibition," J. Acoust. Soc. Am. **20**, 536–544 (1948).

[2] J. C. R. Licklider, "The Influence of Interaural Phase Relations upon the Masking of Speech by White Noise," J. Acoust. Soc. Am. **20**, 150–159 (1948).

[3] J. L. Flanagan and B. J. Watson, "Binaural Unmasking of Complex Signals," J. Acoust. Soc. Am. **40**, 456–468 (1966).

[4] E. D. Schubert, "Importance of Frequency Range in Dichotic Speech," J. Acoust. Soc. Am. **31**, 854A, (1959).

[5] E. D. Schubert, and M. C. Schultz, "Some Aspects of Binaural Signal Selection," J. Acoust. Soc. Am. **34**, 844-849 (1962).

TABLE I. Summary of data. Mean thresholds and 50% intelligibility levels averaged over three tests and four subjects are shown The standard errors were estimated from an analysis of variance carried out on the data for each condition.[a]

	Detectability			Intelligibility		
Condition	Threshold[b]	Standard error	BMLD	50% level[b]	Standard error	BILD
S0N0	−37.8	1.19	...	−19.6	3.67	...
Sπ0/500N0	−49.8	1.06	12.0	−21.7	2.38	2.1
S0π/500N0	−43.8	1.18	5.9	−21.6	2.63	2.0
S0Nπ0/500	−44.2	1.18	6.4	−20.4	3.66	0.8
S0Nu0/500	−37.0	1.03	−0.9	−17.8	4.91	−1.8
$S\Delta t_{1.6}N0$	−49.9	0.48	12.0	−22.9	4.12	3.3
$S\Delta t_{10}N0$	−47.9	0.67	10.1	−22.6	3.65	3.0
SπN0	−50.7	1.18	12.8	−25.3	3.59	5.7
S0N0	−35.1	0.92	...	−23.0	2.26	...
Sπ0/250N0	−40.6	0.77	5.5	−24.4	2.38	1.4
S0π/250N0	−48.9	1.34	13.9	−29.0	2.78	6.0
Sπ0/1000N0	−49.0	1.02	14.0	−23.6	3.15	0.6
S0π/1000N0	−34.8	1.08	−0.2	−21.5	2.29	−1.5
$S\Delta t_{0.5}N0$	−46.6	0.39	11.6	−25.8	3.48	2.8
$S\Delta t_{5.0}N0$	−47.0	1.35	12.0	−22.5	5.86	−0.5
S0Nu	−38.4	1.43	3.4	−23.4	3.45	0.4

[a] All values in decibels.
[b] *re*: 103 dB SPL average level per word. Spectrum level of noise = 49.5 dB.

the binaural gain for low-frequency bandlimited speech was substantially greater than that for speech bandlimited to the intermediate or high-frequency regions, and almost equal to that for broadband speech. In the present investigation the speech signal was not band limited, but portions of the speech spectrum were subjected to a 180° phase reversal. Other stimulus transformations that were investigated included a 180° phase reversal of a band of the noise; decorrelation of a band of the noise; and a large interaural time delay applied to the speech. In all cases, both the release from masking for detection and gain in intelligibility were measured.

I. DEFINITIONS

There are at least two ways in which improvements in intelligibility may be quantified. One method is to measure the gain in percent intelligibility for a given signal-to-noise (S/N) ratio. The other is to measure the reduction in S/N ratio for a given percent intelligibility. The latter method is used here, since it is analogous to a binaural masking-level difference. Several operational definitions follow:

- Detection threshold: that signal level at which the listener, under a given set of conditions, and maintaining a fixed criterion, reports the signal to be present for 50% of his judgments (i.e., "signal present" or "signal absent").

- *p*% intelligibility level: that signal level at which the listener, under a given set of conditions, and maintaining a fixed criterion, correctly identifies *p*% of the words presented.

- Binaural masking level differences (BMLD): the difference in detection thresholds (in decibels) between two binaural conditions.

- Binaural intelligibility level difference (BILD): the difference in *p*% intelligibility levels (in decibels) between two binaural conditions. Unless stated otherwise, the 50% intelligibility level is implied.

II. NOMENCLATURE

The following nomenclature identifies the various experimental conditions:

S0—signal in phase at both ears over entire frequency band.

Sπ—signal 180° out of phase over entire frequency band (i.e., signal to one ear reversed in polarity).

N0—noise in phase over entire frequency band.

Nπ—noise 180° out of phase over entire frequency band.

Suffix 0*π*/*fd* indicates low frequencies in phase, high frequencies 180° out of phase; *fd* is the frequency dividing the two bands.

For example,

S0π/250—signal in phase for all frequencies up to 250 Hz, signal 180° out-of-phase for all frequencies above 250 Hz.

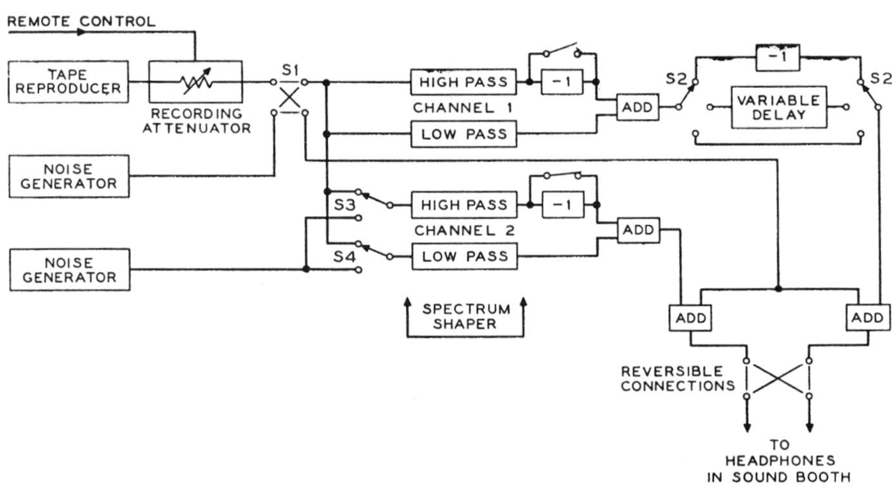

Fig. 1. Layout of equipment. Each spectrum shaper consists of high-pass and a low-pass filter pair. The output of the high-pass section can be reversed in phase prior to being added to the output of the low-pass section. In Channel 1 the combined output can also be reversed in phase or delayed as required.

Suffix *u* indicates zero correlation, e.g.,

Nu—noise uncorrelated over all frequencies.

Nu0/500—noise uncorrelated for frequencies up to 500 Hz, noise in phase for all frequencies above 500 Hz.

Suffix Δt_x indicates an interaural delay,

x—magnitude of delay in milliseconds.

S$\Delta t_{1.6}$—relative interaural delay of 1.6 msec for the signal (over the entire frequency band). The ear receiving the delayed signal was chosen at random and is not specified.

III. APPARATUS AND PROCEDURE

The investigation was carried out in two parts (Table I). In the first experiment, detection thresholds and 50% intelligibility levels were measured for the S0N0, Sπ0/500N0, S0π/500N0, S0Nπ0/500, S0Nu0/500, S$\Delta t_{1.6}$N0, SΔt_{10}N0, and SπN0 conditions. In the second experiment, the measurements were repeated for the S0N0, S0π/250N0, Sπ0/250N0, S0π/1000N0, Sπ0/1000N0, S$\Delta t_{0.5}$N0, S$\Delta t_{5.0}$N0, and S0Nu conditions.

A block diagram of the apparatus is shown in Fig. 1. The test material was recorded on magnetic tape and played back through an Ampex PR10 recorder. The signal was passed through an automatic recording attenuator (Grason–Stadler Model E3262) and then routed via Switch S1 either to the spectrum shaper or directly to the subject's headphones (Telephonic TDH39). The recording attenuator was controlled by the experimenter. The masking noise was produced by a General Radio model 1390B noise generator and its output could similarly be routed via switch S1 to either the spectrum shaper or directly to the headphones. The noise was bandlimited to 4800 Hz and presented at a pressure spectrum level of 49.5 dB.

The spectrum shaper consisted of two matched channels. Each channel consisted of two complementary high-pass and low-pass filters. Each filter was made up of two Allison-type 2BR units in cascade yielding an attenuation rate approaching 72 dB/oct in the stop band. The output of the high-pass filter in Channel 1 was reversed in phase (using a Philbrick-type K2X operational amplifier) and added to the output of the low-pass filter in that channel. Since the passbands of the two filters are contiguous the amplitude spectrum for the channel is reasonably flat (within ± 1.5 dB).

The phase response of the channel, however, undergoes a sharp 180° transition at the dividing frequency *fd*. The output of Channel 1 could also be delayed or subjected to a second phase reversal. Two Audio-Precision model DL-0470-400/125 delay lines were used in series. Each delay line provided a maximum delay of 5 msec with a frequency response flat within ± 1 dB

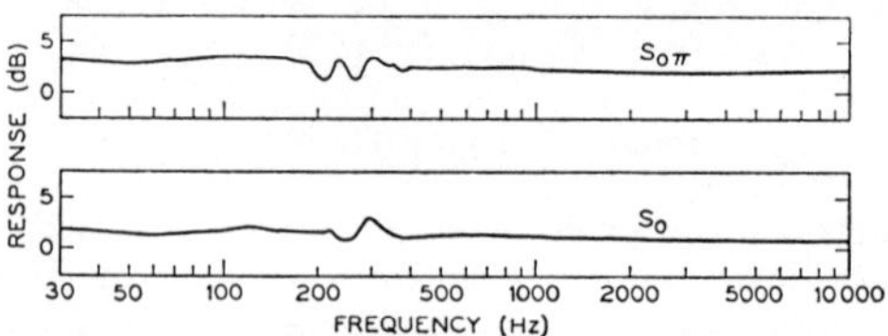

Fig. 2. Typical amplitude–response characteristic. The amplitude–response characteristic for the S0π/150 condition is shown in the upper half of the figure. The response characteristic for the full-band condition is shown in the lower half. The ordinate indicates the over-all difference in gain between channels (in decibels).

TABLE II. Over-all analysis of variance. Separate analyses were carried out for each experiment and also for the detectability and the intelligibility data. Differences between conditions and between subjects were highly significant in all cases. The $S\Delta t_{5.0}N0$ condition has been omitted from the intelligibility data of Expt. 2, hence this analysis involves fewer degrees of freedom.[a]

	Detectability			Intelligibility		
Factors	*df*	Mean square (dB)2	Signif. level	*df*	Mean square (dB)2	Signif. level
Conditions (C)	7	351.27	<0.001	7	61.8	0.005
Subjects (S)	3	73.73	0.001	3	126.8	0.005
Time-order (T)	2	0.07		2	5.3	
Interaction C×S	21	1.76	0.1	21	15.1	
Interaction S×T	6	1.19		6	14.6	
Interaction C×T	14	0.76		14	11.4	
Interaction C×S×T	42	1.04		42	13.2	
Error variance assuming no time order effect.	64	0.96		64	12.7	
Conditions (C)	7	438.84	<0.001	6	70.7	0.001
Subjects (S)	3	70.37	0.01	3	117.1	0.001
Time-order (T)	2	2.79		2	9.2	
Interaction C×S	21	2.43	0.05	18	9.8	
Interaction S×T	6	1.25		6	8.8	
Interaction C×T	14	0.68		12	9.2	
Interaction C×S×T	42	1.17		36	8.1	
Error variance assuming no time-order effect.	64	1.12		56	8.47	

[a] *df*—degrees of freedom.

up to a frequency of 5000 Hz. Channel 2 was identical to Channel 1 except that the outputs of the two filters were added directly without phase reversal, i.e., the operational amplifier was bypassed. Since the experiment is critically dependent on interchannel differences, the two channels were carefully matched. Typical calibration curves are shown in Figs. 2 and 3. Interchannel amplitude differences are within ±1.3 dB in the vicinity of *fd* and within ±0.1 dB elsewhere.

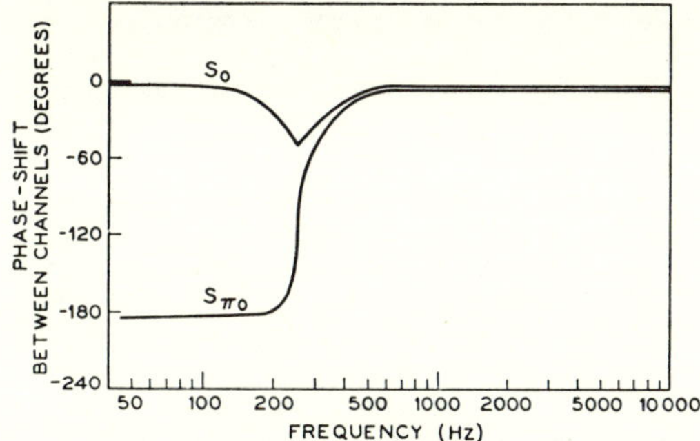

FIG. 3. Typical phase–response characteristic. The interchannel phase difference for the $S\pi0/250$ condition is shown by the lower curve. The upper curve shows the interchannel phase difference when using the spectrum shapers without phase reversal.

Roughly 90% of the 180° phase reversal takes place within a band from approximately 0.8 *fd* to 1.3 *fd* (i.e. within $\frac{1}{3}$ oct above and below the dividing frequency). The interchannel phase response using the spectrum shapers without phase reversal shows a peak approaching 45° in the region of *fd*.

By permutations of Switches S1, S2, S3, and S4 it was possible to set up any of the desired experimental conditions. For the case of uncorrelated noise, a second noise generator of the same type was used and its output was routed through Channel 2. The uncorrelated noise was routed through only the low-pass section of this channel for the S0Nu0/*fd* condition.

Two lists of 50 single CNC words[6] were recorded by a male speaker (General American accent). The words were adjusted in level to a rectified average value of 103 dB SPL measured over the duration of the word. The adjustment process was carried out by digital computer. For each test, 75 words selected at random from the ensemble of 100 were used. The words were presented at three-second intervals. For the intelligibility measurements, the subject was required to repeat each word immediately on hearing it, scoring only for correct repetitions. For the detection-threshold measurements, the subject was required to state whether or not

[6] G. E. Peterson and I. Lehiste, "Revised CNC Lists for Auditory Tests," J. Speech Hearing Disorders, **27**, 62-70 (1962).

a word had been presented during a specified 2-sec observation interval. Warning lights were used to prepare the subject and to mark out the observation interval. Control presentations with no signal present were made in order to estimate the false-alarm rate.

In both the detectability and intelligibility trials, the signal level was controlled by the experimenter according to a simple sequential strategy. Details of the technique are given elsewhere.[7] The purpose of the strategy was twofold: (1) to estimate the 50% level of the response curve rapidly and efficiently, and (2) to restrict data to the symmetric region of the response curve. The latter requirement was of particular importance for the intelligibility measurements, since the intelligibility function tended to flatten at high S/N ratios, seldom exceeding 80% intelligibility.

Four subjects were used, with three replications per condition. Measurements were carried out in random order to protect against learning effects or other regular trends. Within each experimental condition, however, the tests were recorded in sequence thus allowing a subsequent check for possible learning or other time-order effects. The reference S0N0 condition was repeated for both experiments. Each of the subjects was subjected to a preliminary training period of about 10 tests.

IV. RESULTS

The results for both experiments are summarized in Tables I and II. Standard errors were estimated for each experimental condition in order to check the homogeneity of the data. Cochran's test for the largest of a set of variances[8] indicated that the estimated variance for the $S\Delta t_{5.0}N0$ intelligibility data is significantly larger (at the 0.05 level) than that which could reasonably have occurred by chance. There was no reason to expect the error variance for this condition to differ from the rest and it is possible that this particular set of data may have been corrupted by extraneous nonrandom errors. As pointed out later, there are other reasons for suspecting the validity of the $S\Delta t_{5.0}N0$ intelligibility data. No significant heterogeneity was observed among the remaining data.

The observations for each experiment were pooled, and an analysis of variance was carried out on each set of data (Table II). The $S\Delta t_{5.0}N0$ condition was omitted from the intelligibility data of Expt. 2. Had this condition been included, the residual mean square would have been increased by about 15%, but with no marked change in the relative significance of the various factors. Differences between subjects were found to be highly significant for both the detectability and intelligibility data. For detectability, the relative magnitude of these

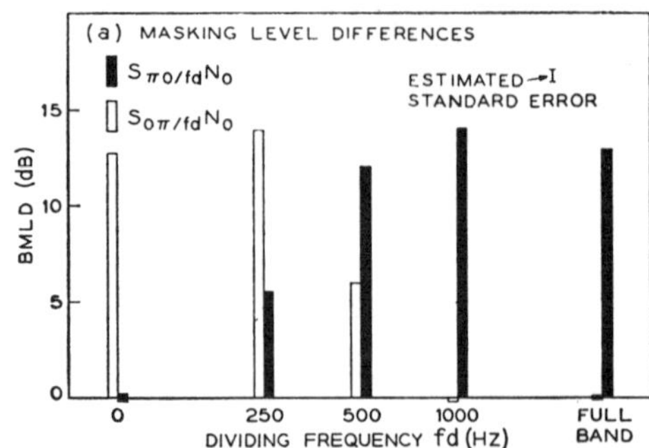

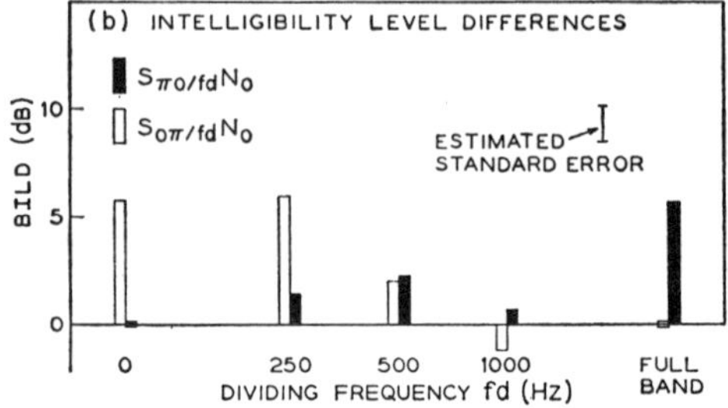

FIG. 4. Variation of BMLD and BILD with dividing frequency BMLD's are shown in the upper diagram, BILD's in the lower diagram. The shaded bars are for conditions of the form $S\pi 0/fdN0$, where fd is the dividing frequency. The unshaded bars are for conditions of the form $S0\pi/fdN0$.

differences was substantially less than the variation between conditions; for intelligibility, however, these differences were comparable. Interactions between subjects and conditions were negligible for the intelligibility data, but not for the detectability data where the F ratio exceeded the 0.1 and 0.05 significance levels, respectively, for the two experiments. This interaction reflects the fact that the change in the size of the binaural masking-level difference (BMLD) from condition to condition is greater for some subjects than others. On average, the range of variation in BMLD between subjects and within conditions was on the order of 2 dB and may be regarded as a second-order effect. If a similar effect exists with intelligibility-level differences (BILD), it was swamped by the larger inherent variability of the intelligibility data.

No significant learning effects or other gradual changes with time were observed within either experiment. A small, but statistically significant difference in both the detection threshold and 50% intelligibility levels between the two experiments was observed for the control S0N0 condition. The data for the two experiments were therefore not combined and all binaural level differences were computed relative to the S0N0 condition for the given experiment.

The observed BMLD's were considerably larger than the corresponding BILD's. In considering the statistical

[7] H. Levitt and L. R. Rabiner, "Use of a Sequential Strategy in Intelligibility Testing," J. Acoust. Soc. Am. 42, 609–612 (1967).

[8] W. G. Cochran, "The Distribution of the Largest of a Set of Estimated Variances as a Fraction of Their Total," Ann. Eugenics **11**, 47–52 (1941).

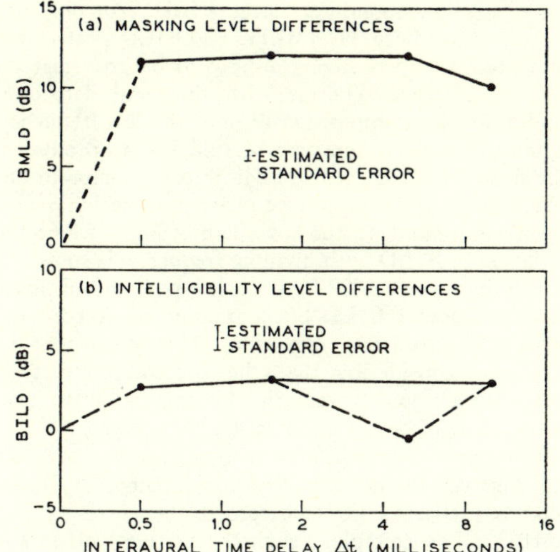

FIG. 5. Variation of BMLD and BILD with interaural time delay. BMLD's are shown in the upper figure, BILD's in the lower figure. The data are for conditions of the form $S\Delta t_x N0$. The value obtained for the $S\Delta t_{5.0}N0$ condition is considered to be unreliable

significance of the measured BMLD's and BILD's it is necessary to consider that as many as seven comparisons between means are made for each set of data, i.e., each condition against the S0N0 condition. Using the procedure derived by Dunn[9] it was found that for the detectability data a difference between means of 1.1 dB was significant at the 0.1 level; for the intelligibility data the corresponding difference was 3.4 dB. The SπN0, Sπ0/500N0, Sπ0/1000N0, S0π/250N0, $S\Delta t_{1.6}N0$, $S\Delta t_5N0$ and $S\Delta t_{10}N0$ conditions all gave rise to a large BMLD in the range 10–14 dB. Moderately large BMLD's on the order of 6 dB were obtained for the S0π/500N0, S0Nπ0/500 and Sπ0/250N0 conditions. For the S0Nu condition the improvement was approximately 3 dB. A small, negative difference was observed for the S0Nu0/500 and S0π/1000N0 conditions, although in both cases the values did not differ significantly from zero.

The variation in BMLD with the dividing frequency *fd* is shown in Fig. 4(a). For low signal frequencies out of phase the BMLD rises rapidly with *fd*, virtually reaching the maximum release from masking at *fd* = 500 Hz. For low frequencies in phase, however, the BMLD begins to decrease at 500 Hz. virtually disappearing at *fd* = 1000 Hz. The variation in BMLD with relative interaural time delay is shown in Fig. 5(a). The release from masking appears to be relatively independent of interaural time delay over the range investigated (0.5 msec–10 msec). Below $\Delta t = 0.5$ msec, the BMLD presumably falls to zero as shown by the dotted line.

No false alarms were obtained in any of the catch trails, indicating that the subjects were using a fairly strict criterion for detection.

The intelligibility data were more difficult to interpret owing to the greater variability of the data and the relatively small magnitude of the intelligibility level differences. Nevertheless, the SπN0 and S0π/250N0 conditions gave rise to highly significant BILD's of roughly 6 dB. The $S\Delta t_{0.5}N0$, $S\Delta t_{1.6}N0$, and $S\Delta t_{10}N0$ conditions gave rise to BILD's on the order of 3 dB, a value bordering on statistical significance (at the 0.2 level). The measured BILD's for the remaining conditions were not statistically significant. The dependence of the BILD on the dividing frequency *fd* is shown in Fig. 4(b). For low frequencies out of phase, the BILD appears to increase slowly with width of the out-of-phase band. For high frequencies out of phase, the BILD appears to decrease relatively rapidly with *fd*.

The curve of BILD versus interaural time delay Δt is virtually flat showing a small BILD of roughly 3 dB over most of its range. The small, negative BILD obtained for the $S\Delta t_{5.0}N0$ condition is believed more likely to have been a result of experimental error than a real effect. Not only was there no corresponding drop in the BMLD for this condition, but independent data obtained by Schubert[10] under similar experimental conditions showed no significant change in intelligibility over a range of interaural delay of from 1 to 7 msec. Furthermore, the estimated standard error for this condition was found to be unusually high, providing an additional reason for suspecting the validity of this measurement.

V. DISCUSSION

The data on release from masking for detection generally supported the hypothesis that BMLD's for speech in broad-band, Gaussian noise are dependent primarily on interaural phase opposition in the frequency region below about 500 Hz. The BMLD for the Sπ0/500N0 condition was virtually as large as that for the SπN0 case. Furthermore, for the Sπ0/250N0 condition the BMLD is much smaller, emphasizing the importance of interaural phase information in the 250 Hz–500 Hz region. The release from masking was nearly 6 dB less for the S0Nπ0/500 condition than for the Sπ0/500N0 condition—a result that compares favorably with the 6 dB difference observed by Hirsh[1] between the SπN0 and S0Nπ conditions for a 200-Hz tone at a similar noise level. Here again, the data are consistent with the hypothesis that the BMLD may be attributed primarily to interaural phase opposition between signal and noise in the low-frequency region.

An unexpected result was that decorrelating the low-frequency noise components did not appear to produce

[9] O. J. Dunn, "Multiple Comparisons Among Means," J. Am. Statist. Assoc. 56, 52–64 (1961).

[10] E. D. Schubert, "Some Preliminary Experiments on Binaural Time Delay and Intelligibility," J. Acoust. Soc. Am. 28, 895–901 (1956).

a significant BMLD. The observed threshold for the S0Nu0/500 condition was in fact higher than that for the S0N0 case, although the difference was not statistically significant. Subsequent measurements in Expt. 2 using full-band uncorrelated noise, however, gave rise to a 3-dB improvement in detectability, which is comparable to the BMLD observed by Robinson and Jeffress[11] for a 500-Hz tone in uncorrelated noise. No obvious explanation could be found for the lack of a BMLD for the S0Nu0/500 condition and further investigation is recommended.

Although low-frequency interaural phase information (the S0Nu0/500 condition excepted) is of primary importance in establishing a BMLD, high-frequency interaural phase information is not unimportant. Comparatively large BMLD's were obtained with interaural phase opposition in only the high-frequency region. The relative importance of high-frequency interaural phase information in the absence of low-frequency information is shown by the unshaded bars in the upper half of Fig. 4. The unshaded bars depict the BMLD's for conditions of the form S0π/*fd*N0. Compared to the complementary condition where the phase opposition occurs in the low-frequency region, as depicted by the shaded bars, the BMLD disappears at a relatively high value of the dividing frequency, *fd*. At *fd* = 500 Hz, for example, the BMLD for the low-frequency band out of phase approaches the maximum value; the corresponding BMLD for the high-frequency band out of phase, however, is very much greater than the minimum value, being almost 6 dB. The near-zero BMLD obtained for the S0π/1000N0 condition is presumably due to the relatively low level of the speech spectrum in the high-frequency region.

Release from masking (for detection) appears to be relatively independent of interaural time delay ($\Delta t > 0.5$ msec). The BMLD is large, approaching that for the SπN0 condition over most of the measured range. The result is similar to that observed by Flanagan and Watson[3] for low-pass filtered pulses at a repetition rate of 10 pps (pulses per second). The comparison further supports the notion that, with respect to the gain in detectability of speech in broadband Gaussian noise, it is the low-frequency region of the spectrum that is dominant. It should be noted that the spectrum density of the masking noise in Flanagan and Watson's experiments was roughly 15 dB less than that used here. For the high spectrum levels used in these experiments, a 15-dB difference in masker level should not produce too large a change in the release from masking. In comparing the data of the two experiments, differences between subjects are more likely to outweigh the effect of a difference in spectrum level.

The intelligibility data indicate that those conditions that give rise to a large BMLD do not necessarily produce a correspondingly large BILD. Not only are the differences between BMLD's and BILD's extremely large, but the two effects appear to be governed by different factors. Whereas with threshold detection, interaural phase opposition in only the low-frequency region of the spectrum may be sufficient to produce a significant BMLD, substantial improvements in intelligibility require interaural phase information over a much wider band. In the lower half of Fig. 4 where the variation in BILD with dividing frequency is shown, it is seen that even a 1000 Hz wide, low-pass, out-of-phase band produces a BILD but a fraction of that for the full-band, antiphasic condition. This result is not surprising considering that the spectral content of many speech sounds essential for intelligibility (e.g., consonants) is spread out over a wide region.

There does, however, appear to be at least one direct link between the detectability and intelligibility data. Observed BILD's never exceeded the corresponding BMLD's. For example, a slightly negative BMLD was observed for both the S0Nu0/500 and S0π/1000N0 conditions; the observed BILD's for these two conditions were also slightly (but not significantly) negative. Similarly, the BILD for the S0Nπ0/500 condition was less than that for the Sπ0/500N0 condition, as were the corresponding BMLD's. The fact that the speech signal is not subject to any binaural phase distortion in the S0Nπ0/500 condition (as opposed to the Sπ0/500N0 condition) does not appear to have been an advantage.

It is interesting to note that the BILD produced by an interaural time difference is roughly half that for the SπN0 condition, whereas an interaural delay can produce the maximum BMLD. The effect of the interaural delay is to produce large interaural phase differences between signal and noise over regularly spaced frequency bands, with small to negligible phase differences in the interleaving bands. If each of the out-of-phase bands is assumed to make an independent contribution towards improving intelligibility, then by summing the contributions of every second band a BILD of roughly half the maximum value should be obtained. For detection to take place, however, it is presumably sufficient for the signal energy in any one band to exceed the noise energy. This interpretation is consistent with the data of Fig. 4 and explains, at a qualitative level, why interaural phase information over a wide band is required for a substantial gain in intelligibility.

The suggestion that the speech energy in separate frequency bands contribute independently to intelligibility is in accord with the underlying philosophy French and Steinberg's procedure for predicting the intelligibility of speech in noise.[12] The use of the

[11] D. E. Robinson and L. A. Jeffress, "Effect of Varying the Interaural Noise Correlation on the Detectability of Tonal Signals," J. Acoust. Soc. Am. 35, 1947-1952 (1963).

[12] N. R. French and J. C. Steinberg, "Factors Governing the Intelligibility of Speech Sounds," J. Acoust. Soc. Am. 19, 90-119 (1947).

Articulation Index for predicting BILD's is considered in a subsequent paper.[13]

It is important to note that the experimental results were obtained using recordings made by a single male speaker. It seems reasonable to assume that similar results will hold for other male speakers, although some differences may arise in the case of female speech. It should also be noted that broadband, Gaussian noise was used and it would be of interest to determine whether similar results hold for noise having the same long-term spectrum as that of speech.

VI. SUMMARY

Binaural release from masking (SπN0 condition) for the detection of single words in high-level broad-band Gaussian noise is on the order of 13 dB and is determined primarily by interaural phase opposition in the spectral region below about 500 Hz. This result is in accord with the observations of Flanagan and Watson using pulsive stimuli. Interaural amplitude differences were not considered in this investigation.

BILD's were substantially smaller than the corresponding BMLD's. Furthermore, it would appear that the gain in intelligibility is not especially dependent on low-frequency interaural phase information but rather on phase opposition over a much larger portion of the spectrum. A simple, approximate interpretation of the data suggests that interaural phase information in different regions of the spectrum contribute independently towards improved intelligibility. Although simplified, this interpretation may be useful as a first step towards relating BMLD and BILD data.

[13] H. Levitt and L. R. Rabiner, "Predicting Binaural Gain in Intelligibility and Release from Masking for Speech," (to be published).

AUTHOR CITATION INDEX

Abraham, H., 30
Abramson, A. S., 263
Ahumada, A., Jr., 250
Aigner, F., 277
Albernaz, P. L. M., 297
Anderson, C. M. B., 15
Atal, B. S., 262

Bachem, A., 15, 155
Barkhausen, H., 277
Bartlett, N. R., 90
Barnes, R. B., 25
Barton, E. H., 101
Bauch, H., 231
Beasley, W., 305, 309
Bedell, E. H., 19
Behrens, H., 277
Békésy, G. von, 31, 32, 132, 146, 167, 180, 191, 240, 250, 262, 277, 294, 299, 309, 330, 354
Benbassat, C. A., 263
Berancek, L. L., 364
Bergeijk, W. A. van, 331
Bergmann, G., 67
Biddulph, R., 16, 67, 104, 227, 240
Bilger, R. C., 191
Bilsen, F. A., 132, 262, 286
Birdsall, T. G., 56, 57, 180, 250
Blackman, R. B., 30
Blackwell, H. R., 57
Bloch, E., 339
Blodgett, H . C., 15, 45, 67, 330, 358, 359, 361
Boer, E. de, 286, 305
Boer, K. de, 277
Boltzmann, L., 30
Boring, E. G., 56, 67, 321, 330
Bouman, M. A., 304
Bray, C. W., 134, 311
Broadbent, D. E., 262
Bryan, M. E., 16
Bühl, A., 30
Bunch, C. C., 30

Bürck, W., 67, 132, 175, 262, 277
Burger, J. F., 263
Burgtorf, W., 300
Burns, E. M., 132, 134
Buytendijk, F. J. J., 262

Campbell, R. A., 132
Cardozo, B. L., 132
Caruthers, R. S., 288
Chapin, E. K., 146, 305
Chistovich, L. A., 181, 286, 300
Churcher, B. G., 85, 102, 110, 111
Clarke, L. F., 250
Cochran, W. G., 376
Cohen, M. F., 330
Colburn, H. S., 330
Corliss, E. L. R., 67, 286
Corso, J. F., 15, 57
Cotzın, M., 332
Craig, J. H., 286
Cramer, E. M., 132
Creelman, C. D., 133, 286
Cremer, L., 277
Crozier, W. J., 90
Culler, E., 105
Cutting, J. E., 133
Czerny, M., 25

Dallenbach, K. M., 306, 332
David, E. E., Jr., 331
Davies, H., 85
Davis, H., 67, 92, 105, 133, 158, 170, 171, 175, 191, 250, 295, 299, 312, 339
Dean, C. E., 81
Deatherage, B. H., 15, 191, 358, 359
Decker, H., 277
Delezenne, M., 132
Derbyshire, A. J., 295, 339
Dimmick, F. L., 85
Divenyi, P. L., 262
Do, M. A., 331
Doughty, J. M., 67, 132

Dubout, P., 299
Duifhuis, H., 262
Dunn, O. J., 377
Durlach, N. I., 330
DuVerney, J. G., 132

Efron, R., 262
Egan, J. P., 15, 57, 305, 331, 357
Eldredge, D. H., 191
Elliott, L. L., 262, 297, 300
Ellis, A. J., 155, 305

Fano, R. M., 160
Farmer, R. M., 263
Fechner, G. T., 56
Feldman, C. B., 288
Feldtkeller, R., 231
Ferguson, C. V., 331, 355
Fernández, C., 171
Feth, L. L., 263
Filler, A. S., 38, 213
Firestone, F. A., 146, 192, 305
Fisher, R. A., 180
Flanagan, J. L., 286, 331, 372
Fletcher, H., 15, 30, 67, 70, 81, 89, 98, 101, 102, 113, 115, 132, 139, 143, 146, 150, 155, 180, 191, 212, 219, 237, 293, 295, 334, 357
Forbes, A., 339
Fourcin, A. J., 132
Fox, W. C., 56, 57, 250
Franks, J. R., 16
French, N. R., 155, 357, 378
Friis, H. T., 288
Frottorp, G., 180
Fry, T. C., 340

Gabor, D., 67
Gage, F. H., 331
Galambos, R., 158, 250, 295, 312
Gales, R. S., 192, 237, 357, 358
Gardner, M. B., 212, 262, 263, 357
Garner, W. R., 67, 86, 94, 132, 180, 299, 357
Gässler, G., 237
Gebhardt, C. J., 331
Gerbrands, R., 231
Gescheider, G., 262
Gilbert, E. N., 181
Goldberg, J. P., 250
Goldstein, D. P., 331, 332
Goldstein, J. L., 133, 191
Graham, C. H., 90, 102, 108
Gray, C. H. G., 30
Green, D. M., 57, 67, 68, 134, 180, 192, 250, 262, 263, 286, 331
Green, H. C., 155
Greenberg, G. Z., 57
Greenwood, D. D., 192
Griffin, D. R., 331
Guernsey, M., 30
Gulick, W. A., 132
Guttman, N., 15, 331

Hahnemann, 31
Hake, H. W., 357
Hall, J. L., 262
Halverson, H. M., 336, 337
Hamilton, P. M., 180
Harris, C. M., 300
Harris, G. G., 15, 133
Harris, J. D., 300
Hartley, R. V. L., 333, 340
Hawkins, J. E., Jr., 83, 192, 219, 237
Hecht, 31
Heisig, H., 30
Helmholtz, H. L. F. von, 87, 133, 152, 155, 286, 305
Hennelly, E. F., 331, 355
Henning, G. B., 67
Hiesey, R. W., 262
Hilliard, J. K., 263
Hirsh, I. J., 44, 45, 191, 262, 320, 331, 358, 370, 372
Hirst, W., 263
Hoekstra, A., 133
Hood, D. C., 16
Hornbostel, E. M. von, 321, 334
Houtsma, A. J. M., 133, 134
Hsieh, R., 250
Huffman, D. A., 250
Huggins, W. H., 132, 361
Huising, H. C., 30

Inglis, A. H., 30
Ivanova, V. A., 181, 286, 300

Jeffress, L. A., 15, 45, 46, 67, 250, 286, 313, 330, 331, 332, 358, 359, 361, 378
Jenkins, R. A., 286
Jenkins, R. T., 30
Jenkins-Lee, J. E., 133
Jestead, W., 67, 68
Jones, R. C., 57

Karlin, J. E., 56, 82, 250
Kay, L., 331
Kelly, W. J., 263
Kiang, N. Y. S., 250
King, A. J., 85
Klemm, O., 331
Klensch, H., 368
Klumpp, R. G., 305, 359

Knudsen, V. O., 67, 69, 81, 85
Kodman, F., Jr., 250
Koenig, W., 331, 368
Kopp, G. A., 155
Kotowski, P., 67, 132, 175, 262, 277
Kovaly, J. J., 250
Krantz, D. H., 250
Kranz, F. W., 30
Kubovy, M., 133
Kucharski, P., 133
Kuttruff, K., H., 262

Ladd, G. T., 321
Ladefoged, P., 262
Lamoré, P., 192
Lane, C. E., 30, 143, 212, 357
Langenbeck, B., 30
Langmuir, I., 331, 355
Larsen, M. J., 305
Lawrence, M., 251, 305, 311
Lawson, J. L., 360
Lehiste, I., 375
Leshowitz, B., 250, 263
Levine, M., 15
Levitt, H., 376
Lewis, D., 67, 192, 305
Lichte, H., 67, 132, 175, 262, 277
Licklider, J. C. R., 44, 45, 57, 67, 133, 240, 305, 311, 313, 331, 358, 361, 370, 372
Lien, A., 277
Lindsay, R. B., 12, 325
Lisker, L., 263
Lochner, J. P. A., 263
Lorente de Nó, R., 44, 158
Lübcke, E., 277
Luce, R. D., 57, 250
Lummis, R. C., 262
Lurie, M. H., 105
Lüscher, E., 263, 300

McAuliffe, D. R., 171
McClellan, M. E., 133, 263, 286
McCulloch, W. S., 156
McFadden, D., 331
McGill, W. J., 250, 286
McGregor, D., 107
McKey, M. J., 57
Makita, Y., 180
Marill, T. M., 250
Markowitz, J., 250
Marks, L. E., 67
Mathes, R. C., 286, 287, 305
Mathews, M. V., 250, 286
Mayer, H. F., 277
Mayer, A. M., 201

Meesters, A., 262
Melrose, J., 250
Mersenne, M., 192
Meyer, E., 30
Meyer, M. F., 155
Michaels, R. M., 180
Miller, G. A., 67, 86, 94, 157, 164, 172, 180, 263, 299, 301, 321, 357
Miller, R. L., 286, 287, 305
Mimpen, H. M., 15
Minton, 30
Mitchell, S., 94
Miyatani, S., 180
Montgomery, H. C., 30
Moore, B. C. J., 133
Morgan, C. T., 83
Morse, P. M., 39
Moses, F. L., 250
Moushegian, G., 313
Munson, W. A., 15, 56, 67, 89, 115, 191, 212, 237, 250, 263, 357
Musick, J. E., 359

Neisser, U., 263
Newman, E. B., 114, 319
Nieder, P. L., 133
Nixon, J. C., 263
Nordmark, J. O ., 15, 263, 331
Nyquist, H., 26

Obusek, C. J., 263
Ohm, G. S., 133
Olson, R. M., 85

Patterson, J. H., 263
Patterson, R. D., 192
Panzerbieter, H., 277
Penner, M. J., 263
Peterson, G. E., 375
Peterson, W. W., 56, 57, 250
Petzold, 277
Pfafflin, S. M., 250, 286
Pierce, A. H., 333
Pierce, J. R., 181, 309
Piercy, J. E., 16
Pieron, H., 321
Pirodda, E., 300
Pitts, W., 156
Plomp, R., 15, 133, 192, 300, 304
Pollack, I., 44, 133, 181, 250, 299, 316
Pores, E. B., 68
Port, E., 300
Potter, R. K., 155
Pratt, C. C., 106
Prothe, W. C., 250
Pruzansky, S., 15

Pumphrey, R. J., 15

Raab, D. H., 250, 286, 300
Rabiner, L. R., 376
Raiford, C. A., 263
Rasmussen, G. L., 250
Rawnsley, A. I., 300
Rayleigh, Lord, 30, 331
Rechten, A., 277
Reich, M., 277
Resnick, S. B., 263
Révész, G., 155
Rice, S. O., 163, 364
Riesz, R. R., 30, 85, 114, 219, 357
Ritsma, R. J., 15, 133
Robertson, R. M., 331
Robinson, D. E., 46, 331, 378
Ronken, D. A., 133, 250
Rosenblith, W. A., 157, 158, 240, 312
Rosenzweig, M. R., 158, 312, 319
Ross, D. A., 38
Roush, R. G., 96, 175
Rubin, H., 300
Rudmose, W., 15
Rutherford, W. A., 133

Samoilova, I. K., 297, 300
Sandel, T. T., 45
Savart, F., 15
Schaefer, V. J., 331, 355
Schafer, T. H., 180, 192, 237, 357
Schouten, J. F., 133, 150, 157, 158, 172, 305, 311
Schroeder, M. R., 133, 262, 305
Schubert, E. D., 262, 263, 331, 372, 377
Schulman, A. I., 57
Schultz, M. C., 372
Seebeck, A., 133
Sersen, E. A., 68
Sewall, S. T., 250
Shaw, E. A. G., 15, 16, 286
Shaxby, J. H., 331
Sherrick, C. E., 297
Sherwin, C. W., 250
Shewmaker, C. A., 180, 192, 237, 357
Shipley, E. F., 57
Shower, E. G., 16, 67, 104, 227, 240
Siebert, W. M., 133, 251
Sivian, L. J., 30, 40, 45, 213, 335, 340
Smith, M., 56, 251
Small, A. M., Jr., 133, 134, 263, 286
Snow, W. B., 101, 333, 337
Spence, K. W., 67
Stein, H. J., 300
Steinberg, J. C., 155, 263, 333, 337, 357, 378
Stenzel, H., 277
Stephens, S. D. G., 331
Steudel, U., 277
Stevens, K. N., 180
Stevens, S. S., 57, 67, 83, 85, 92, 101, 102, 105, 108, 109, 133, 158, 175, 180, 192, 219, 231, 232, 237, 240, 251, 299
Stewart, G. W., 68, 133, 210, 331, 333, 340
Strutt, M. J. O., 277
Stumpf, C., 106
Stumpp, H., 277
Supa, M., 332
Swan, C. N., 30
Swets, J. A., 56, 57, 192, 250, 251, 286

Tanner, W. P., Jr., 56, 57, 180, 192, 251
Tasaki, I., 312
Taylor, M. M., 286
Taylor, R. W., 45, 67, 330
Taylor, W. G., 157, 172, 321
Tempest, W., 16
Teranishi, R., 16
Thiessen, G. J., 286
Thomas, E. C., 250
Thompson, P. O., 180, 192, 237, 357
Thurlow, W. R., 134, 286
Thurstone, L. L., 251
Titchener, E. B., 106, 114
Tobias, J. V., 192
Toepler, A., 30
Tonndorf, J., 312
Townsend, T. H., 332
Trimble, O. C., 333
Trimmer, J. D., 146, 192, 305
Troger, J., 31
Troland, L. T., 320
Turnbull, W. W., 134, 175, 180

Uhlenbeck, G. E., 360

Vance, T. F., 81
Viemeister, N. F., 132, 134
Volkmann, J., 83, 85, 240

Waetzmann, E., 30
Wallach, H., 319, 332
Ward, W. D., 16
Warncke, H., 277
Warren, R. M., 67, 263
Warren, R. P., 263
Watanabe, T., 250
Watson, B. J., 331, 372
Watson, C. S., 16, 263
Wead, C. K., 30
Webster, A. G., 30
Webster, F. A., 331, 332, 358, 361
Wegel, R. L., 16, 30, 70, 139, 143, 202, 212, 357

Wente, E. C., 137
Wertheimer, M., 321, 334
Wever, E. G., 134, 158, 170, 172, 251, 311
White, S. D., 40, 45, 213, 335, 340
Whitfield, I. C., 251
Whittle, L. S., 15
Whitworth, R. H., 313, 332
Wicke, R. W., 134
Wien, M., 30
Wiener, F. M., 15, 38, 213
Wiener, N., 155, 159
Wier, C. C., 67, 68, 134
Wilbanks, W. A., 361
Wilcott, R. C., 358
Wilson, E. A., 56, 251
Wilson, J. G., 30
Windle, W. F., 250
Wood, C. L., 45
Woodworth, R. S., 45, 321, 332
Wroton, H. W., 263

Yantis, P. A., 305
Yeowart, N. S., 16

Zwicker, E., 180, 231, 238, 239, 240, 263
Zwislocki, J. J., 16, 68, 263, 300

SUBJECT INDEX

Absolute threshold, 9, 44–47
  and temporal integration, 100
  theoretical, 25
Amplitude distortion. *See* Nonlinearity
Amplitude spectrum. *See* Spectrum
Anechoic room, 19
Audiogram, noise, 227
Auditory nerve firing pattern, 246–247
Aural harmonic, as phase clue, 311. *See also* Beats, "best"
Autocorrelation, 159–160
  and frequency analysis, 160
  neural model, 155–157

Backward masking, 260, 285–286, 297–298, 303
  dichotic, 298
  and neural delays, 295
Bandwidth
  of critical band, 239
  of masking noise, 229
Basilar membrane, 246
  and critical bands, 230
  and periodicity pitch, 167
  position of peak response, 230
Beats
  "best" beats, 126, 146–149, 186–187, 207, 311
    in opposite ears, 210
  and masking, 205–206, 212
  of mistuned consonance, 187
  optimum rate, 72
  and pitch, 125
  use for $\Delta I/I$, 70–71
Binaural inhibition, 327, 358
Binaural localization. *See* Lateralization; Localization, auditory
Binaural masking level difference. *See* Masking level difference
Binaural pitch, 131–132
Bisection of tonal interval, 106
Browian motion
  in air, 25
  in auditory system, 9

Cancellation
  of fundamental, 151
  of second harmonic, 148
Click pitch, 129, 173–175
Cochlear nucleus, 159
Comma, musical, 123
Critical band, 188–189, 219, 228–230, 255
  and jnd for frequency, 228, 230
  from loudness match, 233–237
  from masking measures, 238
  and mel scale, 240
  from phase relations, 238
  and temporal integration, 98
  from threshold measures, 237
Critical delay time, 265
Critical ratio vs. critical band, 189, 237, 239
Cubic difference tone ($2f_1-f_2$), 190

d'
  definition, 50
  invariance, 52
Deafness, 222
Decibels and loudness, 112(fig.)
Difference limen (DL), 104–105, 112, 114–118, 301
Difference tone (f_2-f_1), 135, 144–145, 149, 212. *See also* Nonlinearity
Diffraction by head, 37
Distortion. *See also* Nonlinearity
  cubic, 190
  difference tone, 212. *See also* Missing fundamental
  harmonic, 146
  temporal, 255–256
Duration
  and integration, 93–95
  and jnd in frequency, 176–178
  relation to other parameters, 63–64

Ear, mechanics of, 245–246
Ear canal, 10, 11, 29, 40, 223
  resonance, 35, 39
Echo perception
  and angle of incidence, 275

and intensity, 273
with large delays, 270
and loudness, 275
and room reverberation, 276
with small delays, 267
and speed of speaking, 272
and timbre, 274
Echo suppression, 256, 267–270
Eighth nerve, 157, 223, 246
E/N_0, 52, 247, 248
Energy of sound, 222
in detection model, 52, 247
Equalization-Cancellation theory, 327
Equal loudness contours, 11
Excitation pattern, 224–227
cochlear position, 230

False alarm, 50, 242, 244
Fechner's law, 65, 90, 92
Filter
auditory, 190
as model, 188, 190, 359
pulsed response, 171
Flutter frequency, 162–164
Fourier analysis, 146, 152, 160
of short tones, 95
Frequency discrimination, 79–80. *See also* Just noticeable difference
and critical bands, 229, 239
dichotic, 329
Frequency position in chochlea, 227, 230
Frequenzgruppe, 231, 237

Gaussian noise and detection, 247

Hair cells, 246
Harmonic distortion, 146. *See also* Nonlinearity
Harmonics
audibility, 152
perceptual isolation, 13, 185
Hearing loss
permanent, distribution in population, 222
and sound pressure, 222

Inner ear, 223, 246
spectrum, 144
Intelligibility
binaural, 328
and frequency region, 372
vs. detectability, 376–379
in German, 271
homophasic vs. antiphasic, 326
and localization, 370

Intensity, of sound, 19, 221
effect on echo perception, 273–274
Intensity coding in auditory fibers, 112, 224
Interaural correlation
effect of, 46–47
and MLD, 359
Interaural differences, 45
and binaural pitch, 131–132
for clicks, 321
and localization, 337–339
in phase, 327
in tonal masking, 209
Interference, of sound waves. *See* Beats; Cancellation

Just noticeable difference, 61–63
and cochlear mechanics, 228
comparison, 85(fig.)
and critical bands, 228–229, 329
and dichotic signals, 329
for frequency, 79, 80
and place theory, 105
for intensity, 73–74, 219
for noise gap, 301–303
for periodicity pitch, 127
for pitch of short tones, 129–130, 177–178
for white noise, 63, 85, 181

Lateralization, 325
of clicks, 321–330
Likelihood ratio, 49, 50, 244
Localization, auditory
and intelligibility, 370
and lateralization, 325
and masking, 367
phase in, 337
and position of source, 339
and reverberation, 343
and sound complexity, 341
Logon, 63, 64
Loudness, 5
and critical band, 233–237
and dichotic listening, 329
effect of echo on, 269–270
and masking, 90–92
and nerve impulses, 224, 250
of physiological noise, 42
scale, 65–66

Masking. *See also* Backward masking
binaural, 209–211
of clicks by clicks, 285–286
comparison of tone and noise, 215–217
definition, 202
of high frequency by low, 196–198

interaural, 209
and loudness, 90–92
by noise bands, 229–230
of noise by noise, 88
pattern, 187, 204, 206, 213, 225
by pulse trains, 290–296
of pure tones by noise, 89
remote, 188
variability of measures, 218
Masking level difference, 45, 327
for complex sounds, 328
and frequency, 359
hierarchy, 358, 365
and interaural correlation, 359
and interaural phase, 358, 363–364
and interaural time difference, 359, 366
neural model for, 361
role of randomness, 361
and signal duration, 359
for speech, 326, 328, 329, 370
Mel scale of pitch, 104
and critical bands, 240
Middle ear, 246
Minimum audible field and pressure, 9, 18
binaural M.A.F., 23
difference in, 9, 28–30
Missing fundamental, 124, 131, 150–152, 158. *See also* Periodicity pitch; Residue
Missing 6dB, 9
Mis-tuning of musical intervals, 122–124

Neural response, latency of, 295
Noise
audiogram, 227
internal, 248, 249
jnd for, 63, 85, 181
Noise level, 223
Nonlinearity, 124, 135, 143–145, 207–209
middle ear, 125, 161
power series, 208. *See also* Harmonic distortion

Observer efficiency, η, 52
Observer's response criterion, 48–49, 242
Octave errors, 171
Ohm's acoustic law, 124, 161, 185
Operational definition, 61, 107–108
Outer ear, 223–224, 245
sound pressure in, 36–39

Periodicity pitch, 125, 126
from interrupted noise, 127, 157, 165–167
and tonality, 127–128
jnd for, 127
matched to other signals, 165–166
Phase
in binaural localization, 337
change in, discrimination of, power, 282. *See also* Just noticeable difference
and critical band, 238
interaural, 131, 132
of internal tone, 147, 187
of masking signal, 249
of neural firing, 246
spectrum, 284
Phase discrimination
and aural harmonic, 311
for click pairs, 281
dichotic, 313
Helmholtz's dictum, 305
listener differences, 310–311
and pitch change, 312
for steady tones, 261, 308–313
Physical correlate theory, 66
Physiological noise, 5, 10–11, 87
intensity, 41–42
interaural relation, 47
loudness of, 42
in signal detection, 248
source, 42–43
spectrum, 41
Pitch. *See also* Just noticeable difference
and basilar mechanics, 105, 122
of clicks, 173–175
function, in mels, 104
of inharmonic partials, 141
lower limit, 12–13, 104
and musical intervals, 106
and musical listening, 121–122
residue, 14
of short sounds, 128–130, 174
jnd for, 129–130, 178–179
tone vs. click, 63
upper limit, 14, 104
of musical pitch, 14
Place theory
and jnd in pitch, 105
vs. neural periodicity, 125–126
and time-frequency uncertainty, 130–131
Poisson process, in detection, 247, 249
Power, acoustic, 19, 26
Power discrimination, 282
Power law, loudness, 65–66, 91, 250
Power series nonlinearity, 208
Power spectrum, 279, 284
Precedence effect, 268, 326, 348–355
Pressure, acoustic, probe for measuring, 32–33
effect on canal field, 38

Psychometric function
  basis, 48–49
  effect of uncertainty, 52
  for noise, 86

Quantal theory
  for discrimination, 85–86, 90–91, 249
  for threshold, 55

Rayleigh's theory of localization, 325
Receiver operating characteristic, 50, 243
Repetition pitch, 256, 283
Residue, 126, 157, 311, 313. *See also* Missing fundamental; Periodicity pitch
Resonance
  of basilar membrane, 295
  of ear canal, 39
Response matrix, 242
Reverberation
  and decay of sensation, 304
  and single echo, 276
Root mean squared pressure, 19, 26

Saturation, of auditory fibers, 250
Scales
  loudness, 111
  pitch, 104
  sensory, 102
Schouten's experiments, 126
Second-choice experiment, 51
Seebeck's siren, 124, 126
Sensation
  decay of, 260, 299–300, 303–304
  level (SL), 90, 91, 112
Signal, known exactly, 51
Single vs. double click, 257–258
Sones, 65, 92, 113, 117
Sound field, 19
Speaking and echo, rate of, 272–273
Spectrum
  analysis, cochlear, 157, 226
    and autocorrelation, 160
    perceptual, 185
  of musical sounds, 136, 142
  as pitch clue, 127, 131
  of tone pips, 170–171
  of tone-pulse trains, 292–294
  of white noise, 161

Temporal integration
  and absolute threshold, 100
  and critical bands, 98
  defined, 93
  for different signals, 94
  lower limit, 98
Temporal order, 261–262
  of click and noise, 317
  of click and tone, 318–319
  of noise and tone, 317–318
  in speech sounds, 314
  of tone bursts, 255
  of tone onset, 315–316
Temporary threshold shift, 2, 259, 299–300. *See also* Backward masking
Threshold
  of audibility, theoretical limit, 25
  of click lateralization, 347
  and critical band, 237
  of pain, 12
  of temporal distortion, 255, 264
  theories, 53–56, 243–245
  of tone pitch and click pitch, 174
Timbre, effect on echo, 274–275
Time constant, 64, 179, 249, 255, 304
Time-frequency uncertainty, 63, 130, 177
Time-intensity trade, 295, 330
Time separation pitch, 126, 256, 283
Tonal attributes, 61

Volley principle, 158, 172

Warble tones, 22
Weber fraction, 69, 249
  and localization, 340
  for noise, 85, 87
White noise
  description, 82
  threshold for, 82–83

About the Editor

EARL D. SCHUBERT was born in Fostoria, Ohio, on November 8, 1916. He completed his undergraduate studies in music at Manchester College in 1938. He also holds a Master's Degree in music from the University of Iowa. After a period of military service, he completed a Ph.D. in psychology at the University of Iowa in 1948.

Between 1948 and joining the Stanford faculty in 1964, he taught and engaged in auditory research at the University of Michigan, the University of Iowa, Western Reserve, and Indiana University. He has maintained an active interest in the academic and editorial activities of the Acoustical Society of America and was previously active in the educational functions of the American Speech and Hearing Association.

Within audition, Professor Schubert's research interests have ranged from measurement of cochlear travel time to perception of musical intervals, centering primarily on speech perception and the perception of pitch. His writing has appeared mostly in the *Journal of the Acoustical Society of America* with an occasional chapter in larger collections.